A Comprehensive Re[...] the Certification and Recertification Examinations for Physician Assistants

FOURTH EDITION

Published in Collaboration with AAPA and PAEA

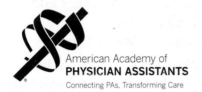
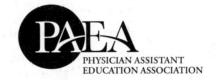

Volume Editor

Claire Babcock O'Connell, MPH, PA-C

Associate Professor
University of Medicine and Dentistry of New Jersey
School of Health Related Professions
Physician Assistant Program
Piscataway, New Jersey

Consulting Editor

Sarah F. Zarbock, PA-C

Medical Writer and Editor
Editor in Chief of JAAPA
Lakeville, Connecticut

Wolters Kluwer | Lippincott Williams & Wilkins
Health
Philadelphia · Baltimore · New York · London
Buenos Aires · Hong Kong · Sydney · Tokyo

Acquisitions Editor: Charles W. Mitchell
Product Manager: Sirkka E. Howes
Marketing Manager: Christen Melcher
Production Vendor Manager: Alicia Jackson
Manufacturing Coordinator: Margie Orzech
Design Coordinator: Stephen Druding
Compositor: MPS Limited, A Macmillan Company.

Fourth Edition

Copyright © 2010, 2007, 2004, 1999 Lippincott Williams & Wilkins, a Wolters Kluwer business.

| 351 West Camden Street | 530 Walnut Street |
| Baltimore, MD 21201 | Philadelphia, PA 19106 |

Printed in China

9 8 7 6 5 4 3 2 1

Library of Congress Cataloging-in-Publication Data

A comprehensive review for the certification and recertification examinations for physician assistants / volume editor, Claire Babcock O'Connell; consulting editor, Sarah F. Zarbock. — 4th ed.
   p. ; cm.
   Includes index.
   Published in collaboration with AAPA and PAEA.
   ISBN 978-1-60547-726-8
   1. Physicians' assistants Examinations, questions, etc. I. O'Connell, Claire Babcock. II. Zarbock, Sarah F. III. American Academy of Physician Assistants. IV. Physician Assistant Education Association.
   [DNLM: 1. Physician Assistants—Examination Questions. 2. Certification—Examination Questions. W 18.2 C7385 2010]
   R697. P45C66 2010
   610.76—dc 22

2009035860

DISCLAIMER

Care has been taken to confirm the accuracy of the information present and to describe generally accepted practices. However, the authors, editors, and publisher are not responsible for errors or omissions or for any consequences from application of the information in this book and make no warranty, expressed or implied, with respect to the currency, completeness, or accuracy of the contents of the publication. Application of this information in a particular situation remains the professional responsibility of the practitioner; the clinical treatments described and recommended may not be considered absolute and universal recommendations.

The authors, editors, and publisher have exerted every effort to ensure that drug selection and dosage set forth in this text are in accordance with the current recommendations and practice at the time of publication. However, in view of ongoing research, changes in government regulations, and the constant flow of information relating to drug therapy and drug reactions, the reader is urged to check the package insert for each drug for any change in indications and dosage and for added warnings and precautions. This is particularly important when the recommended agent is a new or infrequently employed drug.

Some drugs and medical devices presented in this publication have Food and Drug Administration (FDA) clearance for limited use in restricted research settings. It is the responsibility of the health care provider to ascertain the FDA status of each drug or device planned for use in their clinical practice.

To purchase additional copies of this book, call our customer service department at **(800) 638-3030** or fax orders to **(301) 223-2320.** International customers should call **(301) 223-2300:**

Visit Lippincott Williams & Wilkins on the Internet: http://www.lww.com. Lippincott Williams & Wilkins customer service representatives are available from 8:30 am to 6:00 pm, EST.

Dedication

In memory of my parents, Thomas G. Babcock, Jr.
and Claire Smith Babcock, RN, MEd
—*Claire Babcock O'Connell*

To the Physician Assistant profession: joining it was life-transforming.
—*Sarah F. Zarbock*

Preface

Taking certification and recertification examinations are a fact of life for physician assistants (PAs). The certification examination is taken upon graduation from an accredited physician assistant program, and the recertification examination is taken every 6 years thereafter. The National Commission on the Certification of Physician Assistants (NCCPA), using test data from the National Board of Medical Examiners (NBME) as well as the experience and aptitude of test-item writers, develops the two examinations and refines them on an annual basis to keep current with clinical practice and medical advances.

Traditionally, test-preparation books have consisted of practice questions, answers, and explanations. This format provided the opportunity for both new and experienced PAs to improve their test-taking skills by becoming more accustomed to the test experience, and, by reading the answers and explanations provided with each question, the candidate could learn from his or her successes and mistakes.

The last three editions of this test-preparation book included both a pretest and a posttest on an enclosed CD-ROM in a format that simulates the NCCPA exam. This edition continues to include both a pretest and a posttest. The pretest continues to be available in printed format; however, the posttest as well as the pretest are now available online to simulate the computer format of the certification and recertification examinations. Both tests have been written by experienced, NBME-trained PA educators and compiled using the proportions per subject area and skill areas as delineated in the NCCPA guidelines. Each test question also is written according to the NCCPA structure for multiple-choice format, an especially important feature of the last three editions. For further information and explanation of the NCCPA subject and skill areas, see http://www.nccpa.net.

In addition to the practice questions and answers, this book provides, in a condensed outline format, all the necessary information not only to take and successfully complete either of the tests but also to refer to, on a day-to-day basis, in clinical practice. Each chapter has been completely reviewed and rewritten to reflect changes in clinical practice. The test items, both pretest and posttest, are completely new, making the fourth edition even more comprehensive and able to be used as a quick and easy-to-read reference. In other words, this book is a practical, "real-time" educational tool for busy practitioners—a handy resource to be used on the front line of patient care.

The chapters are carefully formatted to give general characteristics of diseases (e.g., incidence, pathophysiology, prognosis), clinical signs and symptoms, diagnostic and laboratory evaluation, and treatment. These chapters, as well as the accompanying questions and their explanations, closely mirror the body of knowledge that is tested on the certification examinations and is needed for the reality of clinical practice. Regardless of their practice setting, PAs can use this book to review and test themselves on the material most likely to be included in either examination. For instance, more extensive information and questions are provided in cardiology because patients with cardiac problems are more common in clinical practice.

The American Academy of Physician Assistants (AAPA) and the Physician Assistant Education Association (PAEA) have continued their close collaboration in the development of this book. This partnership serves to enhance the value and credibility of the book and to ensure that it meets certification and continuing medical education needs of the PA constituency.

We believe that you will find this book helpful in preparing to take either of the NCCPA examinations. Equally important however, we hope that you use this book as a quick and valuable reference in clinical practice. We encourage you to make the book a permanent addition to your library not only upon graduation and every 6 years thereafter but also on a daily basis for the most important use of all—providing quality care to your patients.

Contributors

Frank Acevedo, PA-C, MS
Associate Director/Academic Coordinator, New York
Institute of Technology
Assistant Professor
Department of Physician Assistant Studies
Old Westbury, New York

Edward D. Huechtker, PhD, MPA, PA-C
Chair, Department of Critical Care
University of Alabama at Birmingham
Acting Chair, Department of Diagnostic and Therapeutic
Sciences
School of Health Professions
Birmingham, Alabama

Jennifer Joseph, MS, PA-C
Assistant Professor
University of Medicine and Dentistry of New Jersey
School of Health Related Professions
Physician Assistant Program
Piscataway, New Jersey

Kathy Kemle, MS, PA-C
Assistant Professor
Mercer University School of Medicine
Department of Family Medicine
Assistant Director, Geriatrics Division
Medical Center of Central Georgia
Macon, Georgia

Gertrude Lafavour, MD
Associate Professor of Medicine
University of Medicine and Dentistry of New Jersey
Associate Chief, Division of Nephrology
Robert Wood Johnson Medical School
Piscataway, New Jersey

Susan LeLacheur, DrPH, PA-C
Assistant Professor
The George Washington University
School of medicine and Health Sciences
Physician Assistant Program
Washington, DC

William H. Marquardt, MA, PA-C
Associate Professor
Associate Dean for Physician Assistant Education
Nova Southeastern University
Physician Assistant Department
Fort Lauderdale, Florida

Matthew A. McQuillan, MS, PA-C
Associate Professor
University of Medicine and Dentistry of New Jersey
School of Health Related Professions
Physician Assistant Program
Piscataway, New Jersey

Claire Babcock O'Connell, MPH, PA-C
Associate Professor
University of Medicine and Dentistry of New Jersey
School of Health Related Professions
Physician Assistant Program
Piscataway, New Jersey

Nancy E. Orr, PA-C
Retired Academic Coordinator
Physician Assistant Program
Cuyahoga Community College
Parma, Ohio

Patti Pagels, MPAS, PA-C
Assistant Professor
University of Texas Southwestern Medical Center
Department of Family Medicine
Division of Community Medicine
Dallas, Texas

Lori Parlin Palfreyman, MS, PA-C
Assistant Professor
University of Medicine and Dentistry of New Jersey
School of Health Related Professions
Physician Assistant Program
Piscataway, New Jersey

Rebecca Lovell Scott, PhD, PA-C
Academic Coordinator, Associate Clinical Professor
Northeastern University
Physician Assistant Program
Boston, Massachusetts

Melanie Trecartin, MS, PA-C
Assistant Professor
University of Medicine and Dentistry of New Jersey
School of Health Related Professions
Physician Assistant Program
Piscataway, New Jersey

Eric H. Vangsnes, PhD, PA-C
Associate Professor
Western Michigan University
Chair and Program Director, Physician Assistant Program
Kalamazoo, Michigan

Reviewers

Frank Acevedo, PA-C, MS
Assistant Professor
New York Institute of Technology
Department of Physician Assistant Studies
Old Westbury, New York

Phyllis L. Barks, MPH, PA
Assistant Professor
Oregon Health & Science University
School of Medicine
Division of Physician Assistant Education
Portland, Oregon

Robert Baye, MPAS, PA-C
Assistant Professor
Louisiana State University Health Sciences Center
Physician Assistant Program
Shreveport, Louisiana

Kenneth W. Betzing, MPAS, PA-C
Assistant Professor
Louisiana State University Health Sciences Center
School of Allied Health Professions
Physician Assistant Program
Shreveport, Louisiana

Mark Freeman, MBA, MEd, PA-C
Assistant Professor
Duquesne University
Department of Physician Assistant Studies
Pittsburgh, Pennsylvania

Sheryl L. Geisler, MS, PA-C
Associate Professor
University of Medicine and Dentistry of New Jersey
School of Health Related Professions
Physician Assistant Program
Piscataway, New Jersey

Valeri Houck, MS, PA-C
Crystal River, Florida

Jennifer Joseph, MS, PA-C
Assistant Professor
University of Medicine and Dentistry of New Jersey
School of Health Related Professions
Physician Assistant Program
Piscataway, New Jersey

Dawn LaBarbera, PhD, PA-C
Associate Professor and Chair
University of Saint Francis
School of Health Sciences
Department of Physician Assistant Studies
Fort Wayne, Indiana

Ellen D. Mandel, DMH, MPA, PA-C, RD
Associate Professor
Seton Hall University
School of Health and Medical Sciences
Physician Assistant Program
South Orange, New Jersey

Matthew A. McQuillan, MS, PA-C
Associate Professor
University of Medicine and Dentistry of New Jersey
School of Health Related Professions
Physician Assistant Program
Piscataway, New Jersey

Patti Pagels, MPAS, PA-C
Assistant Professor
University of Texas Southwestern Medical Center
Department of Community and Family Medicine
Dallas, Texas

Lori Parlin Palfreyman, MS, PA-C
Assistant Professor
University of Medicine and Dentistry of New Jersey
School of Health Related Professions
Physician Assistant Program
Piscataway, New Jersey

Harry Pomeranz, MS, PA-C
Assistant Professor
Instructor in Surgery
Weill Cornell Medical College
Physician Assistant Program
New York, New York

Jill Reichman, MPH, PA-C
Associate Professor
University of Medicine and Dentistry of New Jersey
Associate Director, Physician Assistant Program
School of Health Related Professions
Piscataway, New Jersey

Christina M. Robohm, MS, PA-C
Assistant Professor
University of Colorado at Denver and
Health Sciences Center
Child Health Associate, Physician Assistant Program
Aurora, Colorado

Cathy Ruff, MS, PA-C
Assistant Professor
University of Colorado at Denver
Child Health Associate, Physician Assistant Program
Aurora, Colorado

Carol J. Sadley, MEd, PA-C
Associate Professor
University of Medicine and Dentistry of New Jersey
School of Health Related Professions
Physician Assistant Program
Piscataway, New Jersey

Rebecca Lovell Scott, PhD, PA-C
Academic Coordinator, Clinical Associate Professor
Northeastern University
Physician Assistant Program
Boston, Massachusetts

Heidi Schulz, MS, PA-C
Emergency Medical Associates
Livingston, New Jersey

Melanie Trecartin, MS, PA-C
Assistant Professor
University of Medicine and Dentistry of New Jersey
School of Health Related Professions
Physician Assistant Program
Piscataway, New Jersey

Marianne Vail, MS, PA-C
Assistant Professor
Massachusetts College of Pharmacy and Health Sciences
School of Health Sciences
Physician Assistant Studies
Boston, Massachusetts

Eric Vangsnes, PhD, PA-C
Associate Professor
Western Michigan University
Chair and Program Director, Physician Assistant Program
Kalamazoo, Michigan

Erich Vidal, MS, PA-C
Assistant Professor
University of Medicine and Dentistry of New Jersey
School of Health Related Professions
Physician Assistant Program
Piscataway, New Jersey

Dipali Yeh, MS, PA-C
Instructor
University of Medicine and Dentistry of New Jersey
School of Health Related Professions
Physician Assistant Program
Piscataway, New Jersey

Acknowledgments

Once again, the effort required to revise and update this comprehensive review has been tremendous. However, the assistance, support, and encouragement from excellent colleagues have guided those efforts and succeeded in producing a high-quality text and review book. I am indebted to my program directors, Ruth Fixelle and Jill Reichman, and my fellow faculty at the University of Medicine and Dentistry of New Jersey. Their confidence in me has been a constant presence throughout my career as a physician assistant and educator. I am also grateful to the contributing authors, item writers, and reviewers; the personnel at Lippincott Williams & Wilkins; and the leadership of the Physician Assistant Education Association and American Academy of Physician Assistants. Sarah F. Zarbock continues to be an excellent mentor and instrumental in guiding me throughout such a large task— and I thank her for diligence and inspiration. Finally, I wish to thank my family for their endless patience and constant support and love.

—*Claire Babcock O'Connell*

Developing a fourth edition is just as exciting, challenging, and rewarding as beginning from scratch for the first edition. In addition to working with many of the same authors, I had the opportunity to meet some wonderful new and dedicated colleagues. Claire Babcock O'Connell, my coeditor, continues to be at the top of my list. She helped immeasurably in finding new authors, reviewing manuscripts, providing feedback and encouragement, and authoring one of the chapters. Claire combines a level of patience and hard work that is extraordinary, and she has a unique ability in helping authors stay on track. Needless to say, I feel very fortunate to have teamed up with her again. I am also indebted to all the authors—both who revised and updated their chapters and who just came on board. All these efforts were accomplished in their "spare" time—that is, when they were not working in their clinical practices, teaching PA students, or participating in professional activities. I am especially grateful to Greg Thomas, Vice President, Clinical and Scientific Affairs, and Ken Brady, Director, Strategic Business Development and Marketing, at the AAPA. They continually provided encouragement and managed the behind-the-scenes aspects that were crucial to developing this fourth edition. I want to give special thanks to my colleagues at Lippincott Williams & Wilkins. Charley Mitchell, Publisher, enthusiastically supported the need for a fourth edition and carefully shepherded the proposal until its acceptance. The baton was then passed to Kelley Squazzo, Senior Product Manager, who worked diligently and patiently to guide us through the process, and to Sirkka Howes, Associate Product Manager, who took on the project in its last stages, readying it for release to the production team. I would also like to thank my family, friends, and PA colleagues—all of whom helped me take some of the important steps along the way. The PA profession continues to open an extraordinary number and variety of doors. I hope this book continues to help all of us do what we love to do.

—*Sarah F. Zarbock*

Contents

Pretest

Directions: Each of the numbered items or incomplete statements in this section is followed by a list of answers or completions of the statement. Select the ONE lettered answer or completion that is BEST in each case.

1. Physical exam of a 60-year-old male reveals perioral cyanosis with a normal respiratory rate and no use of accessory muscles. Chest percussion is resonant; auscultation demonstrates wheezes and coarse rhonchi that change in location and intensity after a cough. What is the most likely diagnosis?
   A. chronic asthma
   B. chronic bronchitis
   C. community-acquired pneumonia
   D. emphysema

2. A patient admitted to the ICU after a motor vehicle accident has become oliguric. BUN and creatinine are rising. The presence of which of the following indicates a need for urgent dialysis?
   A. blood pH 7.30
   B. pigmented granular casts
   C. seizures
   D. hyperphosphatemia

3. Which of the following is an indication to begin early screening for prostate cancer?
   A. African American race
   B. cigarette smoking
   C. history of cryptorchidism
   D. low sperm count

4. A pregnant 22-year-old female presents with vaginal discharge that has been present for 2 days. Speculum exam reveals an inflamed edematous cervix with a mucopurulent discharge. Wet prep is negative for clue cells, motile flagellae, and hyphae. What is the most appropriate treatment?
   A. ceftriaxone
   B. clindamycin
   C. ciprofloxacin
   D. metronidazole

5. An 8-year-old boy is being evaluated for short stature. His mother reports that he has gained weight over the last year, but he has little or no energy, sleeps more than normal, and complains of being cold all the time. His growth curve demonstrates that he has fallen from the 50th percentile to the 5th percentile for height, but his weight has increased from the 50th percentile to the 90th percentile for weight. On physical exam, he is obese, has immature facies, thin hair, and slow reflexes. What is the most likely cause of this child's symptoms?
   A. acromegaly
   B. Cushing's syndrome
   C. dwarfism
   D. hypothyroidism

6. During a wilderness emergency medicine training course, conducted in a remote location, a member of the group begins choking on a piece of food. The patient has lost the ability to cough and seems unable to breathe. What is the next best step in management?
   A. blind sweep of the oral cavity
   B. emergent cricothyrotomy
   C. emergent tracheostomy
   D. initiate Heimlich maneuver

7. Where is thyroid-stimulating hormone produced?
   A. anterior pituitary
   B. zona fasciculata
   C. posterior pituitary
   D. zona glomerulosa

8. A 3-year-old female presents with rough, erythematous pruritic lesions on her cheeks and antecubital fossae. The family history is significant for asthma. Which of the following measures would be beneficial in the management of her condition?
   A. avoid moisturizers
   B. dehumidifier in bedroom
   C. frequent bathing
   D. wear cotton clothing

9. A 15-year-old girl reports that she has never had menses. She is short in stature and has a webbed neck and wide-spaced nipples. Initial lab work shows a high FSH. Which of the following is best to confirm diagnosis?
   A. estrogen levels
   B. karyotype
   C. LH levels
   D. ultrasonography

10. Which of the following women is most likely to develop breast cancer?
    A. 30-year-old Japanese woman with a history of menarche at age 14
    B. 40-year-old African American woman currently on birth control pills
    C. 50-year-old Indian woman who had her first pregnancy at age 17
    D. 60-year-old white woman whose mother had breast cancer

11. A 12-year-old male has been limping for the past 2 months. Exam reveals a moderately obese young male in no acute distress who complains of pain in his left hip region. There is a limitation of internal rotation of the hip with a 2-cm left limb discrepancy as compared to the right. What is the most appropriate diagnostic test?
    A. AP and lateral radiographs of the left hip
    B. AP pelvic films
    C. frog leg view of both hips
    D. weight-bearing MRI of the left hip

12. A 6-year-old presents with intermittent episodes of wheezing. Exam reveals expiratory wheezing but no rales or rhonchi. She is developing well and is cooperative with the exam. She responds well to an albuterol treatment. What is the most effective method to monitor symptoms at home?
    A. peak expiratory flow rate
    B. respiratory rate
    C. pulse oximetry
    D. blood pressure

13. A woman with a history of cervical conization and a second trimester miscarriage due to cervical dilation presents after a positive pregnancy test. Last menstrual period was 8 weeks ago and she desires pregnancy. What is the current treatment of choice?
    A. bed rest
    B. cerclage
    C. pessary
    D. tocolytic medications

14. A 20-year-old presents for removal of sutures that were placed following a knife wound he received in a street brawl. The patient has a history of alcohol and cocaine abuse and multiple arrests for driving under the influence, assault, and burglary. He has a long history of disruptive behavior and dropped out of high school. He has not been able to hold a job. When you question the patient about his life, he tells you that he sees no reason to change his lifestyle because he likes things the way they are. This patient most likely has what personality disorder?
    A. antisocial
    B. borderline
    C. paranoid
    D. schizoid

15. What is the best method to confirm fetal death?
    A. measuring HCG level since it drops immediately
    B. serial pelvic exams to monitor the regression in the size of the uterus
    C. serial titers of fetal growth hormone
    D. ultrasonography to assess fetal heart movement

16. A 37-year-old complains of diplopia and difficulty swallowing. Exam reveals ptosis and weakness of the extraocular muscles but no nystagmus. Rapid improvement after administration of what medication will confirm the suspected diagnosis?
    A. aminoglycoside
    B. corticosteroids
    C. edrophonium
    D. guanidine

17. A patient diagnosed with Parkinson's disease displays signs of bradykinesia. Which of the following drugs would be least helpful?
    A. amantadine
    B. anticholinergics
    C. levodopa
    D. selective monoamine oxidase inhibitors

18. An otherwise healthy 22-year-old presents with mild jaundice. Which of the following additional historical factors best supports a diagnosis of Gilbert's disease?
    A. family history of recurrent jaundice
    B. family history of sickle cell trait
    C. history of fatty food intolerance
    D. recent fever, malaise, and myalgias

19. A 3-week-old male is brought to the clinic due to nonbilious vomiting that has continued for 1 week. Emesis has become more frequent and is now projectile. The infant is observed being bottle fed during the interview and appears hungry with a good suck. What physical finding will most likely be found in this patient?
    A. abdominal distention
    B. abdominal wall muscle rigidity
    C. olive-shaped abdominal mass
    D. sausage-shaped abdominal mass

20. What organism is responsible for the vast majority of cases of acute infective endocarditis in patients with native valves?
    A. *Streptococcus viridans*
    B. *Staphylococcus aureus*
    C. enterococci
    D. *Pseudomonas aeruginosa*

21. A 38-year-old patient has an older brother who was diagnosed with colon cancer at age 43 years. What is the recommended schedule for colorectal screening for this patient?
    A. screening colonoscopy at 40 years of age
    B. screening colonoscopy at 50 years of age
    C. screening flexible sigmoidoscopy at 40 years of age
    D. screening flexible sigmoidoscopy at 50 years of age

22. An otherwise healthy 70-year-old presents with a painful vesicular eruption spread throughout the left mid lower back. Which of the following would best confirm the suspected diagnosis?
    A. complete a Tzanck smear
    B. measure IgG for varicella
    C. obtain a fungal culture
    D. perform PCR of skin scraping

23. Which of the following is an important concern with the continued administration of proton pump inhibitors (PPIs) or H_2 receptor blockers?
    A. antacids should not be used within 30 minutes of administration of PPI or H_2 receptor blockers
    B. poor compliance occurs because they need to be taken four times a day with food
    C. they alter the absorption of pH-dependent drugs
    D. they potentiate CNS depression with alcohol use

24. A 24-year-old male, status post tetralogy of Fallot surgical repair 20 years ago, continues to exhibit signs of mild pulmonary hypertension. Currently not a surgical candidate, which of the following would slow the progression of his pulmonary hypertension?
    A. corticosteroids
    B. prostacyclin
    C. sildenafil
    D. supplemental oxygen

25. A 45-year-old male presents with an erythematous, swollen elbow. Exam reveals tenderness, limited range of motion, warmth of the overlying skin, and mild excoriations. He is febrile; WBC count is 23,000 with increased bands. Radiography is negative for fracture or foreign body. What is the best initial course of action?
    A. dicloxacillin 500 mg four times a day for 10 days
    B. injection of intra-articular glucocorticoids
    C. penicillin 500 mg four times a day for 10 days
    D. warm soaks, rest, and NSAIDs prn

26. A 32-year-old male presents for a routine physical. He takes no medications, exercises one to two times a week, and eats a fairly healthy diet. He does not smoke and has three to four alcohol drinks on the weekends. His family history is significant for a parent with myocardial infarction at the age of 72 years. His review of systems is essentially negative and physical exam is unremarkable. Fasting lipid panel: total cholesterol 154 mg/dL; triglycerides 78 mg/dL; HDL 24 mg/dL; LDL 109 mg/dL. When should the next fasting lipid profile be obtained on this patient?
    A. 1 year
    B. 3 years
    C. 5 years
    D. 7 years

27. A 52-year-old female presents with 2 months of pain and stiffness in her hands and fingers, along with malaise and a 5-lb weight loss. On examination, she has swelling and tenderness of her MCP and PIP joints. Lab work reveals the presence of anti-CCP antibodies. What is the most effective treatment to prevent bone erosion?
    A. calcium channel blockers
    B. disease-modifying antirheumatic drugs (DMARDs)
    C. high-dose corticosteroids
    D. nonsteroidal anti-inflammatory drugs (NSAIDs)

28. A 23-year-old female presents with a recent development of longer and heavier than normal menses and a rash on her lower extremities. The only thing she can recall of any significance regarding her recent medical history is that she had a sore throat several weeks ago. Exam reveals red to purple hemorrhages that are pinhead sized overlying her shins and ankles; the lesions do not blanch with pressure. Platelet count is 40,000/mm³; the remainder of the CBC and differential is normal. An antistreptolysin O is negative as is a pregnancy test. Which of the following treatments would be most appropriate in this case?
    A. dexamethasone
    B. intravenous immunoglobulin (IVIG)
    C. penicillin VK
    D. ticlopidine (Ticlid)

29. A 7-year-old male presents with a history of frequent respiratory infections with recurrent pulmonary infiltrates and failure to thrive. His cough is persistent and productive of thick, green sputum. A recent sputum culture was positive for *Haemophilus influenzae* and *Staphylococcus aureus*. Which of the following laboratory results is pathognomonic for his condition?
    A. abdominal flat plate showing small intestinal air–fluid levels and small colon
    B. chest radiography revealing hyperinflation and small airway obstruction
    C. elevated sweat chloride levels
    D. irreversible changes in FVC and FEV_1

30. A patient with a history of hypertrophic subaortic stenosis presents with fever, dyspnea, and joint and back pains. Exam reveals a III/VI systolic murmur, conjunctival petechiae, and exudative lesions in the retina. What is the name of these retinal lesions?
    A. Auspitz's sign
    B. Janeway's lesions
    C. Osler's nodes
    D. Roth's spots

31. A 26-year-old female describes several episodes of weakness and numbness of her extremities. Each episode comes on acutely and resolves without residua in 1 to 3 days. Today she presents with imbalance in her gait. What diagnostic study would be most beneficial at this time?
    A. cerebrospinal fluid analysis
    B. computed tomography of the head
    C. magnetic resonance scan of head
    D. visual evoked potentials

32. A 30-year-old female is scheduled to undergo a breast biopsy in the next few days. She gives a history of a mild bleeding disorder that runs in her family. Platelet count, PT, and PTT are normal. Which of the following medications should be administered prior to undergoing this procedure?
    A. cryoprecipitate
    B. desmopressin acetate
    C. factor VIII concentrate
    D. fibrin sealant (Tisseel)

33. A 62-year-old male requests sleeping pills. His sleep is often disturbed by drenching sweats requiring him to change his pajamas two to three times per night. He has daytime fatigue, which he attributes to his poor sleep. On physical examination, he is tender over the sternum and his spleen is easily palpable. A complete blood count is remarkable for a WBC count of 165,000/μL with a left shift. Both basophils and eosinophils are noted on peripheral smear. He has no red cell abnormalities and his platelet count is within normal limits. PCR demonstrates presence of the *bcr/abl* gene. What is the most likely diagnosis?
    A. acute lymphoblastic leukemia
    B. acute myeloid leukemia
    C. chronic lymphocytic leukemia
    D. chronic myeloid leukemia

34. A 14-year-old male presents with anterior knee pain and swelling that gets worse after soccer games. The patient reports no trauma to the knee. On exam, knee range of motion is normal but the patient is tender to palpation over the tibial tubercle. What is the most likely diagnosis?
    A. chondromalacia patella
    B. medial collateral ligament tear
    C. Osgood–Schlatter disease
    D. prepatellar bursitis

35. A 68-year-old female presents with rapid onset of significant eye pain and visual loss. She notes that lights appear to have "halos." Exam reveals a red eye, steamy cornea, and dilated, nonreactive pupil. What is the initial treatment option?
    A. IV acetazolamide
    B. IV mannitol
    C. topical pilocarpine
    D. topical latanoprost

36. A neonate is found to have right ventricular hypertrophy, right ventricular outflow obstruction, and an over-riding aorta via cardiac imaging. What additional finding would you expect to see in this child?
    A. atrial septal defect
    B. discrepancy in upper and lower extremity blood pressure
    C. left bundle branch block
    D. ventricular septal defect

37. A 26-year-old female presents with a history of recent deterioration of her health. A month ago she got fired from her job for making careless errors and being disorganized. In the last month, she has started to lose weight and talk about family members who are "against" her and poisoning her food. Most recently, she has started to perform stereotypical movement of cleaning the countertops, although she was not actually cleaning. Her family is very concerned about her condition. When you examine the patient, she is laughing and does not answer your questions. What is the most likely diagnosis?
    A. anorexia nervosa
    B. bipolar disorder
    C. histrionic personality disorder
    D. schizophrenia

38. A 40-year-old tennis player complains of 3 weeks of right elbow pain, in the absence of any trauma. He denies any other joint pain or systemic symptoms. He is afebrile. Exam reveals tenderness over the lateral epicondyle, but no erythema or edema. Active wrist extension produces pain. Which of the following is the best initial treatment?
    A. ice and rest
    B. forearm splint
    C. oral corticosteroids
    D. surgical management

39. A 68-year-old female presents for health maintenance. She experienced natural menopause 15 years ago. She is healthy and does not have a significant past medical history. She takes 1,000 mg of calcium per day. Her 74-year-old sister has osteoporosis. The patient's bone mineral density T score is found to be −2.6 SD. She is placed on weekly medication. What is the mechanism of action of this medication?
    A. activation of bone remodeling
    B. impairment of osteoclast function by action on the calcitonin receptor
    C. inhibition of bone resorption by impairment of osteoclast function
    D. regulation of calcium absorption from the gastrointestinal tract

40. A 69-year-old male with a 120-pack-year smoking history presents with painless hematuria for 2 days. He also describes frequency and dysuria as well as mild flank pain. He is afebrile and denies a history of recent upper respiratory tract infection. Urine dip is positive for blood. Which of the following is the most likely diagnosis?
    A. benign prostatic hyperplasia
    B. IgA nephropathy
    C. renal cell carcinoma
    D. Wegener's granulomatosis

41. A 42-year-old complains of steady, severe right upper quadrant pain that radiates to the right scapula. This type of pain is associated with disorders of which of the following?
    A. spleen
    B. gallbladder
    C. esophagus
    D. ascending colon

42. A 24-year-old male presents after a day of snowboarding with wrist pain and swelling. An initial x-ray of the wrist appears negative; a scaphoid fracture is considered. What exam finding will help confirm this diagnosis?
    A. dorsal angulation of the wrist
    B. pain over the anatomic snuffbox
    C. pain with ulnar deviation of the wrist
    D. volar angulation of the wrist

43. A lactating female presents complaining of redness, swelling, and tenderness of the upper outer quadrant of the left breast. Temperature is 101.0°F. The left breast nipple appears fissured with surrounding erythema and induration. The area is warm and tender to touch. What is the most appropriate treatment?
    A. dicloxacillin
    B. metronidazole
    C. penicillin
    D. vancomycin

44. A 62-year-old male who has not had medical care for many years was seen 2 days ago at the emergency room for chest pain that was diagnosed as angina pectoris. At follow-up today, he admits to multiple poor health habits: cigarette smoking since age 12, consumption of three to four beers daily, a diet of fast food three times a day, five to seven cups of regular coffee per day, and virtually no exercise. What is the single most important lifestyle modification that he should make?
    A. abstinence from alcohol
    B. cessation of smoking
    C. dietary modifications
    D. increasing exercise

45. When instructing a patient on good lifting mechanics and back care, which of the following should be included?
    A. always use legs for lifting any object
    B. do not stretch after heavy lifting
    C. when lifting objects less than 50 lb, always bend at the waist
    D. when working out at the gym, use heavy weights for low back workout

46. Patients with glucose-6-phosphate dehydrogenase (G6PD) deficiency should be counseled to avoid which class of antibiotic therapy, as it may provoke a hemolytic crisis?
    A. cephalosporins
    B. fluoroquinolones
    C. sulfonamides
    D. tetracyclines

47. Which of the following is the only intervention documented to improve survival in a patients suffering from chronic obstructive pulmonary disease (COPD)?
    A. long-acting anticholinergics
    B. oxygen on a continuous basis
    C. patient-initiated COPD action plans
    D. smoking cessation

48. A 26-year-old is brought to the emergency department by colleagues who state she is acting as if intoxicated. She denies any use of alcohol or drugs but states that her legs have become weak and tingling, causing progressively worsening difficulty walking for 2 days. She thought perhaps she had slept on them wrong as she has also been severely fatigued. Exam reveals tachycardia, an irregular rhythm, and hypotension. As she is waiting for medical consult, she becomes more fatigued and experiences incontinence of urine. What is the next step in management?
    A. admit to intensive care unit
    B. admit to reverse isolation unit
    C. amiodarone
    D. prednisone

49. A 43-year-old male presents with a few weeks of shoulder pain with activity. He also states it wakes him up at night when he rolls on that side. On exam, the patient has painful range of motion, especially on abduction, but does not appear to have any weakness of the shoulder. What is the first step in managing this patient?
    A. activity modification and NSAIDs
    B. corticosteroid injection
    C. immobilization for 2 to 4 weeks
    D. surgical rotator cuff repair

50. A patient has a blind right eye. If sympathetic and parasympathetic innervation is intact, which of the following responses would occur?
    A. A light directed at the left eye will cause both pupils to constrict.
    B. A light directed at the right eye will cause both pupils to dilate.
    C. A light directed at the left eye will cause only the left pupil to constrict.
    D. A light directed at the right eye will cause only the left pupil to dilate.

51. A 36-year-old schoolteacher presents with an acute onset of fever, chills, malaise, headache, and congestion. She is coughing and sneezing. Conjunctivae are injected; pharyngeal mucosa is edematous and injected. What is expected on examination of the lungs?
    A. clear lung fields with good air exchange
    B. diffuse expiratory wheezes
    C. dullness and rhonchi at the bases
    D. scattered crackles and inspiratory wheeze

52. A 78-year-old female presents with low back pain that radiates to both legs. She states her legs get weak when she walks at the mall. What is expected on physical exam?
    A. a positive straight leg raise
    B. normal neurologic exam
    C. paraspinal muscle spasms
    D. point tenderness over L5-S1 spinous processes

53. A woman presents complaining of irregular menses and infertility for 1 year. Pelvic ultrasonography reveals multiple smooth, pearl-white ovarian cysts characterized as "oyster ovaries." Which of the following lifestyle modifications would be best at preventing further cysts from reoccurring?
    A. decrease alcohol intake
    B. moderate weight lifting
    C. smoking cessation
    D. weight loss

54. A basketball player presents after being struck above the eye with an opponent's elbow. Exam is significant for bruising around the eye as well as bleeding into the anterior chamber. Computed tomography is negative for fracture. What is the most appropriate treatment?
    A. NSAIDs to reduce pain and swelling
    B. rest and close ophthalmologic follow-up
    C. surgical intervention
    D. vitamin K to induce clotting

55. An 18-year-old water skier presents with left ear pain with pruritus and discharge. Exam reveals pain on auricular manipulation as well as redness and swelling of the ear canal with purulent debris. The tympanic membrane is intact. What is the most appropriate management?
    A. oral fluoroquinolone
    B. otic antibiotic/anti-inflammatory drops
    C. surgical intervention
    D. use of an ear wick with otic drops

56. Radiculopathy due to herniation of the intervertebral disc at L5-S1 would lead to motor deficit of which area?
    A. dorsiflexors
    B. multiple areas
    C. plantar flexors
    D. quadriceps

57. A 7-year-old presents with his parents who are complaining that for the last 9 months the child has been having increasing difficulty in school. He has consistently been inattentive in school, has difficulty following directions, cannot stay on task, is easily distracted, and is often forgetful about what he is assigned to do. At home he does not listen to his parents. What is the most likely diagnosis?
    A. Asperger's syndrome
    B. attention-deficit disorder
    C. disruptive behavior disorder
    D. hyperkinetic conduct disorder

58. A 55-year-old female presents with sudden onset of dyspnea and chest pain. She is afebrile but is not coughing. She is a smoker with a 30-pack-year history. She returned to the United States from Australia 5 days ago. She is tachycardic. Exam of the heart and lungs is normal. What is the most likely diagnosis?
    A. congestive heart failure
    B. emphysema
    C. pleurisy
    D. pulmonary embolus

59. A patient is 2 days post bilateral ureterosigmoidostomy for bladder resection due to cancer. He complains of increasing shortness of breath. The patient denies cough, chest pain, or fever. Physical examination is unremarkable except for an increased respiratory rate of 30/minute. Labs include Na 132 mEq/L, K 5.6 mEq/L, Cl 127 mEq/L, and CO_2 20 mEq/L. Arterial blood gas reveals pH 7.28, PO_2 98 mm Hg, PCO_2 22 mm Hg, and HCO_3 13 mEq/L. What is the most likely acid–base status?
    A. metabolic acidosis
    B. metabolic alkalosis
    C. respiratory acidosis
    D. respiratory alkalosis

60. A 23-year-old male prostitute presents seeking treatment for recurrence of a nonpainful perianal rash. He gives a history of a similar rash that was treated with multiple "freezing" treatments and a prescription for a gel that he used a couple of times. What is expected on physical exam?
    A. discrete papules, 2 to 5 mm in diameter, slightly umbilicated, flesh colored, and dome shaped
    B. discrete, small (<4 mm), skin-colored to dark brown pedunculated lesions
    C. numerous pale pink, discrete lesions with narrow to wide projections on a broad base with a smooth or velvety, moist surface.
    D. small groups of vesicles that erode, crust, and heal in 10 to 14 days

61. Which of the following factors carries the highest risk for promoting development of microvascular disease of the feet in a patient with diabetes?
    A. cigarette smoking
    B. high-fat diet
    C. hot water soaks
    D. ill-fitting shoes

62. A 29-year-old male presents with numerous tender, follicular pustules across his buttocks and upper thighs. He reports hot tubbing with friends 3 days prior at a resort hotel. What organism is the most likely cause of his symptoms?
    A. human papillomavirus
    B. *Pseudomonas aeruginosa*
    C. *Staphylococcus aureus*
    D. varicella-zoster virus

63. An elderly patient with diabetes mellitus type 2 presents with mouth irritation. Exam reveals creamy white, curd-like patches which are easily scraped off revealing erythematous buccal mucosa. What is the most appropriate treatment?
    A. acyclovir
    B. fluconazole
    C. penicillin
    D. prednisone

64. A 73-year-old male with a history of uncontrolled hypertension presents with hemiparesis, hemisensory loss, and aphasia. Presence of which of the following best supports a diagnosis of middle cerebral artery occlusion?
    A. alexia
    B. homonymous hemianopia
    C. Horner's syndrome
    D. vertigo

65. A 12-year-old male woke suddenly this morning with severe scrotal pain and edema of the scrotal sac that has continued for 2 hours. He has had similar pain before, but it subsided without intervention. Physical examination reveals a tender, swollen, retracted testis. A routine urine exam is normal. Which of the following is the most appropriate next step?
    A. scrotal support and ice packs
    B. immediate surgical intervention
    C. initiation of antibiotic therapy
    D. Tc99 pertechnetate scan

66. A child who resides with someone who has been newly diagnosed with active tuberculosis has a negative initial skin test. Which of the following is the most appropriate next step in the management of this child?
    A. Repeat the skin test in 6 months.
    B. Start the child on isoniazid therapy.
    C. Obtain a chest x-ray.
    D. Obtain sputum cultures.

67. A 75-year-old with a history of Parkinson's disease presents with minimally pruritic facial lesions present for 1 week. Exam reveals scattered discrete macules approximately 1 cm in size with an orange-red greasy scale on the cheeks and nasolabial folds. What is the most appropriate treatment?
    A. benzoyl peroxide gel
    B. hydrocortisone cream
    C. metronidazole gel
    D. mupirocin ointment

68. A 26-year-old female is being placed on hydroxychloroquine (Plaquenil) for systemic lupus erythematosus. Which of the following needs to be completed at least annually as part of regular monitoring for medical side effects?
    A. kidney function tests
    B. liver function tests
    C. retinal exams
    D. upper GI endoscopy

69. A 49-year-old female reports that when she tried recently to donate blood on behalf of a friend, she was refused because of a low hemoglobin level. Today her hemoglobin level is 11 g/dL. She has had mild fatigue for the past several months, but otherwise feels well. She takes no medications on a regular basis. She is most likely to have a history of which of the following?
    A. alcohol abuse
    B. familial anemia
    C. heavy menses
    D. poor diet

70. A 34-year-old female presents with pain along the radial aspect of her wrist. On exam, there is tenderness over the abductor pollicis longus and the extensor pollicis brevis tendons. Which of the following describes the special provocative maneuver that should be done to diagnose the most likely cause for this pain?
    A. arm extended and externally rotated with the patient opening and closing hands for 3 minutes
    B. enclose the thumb in the palm and deviate the wrist in an ulnar direction
    C. passively flex both wrists and hold for 60 seconds
    D. percuss over the ulnar nerve at the elbow

71. A 45-year-old obese female presents for routine gynecologic exam. She complains of heavy, prolonged menstrual periods for the past year. Pelvic exam and TSH are normal. What is the most appropriate next step?
    A. colposcopy
    B. endometrial biopsy
    C. hysterosalpingography
    D. hysteroscopy

72. An elderly male presents with unilateral hearing loss for 1 day. He denies URI symptoms, fever, or ear pain or discharge. He further denies any dizziness or headaches. Physical exam reveals normal balance, negative Romberg, but evidence of conductive hearing loss in the affected ear. What is the most likely diagnosis?
    A. barotrauma
    B. cerumen impaction
    C. eustachian tube dysfunction
    D. otitis media

73. Over the past year, a 21-year-old female has developed amenorrhea and has had milky discharge from her left nipple. She is not taking any medications. She is sexually active but does not wish to become pregnant. Serum HCG is negative. Serum prolactin is 300 mg/dL; MRI reveals a 3-mm mass in the pituitary. Which of the following is the most appropriate therapy at this time?
    A. bromocriptine (Parlodel)
    B. monthly injections of medroxyprogesterone
    C. sequential birth control pill
    D. transphenoidal resection of the tumor

74. A 35-year-old male who is HIV positive with a CD4 count less than 200 cell/μL has had a headache, low-grade fever, lethargy, and confusion for the past 3 weeks. Microscopic examination of the CSF prepared with India ink reveals budding yeasts with prominent capsules. What is the most likely diagnosis?
    A. candidiasis
    B. cryptococcosis
    C. histoplasmosis
    D. pneumocystis

75. A patient complains of difficulty seeing at night. Exam reveals dry conjunctivae with white patches. These findings are consistent with a deficiency of what vitamin?
    A. A
    B. B_{12}
    C. D
    D. niacin

76. A 39-year-old female with a history of poorly controlled hypertension presents with fever, productive cough, and myalgias and is diagnosed with pneumonia. Which of the following medications should be avoided by this patient?
    A. acetaminophen
    B. macrolide antibiotics
    C. nonsteroidal anti-inflammatory drugs
    D. penicillin

77. A 68-year-old male presents with recurring right upper quadrant abdominal pain that radiates to the right scapula. He also complains of fever. Physical exam reveals icteric sclerae, jaundice, and tenderness in the right upper quadrant and epigastrium. Labs show increased ALT, AST, alkaline phosphatase, serum bilirubin, and WBC. Ultrasonography shows dilated bile ducts. What is the most likely diagnosis?
    A. cholangitis
    B. choledocolithiasis
    C. hepatitis
    D. pancreatic carcinoma

78. A 52-year-old male with diabetes seeks medication to combat erectile dysfunction. If a phosphodiesterase-5 (PDE-5) inhibitor is prescribed, the patient should be warned of which of the following likely side effects?
    A. constipation
    B. hypotension
    C. increased risk of prostate cancer
    D. urinary retention

79. A 21-year-old male is brought to the emergency department by his fraternity brothers because he is complaining about his heart "trying to jump out of my chest." He had consumed a large amount of alcohol over the course of the day. He is obviously intoxicated and quite anxious. ECG shows erratic atrial activity with irregular ventricular response. What is the most likely diagnosis?
    A. atrial fibrillation
    B. atrial flutter
    C. paroxysmal supraventricular tachycardia
    D. ventricular premature beats

80. Which of the following medications is likely to produce wheezing and cough in a patient with a history of asthma?
    A. lisinopril (Prinivil)
    B. olopatadine (Patanol eye drops)
    C. ranitidine (Zantac)
    D. timolol (Timoptic eye drops)

81. A 16-year-old presents to the emergency department with productive cough, hemoptysis, and pleuritic chest pain. Chest x-ray reveals dilated and thickened bronchi that appear as tram tracks and ringlike markings. Which of the following is most likely in this patient's history?
    A. exposure to asbestos
    B. family history of sarcoidosis
    C. history of hyaline membrane disease
    D. recurrent purulent pulmonary infections

82. A 24-year-old generally healthy female presents with a concern about a rash on her face that began 2 months after initiating oral contraceptives. She denies history of diabetes or sun exposure. What is the most likely appearance of her rash?
    A. diffuse brown areas of hyperpigmentation
    B. round, atrophic, hyperpigmented lesions
    C. small red or light brown macules
    D. uniform pale brown macules varying in size

83. Which of the following is the recommended initial treatment for obstructive sleep apnea in adults?
    A. continuous positive airway pressure (CPAP)
    B. mandibular repositioning devices
    C. tonsillectomy
    D. uvulopharyngopalatoplasty

84. A patient has a 4-mm flat lesion on her posterior lower thigh. Its color is variegated purple and black and it has well-demarcated margins. What is the preferred evaluation method?
    A. excisional biopsy
    B. KOH prep
    C. punch biopsy
    D. Wood's lamp assessment

85. A 34-year-old female presents with an outbreak of grouped vesicular lesions on erythematous bases along the vermillion border. What patient education information would be important in minimizing the risk of recurrent outbreaks?
    A. avoid use of lipstick
    B. increase dairy intake
    C. prophylactic topical antibiotics
    D. routine use of sunblock

86. Which of the following is associated with the greatest increased incidence of malignant transformation?
    A. colonic strictures
    B. regional enteritis
    C. toxic megacolon
    D. ulcerative colitis

87. A 28-year-old female presents with elevated blood pressure, measured at the local pharmacy, over the last few weeks. Her father has a history of polycystic kidney disease. She denies any symptoms. Vitals include a blood pressure of 148/110 mm Hg measured in the right arm while sitting. This reading is verified in the opposing arm after 30 minutes. Exam is unremarkable. Urinalysis reveals microscopic hematuria. Which of the following diagnostic studies should be performed at this point?
    A. computed tomography
    B. creatinine level
    C. magnetic resonance imaging
    D. ultrasonography

88. A 25-year-old sustained significant blunt force trauma to the chest in a motor vehicle accident. He arrived at the emergency department on supplemental oxygen. An initial evaluation, including chest x-ray, revealed three rib fractures but no other injuries. Suddenly, the patient reports severe shortness of breath. Vital signs at this time are BP 106/66, pulse 20, SaO_2 85%. What is the next best step in management of this patient?
    A. increase supplemental oxygen
    B. intubate immediately
    C. order a STAT CT scan of chest
    D. perform an immediate needle decompression

89. Physical exam of a patient with a "red eye" reveals a homogeneous, sharply demarcated, red area lateral to the iris in the left eye. The cornea remains clear and the pupil is not affected. The patient denies pain and has a visual acuity of 20/20. What is the most likely cause?
    A. acute iritis
    B. conjunctivitis
    C. glaucoma
    D. subconjunctival hemorrhage

90. A 12-year-old girl is found to have elevated blood pressure readings on three separate occasions. Her blood pressure is normal in her legs but femoral pulsations are weak. ECG demonstrates left ventricular hypertrophy. What is the most likely cause of her hypertension?
    A. coarctation of the aorta
    B. pheochromocytoma
    C. tetralogy of Fallot
    D. ventricular septal defect

91. A 45-year-old Caucasian male presents after fasting glucose returns greater than 126 mg/dL for the second time. He has no complaints. His visual acuity is 20/20 in both eyes. When should this patient be referred for formal ophthalmologic evaluation?
    A. immediately upon diagnosis
    B. within 1 year
    C. within 5 years
    D. when he develops visual symptoms

92. A 25-year-old female presents complaining of acute episodes of feeling fearful accompanied by shaking, shortness of breath, nausea, and dizziness. She states that these episodes have occurred several times in the last 2 months and now she worries constantly that she will have "an episode." She is concerned that she is "losing it" and has been avoiding big social gatherings for the last month. What is important to include in patient education for this patient?
    A. avoiding large social gatherings will be helpful
    B. treatment with a tricyclic antidepressant will be helpful
    C. the overall prognosis is not good and she should expect hospitalization
    D. there is an increased chance that she may also develop a severe depression

93. A 50-year-old female presents with acute onset of dyspnea and pleuritic chest pain. She is recovering from hip replacement surgery performed 3 weeks ago. Heart rate is 106. The right leg is swollen and there is pain with palpation of the deep veins. Which of the following diagnostic studies is the best next step to secure diagnosis?
    A. D-dimer blood level
    B. perfusion–ventilation scintigraphy
    C. pulmonary angiography
    D. spiral CT of the chest

94. A 35-year-old male presents for routine physical exam. His last exam was over 16 years ago and he recalls being told that his serum triglyceride level was extremely high. He ignored advice for a cardiac evaluation. What eye finding is likely to be found in this patient?
    A. blue cast to the sclera
    B. green rimming to the iris
    C. pterygium
    D. white cast to the retinal venous bed

95. A generally healthy prepubescent 10-year-old female presents with concerns of recent nonpruritic hair loss on her scalp. She denies trauma, recent illness, fever, or endocrine disorders. What is the most likely physical feature of her hair loss?
    A. 20% to 50% of hair loss with large numbers of hairs with white bulbs after gentle tugging
    B. several 1- to 4-cm oval patches of hair loss with smooth skin and short stubs of new hair
    C. patchy areas of hair loss with fine scale and no inflammation
    D. triangular frontal–temporal recession of hair

96. A 58-year-old complains of headaches, dizziness, and generalized pruritis, especially after showering. Labs reveal hematocrit of 59% with normal RBC morphology and mildly elevated WBC count. Which of the following is considered the mainstay of management?
    A. daily low-dose aspirin
    B. low-salt diet
    C. splenectomy
    D. therapeutic phlebotomy

97. A 35-year-old male underwent gastric bypass surgery 1 year ago and has lost 130 lb. Since his surgery, he has eaten primarily vegetables and fruits. He comes to the office today because his feet sometimes feel "odd," like novocaine wearing off. Which of the following is most likely to be present on neurologic examination?
   A. decreased vibratory sense
   B. hyperactive deep tendon reflexes
   C. impaired two-point discrimination
   D. positive palmar drift

98. A 65-year-old is brought in by his daughter because she is worried that he seems depressed, fatigued, and has lost some weight. The patient describes vague diffuse epigastric pain for 2 months, which started after a couple of weeks of mild diarrhea. He has a 15-lb unintentional weight loss and no appetite. He is not interested in his usual activities. Social history is positive for heavy tobacco and alcohol use. What is the most likely diagnosis?
   A. anemia
   B. depression
   C. diabetes mellitus
   D. pancreatic carcinoma

99. An 8-month-old male infant has had rhinorrhea, sneezing, cough, and low-grade fever for 2 days. On exam, there is nasal flaring, tachypnea, retractions, and wheezes. Chest radiography reveals air trapping and peribronchial thickening. What is the most likely diagnosis?
   A. acute bronchiolitis
   B. asthma exacerbation
   C. cystic fibrosis
   D. viral pneumonia

100. A 79-year-old male with a history of hypertension, controlled with hydrochlorothiazide, and mild COPD presents with dyspnea. He states it began 2 days ago on exertion and has progressed over the last 12 hours to dyspnea at rest. Physical exam reveals 2.1 cm JVD and 2+ pitting edema to the ankles. Which of the following is most likely to be found on cardiac exam?
   A. an ejection click
   B. the presence of a thrill
   C. a third heart sound (S_3)
   D. a fourth heart sound (S_4)

101. A 38-year-old male presents for evaluation of an irritation to his left eye. He works as a miner in a phosphate mine in Florida. Safety regulations at work require the use of a hard hat but not eye protection. Physical examination reveals a fleshy triangular encroachment of the conjunctiva onto the nasal side of the cornea. Visual acuity is 20/20. What is the most likely diagnosis?
   A. ectropion
   B. entropion
   C. pinguecula
   D. pterygium

102. Which of the following is the most frequent site of breast cancer?
   A. lower inner quadrant
   B. lower outer quadrant
   C. upper inner quadrant
   D. upper outer quadrant

103. A 35-year-old female undergoes a dilation and curettage for irregular menstrual bleeding. The endometrial curettings are consistent with the secretory phase of the menstrual cycle. What is the correct interpretation of these results?
   A. the endometrium is under predominantly estrogen stimulation
   B. the patient has ovulated
   C. the patient is entering premature menopause
   D. the patient is taking oral contraceptives

104. An elderly patient is admitted for probable heart failure. Which of the following signs indicates right heart failure?
   A. elevated jugular venous pressure
   B. marked hypotension
   C. perivascular and interstitial edema on chest x-ray
   D. three-pillow orthopnea

105. Which of the following is most characteristic in the presentation of acute mesenteric arterial occlusion?
   A. absence of bowel sounds
   B. intense abdominal pain
   C. bloody diarrhea
   D. peritoneal signs

106. A 58-year-old complains of nausea, "coffee grounds" emesis, and dark tarry stools. There is a history of heavy alcohol use and NSAID exposure secondary to a painful musculoskeletal condition. The patient denies melena. What is the diagnostic test of choice?
   A. abdominal computed tomography
   B. colonoscopy
   C. upper endoscopy
   D. upper gastrointestinal series

107. A 16-year-old girl is brought in by her mother who is concerned that she appears to be losing weight. The mother reports the girl has been on "every diet known" since she was 12 and most recently has refused to eat anything except whole grains, fruits, and vegetables. The girl says that she has lost weight because she has very little appetite, that she has intermittent bouts of diarrhea, and that she is happy about the 10 lb she has lost since starting her new "earth friendly" diet. When asked if she ever has numbness or tingling in her feet, she replies "sometimes." What is the expected finding on peripheral blood smear?
   A. hypersegmented neutrophils
   B. microcytosis
   C. target cells
   D. thrombocytosis

108. A 28-year-old woman describes mild to moderate pelvic pain during the second half of her menstrual cycle with relief upon menses; she also complains of dyspareunia. Laparoscopy shows endometrial implants on the peritoneal walls. The patient would like to maintain her fertility but is not attempting pregnancy at this time. What is the best initial treatment?
   A. aromatase inhibitor
   B. danazol
   C. leuprolide acetate
   D. oral contraceptive

109. A 2-year-old boy presents after two hours of paroxysmal coughing. His mother states he had a gagging episode at lunch, just prior to the cough. Stridor is noted on exam, as well as unilateral wheezing. He has no significant past medical history. Which of the following is highest on the differential diagnosis?
     A. angioedema
     B. epiglottitis
     C. foreign body
     D. laryngotracheobronchitis

110. Which of the following is the typical presentation of nonbullous impetigo?
     A. edematous, red, indurated spreading lesion
     B. inflammatory hot lesion with diffuse erythema
     C. vesicopustular lesion that follows a dermatome
     D. vesicular honey-colored crusted superficial lesions

111. A 36-year-old female who has rheumatoid arthritis is found to be mildly anemic. Which of the following laboratory results is more consistent with anemia of chronic disease than with iron deficiency anemia as her problem?
     A. decreased serum iron
     B. decreased transferrin saturation
     C. normal reticulocyte count
     D. increased serum ferritin

112. An 82-year-old female with a history of severe coronary artery disease is found unresponsive, apneic, and pulseless. What cardiac rhythm disturbance most often causes this presentation?
     A. atrial fibrillation
     B. complete heart block
     C. bundle branch block
     D. ventricular fibrillation

113. A 47-year-old female presents with productive cough and fever. Exam reveals diffuse bronchial breath sounds, rhonchi, and bronchophony in the right middle lobe. What is expected on chest x-ray?
     A. cavitary lesions
     B. diffuse interstitial infiltrates
     C. lobar consolidation
     D. patchy diffuse infiltrates

114. A 28-year-old female who recently began a job with a banking firm complains of headaches that interfere with her ability to concentrate. The headaches typically begin midday and progress unless she takes ibuprofen. She describes the pain as a tightness around the forehead, occiput, and neck. Which of the following characteristics or symptoms is most likely also present?
     A. nausea
     B. phonophobia
     C. pulsatile pain
     D. unilateral pain

115. A 75-year-old male with a history of essential hypertension and hyperlipidemia reports insidious onset of fatigue and dyspnea, as well as recent episodes of exertional syncope. Which of the following is most likely to be found on physical exam?
     A. accentuated S_1 with an opening snap following S_2, heard best at the left sternal border and apex
     B. a diastolic rumbling murmur heard best at the left lower sternal margin and the xiphoid, augmented during inspiration
     C. a low-pitched, blowing decrescendo diastolic murmur, heard best at the third left intercostal space along the left sternal border
     D. a systolic ejection murmur that peaks at mid-systole, heard best at the second intercostal area with radiation to the neck and apex

116. A 50-year-old presents after an apparent suicide attempt from drug ingestion. History is unobtainable. The patient's blood pressure is 130/70 mm Hg. He is tachycardic and displays rapid deep breathing. Laboratory results are as follows:

Na^+	140 mEq/dL
K^+	4.0 mEq/dL
Cl^-	105 mEq/dL
HCO_3^-	10 mEq/dL
Creatinine	1.0 mg/dL
Glucose	120 mg/dL
Serum pH	7.12

     Which of the following drugs was most likely taken?
     A. aspirin
     B. lithium
     C. phenobarbital
     D. acetaminophen

117. A 60-year-old with a 40-year history of alcohol dependence presents stating he "finally quit" drinking yesterday. On physical exam, there is a tremor, tachycardia, tachypnea, and a blood pressure of 150/90. He complains of feeling nervous and is unable to sleep. What is the treatment of choice?
     A. a benzodiazepine every 4 to 6 hours
     B. a daily dose of lithium carbonate
     C. a daily dose of a tricyclic antidepressant
     D. a twice-daily dose of valproate (Depakote)

118. Which of the following physical examination findings is most characteristic of a varicocele?
     A. lying supine decreases the size of the mass
     B. elevation of the testis decreases the pain
     C. "high lie" of the painful testis
     D. small, firm, palpable lump on the testis

119. A patient complains of intermittent epigastric and left upper quadrant pain, weight loss, gaseous abdominal distention, flatulence, and large, greasy, foul-smelling stools. He has a history of alcohol and tobacco abuse. Laboratory testing shows increased serum amylase and lipase as well as glucosuria. What is the most sensitive imaging technique to evaluate the suspected diagnosis?
     A. abdominal computed tomography
     B. abdominal ultrasonography
     C. abdominal plain-film radiography
     D. endoscopic retrograde cholangiopancreatography

120. A sexually active 19-year-old female presents with clusters of painful vesicles with erythematous bases on her vulva and cervix, accompanied by a temperature of 100.0°F and mild malaise. She reports a similar outbreak occurred last month and resolved in 7 days. Microscopic examination of cells from the basement of a blister is likely to reveal which of the following?
    A. Gram-negative rods
    B. Gram-positive cocci in clusters
    C. hyphae and buds
    D. multinucleated giant cells

121. A screening tuberculin skin test (PPD) is placed on a hospital orderly. Two days later, an area of 10-mm induration is noted. The last PPD, placed 18 months ago, was negative. Which of the following statements is true concerning this patient?
    A. The patient has latent tuberculosis.
    B. The patient is infectious.
    C. Pharmacotherapy is not needed.
    D. The patient should be in respiratory isolation.

122. A 36-year-old nulliparous female complains of lower abdominal pressure, bloating, heavy vaginal bleeding, and dysmenorrhea for the past 1 year. On physical exam, the uterus is enlarged with multiple, nontender, discrete, firm irregular masses. What is the most likely diagnosis?
    A. endometrial polyps
    B. endometriosis
    C. uterine carcinoma
    D. uterine leiomyomas

123. A slender elderly female has a long history of untreated elevated serum calcium. Which of the following historical findings is most likely also present due to her known abnormal serum calcium?
    A. DEXA score of −0.6 SD
    B. dyspnea on exertion
    C. loss of thirst
    D. nephrolithiasis

124. While working in a rural clinic, you are asked to assist with the delivery of a 29-year-old multipara. She successfully delivers a baby boy; a continuous, rough, machinery-like murmur is heard on cardiac auscultation of this newborn. What is the drug of choice to administer to the newborn?
    A. ampicillin
    B. β-blocker
    C. heparin
    D. indomethacin

125. A 5-year-old male presents with crusting facial lesions present for 3 days. The mother reports that prior to the development of the facial lesions, her son was scratching at insect bites. Exam reveals confluent erosions with honey-colored crusts below the left nares and cheek. Temperature is 99.8°F. Which of the following is the most appropriate treatment?
    A. acyclovir
    B. cephalexin
    C. doxycycline
    D. hydrocortisone

126. A 50-year-old male presents for routine health maintenance. He states that he could "stand to lose a few pounds" but is otherwise in good health. Past medical history and family history reveal no risk factors. Exam reveals abdominal obesity (waist circumference 45 inches) and blood pressure of 142/90. What additional finding would confirm a diagnosis of metabolic syndrome?
    A. fasting glucose 98 mg/dL
    B. HDL cholesterol 45 mg/dL
    C. LDL cholesterol 120 mg/dL
    D. triglycerides 200 mg/dL

127. A 42-year-old female presents for the third time in the past month complaining of palpitations and a "racing heart." Prior episodes have been successfully treated with adenosine. What definitive treatment should be employed now?
    A. calcium channel blocker
    B. cardioversion
    C. radiofrequency ablation
    D. vagal maneuvers

128. A 31-year-old female complains of chest fullness after eating and progressive dysphagia of solids and liquids over the last 9 months. She has noted a nocturnal cough and also complains of substernal chest pain unrelated to meals. She has had a 10-lb unintentional weight loss. Physical examination is normal. A barium swallow study reveals esophageal dilation with peristalsis appearing diminished or absent in the distal two-thirds. Which of the following is used to confirm the diagnosis?
    A. esophageal manometry
    B. computed tomography
    C. upper endoscopy
    D. 24-hour pH probe

129. What is the first step in the pathogenesis of atherosclerosis?
    A. connective tissue deposits
    B. fatty streak
    C. fibrous capsule formation
    D. small pools of extracellular lipid

130. A patient presents with dull, aching epigastric pain. There is some relief after eating or with antacids. Rapid urease test is positive. Which of the following is a complete recommended treatment regime?
    A. amoxicillin, bismuth subsalicylate, and proton pump inhibitor
    B. amoxicillin, clarithromycin, and proton pump inhibitor
    C. clarithromycin, tetracycline, bismuth subsalicylate
    D. proton pump inhibitor alone

131. A 51-year-old presents for evaluation of involuntary movements of the left hand, which occur only at rest. The symptom has been obvious to his wife for 2 months. Exam reveals a resting tremor, a significant lack of arm movement while walking, and cogwheeling of the shoulder joints with passive ROM. What is the most likely diagnosis?
    A. Creutzfeldt–Jakob syndrome
    B. Huntington's disease
    C. multiple sclerosis
    D. Parkinson's disease

132. Which of the following patients should be referred for audio-logic testing?
     A. 8-year-old male with otitis media
     B. 34-year-old male with history of tympanocentesis as a child
     C. 54-year-old female with chronic cerumen impaction
     D. 68-year-old healthy female

133. Which of the following glucose-lowering agents acts by decreasing insulin resistance and increasing glucose utilization?
     A. acarbose (Precose)
     B. glipizide (Glucotrol)
     C. metformin (Glucophage)
     D. pioglitazone (Actos)

134. A 23-year-old female presents with fever, chills, and flank pain associated with frequency and dysuria. Physical exam reveals CVA tenderness. What is the best treatment regimen?
     A. ceftriaxone 250 mg IM once
     B. ciprofloxacin 750 mg twice daily for 21 days
     C. doxycycline 100 mg twice daily for 10 days
     D. gentamicin 80 mg IM once

135. A 60-year-old male is found to have a new systolic ejection murmur during his annual physical exam. The murmur is heard best in the right second interspace and radiates to his neck. Imaging reveals a calcified, bicuspid aortic valve. Other aspects of the physical exam are normal. Which of the following is indicated at this time?
     A. bovine valve replacement
     B. cardiac catheterization
     C. echocardiography
     D. temporary valvuloplasty

136. A hunter in northwestern Florida, not previously vaccinated for rabies, is attacked and bitten by an aggressive fox. The fox could not be captured. The hunter presents to the emergency department with painful bite lesions on the right hand, upper arm, and anterior chest. He has no other symptoms. Which of the following measures is the appropriate treatment for this patient?
     A. administration of human rabies immune globulin and equine rabies antiserum
     B. cleansing, debridement, and suturing of his wounds
     C. human rabies immune globulin and vaccination with human diploid cell vaccine today and on days 3, 7, 14, and 28
     D. three intramuscular injections of human diploid cell vaccine today, day 7, and day 21 or 28

137. Which of the following is more likely to occur in emphysema-predominant COPD compared to chronic bronchitis–predominant COPD?
     A. dyspnea with exertion
     B. peripheral edema
     C. productive cough
     D. weight loss

138. A 43-year-old female complains of brief episodes of lancinating facial pain that start at the left side of her mouth and radiate to the eye and ear. Which of the following most likely triggers episodes?
     A. chewing
     B. fever
     C. herpetic outbreak
     D. sleep deprivation

139. The risk of developing endometrial cancer can be significantly reduced by the administration of which of the following?
     A. cyclic oral progesterones
     B. estrogen patch
     C. GNRH agonist intramuscularly
     D. oral testosterone

140. A 78-year-old female presents with stiffness of the pelvic and shoulder girdle that has been ongoing for 3 to 4 weeks. Patient denies any headache, jaw claudication, or visual disturbances. ESR is 107. What is the recommended treatment for this patient?
     A. cyclophosphamide
     B. high-dose prednisone
     C. low-dose prednisone
     D. methotrexate

141. A 20-year-old female complains of a pruritic rash for 2 weeks. She noticed one single lesion on her trunk that preceded a generalized eruption of lesions by 1 week. Exam reveals multiple scaling pinkish oval papules and plaques that range in size from 1 to 2 cm, distributed along the cleavage lines of the anterior and posterior trunk. There are a few scattered lesions on the proximal aspect of the arms and legs. The palms and soles are spared. What is the most likely diagnosis?
     A. lichen planus
     B. pityriasis rosea
     C. secondary syphilis
     D. tinea corporis

142. A 70-year-old female reports feeling weak with mild shortness of breath for 1 day. ECG reveals ST elevations and new Q waves in leads II, III, and AVF. What is the most likely diagnosis?
     A. anterior wall infarction
     B. inferior wall infarction
     C. lateral wall infarction
     D. posterior wall infarction

143. On gynecologic examination of a woman in her sixties, which of the following would be considered normal findings?
     A. graying, straight pubic hair and enlarged labia
     B. no pubic hair except for fine hair similar to that on the abdomen
     C. sparse pubic hair, smaller labia and clitoris
     D. thick, dark, curly pubic hair from inner thighs to just below the umbilicus

144. A 52-year-old female presents complaining of constant lower extremity pain. Physical exam reveals dilated, tortuous, elongated veins of her right thigh and leg, most of which are less than 4 mm in diameter. Which of the following interventions is indicated for definitive treatment for this patient?
     A. compression sclerotherapy
     B. greater saphenous vein stripping
     C. leg elevation with bed rest
     D. sequential compression devices

145. The course of schizophrenia is quite variable; however, there are predictive factors associated with a better or poorer course and outcome. Which of the following epidemiologic parameters is predictive of a better outcome for a patient diagnosed with schizophrenia?
     A. age of onset 20 years or older
     B. insidious onset of symptoms
     C. slow rate of progression of illness
     D. low socioeconomic status

146. An 85-year-old female complains of indigestion. She has episodes of feeling "gassy" and feels pressure in the epigastric area after she climbs stairs or walks more than one block. The discomfort she feels is relieved if she sits and rests for 5 to 10 minutes. A resting ECG today demonstrates an old anterior infarction. What ECG finding during one of these episodes would confirm the suspected diagnosis?
    A. development of new Q waves
    B. downsloping ST-segment depression
    C. peaked T waves
    D. presence of U waves

147. A patient presents with low back pain that radiates to the thighs. X-ray shows blurring of the sacroiliac joints; lab work reveals a positive HLA-B27. Which of the following is the likely demographic of this patient?
    A. black male, age 17
    B. black female, age 62
    C. white female, age 42
    D. white male, age 21

148. A 76-year-old female presents with a 2-day history of headache and jaw pain which is exacerbated by chewing. Erythrocyte sedimentation rate is 60 mm/hr. What is the immediate treatment?
    A. cyclophosphamide
    B. fluid resuscitation
    C. oral prednisone
    D. pulsed methylprednisolone

149. A 6-year-old presents with cold symptoms and "pinkeye" for 2 days. Exam reveals red conjunctiva, watery eye discharge, clear rhinorrhea, and a tender preauricular adenopathy. What is the most likely diagnosis?
    A. bacterial conjunctivitis
    B. inclusion conjunctivitis
    C. keratoconjunctivitis sicca
    D. viral conjunctivitis

150. A 25-year-old female G_3P_{0020} presents at 11 weeks gestation with vaginal bleeding and mild cramping. Her previous two pregnancies ended in spontaneous miscarriage at 9 weeks. Examination reveals a moderate bright red flow from the cervical os; the cervix is closed. Palpation reveals an 8-week uterus. What is the diagnosis at this time?
    A. habitual abortion
    B. incomplete abortion
    C. inevitable abortion
    D. threatened abortion

151. A 58-year-old obese female with stable exertional angina presents with an irregular, pruritic, weeping lesion just above the medial malleolus. The surrounding skin is hyperpigmented and slightly edematous. What is the most important intervention to minimize the incidence of similar lesions in the future?
    A. compression stockings
    B. daily topical steroids
    C. lower extremity elevation
    D. regular aerobic exercise

152. A patient presents with dyspnea and cough. Exam reveals low-grade fever, tachycardia, tachypnea, and a pericardial friction rub. There is no edema or jugular venous distention. What other finding is most likely present on exam?
    A. hepatomegaly
    B. orthostatic hypotension
    C. pulsus paradoxus
    D. scattered wheezes

153. A 54-year-old obese African American male with a 40-pack-year history of smoking and regular alcohol use presents with a 3-month history of progressive solid food dysphagia. He has a 10-lb unintentional weight loss. He denies heartburn, melena, or change in bowel habits. What is the most likely diagnosis?
    A. achalasia
    B. esophageal adenocarcinoma
    C. esophageal squamous cell cancer
    D. esophageal stricture

154. A 56-year-old female with no significant past medical history presents complaining of weakness and dyspnea for 2 days. Vitals include a pulse of 42 bpm and a BP of 162/50 mm Hg. ECG reveals irregularly spaced P waves in relation to wide, slow QRS complexes. What is the initial management for this patient?
    A. atropine given intravenously
    B. IV fluid bolus
    C. synchronized cardioversion
    D. temporary pacemaker

155. A 66-year-old female presents with a general complaint of malaise and a throbbing left temporal headache for the past 8 hours. Exam reveals prominent pulsation of the left temporal artery with associated scalp tenderness. Which of the following would be most diagnostic?
    A. color duplex sonography of temporal artery
    B. erythrocyte sedimentation rate
    C. rheumatoid factor level
    D. temporal artery biopsy

156. A patient complains of penile pain after being unable to return his foreskin to its usual position. Which of the following is the diagnosis?
    A. epispadias
    B. hypospadias
    C. paraphimosis
    D. phimosis

157. A patient presents for removal of impacted cerumen in his left ear. He complains of decreased hearing in the affected ear. The Weber test performed on this patient would have which of the following results?
    A. sound would be heard through air longer than through bone in the left ear
    B. sound would be heard through bone longer than through air in the left ear
    C. sound would lateralize to the left ear
    D. sound would lateralize to the right ear

158. A 12-year-old presents with acute onset of dyspnea and wheezing. He reports similar episodes over the past few months. He is not on any medications. Physical exam reveals a respiratory rate of 30, normal blood pressure, no rash, clear throat, and diffuse expiratory wheezing. What is the most likely diagnosis?
   A. anaphylaxis
   B. asthma
   C. cystic fibrosis
   D. toxoplasmosis

159. A 26-year-old asymptomatic female presents for her annual women's health exam. Examination of the external genitalia reveals a few flesh-colored, raised lesions with rough surfaces at the posterior introitus and adjacent labia. What is the most likely etiology?
   A. cytomegalovirus
   B. Epstein–Barr virus
   C. herpes simplex II virus
   D. human papillomavirus

160. A 43-year-old presents for evaluation of involuntary movements. He describes fidgetiness and restlessness, which has progressed to fluid involuntary movements of his upper extremities. His wife has noticed that he is irritable and moody and not wanting to spend time with friends. His father also suffered from the same condition. What type of genetic abnormality is responsible for this condition?
   A. abnormal number of sex chromosomes
   B. deletion of a short arm
   C. transmutation
   D. trinucleotide repeat

161. The parents of a 6-year-old girl inquire as to her risk of developing type 1 diabetes mellitus. Which of the following factors, if present, places her at greatest risk of developing the disease?
   A. a sibling with type 1 diabetes mellitus
   B. body mass index >90th percentile
   C. early introduction of cereals to diet
   D. formula feeding

162. A 50-year-old female is being managed for osteoarthritis of the knees. The pain has become continuous and is even bothersome at night. Which of the following medications is the best option?
   A. acetaminophen (Tylenol)
   B. capsaicin cream
   C. naproxen (Naprosyn)
   D. hydrocodone (Vicodin)

163. A 25-year-old African American female presents with dry cough and dyspnea for 4 weeks. She has become increasingly fatigued. She also complains of occasional blurred vision with increased tearing. She has no significant past medical history. A few scattered maculopapular lesions are noted on her trunk. Chest radiography reveals bilateral hilar adenopathy. What is the most likely diagnosis?
   A. interstitial lung disease
   B. *Pneumocystis jiroveci* (nee *carinii*)
   C. sarcoidosis
   D. tuberculosis

164. A young child presents with right ear pain and pressure, decreased hearing acuity, and a mild fever for 2 days. Physical exam reveals a reddened tympanic membrane with decreased mobility. What is the most likely diagnosis?
   A. acute otitis media
   B. barotrauma
   C. mastoiditis
   D. osteoma

165. A 56-year-old male presents with medial right elbow pain for the past 2 months. He states he started playing golf again after taking a few years off. What is expected on exam?
   A. bulging of the biceps muscle
   B. pain with a valgus stress of the elbow
   C. pain with resisted wrist extension
   D. pain with resisted wrist flexion

166. Occlusion of which of the following arteries is most likely to result in an anterior wall infarction?
   A. left anterior descending
   B. right coronary
   C. left circumflex
   D. left marginal

167. A 28-year-old male presents with a mass in the left testis. The mass is firm, 0.75 cm in size, and does not transilluminate. What blood tests should be ordered at this time?
   A. AFP and βHCG
   B. CA 15-3 and CA 125
   C. FSH and LH
   D. PSA and CEA

168. A 25-year-old male presents to the clinic complaining of sudden onset of dysuria, urinary frequency, shaking chills, and low back and perineal pain. Which of the following physical examination techniques is contraindicated at this time?
   A. expression of penile discharge
   B. palpation of the abdomen with Valsalva
   C. percussion of the urinary bladder
   D. digital rectal examination of the prostate

169. A 15-year-old female complains of abdominal pain that started 12 hours ago after her birthday party where she ate pizza, soda, and birthday cake. The patient has no appetite this morning and she feels warm. LMP was 3 weeks ago. Abdominal exam reveals right lower quadrant tenderness without rebound. In addition to laboratory studies, what is the imaging study of choice?
   A. abdominal computed tomography
   B. endoscopic retrograde cholangiopancreatography
   C. flat plat of abdomen, kidneys, ureter, bladder
   D. pelvic ultrasonography

170. A 27-year-old female presents with numbness and tingling in her right hand specific to the thumb, index and middle finger. The symptoms are more pronounced when working on the computer keyboard at work. She states she occasionally wakes at night with similar symptoms that also include forearm pain. Physical exam is normal. What reasonable recommendation could be made to slow or halt progression of this disease?
   A. ibuprofen when pain is severe
   B. modify computer use and wear wrist splints
   C. topical capsaicin twice daily
   D. surgical release of the carpal tunnel

171. A 30-year-old with asthma reports using levalbuterol (Xopenex) daily. He awakens with wheeze, necessitating use of the inhaler about four nights per month. Exam finds no current wheezing and the patient is not in respiratory distress. He is on no other medications for his asthma. According to current guidelines, which of the following should be initiated at this time?
    A. inhaled long-acting β-agonist
    B. inhaled steroid plus a long-acting β-agonist
    C. nebulized short-acting β-agonist
    D. oral steroid tapering dose

172. A 62-year-old male with a history of coronary artery disease and hypertension presents with altered mental status for 2 hours. Blood pressure is 220/120 mm Hg and papilledema is noted on fundoscopy. Which of the following should be started immediately?
    A. enalapril
    B. hydralazine
    C. labetalol
    D. nitroglycerin

173. When performing a pelvic exam, which of the following cervical changes would be consistent with pregnancy?
    A. erythematous cervix
    B. cyanotic cervix
    C. multiparous cervix
    D. strawberry cervix

174. A 26-year-old is diagnosed with constipation-dominant irritable bowel syndrome (IBS). She has presented numerous times to the local urgent care center due to abdominal pain and inability to pass stool. What is the initial treatment?
    A. anticonstipation agents such as osmotic laxatives
    B. antispasmodic (anticholinergic) agents
    C. high-fiber diet and fiber supplementation
    D. serotonin antagonist such as alosetron

175. A 56-year-old male complains of a nonhealing lesion on his left cheek. Examination reveals a 6-mm pearly papule with surface telangiectasias and a central erosion. What is the most appropriate next step in management?
    A. curettage
    B. electrodesiccation
    C. excision
    D. shave biopsy

176. How is the diagnosis of polymyositis definitively confirmed?
    A. antinuclear antibodies
    B. electromyography
    C. muscle biopsy
    D. serum aldolase level

177. An adult with diabetes mellitus presents with a rapidly developing sore throat with severe pain on swallowing. Examination of the pharynx reveals some mild erythema. Which of the following is true at this time?
    A. laryngoscopy is contraindicated
    B. needle biopsy is indicated
    C. inpatient treatment is necessary
    D. treatment is mainly supportive

178. A 64-year-old female presents with pain in her knees that has been going on for 2 years. She feels fine on waking but has moderate to severe pain and stiffness after being on her feet all day. On exam, limited range of motion and crepitus are noted in both knees and swelling is noted in all DIP joints and some PIP joints. What is the most likely diagnosis?
    A. acute gout
    B. osteoarthritis
    C. reactive arthritis
    D. rheumatoid arthritis

179. A 56-year-old male is admitted to the critical care unit with sepsis. On day 2, he is noted to have hypokalemia that is refractory to potassium administration. What other electrolyte disturbance should be actively looked for?
    A. hyperglycemia
    B. hypernatremia
    C. hypocalcemia
    D. hypomagnesemia

180. What is the routine schedule for immunization against the hepatitis B virus?
    A. baseline and then 1 and 6 months later
    B. baseline and then 2 and 4 months later
    C. baseline with booster at 2 months
    D. baseline with booster at 6 to 18 months

181. A 2-year-old is brought to the office for follow-up after a battery of tests including a hearing test, EEG, and CT scan, all of which are normal. The child's parents describe delayed speech development. The child has age-appropriate motor skills; however, his language and social development are severely delayed. The parents also note that the child has limited play skills and seems to be particularly sensitive to the environment (noise and motion). Which of the following diagnostic statements is characteristic of the most likely diagnosis?
    A. age of onset is generally before age 3
    B. more than half of the patients also have a seizure disorder
    C. most patients will display hallucinations and delusions
    D. level of intelligence is normal in most patients

182. A 22-year-old female was recently diagnosed with HIV. She has a baseline viral load of 230,000 units and a CD4 count of 150 cells/μL. In addition to starting antiretroviral therapy, which of the following is indicated?
    A. azithromycin (Zithromax) 1,200 mg po weekly
    B. fluconazole (Diflucan) 400 mg po daily for 12 weeks
    C. ganciclovir (Cytovene) 1 g po three times daily for 6 weeks
    D. trimethoprim/sulfamethoxazole (Bactrim) DS 1 po three times weekly

183. A 68-year-old female with 40 pack-years of tobacco use presents for evaluation of gradual painless loss of central vision bilaterally. She also describes distorted images in the lower fields. Which of the following funduscopic examination findings is most consistent with the likely diagnosis?
    A. haphazardly distributed hard drusen with sharply defined edges
    B. hyperemic, swollen optic disc with blurred margins
    C. rings and crescents along the temporal border of the optic disc
    D. venous tapering, flame-shaped hemorrhages, copper wiring

184. A 70-year-old female reports gradual onset of pain and stiffness of the neck and shoulder, now progressing to the hips and thighs. There is morning stiffness and pain on movement. What other disease entity shares the same immunologic features and is also likely to occur in this patient?
A. fibromyalgia
B. osteoarthritis
C. osteomyelitis
D. temporal arteritis

185. A 16-year-old Hispanic female presents to the clinic complaining of severe pain in her right ear. She is on the local high school swim team and has been participating in extra practice sessions. Her ear pain is so severe that she cannot lie on her right side to sleep. On physical exam, the right tragus is tender to palpation. The right ear canal is swollen and has scant white, clumpy discharge. Culture of this discharge would most likely reveal what organism?
A. *Haemophilus influenzae*
B. *Moraxella catarrhalis*
C. *Pseudomonas aeruginosa*
D. *Streptococcus pneumoniae*

186. Which of the following is the most common chest x-ray finding in pneumoconiosis?
A. lobar consolidation
B. diffuse nodular infiltrates
C. solid masses
D. granulomas

187. A patient presents with high fever and increasing left lower quadrant abdominal pain. Exam confirms temperature of 101°F (38.3°C), nondistended abdomen, normoactive bowel sounds, and left lower quadrant tenderness with a palpable mass and direct rebound. Stool is positive for occult blood. What is the initial management?
A. clear liquid diet, broad-spectrum IV antibiotics with anaerobic coverage
B. clear liquid diet, broad-spectrum oral antibiotics with anaerobic coverage
C. NPO, IV fluids, broad-spectrum IV antibiotics with anaerobic coverage
D. NPO, IV fluids, nasogastric tube, broad-spectrum IV antibiotics with anaerobic coverage

188. A 14-year-old male presents with fever, myalgias, arthralgias, carditis, and polyarthritis. ASO titer is positive. What is the treatment of choice to relieve his fever and arthralgias?
A. acetaminophen
B. codeine
C. ibuprofen
D. salicylates

189. A 66-year-old male was found wandering in the streets by the police. There are no signs of trauma. BP 90/54; P 115; R 12. Physical exam reveals mild dehydration as well as decreased mental state without focal neurologic findings. Initial laboratory findings include glucose 750 mg/dL, Na 124 mEq/L, K 3.0 mEq/L, Cl 102 mEq/L, CO_2 37 mEq/L, BUN 63 mg/dL, and creatinine 1.0 mg/dL. Which of the following is the most appropriate first step in treating this patient?
A. glucagon
B. insulin
C. phosphate
D. saline

190. A child exhibits short staring spells at school which are sometimes accompanied by loss of postural tone. Episodes last less than a minute. Electroencephalography reveals bilateral 3-Hz spike-and-wave pattern. What is the medication of choice?
A. carbamazepine
B. ethosuximide
C. phenobarbital
D. phenytoin

191. A 25-year-old sexually active female presents complaining of vaginal pruritus and a malodorous, yellow to greenish, frothy discharge, which has been present for 2 days. Exam reveals vaginal erythema and red maculopapular lesions of the cervix. There is no cervical motion tenderness. What is the most appropriate pharmacologic treatment?
A. ceftriaxone
B. clindamycin
C. fluconazole
D. metronidazole

192. A 22-year-old presents to the office complaining of tingling of the left side of her face and numbness in her left arm for the last 2 days. She denies trauma or previous similar episodes. She admits to being anxious often and more anxious recently due to her new job at the factory that requires her to work very quickly. Further questioning reveals that her mother had symptoms of numbness and weakness of her arm and leg as the patient was growing up. Her mother is fine now and the patient does not know the cause of her mother's problem. Which of the following is most likely to be found on physical exam of this patient?
A. muscle atrophy and weakness of the affected extremity
B. papilledema on funduscopic examination
C. sensory loss that does not conform to the dermatomes
D. visual field deficit in the left eye on repeated tests

193. A 2-year-old was recently taken to a nursing home to visit a relative. A few days after the visit, the relative was diagnosed with influenza. In the last 24 hours, the child has been experiencing high fever, cough, sore throat, and myalgias. The child did not receive a flu vaccine. What treatment is warranted at this time for the child?
A. amantadine (Symmetrel)
B. oseltamivir (Tamiflu)
C. rimantadine (Flumadine)
D. zanamivir (Relenza)

194. A 15-year-old male presents with knee pain for the past 3 weeks. At first, he thought it was a football injury but the pain has not resolved. On exam, a mass is felt on the posterior aspect of the femur. Radiography shows a destructive, lytic lesion of the distal femur with soft tissue involvement. What is the most likely diagnosis?
A. enchondroma
B. osteoid osteoma
C. osteomyelitis
D. osteosarcoma

195. A patient being seen in the emergency department displays suicidal ideation. What additional information will most strongly lead to a decision to hospitalize the patient rather than treat on an outpatient basis?
A. anxious mood
B. depressed mood
C. history of impulsive behavior
D. hypersomnolence

196. A 45-year-old male presents with acute hoarseness for 2 days. He gives a history of cold symptoms that have been resolving. He denies cigarette smoking. What is the most appropriate patient education point?
- **A.** He has an increased risk of leukoplakia of the vocal folds.
- **B.** He likely has a bacterial infection and will require antibiotics.
- **C.** He is at risk for vocal cord paralysis.
- **D.** He should avoid singing or shouting until the voice normalizes.

197. A 22-year-old otherwise healthy male presents complaining of cold sores after going to the beach. Exam reveals several areas of small grouped vesicles on an erythematous base on the vermilion border of the lips. What is the most appropriate treatment?
- **A.** oral acyclovir
- **B.** oral prednisone
- **C.** topical idoxuridine (Herplex)
- **D.** topical penciclovir (Denavir)

198. Ten days after a visit to a strawberry farm, a patient presents with a 9-cm rash in her left axilla. The rash has been slowly expanding since its initial appearance and is characterized by a bright red outer border with partial central clearing. In addition, she complains of headache, fever chills, malaise, and fatigue. What is the most likely diagnosis?
- **A.** Lyme disease
- **B.** measles
- **C.** Rocky Mountain spotted fever
- **D.** dermatophytosis

199. A 22-year-old female presents complaining of progressive lower abdominal pain, fever, and purulent vaginal discharge for 3 days. She denies vaginal bleeding or spotting. Her last menstrual period was 3 weeks ago and described as regular flow. The patient reports sexual intercourse 1 week ago with a new partner. Temperature is 101.3°F. There is diffuse lower abdominal tenderness with guarding to palpation. Speculum exam reveals a mucopurulent cervicitis, bilateral adnexal tenderness without masses, and marked cervical motion tenderness. What is the most likely diagnosis?
- **A.** adnexal torsion
- **B.** ectopic pregnancy
- **C.** pelvic inflammatory disease
- **D.** ruptured functional ovarian cyst

200. A 59-year-old male presents with acute chest pain of 20 minutes duration. The pain is described as crushing and radiating to his left arm and jaw. There is a prior history of angina for the past 2 years for which he is treated with medication. What is the best method to differentiate between an exacerbation of his angina and an acute myocardial infarction?
- **A.** cardiac biomarkers
- **B.** coronary angiography
- **C.** electrocardiography
- **D.** stress testing

201. Which of the following is a potential adverse reaction to isoniazid in the treatment of tuberculosis?
- **A.** glaucoma
- **B.** headache
- **C.** hepatitis
- **D.** hypoglycemia

202. A 43-year-old male presents with a rash on his face which has been progressing for the past 1 month. He reports a history of facial flushing in response to hot foods and alcohol. Physical exam reveals persistent erythema, telangiectasias, and papulopustules on the cheeks bilaterally. What is the most likely diagnosis?
- **A.** acne vulgaris
- **B.** folliculitis
- **C.** rosacea
- **D.** seborrheic dermatitis

203. A 15-year-old girl with no significant past medical history presents to the office for a routine physical. She received all routine vaccines before the age of 10 years. She is not sexually active and not considered high risk for any diseases. Which of the following vaccines should be offered to her at this time?
- **A.** hepatitis A
- **B.** human papillomavirus
- **C.** influenza
- **D.** pneumococcal

204. A 50-year-old female describes a feeling of restlessness and a curious sensory disturbance in her legs at night. These sensations often interrupt her sleep and have led to chronic fatigue and irritability. What is the recommended treatment?
- **A.** anticholinergic medication
- **B.** dopamine agonist
- **C.** phenytoin
- **D.** sleep agent

205. An 18-year-old female presents with a small bump on the dorsal aspect of her wrist. She states it does not really hurt but she thinks it is ugly and wants to know what can be done. On exam, it is soft and mobile. What is the most definitive treatment?
- **A.** antibiotics
- **B.** aspiration and steroid injection
- **C.** physical therapy
- **D.** surgical excision

206. A 20-year-old male complains of increased anxiety in social settings. He realizes that he has been turning down invitations to go out with other people and prefers to be alone where he knows he would not be embarrassed by doing something "stupid." He is currently working at a factory where he works alone and can avoid interaction with other people. He avoids most social contact and has one friend from high school who he sees from time to time. What would be the most effective therapy for this patient?
- **A.** aversion therapy
- **B.** behavior therapy
- **C.** insight-oriented therapy
- **D.** self-help group therapy

207. A 15-year-old male with a history of sickle cell anemia presents with increasing lethargy and generalized pain. Vitals: T 98.2; P 98; R 20; BP 116/74. His lips are slightly dry; he has mildly decreased turgor and 3-second capillary refill. No murmurs, abnormal lung sounds, or abdominal pain are noted on physical exam. Reticulocyte count is increased by twofold; hematocrit and hemoglobin are slightly below his baseline. What is the next best step in management?
- **A.** blood transfusion
- **B.** hydration and analgesics
- **C.** hydroxyurea
- **D.** IV broad-spectrum antibiotics

208. A 34-year woman presents to the emergency department complaining of left lower pelvic pain for 2 hours. History reveals intermittent vaginal spotting for 3 days; LMP was 6 weeks ago. Serum β-HCG is 2,000 mU/mL; ultrasonography shows an empty uterus and 3-cm adnexal mass. Vital signs are normal and patient is stable. What is the best course of management?
    A. laparoscopy
    B. laparotomy
    C. methotrexate
    D. watchful waiting

209. A 15-year-old boy presents with a 2-month history of bilateral knee pain. He runs track and attends practice daily. He describes the pain as dull and aching over the anterior knee, increasing with activity. He did not have any specific injury or limp but has noticed some swelling under the knees. On exam, he is afebrile. He has slight swelling and tenderness bilaterally just below the knees. There is full range of motion and negative special tests of the knee. Radiographs are normal. What is the best management at this time?
    A. knee immobility for 6 to 8 weeks
    B. referral to physical therapy
    C. routine referral to orthopaedic surgery
    D. self-limited activity, ice, and NSAIDs

210. A 62-year-old male diagnosed with GERD is being treated with pantoprazole (Protonix). In addition, he takes methotrexate, atenolol, hydrochlorothiazide, and lorazepam. Which medication is most likely to interact with the pantoprazole?
    A. atenolol
    B. hydrochlorothiazide
    C. lorazepam
    D. methotrexate

211. A 25-year-old male presents complaining of extreme weakness, 20-lb weight loss, light-headedness, and dizziness. On physical exam, he appears ill and his blood pressure is 90/70. He has dark skin and hyperpigmented creases on his palms. Serum sodium is low and potassium is elevated; urea level and serum calcium are both elevated. What is the most likely diagnosis?
    A. Addison's disease
    B. Cushing's syndrome
    C. pheochromocytoma
    D. primary hyperaldosteronism

212. A 73-year-old with chronic renal failure presents with weakness. Potassium level returns at 7.0 mEq/L. What is most likely to be found on ECG?
    A. elevated ST segment in all leads
    B. peaked T waves and shortened QT intervals
    C. prolonged ST segments with flattened T waves
    D. sinus tachycardia with prolonged QT segments

213. A 32-year-old male who underwent radiation for acute lymphocytic leukemia (ALL) 15 years ago presents with a weight gain of 20 lb, puffy eyes, and coarse dry skin. Labs reveal TSH 7.2 μU/mL (normal 0.5 to 5.0) and free T_4 0.3 ng/mL (normal 0.7 to 2.7). Which of the following drugs is indicated?
    A. bromocriptine (Parlodel)
    B. growth hormone
    C. levothyroxine (Synthroid)
    D. propylthiouracil (PTU)

214. A 50-year-old well-developed, normal weight female presents with a history of recurrent renal stones, bone pain, osteoporosis, constipation, and depression. She denies weight loss, muscle spasm, or cardiac problems. Which of the following laboratory results is most consistent with her history?
    A. elevated serum calcium
    B. elevated serum phosphorus
    C. suppressed alkaline phosphatase
    D. suppressed parathyroid hormone

215. A 70-year-old female with a history of atrial fibrillation presents with dyspnea and tachycardia. Blood pressure is 88/60 and cardioversion is recommended. Which of the following needs to be done before cardioversion?
    A. cardiac catheterization
    B. chest radiography
    C. tilt test
    D. transesophageal echocardiography

216. A 23-year-old female presents with a 2-week history of mild greenish, foul-smelling diarrhea. She denies use of laxatives or olestra. There are no sick family members or other contacts. She was treated 3 weeks ago for pyelonephritis after returning from her honeymoon in Mexico. Vital signs are stable and the patient is in no distress. What is the next step in the diagnosis and management of this patient?
    A. aggressive oral rehydration and let the diarrhea resolve on its own with time; no specific tests are needed at this time
    B. bowel rest, oral intake as tolerated with flat carbonated beverages and "BRAT" diet; no specific tests are needed at this time
    C. empiric use of antidiarrheal agents; if no improvement in 3 days, consider stool tests
    D. bowel rest while awaiting results of stool culture, ova and parasites, fecal WBC count, and *Clostridium difficile* toxin

217. A 55-year-old male with a history of coronary artery disease and hypertension presents with sudden onset of searing chest pain radiating to his upper back. BP is 220/166 mm Hg. Chest radiography shows a widened mediastinum. Which of the following medications should be given first?
    A. aspirin
    B. labetalol
    C. nitroglycerin
    D. verapamil

218. A 40-year-old female presents complaining of feeling "down" for the last month. She complains that she is very tired all the time and is now sleeping 9 to 10 hours per night. She states she has no energy to do anything and has stopped going out on weekends with friends due to fatigue and loss of interest. She has also noted a 6-lb weight loss and admits to eating less in the last few weeks. She has had episodes of "sadness" in the past but they were not as severe. The patient denies thoughts of suicide. What is the best pharmacologic treatment for this patient?
    A. carbamazepine (Tegretol)
    B. fluoxetine (Prozac)
    C. lithium carbonate
    D. lorazepam (Ativan)

219. A 33-year-old with a past medical history of prolactinoma and parathyroid adenoma is brought to the emergency department by a family member who found her diaphoretic and confused. Initial laboratory studies reveal a fasting blood glucose of 35 mg/dL. The patient responds rapidly to IV dextrose. All other labs are within normal ranges. Which of the following interventions represents the most appropriate long-term treatment for this patient?
   A. discourage alcohol consumption
   B. encourage small frequent meals
   C. glucagon as needed
   D. refer to an appropriate surgeon

220. A 25-year-old female presents with urinary frequency. Urinalysis reveals pyuria. Presence of which of the following would indicate a diagnosis other than cystitis?
   A. flank pain
   B. dysuria
   C. urgency
   D. nocturia

221. A 19-year-old male college student presents with an asymptomatic rash extending over his upper trunk, shoulders, and neck. The hypopigmented annular lesions vary in size from 4 to 5 cm diameter to larger, confluent areas. There is no visible scale associated with the lesions. What organism is the most likely cause of his symptoms?
   A. *Candida*
   B. *Malassezia*
   C. *Staphylococcus aureus*
   D. *Trichophyton rubrum*

222. A 25-year-old female presents with a low-grade fever and nonproductive cough for 5 days. Physical exam reveals a normal chest, mild pharyngeal erythema, and bullous myringitis. What is the most likely diagnosis?
   A. lung abscess
   B. mycoplasma pneumonia
   C. pneumococcal pneumonia
   D. sarcoidosis

223. A 25-year-old female undergoes echocardiography for nonspecific chest pain and palpitations. Results indicate a floppy mitral valve. What finding was most likely present on physical exam?
   A. fixed split S_1
   B. mid-systolic click
   C. late diastolic rumble
   D. early systolic ejection sound

224. A 35-year-old female with systemic lupus erythematosus presents with purplish blotches under her skin. She has also felt extremely fatigued and increasingly weak. She has no pain. On physical examination, she is noticeably pale, with widely distributed purpura and petechiae, particularly on the extremities. She has no lymphadenopathy or hepatosplenomegaly. Initial laboratory testing shows pancytopenia with decreased reticulocytes. What is the most likely diagnosis?
   A. acute lymphocytic leukemia
   B. aplastic anemia
   C. hairy cell leukemia
   D. immune thrombocytopenia

225. A 55-year-old overweight male smoker complains of cramping pain located in the calf muscles bilaterally. The pain is brought on by exercise and relieved with rest. In addition to smoking cessation, which of the following describes the best conservative care intervention?
   A. low-carbohydrate diet and walking
   B. low-fat diet and swimming
   C. swimming and weight lifting exercises
   D. walking and weight loss

226. A 4-year-old girl presents for a routine checkup. She is new to the practice. Physical examination reveals a harsh, holosystolic grade III/VI cardiac murmur at the left sternal border with wide radiation and fixed split S_2. There is no change with position or respiration. What is the most likely diagnosis?
   A. innocent murmur
   B. aortic regurgitation
   C. patent ductus arteriosus
   D. ventricular septal defect

227. A 43-year-old male presents with choreiform movements and diminished cognitive abilities. What would be the most likely finding in a brain MRI of this patient?
   A. Arnold–Chiari malformation
   B. cerebral atrophy
   C. isolated focal lesion
   D. ring-enhancing lesions

228. A 22-year-old college student has been experiencing low-grade fevers, worsening nonproductive cough, and fatigue for the last 7 to 8 days. Despite his symptoms he has been attending class. The patient reports no significant past medical history. Temperature 100.5°F, BP 110/70, pulse 82, and respiratory rate 20 and unlabored. Lung exam is significant for rales and egophony. What is the best management option?
   A. counsel on rest and fluids and recommend an over-the-counter cough preparation
   B. initiate treatment with a macrolide antibiotic and follow-up in 48 hours
   C. obtain a sputum culture and get a complete blood count prior to any treatment
   D. place on 2 L oxygen by nasal canula and call for transport to the hospital

229. A 49-year-old patient with diabetes type 2 returns for follow-up of a nonfasting cholesterol of 235 mg/dL obtained during a community health fair. Which of the following is the most appropriate response?
   A. give advice on diet and exercise to improve lipid profile
   B. obtain fasting lipid profile
   C. reassure that this is an acceptable nonfasting result
   D. start an HMG-CoA reductase inhibitor

230. A 72-year-old recently widowed female is hospitalized with an acute anterior wall myocardial infarction. Echocardiography reveals left ventricular apical ballooning, yet cardiac catheterization reveals clear coronary arteries. What is the most likely diagnosis?
   A. aortic aneurysm
   B. cardiac tamponade
   C. Prinzmetal's angina
   D. Takotsubo cardiomyopathy

231. A 43-year-old female with a history of cholelithiasis presents with moderate boring epigastric pain that came on suddenly 3 hours ago. The pain radiates to the back and is somewhat relieved by leaning forward. She is nauseous and has vomited twice. Exam reveals abdominal distension and tenderness without rigidity or rebound. What is the recommended management?
    A. aggressive IV rehydration, calcium gluconate, and fresh frozen plasma
    B. enteral nutrition, IV somatostatin, and stent placement across the pancreatic duct
    C. NPO, bed rest, nasogastric suction, and analgesia
    D. parenteral nutrition, antibiotics, and infusion of serum albumin

232. A 42-year-old female presents with dry eyes and dry mouth for the past 2 to 3 months. She states she often feels she has "cotton mouth" and her eyes are always itching and burning. Which of the following exam findings is found in one out of three of the patients with the suspected disorder?
    A. loss of normal skin folds
    B. malar butterfly rash
    C. parotid enlargement
    D. progressive proximal muscle weakness

233. A 36-year-old male presents with purulent nasal discharge, headaches, and maxillary jaw pain for 9 days despite the use of nasal saline lavage. This is the fourth episode of similar symptoms so far this year. What diagnostic modality is most appropriate at this time?
    A. computed tomography of sinuses
    B. magnetic resonance of sinuses
    C. radiographs of the skull
    D. culture and sensitivity of the nasal discharge

234. Following an episode of syncope, a 32-year-old male is diagnosed with long QT syndrome. Should he become ill with a bacterial infection, he should be advised to avoid antibiotic drugs from which of the following classes?
    A. aminoglycosides
    B. β-lactams
    C. macrolides
    D. sulfonamides

235. What muscles form the rotator cuff?
    A. subscapularis, teres major, trapezius, deltoid
    B. supraspinatus, infraspinatus, subscapularis, teres minor
    C. supraspinatus, infraspinatus, triceps, biceps
    D. trapezius, deltoid, triceps, biceps

236. A tall, thin 26-year-old male complains of sudden left-sided chest pain and dyspnea. He is tachycardic and there are decreased breath sounds on the left. Which of the following is the initial diagnostic study of choice?
    A. computed tomography of chest
    B. chest plain radiography
    C. magnetic resonance imaging of chest
    D. electrocardiography

237. A patient presents with chronic bilateral eye irritation and pruritis. The eyes appear "red-rimmed" with scales clinging to the eyelashes. Conjunctivae are clear. What is the most likely diagnosis?
    A. blepharitis
    B. chalazion
    C. ectropion
    D. hordeolum

238. A 66-year-old male presents with productive cough and shortness of breath. While he has had a cough for "years," he notes that his shortness of breath is worsening, particularly when he lifts things above his head. He is able to tolerate walking on a treadmill if he uses the armrests. He has had four respiratory infections in the past 6 months. He has smoked one to two packs of cigarettes per day since the age of 16; he works in a cotton textile mill and lives in a large urban area. Exam reveals an overweight gentleman with nicotine-stained fingernails. He is using his accessory muscles of respiration; there is an expiratory wheeze diffusely over the chest. Which of the following contributed most in the pathogenesis of this condition?
    A. air pollution
    B. cigarette smoking
    C. occupational exposure
    D. respiratory infections

239. A 40-year-old male complains of a 2-month history of moderate dyspepsia. He denies weight loss, nausea or vomiting, hematemesis, melena, and hematochezia. He uses alcohol occasionally and is a nonsmoker. He lost his job as a computer analyst 3 months ago. The *Helicobacter pylori* test results are pending. What empiric treatment is recommended?
    A. H₂ receptor antagonist such as famotidine (Pepcid)
    B. prokinetic agent such as metoclopramide (Reglan)
    C. prostaglandin analog such as misoprostol (Cytotec)
    D. proton pump inhibitor such as lansoprazole (Prevacid)

240. Of the following signs of pregnancy, which is defined as when the uterine body and cervix can easily be flexed against one another?
    A. Chadwick's sign
    B. Goodell's sign
    C. Hegar's sign
    D. McDonald's sign

241. Which of the following presentations is most suggestive of early chronic renal failure?
    A. anorexia, fatigue, and weakness
    B. oliguria, shortness of breath, and chest pain
    C. polyuria, polydipsia, and back pain
    D. nausea, pruritus, and abdominal pain

242. A 58-year-old male with a chronic progressive neurologic disorder is being admitted to a long-term care facility. He is unable to walk. He has difficulty swallowing, chewing, and talking as well as cognitive deficits. Exam reveals stiffness and wasting of both upper and lower limbs but intact sensory functions. Tongue appears wasted and contracted and exhibits fasciculations. What is the most likely diagnosis?
    A. amyotrophic lateral sclerosis
    B. Huntington's disease
    C. multiple sclerosis
    D. syringomyelia

243. A 42-year-old male truck driver presents with recurring rhinitis and watery eyes during the spring months. What is the best treatment for this patient?
    A. desloratadine (Clarinex)
    B. fluticasone (Flonase)
    C. montelukast (Singulair)
    D. diphenhydramine (Benadryl)

244. A mother brings her 5-year-old daughter to the office because of a fever and a fiery red rash on both cheeks for 2 days. The child complains of sore throat and appears tired. What can you tell her about the most likely course of this illness?
    A. The rash will spread distally and include central clearing areas resembling a reticulated or lacy appearance.
    B. The cheek erythema will progress to vesicles before crusting over and healing.
    C. She will likely develop red macules on the buccal mucosa and tongue.
    D. A symmetric polyarthritis will likely develop and last 2 to 3 weeks.

245. A 59-year-old male gives a history of chronic productive cough and dyspnea on exertion, which has progressively worsened over the past 3 years. He is obese and continues to smoke 1.5 packs per day. Physical exam reveals diffuse rhonchi and wheeze which clear somewhat with coughing. What is the recommended treatment?
    A. combined long-acting β-agonist with inhaled corticosteroid
    B. daily, low-dose oral steroids
    C. long-acting β-agonist twice daily
    D. short-acting β-agonist as needed

246. What is the most definitive test for the diagnosis of pulmonary embolus?
    A. arterial blood gas
    B. D-dimer
    C. pulmonary angiography
    D. CT scan with contrast

247. In the evaluation of a stable ambulatory patient with angina, which of the following patients should *not* undergo an exercise/treadmill test?
    A. 45-year-old male with history of non-ST segment elevation myocardial infarction (non-STEMI) 2 months ago
    B. 50-year-old female with a history of recurrent congestive heart failure
    C. 65-year-old ambulatory female, status post right hip arthroplasty 2 years ago
    D. 75-year-old male with significant aortic stenosis

248. A 78-year-old male presents with inability to achieve and maintain an erection rigid enough for sexual intercourse. His wife accompanies him and confirms the absence of nocturnal erections. They are both interested in continuing a fulfilling sex life, and he is willing to undergo the full extent of testing to arrive at an etiology of his erectile dysfunction. Comorbidities include angina treated with nitrates. Which of the following diagnostic tests should be performed first?
    A. arteriography
    B. papaverine injection
    C. trial of sildenafil (Viagra)
    D. tumescent testing

249. A 4-year-old presents with a 2-day history of a barking cough, runny nose, and fever. Exam reveals a red pharynx with no exudate, a temperature of 100.4°F, and scattered wheezes throughout both lung fields. What is the recommended treatment?
    A. antitussive such as dextromethorphan
    B. ceftriaxone IM (Rocephin)
    C. nebulized budesonide (Pulmicort)
    D. nebulized epinephrine

250. A 35-year-old G_2P_{1001} presents at 32 weeks gestation by LMP complaining of painless bright red vaginal bleeding after sexual intercourse. She is new to the United States and has not had previous prenatal care. What is the first step in the management?
    A. cervical exam
    B. ferning test
    C. Kleihauer–Betke test
    D. ultrasonography

251. A 27-year-old female presents with pain in her joints and fatigue for 2 months. Exam reveals raised plaques over her nose and cheeks and multiple ulcers in her mouth. What is the most likely diagnosis?
    A. polymyositis
    B. rheumatoid arthritis
    C. systemic lupus erythematosus
    D. systemic sclerosis

252. A 46-year-old male presents for evaluation of physical changes. He has developed coarse facial features and a large prominent jaw; he states his shoe size has increased by half a size over the last year despite no gain in weight. Which of the following physical exam findings is most likely also to be present?
    A. atrophy of the digits
    B. deepening voice
    C. dry skin
    D. enlarged testes

253. A 53-year-old male presents to the emergency department with a 3-hour history of sharp, pleuritic central chest pain that began at rest. This pain is described as worsening in the supine position and improving whenever he sits up and leans forward. Exam does not reveal a murmur but does reveal a two-phase friction rub heard best at the left lower sternal border. Which of the following would best aid in determining the diagnosis?
    A. cardiac catheterization
    B. cardiac enzymes
    C. electrocardiography
    D. pericardial window

254. Each of the following patients presents with a blood pressure of 150/100 on two separate occasions. For which is a secondary cause most likely?
    A. 26-year-old female at 30 weeks gestation
    B. 30-year-old female with BMI 28 and 10-pack-year history of smoking
    C. 48-year-old male who requires three drugs to reduce the pressure
    D. 50-year-old male who presents for his first physical exam in 10 years

255. A 26-year-old female presents to the emergency department with multiple bruises over her face, arms, and trunk. She tells you that she slipped and tumbled down a flight of stairs. The patient is extremely anxious and her contusions are not consistent with her reported fall. When you question her further, she tells you that her husband sometimes drinks too much and she needs to get home before he wakes up. Checking the patient's medical record, you find that this is her third visit in the last year for similar injuries. Which of the following is most likely true about this patient and her situation?

   A. family therapy is usually not very helpful
   B. leaving her home will reduce her risk of injury and death
   C. pregnancy will increase her risk of abuse
   D. it is unlikely that she grew up in a violent home

256. A 53-year-old female recently diagnosed with infective endocarditis complains of nonpainful erythematous lesions located on her palms and soles. What are these lesions?

   A. erythema marginatum
   B. Janeway lesion
   C. Osler's nodes
   D. Roth's spots

257. A patient presents with irrational fear of eating in public and using public restrooms. After taking a complete history and performing a thorough physical exam, a decision to treat with sertraline (Zoloft) is made. In discussing the treatment plan with the patient, what should be included about medication side effects?

   A. it may cause depression
   B. it may cause sexual dysfunction
   C. it may cause photosensitivity
   D. it may cause xerostomia

258. A 29-year-old roofer presents after sustaining a puncture wound to the bottom of his foot. He states he accidentally stepped on a nail at the job site 1 hour ago. Although he did receive his full vaccine series as a child, he is afraid of needles and has not had any immunizations since entering high school. What is the appropriate tetanus prophylaxis at this time?

   A. tetanus immune globulin and penicillin
   B. tetanus immune globulin and tetanus toxoid
   C. tetanus immune globulin, tetanus toxoid, and penicillin
   D. tetanus toxoid only

259. A 9-year-old with recurrent acute otitis media presents with ear pain and purulent aural discharge. Which of the following organisms is the most likely agent?

   A. *Mycoplasma pneumoniae*
   B. *Haemophilus influenzae*
   C. *Pseudomonas aeruginosa*
   D. *Streptococcus pneumoniae*

260. For which of the following dietary recommendations does evidence exist supporting a decreased risk of colorectal cancer?

   A. avoid simple sugars
   B. supplemental vitamins and minerals
   C. rich in fiber from vegetables and fruits
   D. rich in meat from fowl and beef

261. A patient with chronic bronchitis–predominant COPD is likely to have specific findings on pulmonary function tests. Which of the following is the most typical finding?

   A. after the administration of bronchodilators, the FEV_1 and FVC will increase by 15% to 20%
   B. increased FEV_1 and FVC with normal FEV_1/FVC ratio
   C. reduced FEV_1 and low FEV_1/FVC ratio combined with increased TLC
   D. the FEV_1 and FVC are reduced, as is TLC, but the FEV_1/FVC ratio is normal or increased

262. A mother brings in her 2-year-old son stating he has been crying for 2 hours and refuses to move his right arm. He sits with his elbow fully pronated and has tenderness over the radial head. X-rays appear to be negative. What is the recommended treatment for the suspected diagnosis?

   A. immediate reduction
   B. long-arm cast
   C. referral to an orthopaedic surgeon
   D. sling

263. A 20-year-old female presents after four recent episodes of near syncope. During these episodes, she was mildly short of breath and was aware of her heart beating rapidly but not erratically. When she sat down and put her head between her knees, she felt better and her heart slowed down. She has no personal or family history of cardiac problems. ECG done at this visit is entirely normal. What is the most likely diagnosis?

   A. atrial fibrillation
   B. atrial flutter
   C. paroxysmal supraventricular tachycardia
   D. ventricular premature beats

264. A 15-year-old boy with a history of allergic rhinitis presents complaining of recurrent pruritic skin lesions on his wrists and arms. Physical exam reveals generalized dry skin with scattered weepy red plaques and papules without scaling on the flexor surfaces of the wrists and antecubital fossae bilaterally. What is the most likely diagnosis?

   A. atopic dermatitis
   B. impetigo
   C. psoriasis
   D. seborrhea

265. A 72-year-old G_5P_{4104} has been experiencing a sensation of vaginal fullness and pressure which worsens with straining and coughing. She also has been experiencing urinary incontinence. Physical exam reveals no ulcerations or erosions of the vaginal or vulvar mucosa. With bearing down, a thin-walled, smooth, bulging mass projects from the anterior portion of the vagina. Rectovaginal palpation reveals no septal defect or sacculation. What is the most likely diagnosis?

   A. cystocele
   B. rectocele
   C. uterine prolapse
   D. urethrocele

266. An 18-year-old male presents for further evaluation of elevated blood pressure, which was recently detected at a health fair. Exam today reveals a blood pressure of 156/99 with an associated left infraclavicular systolic murmur and a prominent suprasternal notch pulsation. What is the most appropriate next step in the evaluation of this patient?
    A. cardiac catheterization with pressure gradients
    B. magnetic resonance imaging of the chest
    C. signal-averaged electrocardiography
    D. upper and lower extremity blood pressures

267. A 24-year-old complains of intermittent bouts of low-grade fever, right lower quadrant pain, weight loss, and watery diarrhea. Colonoscopy reveals stellate ulcers and segmental inflammation. What is the initial pharmacologic management?
    A. 5-aminosalicyclic acid (5-ASA) compounds
    B. biologic therapies such as anti-TNF or anti-integrin
    C. corticosteroids
    D. immunomodulating drugs such as mercaptopurine

268. A 45-year-old male who is recuperating from influenza suddenly develops sharp substernal pain in his chest. He cannot get comfortable lying down, but is able to get some relief by sitting forward. He also feels as if he cannot get a deep breath, but has no other symptoms other than residual cough from the flu. On cardiac auscultation, a squeaking sound is heard. His ECG demonstrates ST and T wave changes in all leads. CXR is unremarkable. What is the most likely diagnosis?
    A. acute coronary event
    B. angina pectoris
    C. costochrondritis
    D. inflammatory pericarditis

269. A 62-year-old male is brought to the emergency department after having sustained a syncopal episode at home. Vitals include BP 95/64, P 115, and R 20. He is complaining of lower back pain; exam reveals a femoral pulse discrepancy and pulsatile abdominal mass. What is the most likely diagnosis?
    A. acute myocardial infarction
    B. acute pulmonary embolus
    C. dissecting abdominal aortic aneurysm
    D. Wolff–Parkinson–White syndrome

270. A 46-year-old male presents with acute flank pain and hematuria. This is the third episode in 7 months. After appropriate treatment, he should be encouraged to maintain a diet restricted in which of the following?
    A. bran
    B. carbohydrates and fat
    C. fluids
    D. sodium and protein

271. A 34-year-old male presents with symptoms of painful urethral discharge. History reveals recent intercourse with a new partner without protection. Gram stain is positive for intracellular diplococci. Which of the following is the antibiotic of choice?
    A. ceftriaxone
    B. ciprofloxacin
    C. doxycycline
    D. penicillin G

272. The health consequences of obesity are numerous. What is the recommended healthy body mass index (BMI) range?
    A. 14.5 to 18.4
    B. 18.5 to 24.9
    C. 25 to 29.9
    D. 30 to 34.9

273. Which of the following clinical presentations best describes alcoholic hepatitis?
    A. right upper quadrant pain, tender hepatomegaly, and mildly elevated transaminase levels
    B. acute onset of nausea, jaundice, hepatomegaly, leukocytosis, and moderately elevated transaminase levels
    C. jaundice, bruising, nonpalpable liver, and hypoalbuminemia
    D. severe continuous epigastric abdominal pain radiating to the back, nausea and vomiting, and an elevated serum amylase

274. A 26-year-old asymptomatic female presents for preemployment physical. A mid-systolic click is noted during cardiac auscultation. Echocardiography reveals no abnormalities. Which of the following recommendations should be provided to this patient?
    A. the patient has no physical limitations and should receive routine health advice
    B. the patient requires antibiotic prophylaxis for future dental extractions
    C. the patient requires emergent referral to a cardiac surgeon
    D. the patient should return for monitoring every 3 months

275. A 19-year-old college student, upon hearing that she is failing a required course in her major, suddenly becomes nauseated, sweaty, and pale, and then passes out in the classroom. Examination on site reveals tachycardia and a normal blood pressure. Later evaluation at student health, including lying, sitting, and standing blood pressures, cardiac auscultation, and an ECG, is unremarkable. Nothing like this has ever happened to her before. What is the most likely cause of this episode?
    A. cardiogenic syncope
    B. orthostatic hypotension
    C. paroxysmal supraventricular tachycardia
    D. vasomotor syncope

276. A 39-year-old male has peptic ulcer disease refractory to standard therapy with H_2 receptor blockers and proton pump inhibitors. Fasting serum gastrin concentration level is elevated greater than 1,200 pg/mL and the gastric pH is 2.0. What is the most likely diagnosis?
    A. atrophic gastritis
    B. gastrinoma
    C. gastric outlet obstruction
    D. insulinoma

277. A 30-year-old male presents for routine physical. Family history includes a triple bypass at age 50 years (father) and very high cholesterol (brother, aged 36). Which of the following physical exam findings is most likely to be found in this patient?
    A. pes planus
    B. senile cataracts
    C. tendinous xanthoma
    D. tophi of the ear helix

278. A 42-year-old male with no significant past medical history presents with dull pain in his lower left leg. Exam reveals a tender palpable cord; the pain increases on dorsiflexion. After initial treatment and stabilization, which of the following is recommended?
    A. aspirin therapy for 2 months
    B. lifelong anticoagulation therapy
    C. vena cava filter implantation
    D. warfarin therapy for 6 months

279. A woman presents complaining of irregular vaginal spotting for 2 days. LMP was 9 weeks ago. Serum βHCG is high for gestational age. Uterine ultrasonography reveals grapelike clusters and no fetus. What is the initial treatment of choice?
    A. laparoscopy
    B. methotrexate
    C. suction curettage
    D. watchful waiting

280. A 40-year-old reports close, repeated exposure to a child who tested positive for *Bortadella pertussis*. Currently the patient is experiencing coryza, lacrimation, low-grade fever, and mild dry cough. Which of the following treatments is warranted at this time?
    A. betamethasone
    B. ciprofloxacin
    C. erythromycin
    D. pseudoephedrine plus dextromethorphan

281. A 27-year-old patient with HIV disease presents with loss of appetite and odynophagia. Examination of the buccal mucosa and tongue reveals thick, white plaques somewhat adherent to the underlying mucosa. After scraping the patches with a tongue blade, the surface below appears raw and reddened. What is the most likely diagnosis?
    A. candidiasis
    B. carcinoma
    C. diphtheria
    D. hairy leukoplakia

282. A 40-year-old male presents with hematuria and flank pain. Plain film shows a 2-cm calculus at the renal pelvis. BUN is elevated. Which of the following is the most appropriate intervention?
    A. pyelolithotomy
    B. fluids and analgesia
    C. lithotripsy
    D. allopurinol

283. A 25-year-old female complains of a nontender breast mass that has remained unchanged in size or character through three menstrual cycles. Exam reveals a freely mobile, firm, well-circumscribed, 4-cm oval left breast mass.
    A. breast cyst
    B. fibroadenoma
    C. galactocele
    D. intraductal papilloma

284. A 26-year-old with no significant past medical history presents with 2 days of nonbloody diarrhea and low-grade fever. He denies exposure to sick contacts, use of antibiotics, or ingestion of improperly prepared or stored food. Exam reveals hyperactive peristalsis, diffuse abdominal tenderness, and guaiac negative stool. What is the recommended management?
    A. oral rehydration with fluids containing sodium, potassium, and bicarbonate
    B. sending the stool for fecal white blood cell, stool culture, and ova and parasite testing
    C. starting empiric antibiotic therapy while awaiting stool tests
    D. starting symptomatic therapy with antidiarrheal agents

285. A college student who has been under high stress studying for exams and applying to graduate school presents with facial pain and stiffness. The symptoms first began about 1 week ago. He states his eyes and mouth have become so dry that it is affecting his ability to study or eat. Exam reveals inability to close the left eye and an asymmetric grimace. What is the recommended treatment?
    A. IVIG
    B. low-salt diet
    C. lubricating eye drops
    D. prednisone

286. A 47-year-old construction worker presents for evaluation of a growth on his eye which has been present for "many years." Exam reveals a fleshy, triangular encroachment of the conjunctivae onto the nasal side of the cornea bilaterally that is now affecting his field of vision. What is the best treatment option?
    A. artificial tears
    B. excision
    C. iridotomy
    D. topical NSAIDs

287. A 45-year-old male is diagnosed with acute ST elevation myocardial infarction (STEMI). Blood pressure remains at 90/56 mm Hg despite aggressive fluid resuscitation. Which of the following pressor agents is most appropriate at this time?
    A. dobutamine
    B. epinephrine
    C. milrinone
    D. norepinephrine

288. A patient complains of severe tearing pain followed by throbbing in the anal area during defecation. There is bright red blood on the toilet paper but no blood in the stool. Exam reveals cracked epithelium at the anal verge midline posteriorly. What is the most likely etiology of this diagnosis?
    A. carcinoma
    B. infection
    C. inflammation
    D. straining

289. Currently, there are seven types of serotonin receptors recognized: 5-HT1 to 5-HT7. What is the clinical significance of serotonin?
    A. antidepressant action
    B. antihypertensive action
    C. antiparkinsonian action
    D. regulation of cardiac function

290. Which of the following is most likely to develop within 1 hour of an acute arterial occlusion of the lower extremity?
    A. calf tenderness
    B. erythema
    C. pallor
    D. paralysis

291. A 42-year-old male presents to the office with a monoarticular arthritis involving the left knee. He states the pain began approximately 2 days ago and has been associated with fever and chills. Exam reveals a tender swollen left knee that is erythematous and warm to the touch. What is the best next step?
    A. CT scan of the left knee
    B. diagnostic arthrocentesis
    C. erythrocyte sedimentation rate
    D. plain radiography of the left knee

292. An 18-year-old has a history of asthma. Nasal polyps are discovered. What other condition should be suspected in this patient?
    A. adenocarcinoma
    B. aspirin hypersensitivity
    C. cystic fibrosis
    D. rhinitis medicamentosa

293. A 47-year-old male with no significant past medical history is diagnosed by echocardiography with restrictive cardiomyopathy. Myocardial biopsy reveals deposition of immunoglobulins with light chains. What is the most likely cause?
    A. amyloidosis
    B. chronic hypertension
    C. ethanol abuse
    D. sarcoidosis

294. A 25-year-old known asthmatic presents with an exacerbation. Nebulizer treatment with albuterol is begun. Which test would be most useful to evaluate and monitor through treatment?
    A. chest x-ray
    B. methacholine challenge test
    C. peak expiratory flow rate
    D. pulse oximetry

295. A 14-year-old male presents with sore throat and fever, but denies cough. Exam reveals elevated temperature, tender anterior cervical adenopathy, and pharyngeal exudate. What is the most likely diagnosis?
    A. epiglottitis
    B. mononucleosis
    C. peritonsillar abscess
    D. strep pharyngitis

296. A 16-year-old male is tackled while playing football and lands on his left shoulder. Exam reveals pain and tenderness over the left acromioclavicular joint. How can a diagnosis of an acromioclavicular separation best be made?
    A. left clavicular radiography
    B. MRI of left shoulder
    C. weight-bearing AC joint views
    D. Y view of the left shoulder

297. A patient presents with eye pain and photophobia after getting dust in his eyes while cleaning out the attic. Exam reveals normal visual acuity and no foreign body. What is the most appropriate next step?
    A. application of an ophthalmic antibiotic
    B. follow-up in 48 hours
    C. instillation of fluoroscein
    D. use of eye patching

298. A man with hemophilia A fathers four daughters. The mother of the children does not have or carry the disease. The gene for hemophilia will most likely be transmitted to how many of the daughters?
    A. 1
    B. 2
    C. 3
    D. 4

299. A 72-year-old widowed woman presents to the office with the odor of alcohol on her breath on repeated office visits. When asked about alcohol use, she flatly denies it. Which of the following laboratory studies would best support a diagnosis of alcohol abuse in this patient?
    A. elevated γ-glutamyltransferase (GGTP)
    B. elevated high-density lipoproteins (HDL)
    C. microcytic anemia
    D. reduced transaminase enzymes

300. A 26-year-old female gives a history of severe throbbing unilateral head pain associated with onset of menses. The headache comes on gradually and builds, lasting for several hours. What is the most probable underlying mechanism?
    A. activation of trigeminal nerve
    B. antibodies to acetylcholine
    C. estrogen surge
    D. serotonin deficiency

301. A 22-year-old female complains of cold intolerance. She is 5 ft 4 in and weighs 95 lb. She has not had a normal menses in over a year. Skin is dry and scaly with increased lanugo. Which of the following laboratory abnormalities is most likely to be found in this patient?
    A. elevated cholesterol
    B. increased thyroxin (T_4)
    C. increased follicle-stimulating hormone (FSH)
    D. sinus tachycardia on ECG

302. A 32-year-old male with a history of systemic lupus erythematosus presents with an aching pain in his groin that radiates to his knee. He states the pain gets worse as he walks on it throughout the day. On exam, he has decreased range of motion on internal rotation as compared to the other hip. Radiography of the hip is normal. What is the most likely diagnosis?
    A. avascular necrosis
    B. herniated lumbar disc
    C. osteoarthritis
    D. rheumatoid arthritis

303. A 36-year-old male presents complaining of progressive toenail discoloration. On exam, the toenails are thickened with a yellow-brownish discoloration. The nails are brittle with a chalky texture. KOH preparation of the curetting demonstrates hyphae. What is the most appropriate treatment?
   A. griseofulvin
   B. itraconazole
   C. ketoconazole
   D. terbinafine

304. A 42-year-old female complains of a grayish malodorous vaginal discharge for 2 days. The patient denies vaginal pruritus and pain. On physical exam, the vaginal walls are coated with a nonadherent discharge. The cervix is without lesions and there is no cervical motion tenderness. Wet prep demonstrates clue cells. What is the most likely diagnosis?
   A. atrophic vaginitis
   B. bacterial vaginosis
   C. trichomoniasis
   D. vulvovaginal candidiasis

305. Four women are in labor at term and are having external fetal monitoring performed. Which of the following results should prompt a C-section?
   A. fetal heart rate 100 bpm with late decelerations
   B. fetal heart rate 120 bpm with variability
   C. fetal heart rate 140 bpm with accelerations
   D. fetal heart rate 160 bpm with early decelerations

306. A 14-year-old female presents for a gymnastics camp physical. She is 60 inches tall and weighs 82 lbs and is Tanner 1 in sexual development. She describes her caloric intake as less than 1,000 kcal/day with hours of weight training and gymnastics practice. Which of the following laboratory studies is indicated?
   A. insulinlike growth factor 1
   B. serum cortisol level
   C. serum gastrin level
   D. thyroid function tests

Pretest Explanations

1. The answer is **B** [Pulmonology].
   A. Asthmatics are not cyanotic unless the disease is very severe. They typically have an increased respiratory rate and demonstrate expiratory wheezes rather than rhonchi.
   B. This is the typical picture of chronic bronchitis–predominant COPD.
   C. Patients with pneumonia typically present with productive cough and increased respiratory rate; chest percussion may be dull due to an infiltrate.
   D. Patients with emphysema-predominant COPD display tachypnea, use of accessory muscles, and diminished breath sounds. They typically do not demonstrate rhonchi; cyanosis may develop late in the disease.

2. The answer is **C** [Nephrology and Urology].
   A. Severe acidosis (pH <7.20) is an indication for acute dialysis. Milder acidosis can be managed medically.
   B. Pigmented granular ("muddy") casts indicate acute tubular necrosis as the cause of this patient's acute renal failure.
   C. Uremic complications, such as encephalopathy and seizures, are indications for urgent dialysis.
   D. Hyperphosphatemia may be treated over the short term with phosphate-binding agents such as aluminum hydroxide.

3. The answer is **A** [Nephrology and Urology].
   A. African American race is associated with an increased risk of prostate cancer.
   B. Cigarette smoking is not associated with prostate cancer but is associated with cancers of the mouth, lung, pharynx, esophagus, pancreas, kidney, and bladder.
   C. Cryptorchidism is associated with an increased risk of testicular cancer.
   D. Low sperm count is not associated with an increased risk of prostate cancer.

4. The answer is **A** [Obstetrics/Gynecology, Infectious Disease].
   A. Acute cervicitis caused by *Neisseria gonorrhoeae* can be asymptomatic or associated with a purulent vaginal discharge. The cervix is commonly edematous and inflamed. Ceftriaxone 125 mg is the treatment of choice. Alternative regimens include cefpodoxime or spectinomycin. Doxycycline is given at the same time due to the high prevalence of concomitant Chlamydia infections.
   B. Clindamycin or metronidazole is indicated in bacterial vaginosis, which presents with a malodorous, grayish, nonadherent discharge.
   C. Fluoroquinolones are no longer recommended due to rising resistance.
   D. See B.

5. The answer is **D** [Endocrinology, Pediatrics].
   A. Acromegaly presents in adults with extreme growth, headaches, visual field defects, weakness, soft doughy hands, and amenorrhea in females. It is due to the lack of suppression of growth hormone. Excess growth hormone in children causes gigantism.
   B. Cushing's syndrome is due to increased production of cortisol. Clinical symptoms typically include central obesity, generalized weight gain, rounding of the face, and a dorsocervical fat pad along with other symptoms of glucocorticoid excess.
   C. Dwarfism (achondroplasia) is an autosomal recessive disorder with disproportionately short arms and legs, frontal bossing, and midfacial hypoplasia. It is often diagnosed in utero via prenatal ultrasound.
   D. Deceleration of growth is usually the first clinical manifestation of hypothyroidism in children. Myxedematous changes of the skin, constipation, cold intolerance, decreased energy, and an increased need for sleep develop insidiously. Reflexes may be slowed, especially in the ankles.

6. The answer is **D** [Pulmonology].
   A. Blind sweeps of the oral cavity are not recommended, as they will most likely force the object to lodge deeper into the trachea.
   B. See D. Should the Heimlich maneuver prove unsuccessful, a cricothyrotomy would be the best next step.
   C. See D.
   D. The Heimlich maneuver should be tried before invasive procedures are undertaken, especially in the setting where emergency services and sterile conditions are not available.

7. The answer is **A** [Endocrinology].
   A. Thyroid-stimulating hormone is produced by the anterior pituitary.
   B. Zona glomerulosa secretes aldosterone.
   C. Antidiuretic hormone is secreted from the posterior pituitary.
   D. Zona fasciculata secrets cortisol, androgens, and estrogen.

8. The answer is **D** [Dermatology, Pediatrics].
   A. Skin should be kept well moisturized in atopic dermatitis with regular applications of topical emollients.
   B. Low humidity can exacerbate the symptoms of atopic dermatitis, which is why the condition often worsens in winter.
   C. Frequent bathing should be avoided in persons with atopic dermatitis. Soap should be used sparingly to avoid irritating the skin.
   D. Cotton clothing is preferred for persons with atopic dermatitis. Wools and acrylics should be avoided, as they can exacerbate the condition.

9. The answer is **B** [Obstetrics/Gynecology, Pediatrics].
   A. Estrogen levels will be abnormally low but are not diagnostic.
   B. This is a classic picture of Turner's syndrome (gonadal dysgenesis), which is a frequent cause of primary amenorrhea. Karyotyping will show a 45XO pattern.
   C. LH levels are useful in diagnosing pseudohermaphroditism (XY genotype, XX phenotype) and pituitary tumors but not Turner's syndrome.
   D. Ultrasonography will show a gonadal streak, misshapen functionless ovarian tissue. While present in Turner's syndrome, gonadal streaks are also seen with other genetic mutations and, therefore, are not diagnostic.

10. The answer is **D** [Obstetrics/Gynecology].
    A. While some women develop breast cancer without any risk factors, there are several known factors that increase one's risk of the disease. Industrial countries have an increased incidence but Japan is a notable exception. In addition, the risk increases with age: a 30-year-old woman is at a lower risk than an older woman.
    B. The incidence of breast cancer in African Americans is increasing, but it is still not as high as in whites. Current research shows that oral contraceptive pills do not appear to increase one's risk.
    C. Having one's first pregnancy late in one's reproductive life, not early, is an increased risk for breast cancer.
    D. The strongest risk factors in developing breast cancer are increasing age, white race, and a first-degree relative (mother, sister, daughter) with a history of the disease.

11. The answer is **C** [Rheumatology and Orthopaedics, Pediatrics].
    A. See C.
    B. See C.
    C. Slipped capital femoral epiphysis (SCFE) typically occurs during an adolescent growth spurt; patients are frequently overweight. Typical presentation is with hip pain. The pain may worsen on ambulation or cause a "waddling" gait. Pain may be felt in the hip but may be referred to the thigh or knee. Radiographs of the child in the frog leg position are usually diagnostic and can be utilized to grade SCFE severity.
    D. See C.

12. The answer is **A** [Pulmonology, Pediatrics].
    A. Peak expiratory flow rate can be monitored at home using an inexpensive handheld device.
    B. Respiratory rate is unreliable and too subjective for monitoring asthma.
    C. Pulse oximetry may be normal with mild asthma.
    D. The only blood pressure abnormality related to asthma is pulsus paradoxus, which may occur with severe asthma.

13. The answer is **B** [Obstetrics/Gynecology, Surgery].
    A. The scenario describes incompetent cervix. There is often a history of second-trimester painless cervical dilation and subsequent pregnancy loss, past cervical conization or surgery, cervical injury, or diethylstilbestrol (DES) exposure. Bed rest is not the treatment of choice during the first trimester; it should be initiated after the cerclage is in place and there is subsequent dilation.
    B. A cerclage is a purse string–type stitch around the cervix to stop passive dilation during pregnancy. If no labor occurs, it will stay in place until approximately 36 weeks gestation.
    C. Pessary is used for uterine prolapse not incompetent cervix.
    D. Tocolytic medications are used for the treatment of preterm labor not incompetent cervix. Regular contractions and dilation prior to term would be the definition of preterm labor.

14. The answer is **A** [Psychiatry].
    A. Antisocial personality disorder is characterized by a pervasive pattern of disregard for and violation of lawful behavior, aggressiveness, consistent irresponsibility, and lack of remorse.
    B. Borderline personality disorder is characterized by instability of interpersonal relationships, self-image, and affect including identity disturbance and recurrent suicidal behavior.
    C. Paranoid personality disorder is characterized by pervasive distrust and suspiciousness of others including suspecting others of malevolent behavior without evidence, being unable to confide in others, and bearing grudges.
    D. Schizoid personality disorder is characterized by detachment from social relationships and a very restricted range of emotional expression including being a loner, choosing solitary activities, and having little interest in what others might see as pleasurable.

15. The answer is **D** [Obstetrics/Gynecology].
    A. Serial changes in HCG are needed every 48 hours; changes in HCG are not immediate.
    B. See D.
    C. See D.
    D. The first change noted is the absence of movement followed by the absence of fetal heart tones. Fetal death is best evaluated by ultrasonography. In the case of an equivocal ultrasound, serial HCGs are indicated to evaluate levels over 48 hours.

16. The answer is **C** [Neurology].
    A. Aminoglycosides may exacerbate the symptoms of myasthenia gravis.
    B. Corticosteroids are indicated in patients who do not respond to anticholinesterase medications. They are not used to confirm diagnosis.
    C. Edrophonium is a short-acting anticholinesterase. Patients with myasthenia gravis will have a prompt improvement that lasts for 5 to 10 minutes. This is diagnostic.
    D. Guanidine works to precipitate release of acetylcholine from nerve endings. It is helpful in the treatment of botulism.

17. The answer is **B** [Neurology, Geriatrics].
    A. Amantadine, levodopa, and selective monoamine oxidase inhibitor medications help with all manifestations of Parkinson's disease.
    B. Anticholinergics are helpful in treating the tremor and rigidity but less helpful with bradykinesia. Side effects abound, especially in the elderly, and include dry mouth, nausea, constipation, urinary retention, and confusion and agitation.
    C. See A.
    D. See A.

18. The answer is **A** [Gastroenterology].
    A. Gilbert's syndrome is the most common hereditary hyperbilirubinemia. Bilirubin levels typically do not reach levels higher than 3 mg/dL until the patient develops an intercurrent illness or undergoes a prolonged fast.
    B. Patients with sickle cell disease, not trait, develop chronic jaundice from ongoing hemolysis.
    C. History of fatty food intolerance with jaundice is suggestive of acute cholangitis.
    D. The sudden appearance of jaundice in a previously healthy young person, especially if preceded by a brief prodrome of fever, malaise, and myalgias, is likely to be caused by a viral hepatitis.

19. The answer is **C** [Gastroenterology, Surgery, Pediatrics].
    A. Abdominal distention is a nonspecific finding.
    B. Abdominal wall rigidity may indicate peritonitis such as in appendicitis, which is more commonly seen in older children or adolescents.
    C. Pyloric stenosis most commonly manifests in the first 2 to 4 weeks of life. The typical clinical manifestation is nonbilious vomiting that becomes projectile. An olive-shaped mass may be palpated during or immediately after feeding.
    D. Intussusception most commonly occurs between 6 and 18 months of age. Acute pain, drawing up of the knees, and currant jelly stool are characteristic. A sausage-shaped mass may be found in the upper abdomen.

20. The answer is **B** [Cardiology, Infectious Disease].
    A. *Streptococcus viridans*, enterococci, and a number of other Gram-positive and Gram-negative bacilli, as well as yeasts and fungi, tend to cause a subacute endocarditis. *Streptococcus* is the most common etiology.
    B. *Staphylococcus aureus* tends to cause a rapidly progressive picture of endocarditis. It commonly results in a destructive infection in which patients present with acute febrile illnesses, acute valvular insufficiency, early embolization, and myocardial abscess formation. It is more common in injection drug users.
    C. See A.
    D. See A.

21. The answer is **A** [Gastroenterology].
    A. A family history of adenomatous polyps or colorectal cancer is one of the most important risk factors for colorectal cancer. If a cancer was diagnosed at less than 45 years of age, the relative risk is 3.8 times greater than that without such a family history. The positive family history puts this 38-year-old at a risk comparable to that of an average 50-year-old. Screening typically is done beginning at age 50, but in this patient it should begin by 40 years of age. It is suggested that the best screening is colonoscopy every 5 years in patients with this family history.
    B. Screening colonoscopy at age 50 years is the appropriate schedule in average-risk individuals.
    C. Flexible sigmoidoscopy is an appropriate choice for average-risk patients, beginning at age 50, although it will not screen for proximal lesions.
    D. See C.

22. The answer is **D** [Dermatology, Infectious Disease].
    A. Tzanck smear is commonly done with suspected herpetic outbreaks, but it is less sensitive than a polymerase chain reaction (PCR).
    B. Immunoglobulin titers are not helpful in zoster.
    C. This rash is not likely due to a fungal infection.
    D. Herpes zoster is typically a clinical diagnosis. If testing is deemed necessary, a PCR or direct immunofluoroscopy is the test of choice.

23. The answer is **C** [Gastroenterology].
    A. Waiting 30 minutes before taking antacids is typical with sucralfate, not with PPIs or H_2 blockers. Antacids can be given concomitantly with PPIs and with some H_2 blockers.
    B. Misoprostol (Cytotec), a prostaglandin E1 analog, is used for the prevention of NSAID-induced ulcers. It must be taken four times per day with meals.
    C. PPIs and H_2 receptor blockers lessen the acidity, thereby affecting the absorption of drugs dependent upon an acidic pH. PPIs are typically dosed once per day and H_2 blockers one to two times per day.
    D. Agents such as dicyclomine (Bentyl), used for the treatment of irritable bowel syndrome, can potentiate CNS symptoms with alcohol use.

24. The answer is **D** [Cardiology, Surgery].
    A. Steroids are used in cases of lung inflammation, not for pulmonary hypertension.
    B. Prostacyclin is a potent pulmonary vasodilator. Continuous infusions are beneficial in primary pulmonary hypertension. This patient's pathology is secondary to his heart condition.
    C. Sildenafil (Viagra) is a cGMP-specific phosphodiesterase inhibitor effective in erectile dysfunction. Their use may show improvement in symptoms in up to 25% of patients; however they do not slow progression of the disease.
    D. Oxygen should be provided most hours of the day and night, reducing his O_2 demand, resulting in improved pulmonary hypertension.

25. The answer is **A** [Rheumatology and Orthopaedics, Infectious Disease].
    A. Dicloxacillin is effective against septic arthritis.
    B. Intra-articular injections are a cause of septic arthritis.
    C. *Staphylococcus aureus* is the most common organism in septic arthritis. The prevalence of penicillin resistance precludes its use.
    D. Fever and increased WBC with a left shift indicate septic bursitis. Antibiotics are indicated.

26. The answer is **C** [Endocrinology, Cardiology].
    A. See C.
    B. See C.
    C. In adults with no significant risk factors, fasting lipid profiles should be obtained every 5 years.
    D. See C.

27. The answer is **B** [Rheumatology and Orthopaedics].
    A. Calcium channel blockers are used to treat Raynaud's disease.
    B. DMARDs should be started when rheumatoid arthritis (RA) is first diagnosed to reduce inflammation and pain, preserve function, and prevent deformity.
    C. Low-dose corticosteroids can be used in the treatment of RA but should be reserved for severe or otherwise unresponsive cases due to the high risk of adverse effects. High-dose steroids are most often used for short periods of time in patients with giant cell (temporal) arteritis.
    D. NSAIDs can be used in RA for symptomatic relief but they do not prevent bone erosion or alter the disease process.

28. The answer is **A** [Hematology].
    A. Either dexamethasone or prednisone would be appropriate to treat this mild case of immune thrombocytopenia purpura (ITP). Most cases of ITP occur in young females following mild to moderate viral infections frequently involving the upper respiratory tract.
    B. IVIG is second-line treatment for ITP.
    C. The fact that her antistreptolysin O test is negative rules out the need for antibiotics in this case and most likely would not be helpful weeks after a strep infection has resolved.
    D. Ticlopidine would be contraindicated in this case, as it inhibits platelet aggregation.

29. The answer is **C** [Pulmonology, Pediatrics].
    A. The abdominal flat plate findings described are consistent with meconium ileus, which may be seen in newborns with cystic fibrosis.
    B. Hyperinflation can also be seen in asthmatics.
    C. Elevated sweat chloride values are the key to diagnosis of cystic fibrosis. The values for the chloride (and sodium) concentrations in sweat vary with age, but typically a chloride concentration of greater than 70 mEq/L discriminates between patients with cystic fibrosis and those with other lung diseases.
    D. Pulmonary function testing in patients with cystic fibrosis is highly variable, and abnormal findings are generally irreversible.

30. The answer is **D** [Cardiology, Infectious Disease].
    A. Auspitz's sign is the appearance of bleeding points after removal of a skin plaque, commonly seen in psoriasis.
    B. Janeway's lesions are small hemorrhagic lesions in the skin, seen in endocarditis.
    C. Osler's nodes are painful, red, raised skin lesions, seen in endocarditis.
    D. Roth's spots are exudative retinal lesions, seen in endocarditis.

31. The answer is **C** [Neurology].
    A. Cerebrospinal fluid analysis may show lymphocytosis or increased protein, especially soon after an acute increase in symptoms. Elevated immunoglobulins and oligoclonal bands are common but not diagnostic.
    B. Computed tomography is less helpful than magnetic resonance.
    C. This patient is manifesting symptoms of multiple sclerosis (MS). Magnetic resonance is very helpful in demonstrating multiple demyelinating lesions, which are the diagnostic criteria for MS.
    D. Evoked potentials (visual, auditory, muscular) may be helpful to demonstrate the presence of multiple lesions but are less sensitive than MRI.

32. The answer is **B** [Hematology, Surgery].
    A. Cryoprecipitate is used in emergent situations where blood loss from von Willebrand disease may be profound. It is not the treatment of choice in the situation described.
    B. This patient likely has type 1 von Willebrand disease. Intranasal desmopressin on the day of the procedure will likely control blood loss experienced as a result of the breast biopsy.
    C. Factor VIII could be given if desmopressin fails to control her bleeding during or after the biopsy but would not be a first-line choice for a patient with mild type 1 von Willebrand disease.
    D. Fibrin sealant (Tisseel) is used to control local bleeding and may be useful in some surgeries; it is considered an adjunct to other therapies.

33. The answer is **D** [Hematology].
    A. Acute leukemia is likely to present with bleeding into the skin and mucosae or overwhelming infection. A pancytopenia with circulating blasts is characteristic.
    B. Acute myeloid leukemia is distinguished from acute lymphoblastic leukemia by demonstrating Auer's rods or myeloid enzymes such as peroxidase.
    C. Chronic lymphocytic leukemia is likely to present with lymphadenopathy, hepatosplenomegaly, and isolated lymphocytosis.
    D. The clinical picture plus the presence of the *bcr/abl* gene in the peripheral blood is that of chronic myeloid leukemia.

34. The answer is **C** [Rheumatology and Orthopaedics, Pediatrics].
    A. Chondromalacia patella usually presents with symmetric anterior knee pain that is worse after sitting and going up stairs.
    B. Medial collateral ligament tear is usually caused by abnormal force applied to the knee and presents with pain and knee instability.
    C. Osgood–Schlatter disease presents with anterior knee pain and swelling over the tibial tubercle that is associated with activity. It is caused by fragmentation of the tibial tubercle apophysis from chronic tensile stress.
    D. Prepatellar bursitis in a child is usually caused by trauma that allows hematogenous spread of bacteria into the bursa. It presents with a swollen area anterior to the knee joint and does not interfere with knee range of motion.

35. The answer is **A** [Ophthalmology and Otolaryngology, Geriatrics].
    A. Initial treatment of primary acute-closure glaucoma is control of intraocular pressure. IV acetazolamide followed by oral dosing is usually adequate. Osmotic diuretics, such as mannitol, may also be required, especially in patients with severely elevated intraocular pressure.
    B. See A.
    C. After the intraocular pressure decreases, topical pilocarpine is used to reverse the underlying angle closure. Definitive treatment, however, is with surgery (peripheral iridotomy or iridectomy).
    D. Prostaglandin analogs are often used as first-line therapy in chronic glaucoma.

36. The answer is **D** [Cardiology, Pediatrics, Surgery].
    A. The defect in tetralogy of Fallot is in the ventricle, not the atrium.
    B. Dissimilar blood pressure readings are pathognomonic of coarctation of the aorta.
    C. Although ECG findings are not of great significance, usually right bundle branch block occurs in tetralogy of Fallot.
    D. The finding of ventricular septal defect completes the diagnostic criteria for tetralogy of Fallot.

37. The answer is **D** [Psychiatry].
    A. Anorexia nervosa is an eating disorder associated with weight loss but not with disorganized behavior, delusions, stereotyped movement, or an inappropriate affect.
    B. Bipolar disorder is characterized by episodes of depression and mania.
    C. Histrionic personality disorder is characterized by excessive emotionality, attention seeking, and theatricality.
    D. Schizophrenia may present with disorganized behavior, delusions, stereotyped movement, and an inappropriate affect. This patient most likely has disorganized or paranoid subtype based on the history of the delusions and the inappropriate affect.

38. The answer is **A** [Rheumatology and Orthopaedics].
    A. Rest and ice are the best advice for early treatment of lateral epicondylitis. Application of ice three times daily in conjunction with rest usually provides relief in 1 to 2 weeks.
    B. A variety of braces exist that may reduce movement and irritation of the tendon insertion point. This may be useful if conservative therapy is ineffective.
    C. Oral corticosteroids are not recommended. Injectable corticosteroids may be effective for temporary relief of symptoms not relieved with conservative treatment, but there is very little evidence of long-term benefit.
    D. Surgery may be indicated if there is no resolution after 6 to 12 weeks of therapy or if corticosteroid injections fail.

39. The answer is **C** [Rheumatology and Orthopaedics, Geriatrics].
    A. Parathyroid hormone activates bone remodeling through direct action on osteoblast activity.
    B. Calcitonin suppresses osteoclast activity by direct action on the osteoclast calcium receptor.
    C. Bisphosphonates impair osteoclast function and reduce their numbers by induction of apoptosis.
    D. Calcitriol is a form of vitamin D. This medicine regulates calcium absorption from the GI tract.

40. The answer is **C** [Nephrology and Urology].
    A. Benign prostatic hypertrophy presents with voiding symptoms such as hesitancy, straining, weak stream, and post-void dribbling.
    B. IgA nephropathy typically presents after an upper respiratory tract infection and presents with hematuria and proteinuria.
    C. Renal cell carcinoma is linked to cigarette smoking as a risk factor. It is common in the sixth decade and often presents as painless hematuria with mild flank pain or an abdominal mass.
    D. Wegener's granulomatosis involves the kidneys and the lungs. Renal signs include hematuria, red blood cell casts, and proteinuria.

41. The answer is **B** [Gastroenterology, Surgery].
    A. Left upper quadrant pain that radiates to the left shoulder (Kehr's sign) can be associated with splenic disorders.
    B. Right upper quadrant pain radiating to the right scapula or shoulder is commonly seen in acute cholecystitis.
    C. Esophageal pain commonly radiates to the posterior pharynx, mid-chest, and epigastric area.
    D. Pain in the ascending colon may be referred to the right upper quadrant, right costovertebral angle, and right sacroiliac joint, but does not generally radiate to the scapula.

42. The answer is **B** [Rheumatology and Orthopaedics, Surgery].
    A. Dorsal angulation of the wrist is commonly seen in a Colles' fracture.
    B. Pain over the anatomic snuffbox is often seen in a scaphoid fracture.
    C. Pain with ulnar deviation of the wrist is seen in de Quervain's tenosynovitis.
    D. Volar angulation of the wrist is seen in a Smith's fracture.

43. The answer is **A** [Obstetrics/Gynecology, Infectious Disease].
    A. Mastitis most commonly presents 2 to 4 weeks after the start of breast-feeding. Symptoms include fever and chills followed by redness, induration, and tenderness to an area of the breast. *Staphylococcus aureus* from the infant's oral pharynx is the most common etiologic agent. A penicillinase-resistant antibiotic such as dicloxacillin is considered first line.
    B. Metronidazole is appropriate for infections caused by anaerobes.
    C. Penicillin would not provide appropriate coverage as most of the staphylococcal organisms associated with mastitis are penicillinase producing and, therefore, resistant to penicillin.
    D. Vancomycin is the drug of choice for the treatment of methicillin-resistant staphylococcal infections.

44. The answer is **B** [Cardiology].
    A. Reducing or eliminating his alcohol intake, increasing exercise, and initiating dietary modifications would all be helpful in improving his overall health, including his cardiac health, but do not have as great an impact as smoking cessation.
    B. Smoking is the most important cause of preventable morbidity and mortality and is the leading cause of cardiovascular death.
    C. See A.
    D. See A.

45. The answer is **A** [Rheumatology and Orthopaedics].
    A. Good back mechanics include lifting with the legs, warming up before participating in sports or lifting heavy objects, and getting help if the object is too heavy. It is also recommended to work out regularly with moderate weights and balance lumbar workout exercises with an abdominal workout.
    B. See A.
    C. See A.
    D. See A.

46. The answer is **C** [Hematology].
    A. See C.
    B. See C.
    C. Sulfa-containing drugs, such as trimethoprim–sulfamethoxazole (Bactrim) and nitrofurantoin (Macrodantin), should be avoided in patients with G6PD deficiency, as they can provoke a hemolytic crisis.
    D. See C.

47. The answer is **B** [Pulmonology].
    A. Long-acting anticholinergics such as tioproprium or ipratroprium have been shown to reduce acute exacerbations but they do not improve survival.
    B. Continuous oxygen therapy and in some cases continuous positive airway pressure (CPAP) have been found to favorably impact survival rates in COPD, especially in those patients hypoxic at rest.
    C. Evidence suggests that patient-driven COPD action plans reduce exacerbations but no clear data exist that they improve mortality.
    D. COPD sufferers should be strongly encouraged to stop smoking; however, the behavior change will not improve survival rates.

48. The answer is **A** [Neurology].
    A. This patient likely has Guillain–Barré syndrome (acute idiopathic polyneuropathy), which causes progressive weakness and possibly widespread autonomic dysfunction. Incontinence indicates that her course of disease will probably be severe. She should be admitted to the intensive care unit and provided supportive care including intubation if forced vital capacity begins to become compromised.
    B. Although Guillain–Barré has been linked to infection with *Campylobacter*, an infectious cause has not been established. It is not a contagious disease.
    C. Cardiac arrhythmias are common in Guillain–Barré but this patient will need generalized treatment rather than specific cardiac interventions.
    D. Prednisone is ineffective and may prolong the recovery time.

49. The answer is **A** [Rheumatology and Orthopaedics, Surgery].
    A. Rotator cuff disorders, which include rotator cuff tendinitis, impingement syndrome, subacromial bursitis or partial or full rotator cuff tears, are initially treated conservatively. They are treated first with activity modification, NSAIDs, and physical therapy, next with corticosteroid injections and more physical therapy, and finally with surgical intervention.
    B. See A.
    C. Immobilization is not recommended as the shoulder will stiffen and may become frozen.
    D. See A.

50. The answer is **A** [Ophthalmology and Otolaryngology].
    A. As long as sympathetic and parasympathetic innervation is intact, unilateral blindness does not cause anisocoria. A light directed into the seeing eye causes both pupils to constrict; a light directed into the blind eye does not cause any response in either eye.
    B. See A.
    C. See A.
    D. See A.

51. The answer is **A** [Pulmonology, Infectious Disease].
    A. The lung exam in influenza is generally normal.
    B. Diffuse expiratory wheezes are indicative of bronchospasm (asthma).
    C. Dullness and rhonchi indicate bacterial pneumonia.
    D. Scattered crackles and inspiratory wheeze indicate interstitial disease.

52. The answer is **B** [Rheumatology and Orthopaedics, Geriatrics].
    A. A positive straight leg raise is found in less than 10% of patients with spinal stenosis but is often found in patients with a herniated disc.
    B. Patients with spinal stenosis often have an unimpressive physical exam; less than 25% have diminished reflexes and about 60% have slight proximal muscle weakness.
    C. Paraspinal muscle spasms are usually found in patients with mechanical back pain or lumbar strain.
    D. Point tenderness over the vertebral bodies or spinous processes suggests osteomyelitis or fracture.

53. The answer is **D** [Obstetrics/Gynecology].
    A. Alcohol intake is not related to polycystic ovarian syndrome (PCOS).
    B. Moderate weight lifting is advantageous for a healthy lifestyle but will not help with the treatment of PCOS unless there is accompanying weight loss.
    C. Smoking cessation will not help with the treatment of PCOS.
    D. This woman likely has PCOS, which is often characterized by infertility, hirsutism, and obesity. Forty percent of patients with PCOS are obese. Weight loss is often effective in decreasing the severity of the disease.

54. The answer is **B** [Ophthalmology and Otolaryngology].
    A. NSAIDs and any drugs that affect coagulation should be avoided due to increased risk of secondary hemorrhage.
    B. An injury that causes hyphema has the risk of secondary hemorrhage, which can lead to problematic glaucoma and permanent visual loss. The patient should rest until complete resolution; daily ophthalmologic assessment is recommended.
    C. Surgical intervention may be indicated in blowout fractures.
    D. Vitamin K deficiency in healthy people is very rare. It may be given to reverse the effects of warfarin.

55. The answer is **B** [Ophthalmology and Otolaryngology, Infectious Disease].
    A. In resistant cases, especially with development of cellulitis around the auricle, an oral fluoroquinolone (i.e., ciprofloxacin) is the drug of choice due to effectiveness against *Pseudomonas*.
    B. An antibiotic/anti-inflammatory otic drop is the most appropriate treatment in uncomplicated otitis externa.
    C. In the diabetic or immunocompromised patient, persistent external otitis can develop into osteomyelitis (malignant external otitis). Surgical debridement is needed if medical therapy fails.
    D. If there is significant edema of the ear canal wall, which prevents the entry of drops into the ear, a wick can be placed. Here the tympanic membrane can be visualized, which makes the ear wick unnecessary.

56. The answer is **C** [Rheumatology and Orthopaedics, Surgery].
    A. L4-L5, L5 nerve root, affects dorsiflexion.
    B. Cauda equina syndrome affects multiple areas.
    C. L5-S1, L5 nerve root, affects plantar flexion.
    D. L3-L4, L4 nerve root, affects the quadriceps.

57. The answer is **B** [Psychiatry, Pediatrics].
    A. Asperger's syndrome is a pervasive developmental disorder characterized by impairment of social functioning and interactions. Patients display restricted repetitive and stereotyped patterns of behavior.
    B. Attention-deficit disorder is characterized by inattentive behavior in school and at home.
    C. Disruptive behavior disorder includes oppositional and defiant behaviors rather than inattentive behaviors.
    D. Hyperkinetic conduct disorder includes symptoms of hyperactivity, impulsivity, and aggression.

58. The answer is **D** [Pulmonology, Cardiology].
    A. Congestive heart failure more typically occurs in patients at risk (hypertension, coronary artery disease) and presents with rales on exam.
    B. Emphysema manifests as an insidious progression of dyspnea without chest pain in a long-time smoker. Exam reveals diminished breath sounds and use of accessory muscles.
    C. Pleuritic pain is sharp and exacerbated by cough, sneeze, or deep breathing.
    D. Venous stasis, such as a long plane ride, is an important risk factor for deep venous thrombosis which may progress to pulmonary embolus. Dyspnea and chest pain are the most common symptoms.

59. The answer is **A** [Nephrology and Urology].
    A. Ureterosigmoidostomy may result in a loss of bicarbonate through the urine with resulting normal anion gap, hyperchloremic acidosis. Respiratory compensation leads to hyperventilation.
    B. See A.
    C. See A.
    D. See A.

60. The answer is **C** [Dermatology, Infectious Disease].
    A. Molluscum contagiosum, caused by a self-limited poxvirus infection, may be spread by touching or trauma such as scratching or shaving. They are frequently painless and found grouped as a few lesions or may be more widespread, such as in immunocompromised individuals. Lesions on the face and trunk are common in children; in sexually active adults, lesions appear on the genitals or inner thighs.
    B. Skin tags are common, asymptomatic, benign growths found more commonly in the elderly. They occur most frequently in the axillae, neck, and groin and increase with pregnancy. Treatment is shave–snip and biopsy as clinically warranted.
    C. The history of freezing and gels supports the diagnosis of condyloma acuminata. This infection is caused by the human papillomavirus (HPV). Condyloma acuminata may progress to form painless cauliflower-like lesions in the rectal or perineal areas.
    D. This describes genital herpes caused by herpes simplex virus (HSV), often associated with itching or pain preceding recurrence. Lesions may be hard to find in females as they can be hidden from view in the vaginal canal or labial folds. They may be hidden under the foreskin in uncircumcised males.

61. The answer is **A** [Neurology, Endocrinology].
    A. Cigarette smoking represents the strongest risk for the development of microvascular disease regardless of the presence of diabetes. Tobacco causes vasoconstriction, which compounds the risk of microvascular disease and ischemia.
    B. A high-fat diet contributes to macrovascular disease.
    C. Ill-fitting shoes and hot water soaks contribute to the development of foot ulcers in patients with microvascular disease.
    D. See C.

62. The answer is **B** [Dermatology, Infectious Disease].
    A. Human papillomaviruses (HPV) cause warts, not hot tub folliculitis.
    B. Hot tub folliculitis is caused by *Pseudomonas aeruginosa*, erupting between 1 and 4 days after exposure.
    C. *Staphylococcus aureus* does not cause hot tub folliculitis though it can be the cause of other types of folliculitis, especially in diabetics.
    D. Latent varicella-zoster virus causes herpes zoster which presents in a unilateral, dermatomal distribution.

63. The answer is **B** [Ophthalmology and Otolaryngology, Infectious Disease, Geriatrics].
    A. Acyclovir may shorten the course and decrease postherpetic pain in herpetic stomatitis.
    B. Fluconazole is one of the effective antifungal therapies for candidiasis. Others include ketoconazole, clotrimazole troches, and nystatin mouth rinses.
    C. Penicillin is not indicated with oral candidiasis.
    D. A tapering dose of prednisone may be used to treat aphthous ulcers.

64. The answer is **B** [Neurology, Geriatrics].
    A. Alexia, the inability to understand written words (word blindness), is seen with posterior cerebral artery occlusion.
    B. Middle cerebral artery occlusions often result in homonymous hemianopia.
    C. Horner's syndrome is associated with posterior inferior cerebellar artery occlusion.
    D. Vertigo is more likely with occlusion of any of the major cerebellar arteries.

65. The answer is **B** [Nephrology and Urology, Surgery, Pediatrics].
    A. Ice packs cause further vasoconstriction, thereby increasing the risk of infarction.
    B. Testicular torsion is most common in adolescent boys. It is a surgical emergency. If torsion is complete, a testis can be infarcted in 4 to 6 hours.
    C. Antibiotic therapy has no place in the treatment of torsion.
    D. Delaying surgical intervention beyond 4 to 6 hours can lead to testicular infarction and subsequent infertility. Tc99 pertechnetate scans will confirm the presence of torsion; however, Doppler studies are quicker, less invasive, and just as effective to confirm the diagnosis.

66. The answer is **B** [Pulmonology, Infectious Disease].
    A. Failure to begin prophylactic therapy increases the risk that this child will become infected with tuberculosis.
    B. Even though the child initially has a negative skin test, it is recommended to begin prophylaxis with isoniazid for 3 months. At that time repeat the skin test, and if it is positive, the preventive therapy should be continued for at least 9 months total duration. If the repeat tuberculin skin test is negative, treatment may be discontinued.
    C. Chest x-rays are indicated following a positive skin test.
    D. Sputum cultures are reserved for symptomatic disease.

67. The answer is **B** [Dermatology].
    A. Acne is characterized by open and closed comedomes. It may also present with papular and pustular lesions with cysts and nodules. Benzoyl peroxide gel is an effective topical treatment for mild acne.
    B. Hydrocortisone cream is a topical corticosteroid that is appropriate for first-line treatment of facial seborrhea.
    C. Metronidazole gel is an effective treatment for rosacea.
    D. Mupirocin ointment is an effective topical treatment for impetigo.

68. The answer is **C** [Rheumatology and Orthopaedics].
    A. Hydroxychloroquine does not have renal adverse effects.
    B. Although there are a limited number of cases of abnormal liver function in patients taking hydroxychloroquine, these are extremely rare and regular monitoring in all patients is not recommended.
    C. Hydroxychloroquine is effective against the fevers, arthritis, and mucocutaneous manifestations of systemic lupus erythematosus. Although retinal toxicity is not common, it is dose dependent. Ophthalmologic exam, including visual acuity, slit-lamp, funduscopic, and visual field exam, is recommended at baseline and regularly, dependent on the medication dose.
    D. Hydroxychloroquine may cause GI upset but there is no need for annual endoscopy.

69. The answer is **C** [Hematology, Obstetrics/Gynecology].
    A. Alcohol abuse is more commonly associated with folate deficiency than with iron deficiency anemia.
    B. Familial anemias are usually diagnosed earlier in life.
    C. Iron deficiency anemia is the most common anemia worldwide. In adults in the United States, the most common cause is chronic blood loss.
    D. Although a poor diet may contribute to iron deficiency, the more likely cause in a developed country is blood loss.

70. The answer is **B** [Rheumatology and Orthopaedics].
    A. The elevated stress test is used to diagnose thoracic outlet syndrome.
    B. The Finkelstein's test is used to diagnose de Quervain tenosynovitis which is described in this scenario.
    C. The Phalen's maneuver and the Tinel's sign are used to diagnose carpal tunnel syndrome.
    D. See C.

71. The answer is **B** [Obstetrics/Gynecology].
    A. Colposcopy evaluates the cervix for possible cervical cancer or precancerous changes and is usually done to follow-up an abnormal Pap smear.
    B. In a patient with prolonged heavy menses, endometrial hyperplasia and endometrial cancer must be ruled out. Out of the choices here, endometrial biopsy is the only one that can evaluate the endometrium for both.
    C. Hysterosalpingography evaluates the patency of the fallopian tubes.
    D. Hysteroscopy evaluates abnormal uterine bleeding in the presence of a negative endometrial biopsy or dilation and curettage. It is a more invasive procedure that allows for directed biopsy and would not be the first step in the evaluation of prolonged, heavy bleeding.

72. The answer is **B** [Ophthalmology and Otolaryngology, Geriatrics].
    A. Patients with poor eustachian tube function may be unable to equalize barometric changes on the middle ear when confronted with rapid changes such as with flying, underwater diving, or rapid altitude change. Such barotrauma may present with ear pain and hearing loss related to those activities.
    B. Cerumen impaction is more common in the elderly due to age-related changes, such as the production of a drier wax and coarse hair in the ear canal. In many cases, it is self-induced due to incorrect ear cleaning methods. It is the most common cause of acute unilateral hearing loss.
    C. In eustachian tube dysfunction, the tube does not open properly when necessary, resulting in trapped air and negative pressure. Patients will present with ear fullness and mild to moderate hearing loss. It is commonly associated with viral URIs and allergies.
    D. Acute otitis media presents with otalgia, often associated with a URI. It is common in infants and children but it can occur in adults as well. Symptoms include ear pain, aural pressure, impaired hearing acuity, and fever. Physical exam findings include redness and decreased mobility of the tympanic membrane.

73. The answer is **A** [Endocrinology, Neurology].
    A. Bromocriptine (Parlodel) is a dopamine agonist which is the initial treatment of choice for prolactinomas. This will lead to a drop in serum prolactin and shrinkage of the microadenoma.
    B. See C.
    C. Sequential contraceptives may need to be started after therapy with a dopamine agonist, as her fertility will return while on therapy.
    D. Transphenoidal surgery is reserved for macroadenomas (>3 cm). This patient has a microadenoma and surgery is not recommended unless there is risk of stroke or compromise of the visual fields.

74. The answer is **B** [Infectious Disease, Neurology].
    A. Disseminated candidiasis may include infection of the brain in immunocompromised individuals. The organism would not display a capsule on staining.
    B. Infections caused by *Cryptococcus neoformans* have predominant CNS manifestations. The spectrum of disease consists predominantly of meningoencephalitis and pneumonia. A diagnosis of cryptococcosis requires demonstration of *C. neoformans* in normally sterile tissues. Visualization of the capsule in CSF mixed with India ink is a useful rapid diagnostic technique.
    C. Histoplasmosis is a fungal infection that is most commonly seen in immunocompromised hosts. It is mainly a pulmonary infection but may also cause disease of the retina.
    D. Pneumocystis is a common pathogen in patients with HIV disease. It is most noted for its effects on the respiratory system.

75. The answer is **A** [Gastroenterology, Ophthalmology and Otolaryngology].
    A. Night blindness is the earliest symptom of vitamin A deficiency. Xerosis is dry conjunctivae and Bitot's spots are white patches on the conjunctivae. In the United States, it is typically related to fat malabsorption syndromes or mineral oil laxative abuse. Food sources are those with β-carotenes such as carrots.
    B. Vitamins B$_{12}$ (cobalamin) and folate deficiencies present early with megaloblastic anemia. Mucosal changes may cause glossitis and diarrhea. In addition, B$_{12}$ deficiency leads to neurologic changes such as decreased vibratory sensation and position sense. B$_{12}$ is present in foods of animal origin and its deficiency is unusual unless one is on a vegan diet. Examples of more rare causes are gastrectomy, surgical resection of the ileum, pancreatic insufficiency, and severe Crohn's disease.
    C. Vitamin D deficiency results in secondary hyperparathyroidism often marked by normal to elevated levels of serum calcium but otherwise patients may be asymptomatic. Major sources of vitamin D are sunlight and fortified milk.
    D. Niacin (nicotinic acid) can be synthesized from the amino acid tryptophan. Major food sources are protein foods and numerous vegetables, cereals, and dairy. Niacin deficiency in the early stages has nonspecific manifestations as with other B vitamins. Advanced deficiency causes pellagra with the triad of diarrhea, dermatitis, and dementia.

76. The answer is **C** [Cardiology, Infectious Disease].
    A. Acetaminophen use is not associated with elevated blood pressure readings.
    B. Macrolides may cause QT prolongation in rare cases, but otherwise do not cause cardiac changes.
    C. NSAIDs are known to produce blood pressure elevations of about 5 mm Hg and should be avoided in hypertensive patients when possible.
    D. Penicillin may be effective in community-acquired pneumonia but resistance is known.

77. The answer is **A** [Gastroenterology, Surgery].
    A. This patient displays the criteria for Charcot's triad for cholangitis: RUQ pain, fever, and jaundice.
    B. This patient's abdominal pain suggests choledocholithiasis but also meets Charcot's triad, making cholangitis the correct diagnosis.
    C. Acute viral hepatitis has a prodrome of nausea and vomiting, anorexia, and malaise. There can be fever, jaundice, and an enlarged tender liver. Hepatitis can also be caused by autoimmune disease, alcohol use, toxic agents, and drugs. The dilated biliary ducts of this patient suggest obstruction (gallstones) as the etiology.
    D. Pancreatic carcinoma may present with obstructive jaundice (may be painless), along with a palpable gallbladder (Courvoisier's law), upper abdominal pain with radiation to the back, and weight loss.

78. The answer is **B** [Nephrology and Urology].
    A. Constipation does not occur with PDE-5 inhibitors, such as sildenafil (Viagra).
    B. PDE-5 inhibitors can result in a decrease in preload leading to hypotension.
    C. PDE-5 inhibitors are not hormones and therefore do not increase the risk of developing prostate cancer.
    D. Urinary retention is not a side effect of PDE-5 inhibitors.

79. The answer is **A** [Cardiology].
    A. Alcohol excess or alcohol withdrawal may precipitate atrial fibrillation; this presentation is often called "holiday heart."
    B. Atrial flutter is most often seen in persons with COPD or heart disease.
    C. Paroxysmal supraventricular tachycardia (PSVT) is common and occurs in patients without structural disease. It does not have an association with alcohol use.
    D. Ventricular premature beats are usually experienced as a sensation of the heart skipping beats and are more likely with stimulant use than with alcohol.

80. The answer is **D** [Pulmonology].
    A. ACE inhibitors are known to produce cough but not wheezing.
    B. Olopatadine is an antihistamine and is not associated with wheezing.
    C. H$_2$ blockers are not known to trigger asthma or cause wheezing.
    D. β-Blockers, even in the form of eye drops, can cause bronchoconstriction in asthmatics.

81. The answer is **D** [Pulmonology, Pediatrics, Infectious Disease].
    A. Asbestos exposure is linked to mesothelioma and pleuritic plaques.
    B. Sarcoidosis may cause dyspnea but not a productive cough or hemoptysis.
    C. A history of hyaline membrane disease does not predispose to bronchiectasis.
    D. Bronchiectasis notoriously causes recurrent pulmonary infections requiring antibiotics. Cystic fibrosis is a common underlying cause.

82. The answer is **A** [Dermatology, Endocrinology].
    A. Melasma manifests as patterned hyperpigmentation areas of the face and is associated with estrogen such as during pregnancy or administration of estrogen-containing medications.
    B. These lesions indicate diabetic dermopathy, which occurs in men more than in women. They often begin as round to oval, flat-topped, red, scaly papules that may become eroded. Healed lesions may result in epidermal atrophy or hyperpigmentation. Men are affected twice as often as women. These lesions may be initiated by trauma.
    C. These macules describe freckles. They occur predominantly in sun-exposed areas and fade during the winter months. The number varies from a few spots on the face to hundreds, which may coalesce. An autosomal dominant trait, freckles are most often found in individuals with fair complexions.
    D. This describes cafe-au-lait spots that are typically congenital but may occur in about 10% to 20% of normal children. They can be associated with von Recklinghausen's disease (neurofibromatosis).

83. The answer is **A** [Pulmonology].
    A. CPAP is the initial treatment recommended by the American Academy of Sleep Medicine and is usually well tolerated. Evidence is available that use of CPAP improves daytime sleepiness, reduces hypertension, and improves left ventricular function.
    B. Oral appliances are less effective than CPAP in preventing the apnea–hypopnea index and are recommended for snoring or for those patients unable to tolerate CPAP.
    C. Nonsurgical interventions are favored over surgical in most cases. Tonsillectomy and adenoidectomy is an initial intervention in children with obstructive sleep apnea. Newer methods involving ablation of tonsillar tissue may make this a more favorable option in the future.
    D. Uvulopharyngopalatoplasty is removal of the rim of the soft palate and uvula, resulting in an enlarged upper airway. The cure rate of this procedure is 40% to 50%. Patients with enlarged tongues or lower airway defects may derive little or no benefit from this procedure.

84. The answer is **A** [Dermatology].
    A. Any lesion suspected to be malignant melanoma must be biopsied. Excisional biopsy is preferred, especially with small focal lesions. A lesion does not have to meet all criteria (ABCD) to be suspicious.
    B. KOH prep is used to confirm dermatophytosis.
    C. A punch biopsy may be inadequate in suspected melanoma.
    D. Wood's lamp assessment is not helpful in evaluating lesions suspicious of melanoma. It is helpful in dermatophytoses.

85. The answer is **D** [Dermatology, Infectious Disease].
    A. Cosmetic use is not associated with exacerbations of herpes simplex.
    B. Deficient dietary dairy intake is not associated with outbreaks of herpes simplex.
    C. Herpes simplex is a viral disorder; therefore, topical antibiotics are not beneficial.
    D. Regular use of sunscreen can aid in reducing outbreaks of herpes simplex since sun exposure can trigger outbreaks.

86. The answer is **D** [Gastroenterology].
    A. Colonic strictures result from scarring and fibrosis in inflammatory disorders. They have no malignant potential outside of the pathology behind their development.
    B. Although Crohn's disease carries a higher than average risk of malignancy, it is much lower than that seen in ulcerative colitis.
    C. Toxic megacolon is colonic dilation beyond 6 cm; it occurs as a complication of ulcerative colitis and does not carry malignant potential.
    D. Ulcerative colitis carries a higher than average risk of malignant transformation, most notably in patients with pancolitis.

87. The answer is **D** [Nephrology and Urology].
    A. While CT would be useful in imaging the kidneys, it is more expensive than ultrasonography and exposes the patient to radiation. It is indicated if ultrasonography is inconclusive.
    B. An abnormal creatinine level would not be specific for polycystic kidney disease.
    C. MRI may be useful but is much more expensive than ultrasonography.
    D. Ultrasonography offers a relatively fast and noninvasive means of testing for polycystic kidney disease. There are well-established standards with high sensitivities to justify the use of ultrasonography. If ultrasonography is inconclusive, CT would then be indicated.

88. The answer is **D** [Pulmonology, Surgery].
    A. The patient is experiencing a tension pneumothorax. Increasing the supplemental oxygen will not help and may even exacerbate the problem.
    B. Intubation will only delay definitive treatment which is to relieve the tension.
    C. Immediate decompression of the tension pneumothorax is key to this patient's survival. A CT scan will only delay treatment. Once adequate decompression is achieved, CT scan or chest x-ray will be helpful while placing a chest tube.
    D. Immediate needle decompression is the key to this patient's survival, as he is experiencing a tension pneumothorax.

89. The answer is **D** [Ophthalmology and Otolaryngology].
  A. Acute iritis presents with ciliary flush or diffuse redness. Patients complain of moderate, deep, aching pain with decreased visual acuity. The cornea may be clear or slightly cloudy and the pupil may appear small or irregular.
  B. Patients presenting with conjunctivitis show diffuse redness due to dilatation of the conjunctival vessels with redness that tends to be maximal peripherally. The condition typically causes discomfort rather than true pain. Visual acuity is normal. The cornea remains clear. There may be a watery, mucoid, or mucopurulent discharge depending on etiology.
  C. Severe, aching, deep pain accompanies acute glaucoma. Visual acuity is decreased and the cornea is steamy or cloudy. The pupil is dilated and fixed. The redness may be diffuse or present as a reddish violet flush around the limbus.
  D. Leakage of blood outside the vessels secondary to trauma, bleeding disorders, or a sudden increase in venous pressure produce a homogeneous, sharply demarcated red area that fades to yellow and then disappears; this may take days to weeks. This patient's exam is consistent with a subconjunctival hemorrhage.

90. The answer is **A** [Cardiology, Pediatrics, Surgery].
  A. This is the classic description of coarctation of the aorta as a cause of secondary hypertension.
  B. Pheochromocytoma is a cause of secondary hypertension, but presents with flushing, headaches, and fluctuating blood pressures.
  C. Tetralogy of Fallot includes over-riding aorta, pulmonic stenosis, right ventricular hypertrophy, and ventricular septal defect. It is not associated with secondary hypertension. Untreated older children risk pulmonary valve problems and congestive heart failure. After surgical correction, older children are at risk for endocarditis, arrhythmias, and coronary artery disease.
  D. Large ventricular septal defects may cause arrhythmias but are not associated with hypertension.

91. The answer is **A** [Ophthalmology and Otolaryngology, Endocrinology].
  A. Diabetic retinopathy is the leading cause of new blindness among adults aged 20 to 65 years. It increases in prevalence and severity with increasing duration and poorer control of diabetes. In type 1 diabetes, retinopathy is generally not detectable for at least 3 years after diagnosis. In type 2 diabetes, retinopathy is present in up to 20% of patients at the time of diagnosis. Appropriate screening in patients with type 2 diabetes includes examination by an ophthalmologist at the time of diagnosis and yearly thereafter. For patients with type 1 diabetes, screenings should begin 3 to 5 years after diagnosis and continue yearly thereafter. Examinations should be done sooner if ocular symptoms develop.
  B. See A.
  C. See A.
  D. See A.

92. The answer is **D** [Psychiatry].
  A. Avoiding social settings promotes agoraphobia, which may accompany panic attacks.
  B. Tricyclic antidepressants are effective for panic; however, the side effect profile is such that they are rarely used. Mild panic disorders can be treated with psychotherapy alone.
  C. The prognosis of panic disorder with treatment is good.
  D. There is a 40% chance that this patient with panic disorder may experience a severe depression. Patients should be counseled on the symptoms of depression, and antidepressants should be considered as part of the overall treatment plan.

93. The answer is **D** [Pulmonology, Cardiology].
  A. In those with unlikely probability, a D-dimer test should be performed and, if normal, the disease can be safely ruled out.
  B. Although a normal perfusion scan adequately rules out pulmonary embolus (PE) and a high-probability perfusion–ventilation scan adequately rules in PE, the major disadvantages are the high proportion of nondiagnostic test results (~50%) and therefore the need for additional (costly) testing, usually with pulmonary angiography.
  C. The classic gold standard is pulmonary angiography, which is an invasive method requiring expertise. Hence, complementary strategies have evolved to diagnose PE more readily.
  D. At present, the most popular method to identify PE is the multislice spiral CT of the chest. This technique accurately detects PE and, if normal, has been shown to also safely rule out the presence of an embolus. Another advantage is the possibility of detecting an alternative disease in the thorax in those in whom PE is excluded, which may provide an explanation for the presenting symptoms.

94. The answer is **D** [Endocrinology, Ophthalmology and Otolaryngology].
  A. A blue sclera is associated with osteogenesis imperfecta.
  B. Keyser–Fleischer rings (green rimming to the iris) are associated with Wilson's disease.
  C. Pterygia are benign eye findings unassociated with hypertriglyceridemia.
  D. Lipemia retinalis may occur with serum triglyceride levels exceeding 3,000 to 4,000 mg/dL (34.5 to 46 mmol/L). With reflected light, these triglyceride particles produce a white cast to the venous bed of the retina.

95. The answer is **B** [Dermatology].
  A. This hair loss describes telogen effluvium, which often follows 2 to 4 months after an insult such as crash dieting, high fever, or significant illness.
  B. This describes alopecia areata, which often presents acutely with 1- to 4-cm patchy areas of hair loss on the scalp. Areas of hair loss are smooth and a defining point is broken hairs near the scalp surface.
  C. This pattern describes tinea capitis which, depending upon the fungus, may also include short stubs of broken hair with or without purulent discharge.
  D. This pattern describes androgenic alopecia, which occurs more commonly in men.

96. The answer is **D** [Hematology, Geriatrics].
    A. Patients with polycythemia vera should be placed on daily prophylactic aspirin if there are no other contraindications to its use.
    B. Low-salt diets can be especially helpful to those patients with hypertension and should be recommended for patients likely to retain fluid.
    C. If painful splenomegaly is present or there are repeated episodes of thrombosis causing splenic infarction, the patient with polycythemia vera may benefit from therapeutic splenectomy.
    D. The mainstay of treatment for patients with polycythemia vera is periodic therapeutic phlebotomy.

97. The answer is **A** [Hematology].
    A. This man most likely has a vitamin B_{12} deficiency, which affects first the peripheral nerves, leading to paresthesias, and then the posterior columns, leading to difficulty with balance. Decreased vibratory and position sense may be present, although early in the disease neurologic testing may be normal.
    B. Hyperactive deep tendon reflexes suggest a central, rather than a peripheral, problem.
    C. Impairment of two-point discrimination suggests injury rather than peripheral neuropathy.
    D. Palmar drift reflects a problem with muscle weakness.

98. The answer is **D** [Gastroenterology].
    A. Anemia can cause fatigue. Patients using alcohol heavily are more likely to have megaloblastic anemia due to folate deficiency.
    B. Depression can present with weight loss, somatic complaints, and a lack of interest in usual activities but this patient's social history and presentation are highly suspicious for malignancy and must be evaluated before a diagnosis of depression can be made.
    C. Diabetes mellitus type 1 is more likely associated with weight loss but at this patient's age, he would more likely develop type 2 diabetes. New-onset diabetes mellitus type 1 in a patient over 45 years of age should prompt an evaluation for pancreatic cancer.
    D. This is a classic presentation of pancreatic carcinoma with vague epigastric or left upper quadrant pain, weight loss, and depression. Risk factors include heavy alcohol and tobacco use, increasing age, obesity, chronic pancreatitis, prior abdominal radiation, and family history.

99. The answer is **A** [Pulmonology, Infectious Disease, Pediatrics].
    A. These are classic clinical symptoms and signs of acute bronchiolitis. Diagnosis is typically based upon clinical findings.
    B. Asthma typically has a recurrent pattern.
    C. Cystic fibrosis may be associated with poor growth, recurrent pulmonary infections, chronic diarrhea, or a family history of the disease.
    D. Pneumonia is usually associated with an infiltrate demonstrated on chest radiography.

100. The answer is **C** [Cardiology, Geriatrics].
    A. An ejection click is indicative of mitral valve prolapse or aortic stenosis.
    B. Thrills often accompany loud, harsh, or rumbling murmurs such as those of aortic stenosis, patent ductus arteriosus, ventricular septal defect, and mitral stenosis.
    C. An S_3 is highly suggestive of heart failure in adults. An S_3 is due to increased resistance to ventricular filling during passive atrial emptying.
    D. An S_4 occurs when there is increased resistance to ventricular filling during atrial contraction. The causes of an S_4 include hypertensive heart disease, coronary artery disease, aortic stenosis, and cardiomyopathy. It may be present in diastolic failure.

101. The answer is **D** [Ophthalmology and Otolaryngology].
    A. Ectropion (outward turning of the lower lid) is common with advanced age. Surgery is indicated if there is excessive tearing, keratitis, or a cosmetic concern.
    B. Entropion (inward turning, usually of the lower lid) occurs occasionally in older people as a result of degeneration of the lid fascia, or may follow extensive scarring of the conjunctiva and tarsus. Surgery is indicated if the lashes rub on the cornea (trichiasis).
    C. A pinguecula is a yellow, elevated conjunctival nodule that develops typically on the nasal side and can be bilateral.
    D. A pterygium is a fleshy, triangular, vascularized lesion that grows toward the cornea, usually on the nasal side. Risk factors include constant exposure to the wind, sun, sand, or dust. Pterygia become inflamed and may grow. Artificial tears or topical nonsteroidal anti-inflammatory agents may be needed. Surgery is indicated if pterygium becomes severely inflamed, threatens vision, or causes marked astigmatism or severe irritation.

102. The answer is **D** [Obstetrics/Gynecology, Surgery].
    A. See D.
    B. See D.
    C. See D.
    D. About 45% of breast cancers occur in the upper outer quadrant of the breast.

103. The answer is **B** [Obstetrics/Gynecology].
    A. See B.
    B. During the first half of the menstrual cycle, the endometrium is in the proliferative phase, with predominantly estrogen influence. The second half of the menstrual cycle, the secretory phase, occurs only after ovulation has occurred and progesterone becomes predominant.
    C. If a patient has entered premature menopause, she is either not ovulating at all or ovulating irregularly. Thus, proliferative or atrophic endometrium would be noted.
    D. Although oral contraceptives contain progesterone, the endometrium tends to be much thinner than that seen in normal menstrual cycles.

104. The answer is **A** [Cardiology, Geriatrics].
    A. Elevated jugular venous pressure is found in right heart failure.
    B. Marked hypotension, perivascular and interstitial edema, and three-pillow orthopnea indicate left heart failure.
    C. See B.
    D. See B.

105. The answer is **B** [Gastroenterology, Surgery].
    A. Initially, hyperactive bowel sounds are heard.
    B. Acute arterial obstruction causes abrupt, intense abdominal pain which is out of proportion to physical findings.
    C. Abrupt bowel evacuation frequently occurs in intestinal arterial occlusion; however, bloody diarrhea occurs later in the course of the disease following sloughing of the infarcted mucosa.
    D. As ischemia progresses, a tender abdominal mass and peritoneal signs appear.

106. The answer is **C** [Gastroenterology].
    A. See C.
    B. Colonoscopy is indicated for lower GI bleeding. This clinical presentation suggests upper GI bleeding.
    C. An upper endoscopy is the study of choice for suspected upper GI bleeding. Common causes include gastroduodenal ulcers, erosive esophagitis, erosive gastritis, Mallory–Weiss tears, vascular anomalies, portal hypertension, or malignancy.
    D. See C.

107. The answer is **A** [Hematology, Pediatrics, Gastroenterology].
    A. Persons who consume no animal products at all are at risk for vitamin B_{12} deficiency. Hypersegmented neutrophils are among the expected findings on peripheral blood smear.
    B. Vitamin B_{12} deficiency leads to a macrocytic rather than a microcytic anemia.
    C. Target cells are found in a number of anemias, including thalassemia.
    D. Vitamin B_{12} deficiency may lead to thrombocytopenia and leukopenia.

108. The answer is **D** [Obstetrics/Gynecology].
    A. Aromatase inhibitors are being studied for treatment of endometriosis and appear to be useful but are reserved for when other treatments have failed to work.
    B. Danazol is an effective treatment for endometriosis, but because of its side effects (decreased breast size, weight gain, acne, hirsutism, and lowering of voice which can be permanent), it is usually not the first line of treatment.
    C. Leuprolide acetate is an effective treatment for endometriosis but can only be used for up to 6 months because it can cause bone demineralization; therefore, it is not recommended for the initial treatment.
    D. This patient has the classic presentation of endometriosis. The best line of treatment is oral contraceptives. The side affect profile is good and the return of fertility is quick once use is discontinued.

109. The answer is **C** [Pulmonology, Pediatrics].
    A. Angioedema can present at any age. Symptoms have a sudden onset. The patient may exhibit stridor and a hoarse voice and may develop facial edema. It may be associated with ingestion of food causing anaphylaxis.
    B. Epiglottitis is most commonly seen in children 2 to 6 years old. It has a rapid onset, stridor may be present, and the patient may drool and appear toxic.
    C. Airway foreign bodies most commonly occur in children 1 to 3 years old. The classic triad of physical findings is sudden onset of paroxysmal coughing, wheezing, and diminished breath sounds. Stridor may also be present. The history of having choked or gagged raises this diagnosis to the top of the differential.
    D. Croup is most commonly seen in children 6 months to 3 years old. It has an insidious onset and is associated with upper respiratory symptoms.

110. The answer is **D** [Infectious Disease, Dermatology].
    A. Edematous, red, indurated spreading lesion is characteristic of erysipelas.
    B. An inflammatory hot lesion with diffuse erythema is characteristic of cellulitis.
    C. Vesicopustular lesions that follow a dermatome are characteristic of herpes zoster.
    D. Nonbullous impetigo is characterized by vesicular honey-colored crusted superficial lesions.

111. The answer is **D** [Hematology].
    A. Serum iron may be decreased in both iron deficiency and anemia of chronic disease.
    B. Transferrin saturation may be decreased in both.
    C. Reticulocytes are increased in anemia of chronic disease and decreased in iron deficiency anemia.
    D. Serum ferritin is likely to be normal or increased in anemia of chronic disease, but decreased in iron deficiency. Values less than 30 µg/L suggest iron deficiency.

112. The answer is **D** [Cardiology, Geriatrics].
    A. Although atrial fibrillation is very common in the elderly with coronary artery disease, it does not usually result in sudden cardiac death.
    B. Atrioventricular rhythm blocks, including complete heart block, generally have a good prognosis.
    C. Bundle branch blocks have a good prognosis, usually related to the level of underlying cardiac disease. They may also be present in a normal heart, especially right bundle branch block.
    D. Ventricular fibrillation is the most common cause of sudden cardiac death.

113. The answer is **C** [Pulmonology, Infectious Disease].
    A. Cavitary lesions are common in granulomatous disease, such as tuberculosis.
    B. Diffuse interstitial infiltrates are common in *Pneumocystis jiroveci* (nee *carinii*).
    C. Lobar consolidation is typical in pneumococcal pneumonia.
    D. Patchy diffuse infiltrates are common in viral or mycoplasma infections.

114. The answer is **B** [Neurology].
  A. Nausea and possibly vomiting are more typical in migraines than in tension headaches.
  B. Phonophobia is common in both tension headaches and migraines.
  C. Tension headaches are typically generalized, nonpulsatile, and described as tight or viselike.
  D. Migraine headaches are typically unilateral and pulsatile.

115. The answer is **D** [Cardiology, Geriatrics].
  A. This indicates mitral stenosis.
  B. This indicates tricuspid stenosis; patients typically present with right heart failure.
  C. This indicates aortic regurgitation; it is less common since the prevalence of rheumatic heart disease has decreased. Patients typically present in failure.
  D. This is the typical finding in aortic stenosis. This is the most common acquired valve disorder in the elderly, associated with hypertension, elevated lipids, and smoking.

116. The answer is **A** [Endocrinology].
  A. Aspirin overdose, though initially leading to respiratory alkalosis, subsequently causes a high anion gap acidosis.
  B. Lithium does not cause an increase in the anion gap.
  C. Phenobarbital does not cause an increase in the anion gap.
  D. Acetaminophen does not cause an increase in the anion gap.

117. The answer is **A** [Psychiatry].
  A. A benzodiazepine is a key part of the treatment used to prevent delirium tremens in a patient withdrawing from alcohol.
  B. Lithium carbonate is a mood stabilizer used to treat bipolar disorder.
  C. Tricyclic antidepressants are appropriate for the treatment of depression and panic disorders.
  D. Valproate (Depakote) is used in the treatment of bipolar disorder and seizure disorders.

118. The answer is **A** [Nephrology and Urology].
  A. Varicocele is an abnormality of the vein that drains the testis. Palpation reveals a twisted mass along the spermatic cord. It is often described as a bag of worms. Lying supine will enhance drainage of the pampiniform plexus and decrease the size of the mass.
  B. See A.
  C. A high-lying painful testis indicates torsion.
  D. A small, firm, palpable lump indicates a mass.

119. The answer is **D** [Gastroenterology].
  A. Abdominal CT may show more calcifications than visible on a plain abdominal x-ray and may show dilation of ducts and atrophy or other changes in the pancreas. It is not as sensitive as endoscopic retrograde cholangiopancreatography (ERCP).
  B. Abdominal ultrasonography may reveal suggestions of calcifications, dilated ducts, or pseudocysts, but it is not the most sensitive imaging technique.
  C. Abdominal plain films show calcifications in about 30% of patients with chronic pancreatitis but are not the most sensitive imaging choice.
  D. This patient most likely has chronic pancreatitis. ERCP is the most sensitive imaging modality for pancreatitis and can reveal dilated ducts, intraductal stones, pseudocysts, or strictures.

120. The answer is **D** [Infectious Disease, Dermatology].
  A. Gram-negative rods are usually enteric pathogens.
  B. Gram-positive cocci are consistent with staphylococcal or streptococcal infection.
  C. Hyphae and buds are seen on KOH prep with fungal infections.
  D. The clinical presentation is consistent with herpes simplex. A Tzanck smear is a cytologic technique commonly used in the diagnosis of herpes virus infections. Multinucleated epithelial giant cells suggest the presence of herpes virus or varicella virus.

121. The answer is **A** [Pulmonology, Infectious Disease].
  A. A positive PPD indicates exposure to *Mycobacterium tuberculosis*. It does not indicate active infection unless the patient is symptomatic. Induration greater than or equal to 10 mm is considered positive for employees in health care facilities.
  B. Patients with latent tuberculosis are asymptomatic and are not infectious.
  C. Any recent converter (<2 years) of the skin test should be treated with medication.
  D. Respiratory isolation is indicated in active disease.

122. The answer is **D** [Obstetrics/Gynecology, Surgery].
  A. Endometrial polyps arise from the endometrium and create abnormal protrusions into the endometrial cavity. They can cause menorrhagia and spontaneous bleeding during the reproductive years. Ultrasonography will show focal thickening of the endometrial stripe.
  B. Endometriosis is the most common cause of secondary dysmenorrhea due to growth of the endometrium outside of the uterus. The pain of endometriosis may be midcycle, premenstrual, postmenstrual, or continuous. It is typically associated with deep dyspareunia and tender pelvic nodules, especially in the uterosacral ligaments.
  C. Uterine (endometrial) carcinoma presents with abnormal bleeding, typically after menopause. Multiple discrete lesions are not seen.
  D. Uterine leiomyomas (fibroids) are the most common benign neoplasm of the uterus and are composed of smooth muscle cells. Risk factors include family history, nulliparity, ethnicity (more common in African Americans), and higher body mass index. Symptoms include pelvic pressure, bloating, heaviness in the lower abdomen, and lower back pain. Menorrhagia and metrorrhagia may lead to anemia. The uterus will likely be enlarged with palpable, firm, irregular masses.

123. The answer is **D** [Endocrinology, Geriatrics, Nephrology and Urology].
  A. Chronic hypercalcemia due to untreated hyperparathyroidism is associated with diffuse demineralization and cystic lesions, which will cause an abnormal DEXA scan (score <−1.0 SD).
  B. Hyperparathyroidism is not associated with dyspnea.
  C. Most patients with hyperparathyroidism are asymptomatic. Some may report polyuria and polydipsia due to hypercalcemia-induced nephrogenic diabetes insipidus.
  D. Approximately 20% of patients with hyperparathyroidism report a history of kidney stones, mostly the calcium oxalate type.

124. The answer is **D** [Cardiology, Pediatrics, Surgery].
  A. Antibiotics are not indicated in the treatment of patent ductus arteriosus.
  B. β-Blockers will slow the heart rate and, therefore, may be harmful.
  C. Anticoagulants are not indicated and may be harmful in the neonate.
  D. Indomethacin, a prostaglandin inhibitor, is routinely administered to help close a patent ductus arteriosus.

125. The answer is **B** [Dermatology, Infectious Disease, Pediatrics].
  A. Acyclovir is an antiviral beneficial in the treatment of herpes infections. Herpes infections usually present as grouped vesicles that eventually erode and crust.
  B. Cephalexin provides appropriate coverage for impetigo caused by *Staphylococcus* and *Streptococcus* species. Systemic antibiotics are recommended with widespread or complicated infections or if systemic symptoms, such as fever and malaise, are present.
  C. Doxycycline is a reasonable alternative for the treatment of impetigo but is contraindicated for use in children.
  D. Hydrocortisone is contraindicated in infectious lesions.

126. The answer is **D** [Endocrinology, Cardiology].
  A. Fasting glucose greater than 100 mg/dL is one of the criteria for metabolic syndrome.
  B. HDL cholesterol of less than 40 mg/dL in men (<50 mg/dL in women) is part of the criteria.
  C. LDL cholesterol is not included in the diagnostic criteria for metabolic syndrome.
  D. Metabolic syndrome is diagnosed by the presence of three or more of the following criteria: central obesity (waist circumference >40 inches in men, >35 inches in women); triglycerides greater than 150 mg/dL; HDL cholesterol less than 40 mg/dL in men or less than 50 mg/dL in women; elevated blood pressure; and fasting blood glucose greater than 100 mg/dL.

127. The answer is **C** [Cardiology].
  A. Calcium channel blockers do not provide definitive treatment and may cause hypotension and myocardial depression in this patient.
  B. Electrical therapies such as cardioversion are reserved for unstable patients or when oral agents are unsuccessful; furthermore, they are not definitive for this patient.
  C. Radiofrequency ablation is the preferred approach to treat recurrent supraventricular tachycardia.
  D. Vagal maneuvers are performed in the emergent, monitored setting but are not definitive treatment.

128. The answer is **A** [Gastroenterology].
  A. Achalasia is an idiopathic motility disorder that manifests as loss of peristalsis in the distal two-thirds (smooth muscle) of the esophagus and impaired relaxation of the lower esophageal sphincter. Barium esophagography, if done, will reveal esophageal dilation, loss of esophageal peristalsis, poor esophageal emptying, and a smooth, symmetric "bird's beak" tapering of the distal esophagus but does not confirm the diagnosis. The diagnosis is confirmed by esophageal manometry.
  B. Computed tomography does not allow assessment of motility.
  C. Endoscopy may be performed to evaluate the distal esophagus and gastroesophageal junction to exclude a distal stricture or submucosal infiltrating carcinoma.
  D. A 24-hour pH probe is not diagnostic.

129. The answer is **B** [Cardiology].
  A. See B.
  B. The initial step in the pathogenesis of atherosclerosis is development of the fatty streak, which is a subendothelial accumulation of lipids and lipid-laden monocytes. Macrophages then migrate into the subendothelial space and take up lipid ("foam" cells) followed by smooth muscle cells. A fibrous cap forms, the lesion calcifies, and the vessel becomes narrowed.
  C. See B.
  D. See B.

130. The answer is **B** [Gastroenterology, Infectious Disease].
  A. This regime is missing clarithromycin.
  B. This patient has *Helicobacter pylori*–positive peptic ulcer disease. Combination therapy with amoxicillin, clarithromycin, and a proton pump inhibitor (PPI) is one proper option of three accepted regimens. If the patient is penicillin allergic, metronidazole may be substituted for the amoxicillin. Alternative regimens are PPI with bismuth subsalicylate, tetracycline, and metronidazole or PPI with amoxicillin followed by PPI with clarithromycin.
  C. This regimen is missing the PPI.
  D. PPI alone does not eradicate *H. pylori*.

131. The answer is **D** [Neurology].
  A. Creutzfeldt–Jakob is a result of long-standing prion disease. It may manifest with parkinsonian features but dementia and jerking movements of extremities are common.
  B. Huntington's disease manifests with flowing chorea movements and dementia. Family history is key to diagnosing this autosomal dominant disorder.
  C. Multiple sclerosis typically presents with a pattern of relapsing and remitting features. Weakness, numbness, and paresis predominate.
  D. This is a typical presentation of Parkinson's disease.

132. The answer is **D** [Ophthalmology and Otolaryngology, Geriatrics].
   A. A patient who notes hearing loss should be referred for audiometry unless the cause is readily identifiable and treatable (i.e., cerumen impaction, otitis media).
   B. Routine audiologic screening is not recommended for adults with grossly normal hearing, unless there are risk factors (i.e., excessive noise exposure, older age). History of tympanostomy is not a risk factor.
   C. See A.
   D. Once patients have reached 65 years of age, audiologic evaluations should be done every few years.

133. The answer is **D** [Endocrinology].
   A. α-Glucosidase inhibitors, such as acarbose, reduce glucose by delaying glucose absorption.
   B. Glipizide and other sulfonylureas work by increased insulin secretion.
   C. Metformin, a biguanide, lowers glucose by decreasing hepatic glucose production and increasing glucose utilization.
   D. Pioglitazone is a thiazolidinedione and decreases insulin resistance and increases glucose utilization.

134. The answer is **B** [Nephrology and Urology, Infectious Disease].
   A. Ceftriaxone and doxycycline are used to treat sexually transmitted diseases.
   B. Uncomplicated pyelonephritis can be treated in the outpatient setting with a quinolone.
   C. See A.
   D. Gentamicin in a single dose will not provide satisfactory drug levels to eradicate the organism responsible.

135. The answer is **B** [Cardiology, Surgery].
   A. Valve replacement surgery is performed urgently only for symptomatic patients (heart failure, syncope, angina).
   B. This patient requires additional studies, including a cardiac catheterization prior to any plans for future valve replacement surgery.
   C. Although an echocardiography would confirm the valve disease, it is not required prior to surgery.
   D. Balloon valvuloplasty is less effective and associated with high restenosis rates.

136. The answer is **C** [Infectious Disease, Dermatology].
   A. Equine rabies antiserum is not available.
   B. Proper cleansing, irrigation, and debridement of animal bites are essential; these wounds should not be sutured.
   C. Rabies is a viral encephalitis transmitted by infected saliva that gains entry into the body by an animal bite or an open wound. Decision to treat should be based on the circumstances of the bite, including the extent and location of the wound, the biting animal, the history of prior vaccination, and the local epidemiology of rabies. Wounds should be cleaned and debrided as needed. The optimal form of passive immunization is human rabies immune globulin (half dose should be infiltrated into the wound and the remainder administered IM) combined with human diploid cell vaccine given IM in a separate site using a different syringe. The patient should receive additional doses of vaccine on days 3, 7, 14, and 28.
   D. Three injections of human diploid cell vaccine is the recommendation for preexposure prophylaxis for persons at high risk for exposure.

137. The answer is **D** [Pulmonology].
   A. Dyspnea is common in both types, although patients with chronic bronchitis–predominant COPD will experience greater dyspnea with exertion. Predominantly emphysematous patients are more dyspneic in general.
   B. Peripheral edema is more common in chronic bronchitis-predominant COPD.
   C. A productive cough is more common in chronic bronchitis–predominant COPD. Patients with emphysema-predominant COPD have a dry cough.
   D. Weight loss is more common in emphysema-predominant COPD.

138. The answer is **A** [Neurology].
   A. The pain of trigeminal neuralgia (tic douloureux) is triggered by touch, movement such as talking or chewing, or cold drafts.
   B. Fever, herpes lesions, and sleep deprivation have not been associated with episodes of trigeminal neuralgia.
   C. See B.
   D. See B.

139. The answer is **A** [Obstetrics/Gynecology].
   A. The use of oral progesterone, alone or in combination with estrogen, has been found to decrease the risk of developing endometrial hyperplasia, which leads to subsequent endometrial cancer.
   B. The use of estrogen alone has been found to cause endometrial hyperplasia, which leads to endometrial cancer.
   C. GNRH agonists (i.e., Lupron) put a woman into a pseudomenopausal state. These products are often used to treat endometriosis and uterine fibroids. Their use is not implicated in the development of endometrial cancer; however, they should be used for no longer than 6 months at a time due to risk of significant bone demineralization.
   D. Oral testosterone is sometimes prescribed for decreased libido and for the treatment of endometriosis. It is not related to the development of endometrial cancer.

140. The answer is **C** [Rheumatology and Orthopaedics, Geriatrics].
   A. Cyclophosphamide is used in other vasculitides such as Wegener's granulomatosis and microscopic polyangitis.
   B. High-dose prednisone would be indicated if the patient also had signs of giant cell (temporal) arteritis.
   C. Low-dose prednisone is indicated in patients with polymyalgia rheumatica without above-the-neck symptoms of giant cell arthritis.
   D. Methotrexate is indicated in rheumatoid arthritis.

141. The answer is **B** [Dermatology].
- **A.** Lichen planus is an acute or chronic inflammatory dermatosis involving the skin and/or mucous membranes. The lesions are characterized as flat-topped, pink to purple in color, polygonal, pruritic papules most commonly located on the wrists, lumbar region, shins, and scalp.
- **B.** Pityriasis rosea is an acute pruritic exanthematous eruption. A single herald patch typically precedes the generalized exanthem which presents with fine scaling papules and plaques with marginal collarette. The lesions typically link up along the cleavage lines of the skin creating a "Christmas tree" pattern. The lesions are predominantly on the trunk and proximal aspect of the extremities. Rarely lesions may occur on the face.
- **C.** The rash of secondary syphilis is characterized by macules and papules ranging in size from 0.5 to 1.0 cm, round to oval, and pink to brownish-red in color. It appears weeks after the primary chancre. A generalized eruption occurs on the trunk; lesions also occur on the head, neck, palms, and soles. Associated symptoms may include fever, sore throat, malaise, anorexia, and headache.
- **D.** Tinea corporis is a dermatophyte infection caused most commonly by *Trichophyton rubrum*. The lesions are typically ring-shaped plaques with sharp margins and an advancing scaly border with central clearing. The lesions can be single or multiple, may vary in size, and are associated with mild pruritus.

142. The answer is **B** [Cardiology].
- **A.** Anterior wall infarction will likely show Q waves and ST elevation in leads I, AVL, and V2 to V6.
- **B.** Inferior wall infarction will likely show Q waves and ST elevation in leads II, III, and AVF.
- **C.** Lateral wall infarction will likely show ST depressions in leads I, AVL, and V5 to V6.
- **D.** Posterior wall infarction will likely show ST depressions and then elevations in V1 to V3.

143. The answer is **C** [Obstetrics/Gynecology].
- **A.** See C.
- **B.** See C.
- **C.** After menopause, most women note some change in patterns of body hair. Usually, there is a variable loss of pubic and axillary hair. The labia and clitoris become smaller.
- **D.** See C.

144. The answer is **A** [Cardiology, Surgery].
- **A.** Compression sclerotherapy produces permanent fibrosis in small veins. It typically relieves all symptoms.
- **B.** Stripping is reserved for large vessels as a second resort after ablation therapy.
- **C.** Leg elevation and rest are palliative, not definitive.
- **D.** Sequential compression devices are used for nonambulatory patients, usually in the acute care setting, as prophylaxis against thrombosis.

145. The answer is **A** [Psychiatry].
- **A.** Onset of illness at age 20 years or later is associated with a better outcome.
- **B.** Insidious onset, slow rate of progression, and low socioeconomic status are associated with a poorer outcome.
- **C.** See B.
- **D.** See B.

146. The answer is **B** [Cardiology, Geriatrics].
- **A.** Development of new Q waves would indicate a myocardial infarction rather than angina pectoris.
- **B.** Downsloping ST-segment depression is characteristic of angina pectoris.
- **C.** Peaked T waves are associated with hyperkalemia.
- **D.** U waves are associated with hypokalemia.

147. The answer is **D** [Rheumatology and Orthopaedics].
- **A.** See D.
- **B.** See D.
- **C.** See D.
- **D.** The incidence of ankylosing spondylitis is greater in males than in females and usually presents in the late teens or early 20s. Whites are more commonly affected than blacks.

148. The answer is **C** [Cardiology, Geriatrics].
- **A.** Cyclophosphamide is an anticancer chemotherapeutic agent. It is not indicated in giant cell arteritis.
- **B.** Fluids are part of the overall patient management but do not directly help relieve the pathology of giant cell arteritis.
- **C.** Prednisone starting at 60 mg/day is therapeutic and may prevent permanent blindness associated with giant cell arteritis.
- **D.** Pulsed steroids are indicated for critically ill patients with polyarteritis nodosa or patients with giant cell arteritis who have developed visual loss.

149. The answer is **D** [Ophthalmology and Otolaryngology, Infectious Disease, Pediatrics].
- **A.** Bacterial conjunctivitis typically produces a purulent discharge. There is usually minimal irritation and no visual impairment. Preauricular adenopathy is rare.
- **B.** Inclusion conjunctivitis is commonly a sexually transmitted disease in adults, typically chlamydia. The eye is usually affected after exposure to genital secretions. A nontender preauricular adenopathy is common.
- **C.** Dry eye syndrome is common, especially in elderly females. It can be caused by a variety of conditions including lacrimal gland dysfunction, systemic disease (i.e., Sjogren's syndrome), and drugs.
- **D.** Viral conjunctivitis is usually associated with URI symptoms. The conjunctiva is red with copious watery discharge and scanty exudate. Tender preauricular adenopathy is common. Children are affected more often than adults.

150. The answer is **D** [Obstetrics/Gynecology].
- **A.** Although she may eventually be diagnosed as having habitual or recurrent abortions (defined as three or more consecutive spontaneous pregnancy terminations) if she aborts this pregnancy, this is not the correct description at this time.
- **B.** Incomplete abortion refers to the expulsion of some but not all of the products of conception.
- **C.** An inevitable abortion would present with dilation of the cervix without expulsion of the products of conception.
- **D.** Threatened abortion is defined as intrauterine bleeding prior to 20 weeks with a closed cervix.

151. The answer is **A** [Dermatology, Cardiology].
- **A.** Wearing compression stockings will reduce edema, improve venous return, and minimize the risk of future leg ulcers from venous insufficiency.
- **B.** Frequent use of topical steroids can lead to irreversible atrophic skin changes.
- **C.** Leg elevation will improve venous circulation; however, this is only helpful when the patient is sedentary.
- **D.** Regular aerobic exercise is important to promote weight loss but will be less effective than compression stockings as a preventive intervention against venous stasis ulcers.

152. The answer is **C** [Cardiology].
- **A.** Hepatomegaly and scattered wheezes in a patient with dyspnea and cough indicate congestive heart failure.
- **B.** Orthostatic hypotension indicates a volume deficit.
- **C.** Pulsus paradoxus is a classic finding in pericardial effusion.
- **D.** See A.

153. The answer is **C** [Gastroenterology, Surgery].
- **A.** Achalasia is a motility problem in which peristalsis is lost in the distal (smooth muscle) portion of the esophagus and the tone of the lower esophageal sphincter is impaired. Achalasia is associated with an increased risk of esophageal squamous cell carcinoma.
- **B.** Esophageal cancers typically develop in ages 50 to 70 years, with a male to female ratio of 3:1. Adenocarcinoma is more common in whites.
- **C.** Chronic alcohol and tobacco use are strongly correlated with esophageal squamous cell cancer. It is much more common in African Americans than in whites.
- **D.** Strictures are caused by caustic exposure such as occurs with chronic GERD, disordered motility or hiatal hernia.

154. The answer is **D** [Cardiology].
- **A.** Although given in cases of symptomatic bradycardia to increase heart rate, atrioventricular block will not respond to atropine.
- **B.** The fluid/dehydration status of this patient is less important than her cardiac arrhythmia.
- **C.** The patient has a sinus node pacemaker working—just not a normal ventricular response, indicating third-degree/complete atrioventricular block.
- **D.** Patients with complete heart block require temporary pacing until a permanent pacemaker can be implanted.

155. The answer is **D** [Cardiology, Surgery].
- **A.** Color duplex sonography is an investigational procedure. At this time, it is not a practical choice.
- **B.** Erythrocyte sedimentation rate (ESR) is nonspecific and, therefore, not definitive.
- **C.** Rheumatoid factor level is not indicated in temporal arteritis.
- **D.** The clinical appearance of the temporal arteritis may be normal or pulsatile, nodular, enlarged, or tender. A temporal artery biopsy should be made as soon as the diagnosis is entertained, but therapy should never be delayed while awaiting the biopsy. Empiric therapy with steroids should be started with biopsy performed within the following 2 weeks.

156. The answer is **C** [Nephrology and Urology].
- **A.** Epispadias is a congenital defect where the urethral meatus is located on the dorsal aspect of the penis instead of at the tip of the glans.
- **B.** Hypospadias is a congenital defect where the urethral meatus is located on the ventral side of the penis instead of at the tip of the glans.
- **C.** Paraphimosis is the inability to replace the foreskin to its usual position. This can lead to constriction of the glans penis and ultimately to edema or gangrene.
- **D.** Phimosis is the inability to retract the foreskin.

157. The answer is **C** [Ophthalmology and Otolaryngology].
- **A.** In a sensorineural hearing loss, air conduction exceeds bone conduction in the unaffected ear. This is the Rinne's test.
- **B.** See A.
- **C.** Cerumen impaction is a cause of unilateral conductive hearing loss. In a properly performed Weber test, sound will lateralize to the affected ear.
- **D.** See C.

158. The answer is **B** [Pulmonology, Pediatrics].
- **A.** Anaphylaxis will manifest with urticaria, hypotension, and nausea as well as dyspnea.
- **B.** This is a typical presentation of asthma.
- **C.** Patients with cystic fibrosis have chronic productive cough and clubbing.
- **D.** Acute toxoplasmosis presents with fever, dyspnea, and nonproductive cough. It is more common in immunocompromised patients.

159. The answer is **D** [Infectious Disease, Dermatology].
- **A.** Cytomegalovirus and Epstein–Barr virus are not associated with warts.
- **B.** See A.
- **C.** Herpes simplex virus causes grouped vesicles with erythematous bases.
- **D.** Human papillomaviruses selectively infect the epithelium of skin and mucous membranes. These infections may be asymptomatic, produce warts, or be associated with a variety of both benign and malignant neoplasms. Anogenital warts develop on the skin and mucosal surfaces. In women, warts typically first appear at the posterior introitus and adjacent labia.

160. The answer is **D** [Neurology].
- **A.** An abnormal number of chromosome results in sex-linked disorders such as Klinefelter's or Turner's.
- **B.** Deletions and crossovers represent genetic mutations such as in Duchenne muscular dystrophy.
- **C.** Transmutations are thought to be responsible for many diseases including some cancers. Some transmutations are beneficial.
- **D.** Huntington's disease is an autosomal dominant disorder resulting from an expanded and unstable CAG trinucleotide repeat on chromosome 4.

161. The answer is **A** [Endocrinology, Pediatrics].
- **A.** A sibling with type 1 diabetes places a child at 15 times the normal risk for development of type 1 diabetes.
- **B.** A high body mass index may place a child at higher risk for type 2 diabetes.
- **C.** Introduction of cereals before 4 months has been suggested to increase the risk of autoimmunity.
- **D.** Milk-based protein has been shown to increase susceptibility for type 1 diabetes in animal models, but has yet to be shown in human studies.

162. The answer is **C** [Rheumatology and Orthopaedics].
- **A.** Acetaminophen may be effective in treating patients with mild osteoarthritis symptoms.
- **B.** Capsaicin cream may be effective in treating mild osteoarthritis.
- **C.** NSAIDs are the most popular medication for treatment of moderate osteoarthritis. Clinical trials have shown greater improvement of symptoms with NSAIDs compared to acetaminophen.
- **D.** Opiates are quite effective in controlling pain; however, because of the side effects and risk of dependence, these should be reserved for patients unresponsive to other treatments.

163. The answer is **C** [Pulmonology].
- **A.** Persons with interstitial lung disease present with progressive exertional dyspnea or persistent nonproductive cough. Chest radiography reveals a bibasilar reticular pattern.
- **B.** Pneumocystis is an opportunistic pulmonary pathogen that is an important cause of pneumonia in the immunocompromised host. Diagnosis is typically clinical or via histologic staining.
- **C.** Sarcoidosis is more common in young, healthy adults. In the United States, it is more commonly seen in African American women. Most common presenting symptoms are cough, dyspnea, and fatigue. Organ involvement outside the lungs is fairly common; eye and skin symptoms are more common in African Americans. Bilateral hilar adenopathy is classic for stage 1 sarcoidosis.
- **D.** Tuberculosis most often affects the lungs, although other organs are involved in up to one-third of cases. Chest radiography may show typical upper lobe granuloma with cavitation.

164. The answer is **A** [Ophthalmology and Otolaryngology, Infectious Disease, Pediatrics].
- **A.** Acute otitis media is most common in infants and children and presents with the symptoms described.
- **B.** Patients with poor eustachian tube function may be unable to equalize barometric stress on the middle ear (i.e., flying, diving, rapid altitude changes), resulting in barotrauma. They present with severe ear pain and hearing loss.
- **C.** Acute mastoiditis may appear acutely or after several weeks of inadequately treated acute otitis media. Presenting symptoms include postauricular pain and redness with a spiking fever.
- **D.** Bony overgrowths in the ear canal can be an incidental finding. Solitary osteomas have no clinical significance unless they cause obstruction or infection.

165. The answer is **D** [Rheumatology and Orthopaedics, Surgery].
- **A.** Bulging of the biceps muscle is seen in proximal or distal rupture of the biceps muscle.
- **B.** Pain with valgus stress of the elbow is seen in elbow instability or posterior elbow impingement.
- **C.** Pain with resisted wrist extension is seen in lateral epicondylitis.
- **D.** Pain with resisted wrist flexion is seen in medial epicondylitis.

166. The answer is **A** [Cardiology].
- **A.** The left anterior descending artery supplies the anterior free wall of the left ventricle and anterior two-thirds of the interventricular septum.
- **B.** The right coronary artery supplies the posterior portion of the heart and the AV node.
- **C.** The left circumflex artery supplies the posterolateral surface of the heart.
- **D.** The left marginal artery supplies the left lateral wall of the heart.

167. The answer is **A** [Nephrology and Urology, Surgery].
- **A.** AFP and βHCG are common markers used to help identify type of testicular tumor. Nonseminomatous types produce increased levels of both AFP and βHCG; seminomatous types do not produce AFP.
- **B.** CA 15-3 is used to monitor breast cancer and CA 125 is used in the detection of ovarian cancer.
- **C.** FSH and LH are hormones that stimulate cells in the testes to produce spermatozoa and testosterone.
- **D.** PSA and CEA are used to monitor patients with prostate cancer.

168. The answer is **D** [Nephrology and Urology].
- **A.** See D.
- **B.** See D.
- **C.** See D.
- **D.** The major risk of performing a rectal examination in a patient with acute prostatitis is sepsis. It is felt that manipulation of the infected gland may cause dissemination of the pathogen into the blood stream.

169. The answer is **A** [Gastroenterology, Surgery, Pediatrics].
- **A.** An abdominal CT is the imaging modality of choice for evaluation of suspected appendicitis. CT is more sensitive than ultrasonography.
- **B.** ERCP is an imaging modality for evaluation of the pancreas and related structures.
- **C.** A flat plate is not specific to appendicitis. It may be beneficial if ileus or small bowel obstruction is in the differential. Gas-filled loops of small and large intestines may be seen with ileus. Air fluid levels may also be detected.
- **D.** Ectopic pregnancy is in the differential for this patient. If the patient has a positive βHCG, then pelvic ultrasonography would be appropriate. However, the clinical picture indicates appendicitis.

170. The answer is **B** [Rheumatology and Orthopaedics].
   A. Ibuprofen on a PRN basis will only mask the symptoms and will do nothing to slow or halt the disease.
   B. Modification of activity and splint will slow or halt the progression of carpal tunnel syndrome in the early stages of the disease.
   C. Topical capsaicin has shown benefit in patients with mild to moderate osteoarthritis but not carpal tunnel syndrome.
   D. Surgical release is reserved for late stage disease.

171. The answer is **B** [Pulmonology].
   A. Long-acting β-agonist alone is not recommended for persistent asthma.
   B. According to current guidelines, this patient has moderate persistent asthma and requires a combination approach including an inhaled steroid plus a long-acting β-agonist.
   C. His current medication is a short-acting β-agonist, and nebulization offers no advantage over proper inhalation.
   D. Oral steroid tapering dose is reserved for exacerbations unresponsive to inhaled therapies.

172. The answer is **C** [Cardiology].
   A. Enalapril does lower blood pressure very well but takes about 6 hours for peak action.
   B. Hydralazine has less predictable results and is used most often during pregnancy for blood pressure control.
   C. Labetalol has combined β- and α-blocking action and is most potent for rapid blood pressure lowering needs.
   D. Nitroglycerin is indicated for patients who also have chest pain.

173. The answer is **B** [Obstetrics/Gynecology].
   A. An erythematous cervix is indicative of an inflammatory process.
   B. A bluish cervix is indicative of pregnancy (Chadwick's sign).
   C. Multiparous cervix indicates past pregnancy and delivery but not necessarily a current pregnancy.
   D. Strawberry cervix is pathognomonic for *Trichomonas* infection.

174. The answer is **A** [Gastroenterology].
   A. Osmotic laxatives, such as polyethylene glycol or milk of magnesia, may be helpful to decrease straining at defection, improve stool consistency, and increase stool frequency.
   B. Antispasmodics (anticholinergic) agents do not have well-documented efficacy but have been used for bloating or acute pain episodes. They must be used with great caution in the elderly and in those with constipation because of the anticholinergic side effects. Anticholinergic side effects may further increase constipation. To this end, they are not appropriate for constipation-dominant IBS.
   C. A high-fiber diet and fiber supplementation have limited value in irritable bowel syndrome; about half will respond to placebo as well. A subset of patients report increased gas and distention with little change in bowel frequency.
   D. The 5-HT3 antagonist alosetron is for diarrhea-predominant IBS in women refractory to other therapies. It should not be used in those with constipation-dominant IBS.

175. The answer is **D** [Dermatology].
   A. Curettage is not indicated in the initial evaluation of suspected basal cell carcinoma.
   B. Electrodesiccation is not indicated in the initial evaluation of suspected basal cell carcinoma.
   C. Lesions suspicious for basal cell carcinoma should undergo biopsy before excision is attempted.
   D. All lesions suspicious for basal cell carcinoma should undergo either shave or punch biopsy prior to initiating curative treatment.

176. The answer is **C** [Rheumatology and Orthopaedics].
   A. See C.
   B. See C.
   C. Polymyositis is an idiopathic inflammatory myopathy associated with progressive proximal muscle weakness in which the facial and ocular muscles are spared. Although tests such as muscle enzymes, electromyography, and rheumatoid factor may be ordered, they are not diagnostic. Only a biopsy of involved muscle can be utilized as a specific diagnostic test.
   D. See C.

177. The answer is **C** [Ophthalmology and Otolaryngology, Endocrinology].
   A. With epiglottitis (supraglottitis), laryngoscopy is generally safe in adults and may show a swollen, erythematous epiglottis.
   B. Needle aspiration would be indicated in peritonsillar abscess.
   C. Epiglottitis is more common in adults with diabetes. It may be viral or bacterial. Initial treatment is admission and IV antibiotics (ceftizoxime or cefuroxime) and steroids (dexamethasone) until etiology is secured. Examination of the airway is important, and intubation may be necessary.
   D. See C.

178. The answer is **B** [Rheumatology and Orthopaedics].
   A. Acute gout usually presents suddenly and is characterized by extreme pain, redness, and swelling of one joint, most commonly the great toe.
   B. Osteoarthritis (OA) has an insidious onset and gets worse throughout the day. Heberden's nodes (DIP joint) and Bouchard's nodes (PIP joint) are often seen in patients with OA.
   C. Reactive arthritis (Reiter's syndrome) usually occurs after a dysenteric infection (notably *Campylobacter*) or sexually transmitted infection and presents with a classic tetrad of urethritis, conjunctivitis, mucocutaneous lesions, and aseptic arthritis.
   D. Rheumatoid arthritis usually presents with symmetric swelling of multiple joints along with tenderness and pain. Stiffness usually lasts more than 30 minutes in the morning. Patients often have systemic complaints as well.

179. The answer is **D** [Nephrology and Urology].
   A. See D.
   B. See D.
   C. See D.
   D. Hypokalemia can occur in association with a normal or decreased pH. Most commonly hypokalemia is due to increased losses via the gastrointestinal tract. In cases of refractory hypokalemia, magnesium levels should be checked, as magnesium is very important for normal potassium uptake and maintenance.

180. The answer is **A** [Gastroenterology, Infectious Disease, Pediatrics].

 A. Hepatitis B immunization series consists of three shots: baseline and then 1 and 6 months later. It is recommended to begin the series at birth but, if not, the same schedule is to be followed once the series is begun.

 B. Baseline and then 2 and 4 months is the schedule for DTaP, typically starting at age 2 months.

 C. Baseline with booster at 2 months is the schedule for varicella-zoster vaccine in those over 13 years of age.

 D. Baseline with booster at 6 to 18 months is the schedule for hepatitis A vaccine.

181. The answer is **A** [Psychiatry, Pediatrics].

 A. The onset of autism is before 36 months.

 B. Autism is associated with seizures in less than one-third of patients.

 C. Autism is not associated with hallucinations or delusions. It is associated with absence of speech, stereotyped phrases, and failure to develop relatedness.

 D. Autism is almost always associated with subnormal intelligence; intelligence is severely impaired in 70% of patients.

182. The answer is **D** [Infectious Disease, Pulmonology].

 A. Azithromycin is appropriate prophylaxis against *Mycobacterium avium* complex for HIV-positive patients with CD4 counts less than 50 cells/μL.

 B. Fluconazole is effective prophylaxis against cryptococcus infection in HIV-positive patients with CD4 counts less than 200 cells/μL.

 C. Ganciclovir is the preferred drug for prophylaxis against cytomegalovirus infection in HIV-positive patients with CD4 counts less than 100 cells/μL.

 D. Trimethoprim/sulfamethoxazole (TMP–SMX) is the prophylactic drug of choice again pneumocystis infections in HIV-positive patients with CD4 counts less than 200 cells/μL. This patient should start TMP–SMX administration in addition to antiretroviral therapy. Although incidence has dramatically declined following effective prophylactic regimens (HAART), it is still the most common opportunistic infection in HIV-positive patients in the United States.

183. The answer is **A** [Ophthalmology and Otolaryngology, Geriatrics].

 A. Macular degeneration is an important cause of gradual central visual loss in the elderly. Patients often complain of distorted images (metamorphopsia). Funduscopic exam may reveal drusen, which are yellowish round spots of variable size often haphazardly distributed or concentrated at the posterior pole. Drusen represent undigested cellular debris.

 B. A hyperemic, swollen optic disc with blurred margins in the presence of bulging of the physiologic cup indicates papilledema.

 C. Rings and crescents are developmental variations of either white sclera or black retinal pigment. They are typically found along the temporal border of the optic disc.

 D. Funduscopic examination of patients with hypertensive retinopathy may reveal cotton wool patches, copper wiring, silver wiring, flame-shaped hemorrhages, AV nicking or tapering.

184. The answer is **D** [Rheumatology and Orthopaedics, Geriatrics].

 A. See D.

 B. See D.

 C. See D.

 D. Temporal arteritis (giant cell arteritis) and polymyalgia rheumatica are considered two manifestations of the same disease and frequently coexist.

185. The answer is **C** [Ophthalmology and Otolaryngology, Infectious Disease, Pediatrics].

 A. The incidence of otitis media due to *Haemophilus influenzae* has been significantly decreased with vaccination programs. It rarely causes otitis externa.

 B. *Moraxella catarrhalis* is a common pathogen in otitis media.

 C. The majority of cases of otitis externa are caused by *Pseudomonas aeruginosa* or *Proteus* spp. Less common causes include *Staphylococcus aureus*, *Staphylococcus epidermidis*, *Aspergillus*, and *Actinomyces*. Topical antibiotic coverage should include antipseudomonal activity.

 D. Acute otitis media typically follows a viral URI. Viruses can cause the infection or predispose the patient to a secondary bacterial infection. *Streptococcus pneumoniae* is the most common bacterial pathogen.

186. The answer is **B** [Pulmonology].

 A. Lobar consolidation is more common in pneumonia.

 B. The most common findings are diffuse nodular infiltrates, particularly before the disease becomes symptomatic.

 C. Solid masses are more consistent with neoplastic disease.

 D. Granulomas are more common in tuberculosis and other similar diseases.

187. The answer is **C** [Gastroenterology].

 A. This treatment suggestion is a hybrid of approaches containing recommendations for patients with mild and severe diverticulitis.

 B. This is a reasonable approach for patients with diverticulitis who have mild symptoms without signs of peritoneal irritation.

 C. This patient is presenting with severe diverticulitis. This requires hospitalization and bowel rest (NPO), IV fluids, and broad-spectrum antibiotics with anaerobic coverage.

 D. The addition of the nasogastric tube is for severe diverticulitis with ileus.

188. The answer is **D** [Cardiology, Pediatrics, Infectious Disease].

 A. Acetaminophen or ibuprofen would reduce the fever and pain, but they are not the drugs of choice in rheumatic fever.

 B. Codeine may be used to relieve severe pain but should be reserved for such cases.

 C. See A.

 D. Aspirin is the drug of choice in rheumatic fever; it has consistently shown greater anti-inflammatory properties over other NSAIDs.

189. The answer is **D** [Endocrinology, Geriatrics].
  A. Glucagon would further increase the blood glucose.
  B. Insulin is typically not needed unless the glucose is resistant to fluids.
  C. Hypophosphatemia may develop if insulin is given.
  D. Hyperglycemia in the absence of ketosis is common in elderly type 2 diabetics. With mild dehydration, sodium is low but rises as the dehydration worsens. Elevated BUN is key to diagnosis. This patient is presenting with hyperglycemic hyperosmolar state and is dehydrated. Correction of the hypovolemia will reduce the hyperglycemia and thereby allow the kidneys to excrete the glucose.

190. The answer is **B** [Neurology, Pediatrics].
  A. Carbamazepine, phenobarbital, and phenytoin are indicated for tonic–clonic (grand mal) or partial focal seizures.
  B. Absence, or petit mal, seizures are best treated with either ethosuximide or valproic acid. Clonazepam is also effective but can be habit forming.
  C. See A.
  D. See A.

191. The answer is **D** [Obstetrics/Gynecology, Infectious Disease].
  A. Ceftriaxone is recommended for the treatment of *Neisseria gonorrhoeae* infections. The patient may be asymptomatic or present with a mucopurulent cervicitis and a red, swollen, and friable cervix.
  B. Bacterial vaginosis is due to overgrowth of *Gardnerella vaginalis* and other anaerobes. It is associated with a malodorous, grayish, nonadherent discharge, which demonstrates an amine "fishy" odor after alkalization with KOH. Clue cells are seen on wet mount. Treatment options include oral metronidazole or clindamycin cream.
  C. Vulvovaginal candidiasis is associated with pruritus, erythema of the vulva and vagina, and a white, curd-like, nonodorous discharge. Risk factors include pregnancy, diabetes, recent antibiotic use, and occlusive clothing. Wet prep shows budding yeast cells, filaments, and spores. Fluconazole in a single dose is therapeutic.
  D. Trichomoniasis is a sexually transmitted infection associated with pruritus and a malodorous, frothy, yellow to greenish discharge. Red maculopapular lesions may be visible on the cervix. Wet mount will show motile flagellate protozoans. Treatment is metronidazole orally in a single dose.

192. The answer is **C** [Psychiatry, Neurology].
  A. Muscle atrophy and/or true muscle weakness would not be seen in a conversion disorder.
  B. The funduscopic exam would be normal in a conversion disorder.
  C. Sensory loss does not conform to a recognized pattern of distribution in a conversion disorder.
  D. Visual fields are normal or inconsistently abnormal in patients with conversion disorder.

193. The answer is **B** [Pulmonology, Infectious Disease, Pediatrics].
  A. Amantadine and ramantidine are no longer recommended for the early treatment or prophylaxis of influenza because of the resistance that has developed to these two antivirals.
  B. Oseltamivir is recommended for both the treatment and prophylaxis of influenza A or B in children greater than 1 year of age and should be initiated within 48 hours of symptoms suggestive of the flu.
  C. See A.
  D. Zanamivir is not recommended in children under the age of 7 years.

194. The answer is **D** [Rheumatology and Orthopaedics].
  A. An enchondroma is a benign tumor usually found in the small tubular bones of the hands and feet; enchondromas are usually asymptomatic.
  B. Osteoid osteomas are benign tumors that usually present with dull, aching pain that is relieved with NSAIDs. They most commonly occur in the proximal femur.
  C. Osteomyelitis is an infection of the bone and presents with pain, fever, and bone destruction on x-ray.
  D. Osteosarcoma is the most common primary malignant bone tumor and usually presents in the second or third decade of life. Patients are usually male, and present with pain and a mass in the distal femur or proximal tibia.

195. The answer is **C** [Psychiatry].
  A. An anxious or depressed mood is not an indication for hospitalization unless accompanied by other indications.
  B. See A.
  C. History of impulsive behavior, poor social support, and/or a suicidal plan are each reasons to hospitalize a suicidal patient.
  D. Hypersomnolence is commonly seen with depression but is not an indication for hospitalization.

196. The answer is **D** [Ophthalmology and Otolaryngology, Infectious Disease].
  A. Leukoplakia of the vocal folds is often found in patients who smoke. Voice change is insidious.
  B. Acute laryngitis is usually viral.
  C. Vocal cord paralysis is caused by a lesion or damage to the vagus or recurrent laryngeal nerve, which can result from thyroid surgery or cancer, other neck surgery, and lung cancer, among other causes.
  D. Voice rest is appropriate, as continued strong voice use with laryngitis can lead to traumatic vocal cord nodules, polyps, and cysts but not paralysis.

197. The answer is **A** [Ophthalmology and Otolaryngology, Infectious Disease].
  A. Treatment of herpes labialis is not required in immunocompetent patients but is offered to hasten recovery. Oral acyclovir will shorten the duration and severity of symptoms.
  B. Prednisone has a high risk of side effects and is not indicated in benign herpetic lesions in an immunocompetent host.
  C. Topical idoxuridine is indicated for herpetic keratitis.
  D. Topical antivirals, such as penciclovir, are generally not very effective in herpes labialis.

198. The answer is **A** [Infectious Disease, Dermatology].

  A. Lyme borreliosis is caused by a spirochete, *Borrelia burgdorferi*, and is transmitted via deer ticks. Lyme disease is now the most common vector-borne infection in the United States and Europe. Because of the small size of the nymph tick, most patients do not remember the preceding tick bite. After an incubation period of 3 to 32 days, erythema migrans (EM), which may occur at the site of the tick bite or distant, usually begins as a red macule or papule that expands slowly to form a large annular lesion. As the lesion increases in size, it often develops a bright red outer border and partial central clearing. Although EM can be located anywhere, the thigh, groin, and axilla are particularly common sites. Up to 25% of those infected either do not exhibit or miss the rash.

  B. The erythematous, maculopapular rash associated with the measles virus begins at the hairline and behind the ears, spreads down the trunk and limbs to include the palms and soles, and often becomes confluent.

  C. Also caused by a vector-borne spirochete, RMSF presents with macules on the wrist and ankles and spreads to the extremities and the trunk.

  D. Dermatophytosis causes burning, itching and stinging. The rash is characterized by rings composed of advancing scaly borders with central clearing. Systemic symptoms do not occur.

199. The answer is **C** [Obstetrics/Gynecology, Infectious Disease].

  A. Adnexal torsion characteristically presents as acute severe unilateral lower abdominal pain. It may be precipitated by a dull soreness, which represents intermittent twisting and untwisting of the fallopian tube. Patients may also have fever, nausea, and vomiting. Ultrasonography can help to confirm the diagnosis. Surgical intervention is required.

  B. The classic triad of ectopic pregnancy includes amenorrhea, vaginal bleeding, and lower abdominal pain. The diagnosis is facilitated by a positive pregnancy test and confirmed by the absence of intrauterine pregnancy on ultrasonography.

  C. Pelvic inflammatory disease is a sexually transmitted infection of the upper reproductive tract caused most commonly by *Chlamydia trachomatis* or *Neisseria gonorrhoeae*. Symptomatic PID commonly presents as lower abdominal pain and tenderness, abnormal vaginal discharge, and fever. Clinical signs include lower abdominal tenderness, uterine and adnexal tenderness, cervical motion tenderness, and a mucopurulent cervicitis.

  D. Functional cysts may cause pelvic pain, a dull sensation or heaviness in the pelvis. They are usually asymptomatic and can reach sizes of 15 cm in diameter. Typically, functional cysts regress during the next menstrual cycle. They may undergo torsion or rupture causing lower abdominal pain and tenderness and hemoperitoneum. Depending on their size, functional cysts may be palpable on bimanual examination. Pelvic ultrasonography will confirm a cystic lesion.

200. The answer is **A** [Cardiology].

  A. Acute coronary syndrome includes unstable angina and acute myocardial infarction. ECG findings, particularly ST-segment changes, are utilized to classify and determine initial treatment. Cardiac biomarkers allow for a chemical determination of the occurrence of myocardial infarction.

  B. Coronary angiography may be indicated after the MI is confirmed to plan and perform stenting procedures.

  C. See A.

  D. Stress testing is not indicated if acute myocardial infarction is suspected. It is highly valuable in determining the severity of angina but not in the acute setting.

201. The answer is **C** [Pulmonology, Infectious Disease].

  A. Distortions in color perception have been reported in some cases but not glaucoma.

  B. Headache is not a reported side effect of isoniazid.

  C. Patients on isoniazid therapy should have both their hepatic and their renal function monitored. Older patients are particularly at risk for developing drug-induced hepatitis from isoniazid use.

  D. Isoniazid users may experience hyperglycemia while on treatment, especially if they have diabetes.

202. The answer is **C** [Dermatology].

  A. Acne vulgaris is an inflammation of the pilosebaceous glands, mainly affecting the face and upper trunk. It most commonly presents during adolescence and manifests as comedones, papulopustules, nodules, and cysts.

  B. Folliculitis occurs in the upper portion of the hair follicle and is characterized by a follicular papule or pustule surrounded by superficial erythema. Shaving may facilitate the infection. Lesions may occur on the face in the beard areas, scalp, neck, legs, trunk, and buttocks.

  C. Rosacea is a chronic inflammatory disorder of the pilosebaceous glands associated with a vascular component that results in flushing and telangiectasias. It has a peak incidence between 40 and 50 years of age. It is associated with a history of facial flushing in response to heat stimuli and sun exposure.

  D. Seborrheic dermatitis is a maculopapular rash characterized by redness and dry scales or oily, yellowish crusting. Facial lesions occur on the cheeks, nasolabial folds, and eyebrows.

203. The answer is **B** [Obstetrics/Gynecology, Pediatrics, Infectious Disease].

  A. Hepatitis A vaccine is recommended for high-risk groups including people who live or plan to travel to endemic areas, men who have sex with men, those who use street drugs, patients with chronic liver disease, or people who work with primates. This patient does not fall into a high-risk group.

  B. Human papillomavirus vaccine is recommended for all females between 11 and 26 years of age regardless of their current sexual activity. It is a series of three doses; administer the second dose 2 months after the first dose and the third dose 6 months after the first dose.

  C. Influenza vaccine is recommended annually for children aged 6 to 59 months and for children 5 years and older with risk factors such as close contact with the immunocompromised and history of asthma or chronic illness.

  D. Pneumococcal vaccine is recommended to high-risk patients such as those who have chronic illness, are asplenic, or are immunocompromised.

204. The answer is **B** [Neurology].
  A. Anticholinergic medications are helpful in parkinsonism but not in restless leg syndrome. Side effects may include increased restlessness and agitation.
  B. Nonergotamine dopamine agonists, such as pramipexole (Mirapex) or ropinirole (Requip), are recommended in the treatment of restless leg syndrome. They are also helpful in parkinsonism.
  C. Phenytoin is an antiseizure medication.
  D. Sleep agents may overcome the insomnia, but do not treat the underlying disorder.

205. The answer is **D** [Rheumatology and Orthopaedics, Surgery].
  A. Antibiotics are not indicated, as there are no signs of infection.
  B. Aspiration and steroid injection may help but recurrence is common.
  C. Physical therapy is not indicated in the treatment of a ganglion cyst.
  D. Surgical excision is the most definitive treatment for a ganglion cyst. Surgery is recommended if the cyst causes pain, disruption of function, or cosmetic distress.

206. The answer is **B** [Psychiatry].
  A. Aversion therapy is used for alcohol abuse and other disorders where impulsive behavior is involved. It is the application of a noxious stimulus after a behavioral response. It is a very controversial therapy.
  B. Behavior therapy is a broad term used to treat a number of psychiatric illnesses, but it is particularly effective with phobias such as the social phobia demonstrated by the patient in this case.
  C. Insight-oriented therapy may be helpful in many psychiatric illnesses including phobias but is not effective unless combined with behavioral therapy for patients with phobias.
  D. Self-help group therapy, such as Alcoholics Anonymous or Overeaters Anonymous, is helpful to provide support for people coping with the same problem. It is not generally recommended for patients with phobias.

207. The answer is **B** [Hematology, Pediatrics].
  A. Blood transfusions are necessary when the hemoglobin or hematocrit has dropped significantly or the patient is short of breath. It is not necessary in all cases of acute pain in patients with sickle cell disease.
  B. The patient is mildly dehydrated, which can occur during a period of acute sickling or during other complications associated with sickle cell disease. Many times, intravenous or oral fluids along with appropriate pain control are sufficient to correct the problem and bring relief.
  C. Hydroxyurea is used to prevent or reduce the number of episodes of sickling that can lead to more serious complications of sickle cell disease.
  D. In this case, CBC, CXR, and urinalysis may be required to look for an underlying infectious cause but, until additional tests are run, broad-spectrum antibiotics would be out of place.

208. The answer is **C** [Obstetrics/Gynecology, Surgery].
  A. This patient has an ectopic pregnancy. The essentials of diagnosis include positive pregnancy test with unilateral pelvic pain, amenorrhea, and spotting. Nothing will be detected in the uterus via transvaginal ultrasound and the serum β-HCG will be greater than 2,000 mU/mL. While laparoscopy is an option, because the patient is stable, she can be treated medically with methotrexate.
  B. Laparotomy is rarely performed for ectopic pregnancy and reserved for patients who cannot be treated medically and for whom laparoscopy is contraindicated (obese, known severe abdominal adhesions from prior surgeries).
  C. Methotrexate can treat up to 80% of ectopic pregnancies. It is given intramuscularly and the patient must be deemed reliable to return for follow-up and subsequent monitoring.
  D. Watchful waiting without intervention is never the standard of care for an ectopic pregnancy. There is a risk of rupture, hemorrhage, and death.

209. The answer is **D** [Rheumatology and Orthopaedics, Pediatrics].
  A. Knee immobility may be considered in severe cases where symptomatic care and rest do not control the symptoms.
  B. Physical therapy can be considered for assistance with isometric and flexibility exercises in moderate to severe cases that are slow to resolve.
  C. Removal of ossicles from the tibial tuberosity is rarely necessary.
  D. Osgood–Schlatter disease is characterized by pain over the tibial tubercle in a growing child. It occurs during late childhood or adolescence, especially in athletes, and is likely due to repetitive tensile microtrauma. It is more common in males. Rest, restriction of activities, and, occasionally, a knee immobilizer may be necessary, combined with an isometric and flexibility exercise program.

210. The answer is **D** [Gastroenterology, Nephrology and Urology].
  A. Atenolol most commonly interacts with catecholamine-depleting drugs.
  B. Hydrochlorothiazide most commonly interacts with digitalis.
  C. Lorazepam most commonly interacts with other CNS depressants.
  D. Proton pump inhibitors may decrease the excretion of methotrexate.

211. The answer is **A** [Endocrinology].
  A. Common manifestations of Addison's disease reflect decreased glucocorticoids. Symptoms may include weight loss, fatigue, postural dizziness, muscle and joint pain, and gastrointestinal symptoms. Often signs of increased pigmentation are present due to increased production of ACTH. Laboratory abnormalities may include hyponatremia, hyperkalemia, mild metabolic acidosis, azotemia, and hypercalcemia.
  B. Cushing's syndrome is due to increased production of cortisol. Clinical symptoms are typically central obesity, generalized weight gain, rounding of the face, and a dorsocervical fat pad along with other symptoms of glucocorticoid excess.
  C. Pheochromocytoma usually presents with hypertension as well as a triad of headache, palpitations, and sweating.
  D. Hypertension, hypokalemia, and metabolic alkalosis are the main clinical manifestations of hyperaldosteronism.

212. The answer is **B** [Cardiology, Nephrology and Urology].
- **A.** Elevated ST segments in all leads are seen in pericarditis.
- **B.** Peaked T waves are the earliest ECG manifestation in hyperkalemia. As the potassium continues to rise, ECG may show shortened QT intervals, widened QRS, increased PR intervals (AV conduction delay), absent P waves, ventricular fibrillation, to asystole.
- **C.** Prolonged ST segments with flattened T waves are seen in hypokalemia.
- **D.** Sinus tachycardia may also show prolonged QT segments; it is not related to potassium level.

213. The answer is **C** [Endocrinology].
- **A.** Bromocriptine is utilized for treatment of prolactinoma.
- **B.** Growth hormone deficiency causes central obesity but is not associated with thyroid deficiencies.
- **C.** The patient is exhibiting hypothyroidism as indicated by the low free T_4 and elevated TSH; thyroid replacement is indicated.
- **D.** Propylthiouracil is utilized in hyperthyroidism.

214. The answer is **A** [Endocrinology].
- **A.** Primary hyperparathyroidism matches this patient's history, and elevated serum calcium would be expected. Untreated primary hyperparathyroidism results in persistently elevated serum calcium levels as well as an elevated serum parathyroid hormone (PTH). Serum calcium level may need "correcting" in the presence of a low albumin level.
- **B.** Elevated serum ionized calcium level, low serum phosphorus, and normal or elevated alkaline phosphatase characterize hyperparathyroidism.
- **C.** See B.
- **D.** The serum PTH level is elevated in hyperparathyroidism.

215. The answer is **D** [Cardiology, Geriatrics].
- **A.** Cardiac catheterization is invasive and would not be diagnostic or therapeutic.
- **B.** Chest radiography is nondiagnostic.
- **C.** The tilt test is helpful in distinguishing dysautonomy as a cause of syncope.
- **D.** A serious complication of atrial fibrillation is the development of thrombi within the atria secondary to stasis. Evaluation of patients with atrial fibrillation in whom atrial thrombi are suspected requires echocardiography prior to cardioversion. Transesophageal echocardiography is more sensitive than traditional echocardiography.

216. The answer is **D** [Gastroenterology, Infectious Disease].
- **A.** Most cases of mild diarrhea will not lead to dehydration if the patient takes in oral fluids with electrolytes and carbohydrates. More severe cases may benefit from aggressive oral rehydration with special solutions. Intravenous hydration is not commonly needed.
- **B.** Bowel rest is an appropriate measure for diarrhea but is not enough when *C. difficile* is in the differential diagnosis.
- **C.** Empiric use of antidiarrheal agents may be proper in mild diarrhea but not if *C. difficile* is suspected.
- **D.** The most important cause to rule out in this patient is *C. difficile* because of her recent antibiotic use. Antibiotic-associated colitis often requires specific antibiotic treatment (metronidazole, vancomycin).

217. The answer is **B** [Cardiology, Surgery].
- **A.** Aspirin is a first-line medication for myocardial infarction but not dissecting aneurysms.
- **B.** Labetalol is an excellent drug to lower blood pressure quickly and safely in the setting of aortic dissection. Emergent surgical correction is needed.
- **C.** Nitroglycerin is useful in myocardial infarction, as it enhances vasodilation; this may be harmful in patients with dissection.
- **D.** Verapamil is used in patients with contraindications for beta-blocker (such as severe asthma) as a second-line drug choice in dissecting aneurysm.

218. The answer is **B** [Psychiatry].
- **A.** Carbamazepine (Tegretol) is an antiepileptic medication that may be useful in treating bipolar disorder.
- **B.** Fluoxetine (Prozac) is one of many 5-HT reuptake inhibitors (SSRIs) commonly used in the treatment of major depression.
- **C.** Lithium carbonate is a mood stabilizer used to treat bipolar disorder.
- **D.** Lorazepam (Ativan) is a benzodiazepine and may be used to treat anxiety disorders and/or alcohol withdrawal.

219. The answer is **D** [Endocrinology, Surgery].
- **A.** See D.
- **B.** See D.
- **C.** This patient has hypoglycemia most likely secondary to an insulinoma, which will respond to the glucagon immediately; however, this is not a long-term therapy.
- **D.** Referral to an endocrinologist and surgeon for removal of the insulinoma is needed for long-term care or cure.

220. The answer is **A** [Nephrology and Urology, Infectious Disease].
- **A.** Pyelonephritis involves the renal parenchyma and pelvis. Pain of renal origin is usually located in the ipsilateral costovertebral angle. Irritative symptoms in the presence of fever or flank pain indicate inflammation outside the bladder.
- **B.** Dysuria is associated with inflammation along the lower urinary tract and is typically referred to the tip of the penis in men or the urethra in women.
- **C.** Urgency is associated with inflammatory conditions such as cystitis or neurogenic bladder.
- **D.** Nocturia has multiple causes, one of which is irritative pathology of the urinary tract as in cystitis/UTI.

221. The answer is **B** [Dermatology, Infectious Disease].
- **A.** Tinea versicolor is not caused by *Candida*.
- **B.** The patient has tinea versicolor, which is caused by an overgrowth of the yeast organism *Malassezia*, a common skin colonizer of all humans.
- **C.** Tinea versicolor is not caused by bacteria.
- **D.** *Trichophyton rubrum* is the most common cause of tinea corporis.

222. The answer is **B** [Pulmonology, Infectious Disease].
    A. Lung abscess typically presents with severe systemic symptoms and foul-smelling sputum.
    B. Mycoplasma pneumonia is more common in younger people and in crowded conditions. It presents with an insidious cough, typically nonproductive. Bullous myringitis is an uncommon but unique finding.
    C. Pneumococcal pneumonia usually includes a productive cough and dullness to percussion with bronchophony or egophony in a single lobe.
    D. Sarcoidosis affects multiple organs. Hilar adenopathy is common on chest x-ray.

223. The answer is **B** [Cardiology].
    A. See B.
    B. A mid-systolic click is the hallmark of prolapse of the mitral valve. The click may be followed by a mid- to late systolic murmur, indicating mitral valve regurgitation.
    C. See B.
    D. See B.

224. The answer is **B** [Hematology, Rheumatology and Orthopaedics].
    A. Early acute lymphocytic leukemia may present with pancytopenia, but patients will usually have bone pain, lymphadenopathy, and hepatosplenomegaly.
    B. The clinical presentation is most consistent with aplastic anemia.
    C. Patients with hairy cell leukemia will have splenomegaly.
    D. The failure of all cell lines suggests aplastic anemia rather than immune thrombocytopenia.

225. The answer is **D** [Cardiology].
    A. Low-carbohydrate diets have not been recommended by the American Heart Association for cardiovascular disease.
    B. While low-fat diets have been recommended for cardiovascular disease patients, swimming is not the best exercise for weight loss and fitness.
    C. Weight lifting exercises must be undertaken cautiously in patients with cardiovascular disease.
    D. Walking and weight loss have been shown to improve symptoms of peripheral vascular disease.

226. The answer is **D** [Cardiology, Pediatrics].
    A. Innocent murmurs are usually soft (grade I or II), short in duration, and systolic. If a ventricular septal defect is misdiagnosed as an innocent murmur and not corrected, the sequelae of the increased pulmonary artery pressure from the ventricular septal defect can lead to irreversible pulmonary artery hypertension (Eisenmenger's syndrome), resulting in premature death.
    B. The murmur of aortic regurgitation is a diastolic murmur, not a holosystolic murmur.
    C. The murmur of a patent ductus arteriosus is continuous, not holosystolic. The murmur accentuates in late systole.
    D. Ventricular septal defects are typically harsh holosystolic murmurs heard best at the left sternal border. The fixed split S_2 has a louder pulmonary component.

227. The answer is **B** [Neurology].
    A. Arnold–Chiari malformations of the brain most often cause severe headaches that are centered at the back of the head and aggravated by coughing, laughing, or sneezing. Serious complications such as hydrocephalus can develop.
    B. This patient is exhibiting signs and symptoms of Huntington's disease, which is associated with cerebral atrophy on MRI.
    C. Huntington's disease patients do not have focal brain lesions on MRI.
    D. Ring-enhancing cerebral lesions are characteristic of acute toxoplasmosis, which is most common in patients with AIDS.

228. The answer is **B** [Pulmonology, Infectious Disease].
    A. It is possible that the patient has viral pneumonia; however, persistent fever and rales indicates a bacterial etiology.
    B. Best practice for community-acquired pneumonia is to start either a macrolide or doxycycline, as it is most likely streptococcus or mycoplasma.
    C. If the patient was at extremes of age, had comorbidities, or other risk factors, then it might be prudent to obtain a CBC. A sputum culture might be necessary for those at high risk (alcoholics, immunocompromised, recently hospitalized patients), as it may be caused by uncommon respiratory pathogens. Sputum cultures are difficult to obtain and often fail to reveal the microbe responsible; therefore, they are not obtained in uncomplicated cases.
    D. The patient is not in respiratory distress. Neither oxygen nor hospitalization is required for a healthy, immunocompetent patient with community-acquired pneumonia. Outpatient antibiotics with follow-up in 24 to 48 hours is the recommended management in this case.

229. The answer is **B** [Endocrinology, Cardiology].
    A. See B.
    B. A patient with multiple risk factors for coronary artery disease needs a complete lipid profile with an overnight fast.
    C. Nonfasting lipids are unreliable.
    D. See B.

230. The answer is **D** [Cardiology, Geriatrics].
    A. Imaging would show widening of the aorta in aortic aneurysm.
    B. In tamponade, the echocardiography would demonstrate pericardial fluid and additional cardiac pressure changes.
    C. Although coronary arteries are usually clear in Prinzmetal's angina, the ventricular enlargement, if present, would be more uniform.
    D. This is the classic description of Takotsubo cardiomyopathy (literally "octopus bottle") found in postmenopausal women (90% of cases), often occurring after a major discharge of catecholamines.

231. The answer is **C** [Gastroenterology].
- **A.** For severe pancreatitis, such as necrotizing pancreatitis, admission to an intensive care unit for monitoring and aggressive IV rehydration is needed. Calcium gluconate is given if hypocalcemia with tetany is present. Serum albumin or fresh frozen plasma is given for those with hypoalbuminemia or coagulopathy.
- **B.** Enteral nutrition is appropriate for patients with mild acute pancreatitis, although some cannot tolerate it if accompanied by ileus. IV somatostatin is sometimes given in severe acute pancreatitis, but the evidence is not clear. Stent placement across the pancreatic duct is more common, as it seems to decrease the risk of post-ERCP pancreatitis.
- **C.** For mild to moderate acute pancreatitis, the pancreas is rested (NPO and bed rest). When ileus is present (distention, vomiting), nasogastric suction should be employed. Analgesics are an important component of patient care; narcotics are often required.
- **D.** Parenteral nutrition is given to patients with acute severe pancreatitis who have ileus and who will be NPO for 7 or more days. Antibiotics are appropriate if there is an infected necrosis but is controversial in sterile necrosis. Serum albumin or fresh frozen plasma is given for those with hypoalbuminemia or coagulopathy.

232. The answer is **C** [Rheumatology and Orthopaedics].
- **A.** Loss of skin folds is typically seen in systemic sclerosis (scleroderma).
- **B.** Malar rash is most often seen in systemic lupus erythematosus.
- **C.** Parotid enlargement is seen in about 30% of patients with Sjögren's syndrome.
- **D.** Progressive proximal muscle weakness is seen in polymyositis.

233. The answer is **A** [Ophthalmology and Otolaryngology, Infectious Disease].
- **A.** Common presenting symptoms of sinusitis include nasal drainage and congestion, facial pain or pressure, and headache. Most patients are diagnosed on clinical grounds and improve without antibiotic therapy. In the evaluation of persistent, recurrent, or chronic sinusitis, computed tomography is the radiographic study of choice. It provides a rapid and effective assessment of the paranasal sinuses and can be used to monitor therapy.
- **B.** If malignancy, opportunistic infection, or intracranial extension of malignancy or infection is suspected, magnetic resonance with gandolinium is indicated. It is more effective at distinguishing tumor from inflammation and inspissated mucus.
- **C.** It is usually possible to make the diagnosis of acute bacterial rhinosinusitis on clinical grounds alone. Although more sensitive than clinical examination, routine plain radiography is not cost-effective and is not recommended.
- **D.** Endoscopic culture of the affected sinus cavity may provide additional information regarding etiology. Culture and sensitivity of nasal discharge is unlikely to be of any use.

234. The answer is **C** [Cardiology, Infectious Disease].
- **A.** Aminoglycosides, β-lactams, and sulfonamides do not prolong the QT interval.
- **B.** See A.
- **C.** Macrolides and some fluoroquinolones may prolong the QT interval and should be avoided in patients with long QT syndrome.
- **D.** See A.

235. The answer is **B** [Rheumatology and Orthopaedics].
- **A.** See B.
- **B.** The rotator cuff is composed of the supraspinatus, infraspinatus, subscapularis, and teres minor.
- **C.** See B.
- **D.** See B.

236. The answer is **B** [Pulmonology].
- **A.** See C.
- **B.** Most pneumothoraces are identified on chest x-ray. An expiratory film provides the best visualization.
- **C.** An MRI or CT scan is not warranted in a simple pneumothorax.
- **D.** QRS axis and precordial T wave changes may occur with left-sided pneumothoraces, but are nonspecific.

237. The answer is **A** [Ophthalmology and Otolaryngology].
- **A.** Blepharitis is a common chronic bilateral inflammatory condition of the lid margins. Anterior blepharitis involves the eyelid skin, eyelashes, and associated glands. Patients will present with irritation, burning, and itching.
- **B.** Chalazion is a common granulomatous inflammation of a Meibomian gland. It appears as a firm, nontender swelling on the eyelid with redness and swelling of the nearby conjunctiva. It often develops following a partially resolved hordeolum. Treatment is incision.
- **C.** Ectropion is outward turning of the lower eyelid; it is common in the elderly.
- **D.** Hordeolum (stye) is an abscess that presents as a tender, localized, erythematous swelling on the eyelid.

238. The answer is **B** [Pulmonology].
- **A.** Although exposure to high levels of ambient particulate matter and specific occupational dusts and fumes are risk factors for COPD, the magnitude of these effects appears to be substantially less than that of the effect of cigarette smoking.
- **B.** Cigarette smoking is considered a major risk factor for mortality from chronic bronchitis and emphysema. The causal relationship between cigarette smoking and the development of COPD has been proven; although other factors are predictors of development and decline of lung function, smoking is the biggest independent variable.
- **C.** See A.
- **D.** Respiratory infections have been studied as potential risk factors for the development and progression of COPD in adults, the impact of which is controversial. Although respiratory infections are important causes of exacerbations of COPD, the association of adult respiratory infections in the development and progression of COPD remains unproven.

239. The answer is **D** [Gastroenterology].
     A. An H_2 receptor antagonist, such as famotidine, can be useful for mild GERD, PUD, and stress gastritis. Proton pump inhibitors (PPIs) are the preferred agent for moderate to severe GERD, PUD, and functional dyspepsia.
     B. While a prokinetic agent may improve symptoms, the improvement does not relate to gastric emptying. Metoclopramide has a high incidence of neuropsychiatric side effects and, therefore, it is not a recommended therapy in uncomplicated dyspepsia.
     C. A prostaglandin analog, such as misoprostol, is used to mitigate NSAID-associated gastroduodenal ulcers.
     D. This presentation is common in chronic dyspepsia or functional dyspepsia. In patients less than 50 years of age who do not have weight loss, hematemesis, melena, persistent vomiting, or severe or constant pain, empiric treatment with a 4-week trial with a PPI may be initiated. Noninvasive *H. pylori* testing can be conducted. Any of the warning signs should prompt a further investigation with a CBC, electrolytes, thyroid function tests, calcium, and liver enzymes as well as imaging.

240. The answer is **D** [Obstetrics/Gynecology].
     A. Chadwick's sign is congestion of the pelvic vasculature causing bluish or purplish discoloration of the vagina and cervix.
     B. Goodell's sign is softening of the cervix; it develops by the beginning of the second month.
     C. Hegar's sign is widening of the softened area of the isthmus, resulting in bluish cervix and compressibility of the isthmus on bimanual examination; it occurs by 6 to 8 weeks.
     D. McDonald's sign is when the uterine body and cervix can easily be flexed against one another.

241. The answer is **A** [Nephrology and Urology].
     A. Anorexia, fatigue, and weakness are early symptoms of renal failure.
     B. Late symptoms of renal failure include oliguria, dyspnea, chest pain, nausea, vomiting, and abdominal pain.
     C. Polyuria and polydipsia are common manifestations of diabetes; back pain is reported in pyelonephritis.
     D. Nausea, anorexia, pruritus, and abdominal pain suggest hepatobiliary tract obstruction.

242. The answer is **A** [Neurology].
     A. This patient is exhibiting both upper and lower motor neuron disease, which is typical of amyotrophic lateral sclerosis (Lou Gehrig's disease).
     B. Huntington's patients display the fluid involuntary movements of chorea and dementia.
     C. Multiple sclerosis manifests predominantly as weakness and spastic changes. Cognitive deficits are rare.
     D. Syringomyelia involves cavitary destruction within the spinal cord, resulting in both motor and sensory deficits.

243. The answer is **B** [Ophthalmology and Otolaryngology].
     A. Newer-generation antihistamines have lower rates of drowsiness; desloratine is minimally sedating. However, there is still a risk, especially considering his occupation.
     B. Evidence-based reviews show that intranasal corticosteroid sprays are more effective and less expensive than nonsedating antihistamines. They are also nonsedating. However, there may be a delay in relief of symptoms.
     C. Antileukotriene agents alone or with antihistamines can help with rhinorrhea, sneezing, and congestion but may cause drowsiness.
     D. First-generation antihistamines have lower cost, but the highest risk of drowsiness.

244. The answer is **A** [Infectious Disease, Pediatrics, Dermatology].
     A. Erythema infectiosum (fifth disease) is characterized by a "slapped cheeks" appearance followed by a lacy rash on the trunk, neck, and extremities 1 to 4 days later. Mild symptoms of fever, headache, coryza, and malaise often accompany the facial rash.
     B. Vesicles are very rare and atypical in erythema infectiosum.
     C. Mucosal lesions are uncommon in erythema infectiosum.
     D. Arthralgias are uncommon in children with erythema infectiosum; however, they are quite common in adults (especially women) who contract this viral infection caused by parvovirus B19.

245. The answer is **A** [Pulmonology].
     A. Combined long-acting β-agonist with inhaled corticosteroid is the treatment recommended for severe COPD. A short-acting β-agonist and inhaled ipratropium may also be included in the management at this stage of the disease.
     B. Tapered doses of oral steroids may be necessary for acute exacerbations but are not recommended for long-term use.
     C. Long-acting β-agonist is recommended in mild COPD along with as-needed short-acting β-agonist combined with ipratropium.
     D. See C.

246. The answer is **C** [Pulmonology, Cardiology].
     A. Arterial blood gas may show hypoxia and hypocapnia, but is not specific to pulmonary embolus.
     B. A negative D-dimer makes pulmonary embolus less likely, but a positive test cannot confirm a pulmonary embolus.
     C. Pulmonary angiography is the gold standard for diagnosis of pulmonary embolus. It is an invasive procedure and should not be the initial diagnostic study in a patient suspected to have a pulmonary embolus.
     D. Ventilation perfusion scan or a helical CT scan is more commonly used to diagnose pulmonary embolus. If these tests are negative and suspicion of pulmonary embolus remains, an angiography is indicated.

247. The answer is **D** [Cardiology].
     A. Prior myocardial infarction is not a contraindication for stress testing once the patient is stable.
     B. Once a contraindication, exercise stress testing is now considered appropriate for patients with congestive heart failure.
     C. As long as she is ambulatory, hip arthroplasty is not a contraindication to stress testing.
     D. Aortic stenosis remains a significant contraindication to exercise stress testing due to the chance of precipitating a syncopal episode during exercise.

248. The answer is **B** [Nephrology and Urology].
  A. Arteriography is an invasive procedure which should only be performed after other studies suggest a vascular system abnormality.
  B. Papaverine is a vasoactive substance that, when injected into the penis, should cause a rigid erection in those with intact vascular systems. Failure to achieve an erection after injection of a vasoactive substance would then lead to assessment of the vascular system with arteriography in those patients desiring a complete workup.
  C. This patient is currently on nitrates for angina. Addition of sildenafil, even for diagnostic purposes, could lead to hypotension. Therefore, this and similar drugs are contraindicated.
  D. There is no indication for tumescent testing, as they both deny nocturnal erections. Presence of nocturnal erections with the inability to achieve an erection before intercourse would suggest a psychological etiology.

249. The answer is **C** [Pulmonology, Pediatrics, Infectious Disease].
  A. Antitussives, decongestants, and antibiotics are not recommended for treatment of viral croup. Most croup is viral in origin.
  B. See A.
  C. Nebulized budesonide or oral dexamethasone is the recommended treatment for mild to moderate viral croup.
  D. Nebulized epinephrine is reserved for severe symptoms of croup such as audible stridor, cyanosis, or oxygen saturation below 92%.

250. The answer is **D** [Obstetrics/Gynecology].
  A. A cervical exam should never be done on a pregnant patient with bleeding of unknown cause until placental location is determined.
  B. Ferning test is used to diagnose rupture of membranes. If the woman presented after a "gush of fluid" from the vagina, it would be a better choice.
  C. Kleihauer–Betke test is a maternal blood test to check for fetal blood cells in the maternal blood. It is most often used after the mother has sustained a trauma.
  D. This woman has placenta previa until proven otherwise. The hallmark of placenta previa is painless vaginal bleeding during the third trimester. Ultrasonography is the test of choice to determine placental location. It is quick, noninvasive, and inexpensive.

251. The answer is **C** [Rheumatology and Orthopaedics].
  A. Polymyositis presents with progressive weakness of the proximal muscle groups of the upper and lower extremities.
  B. Rheumatoid arthritis may present with joint pains and fatigue but is not usually associated with malar rash and oral ulcers.
  C. Systemic lupus erythematosus (SLE) presents with joint pains in 90% of cases. Fatigue, malar rash, and oral ulcers are also associated with SLE.
  D. Systemic sclerosis (scleroderma) usually presents with thickened skin, fever, malaise, and edema. Over 90% of patients with scleroderma also have Raynaud's phenomenon.

252. The answer is **B** [Endocrinology].
  A. In acromegaly, there is thickening of the soft tissue of the hands and feet.
  B. Hypertrophy of pharyngeal and laryngeal tissue causes voice deepening in acromegaly.
  C. Skin changes in acromegaly include hyperhidrosis and oiliness.
  D. Males with acromegaly may develop atrophy of the testicles.

253. The answer is **C** [Cardiology].
  A. Cardiac catheterization is an invasive procedure. It is not indicated in suspected pericarditis.
  B. Cardiac enzymes would be indicated to rule out a suspected myocardial infarction.
  C. Electrocardiography frequently reveals diffuse ST and T wave changes in pericarditis. This along with the presentation can make the diagnosis.
  D. Pericardial window may be necessary as a therapy for refractory cases.

254. The answer is **B** [Cardiology].
  A. Gestational hypertension is an indication of preeclampsia.
  B. Secondary causes of hypertension are likely in those presenting at an early age, those first exhibiting elevated pressure after the age of 50 years, or those previously well controlled who become refractory to treatment despite multiple medications.
  C. See B.
  D. See B.

255. The answer is **C** [Psychiatry].
  A. Family therapy is effective in treating the problem, usually in conjunction with other social and legal services.
  B. When women leave a home where domestic violence is taking place, the risk of being killed initially increases.
  C. Pregnancy is considered a high-risk period for abuse; 15% to 25% of pregnant women report being abused.
  D. About half of all women who are abused come from a violent home.

256. The answer is **B** [Cardiology, Infectious Disease].
  A. Erythema marginatum is associated with rheumatic fever.
  B. Clinical manifestations of infective endocarditis may include peripheral lesions such as subungual "splinter" hemorrhages, Roth's spots (retinal lesions), Osler's nodes (painful violaceous lesions of the fingers, toes, or feet), or Janeway lesions (painless erythematous lesions of the palms and soles).
  C. See B.
  D. See B.

257. The answer is **B** [Psychiatry].
  A. Sertraline (Zoloft) is an antidepressant and would not cause depression. It is more likely to cause anxiety or nervousness.
  B. Use of sertraline (Zoloft) is often associated with sexual dysfunction.
  C. Sertraline (Zoloft) is not likely to cause a photosensitivity reaction or xerostomia. It is more likely to cause diarrhea or nausea.
  D. See C.

258. The answer is **D** [Infectious Disease].
- **A.** See D. Penicillin is used to treat active disease.
- **B.** See D.
- **C.** See D.
- **D.** *Clostridium tetani* spores are ubiquitous in soil and may germinate when introduced into a wound. Patients presenting with a "dirty wound" require tetanus toxoid if they do not know their most recent immunization status, if they have had less than the three recommended doses of toxoid, or if it has been more than 5 years since the last dose. Immune globulin is recommended if entire immunization status is unknown or if the individual received less than the full initial series in childhood.

259. The answer is **C** [Ophthalmology and Otolaryngology, Infectious Disease].
- **A.** *Mycoplasma pneumoniae*, *Haemophilus influenzae*, and *Streptococcus pneumoniae* are more commonly associated with acute otitis media.
- **B.** See A.
- **C.** *Pseudomonas aeruginosa* is associated with chronic otitis media. Other organisms that are associated with chronic otitis media are *Proteus* and *Staphylococcus aureus*.
- **D.** See A.

260. The answer is **C** [Gastroenterology].
- **A.** Avoiding simple sugars is not known to affect the risk of colorectal cancer but may reduce the risk for obesity and type 2 diabetes.
- **B.** Research evaluating the role of supplements for the prevention of colorectal cancer is ongoing including fiber supplementation, folic acid, vitamin D, calcium carbonate, and antioxidant vitamins, but the results have ranged from no benefit to a possible modest reduction in relative risk. At this time, no definitive recommendations can be made.
- **C.** A generally lifelong diet rich in fiber with vegetables and fruits has been associated with decreased risk of colorectal cancer.
- **D.** A diet rich in fat and red meat is associated with increased risk of colorectal cancer.

261. The answer is **C** [Pulmonology].
- **A.** Reversible bronchoconstriction is characteristic of asthma.
- **B.** An increased FEV_1 and FVC with normal ratio is characteristic of athletes.
- **C.** A reduced FEV_1 and low FEV_1/FVC ratio combined with increased TLC is characteristic of chronic bronchitis.
- **D.** Restrictive lung disease, such as pulmonary fibrosis, will display reduced FEV_1, FVC, and TLC but a normal to increased ratio.

262. The answer is **A** [Rheumatology and Orthopaedics, Pediatrics].
- **A.** Nursemaid's elbow (subluxation of the radial head) is treated with immediate reduction by supinating the elbow and moving it from full flexion to full extension.
- **B.** A long-arm cast is appropriate treatment for forearm fracture or fracture around the elbow.
- **C.** Nursemaid's elbow is best taken care of immediately; it should not be left dislocated or subluxed for a long period of time.
- **D.** A sling can be used for a brief time after the reduction for comfort.

263. The answer is **C** [Cardiology].
- **A.** Atrial fibrillation is more common in older individuals and is associated with an irregular rhythm.
- **B.** Atrial flutter is most often seen in persons with COPD or heart disease.
- **C.** Paroxysmal supraventricular tachycardia (PSVT) is common and occurs in patients without structural heart disease. Paroxysms may be interrupted by maneuvers that increase vagal tone.
- **D.** Ventricular premature beats are usually experienced as a sensation of the heart skipping beats.

264. The answer is **A** [Dermatology].
- **A.** Atopic dermatitis (eczema) is a relapsing disorder characterized by underlying dry skin and pruritus. It is often associated with a personal or family history of atopy. Acutely lesions include erythematous patches and plaques with or without a scale. Lesions can erode and appear moist and crusted. Common sites of atopic dermatitis include the neck, eyelids, forehead, face, wrists, antecubital and popliteal fossae, hands, and dorsa of the feet.
- **B.** Impetigo is a superficial skin infection of the epidermis commonly caused by *Staphylococcus* or *Streptococcus*. The lesions are vesicles, bullae, or pustules that rupture and result in erosions with golden-yellow crusts. Impetigo may arise from minor breaks in the skin.
- **C.** Psoriasis is characterized by well-demarcated red plaques with thick whitish-silver scales. The scales are loosely adherent and easily removed. The classic sites of psoriasis include the extensor surfaces of the knees and elbows, scalp, and sacral–gluteal region. Psoriasis is associated with HLA inheritance.
- **D.** Seborrheic dermatitis is a maculopapular rash characterized by redness and dry scales or oily, yellowish crusting. It occurs in the regions where the sebaceous glands are most predominant: face, scalp, and body folds.

265. The answer is **A** [Obstetrics/Gynecology, Surgery].
- **A.** Cystocele is an anterior vaginal wall defect.
- **B.** Rectocele is a posterior vaginal wall defect.
- **C.** Uterine prolapse presents as a firm, muscular mass in the vagina or protruding from the vagina.
- **D.** Urethrocele is when the urethral mucosa protrudes through the meatus and forms a hemorrhagic, sensitive vulvar mass.

266. The answer is **D** [Cardiology, Pediatrics].
- **A.** Catheterization may be indicated after MRI or CT to definitively measure the gradients in planning for percutaneous stenting.
- **B.** MRI or CT will illustrate the anatomy of the coarctation prior to surgical repair.
- **C.** ECG will reveal left ventricular hypertrophy, but this is not diagnostic.
- **D.** Coarctation of the aorta commonly presents as systemic hypertension. Elevated hypertension reading in the arms with normotensive lower extremities is characteristic. Prominent infraclavicular murmurs or late systolic ejection murmurs located at the base of the heart and heard best over the spinous processes may also be found.

267. The answer is **A** [Gastroenterology].
   A. 5-Aminosalicyclic acid (5-ASA) compounds, while non-specific, are the initial choice for mild inflammatory bowel disease.
   B. Biologic therapies, such as anti-TNF and anti-integrin, are used in patients with refractory or corticosteroid dependent inflammatory bowel disease (IBD). They are costly and have serious to life-threatening side effects beyond the other pharmacologic agents for treating IBD.
   C. Corticosteroids are for short-term management of moderate to severe IBD. They are not the initial treatment for mild IBD.
   D. Immunomodulating drugs, such as mercaptopurine, aza-thioprine, or methotrexate, are used in patients with corti-costeroid-dependent IBD in an effort to decrease or withdraw the steroids.

268. The answer is **D** [Cardiology, Infectious Disease].
   A. The pain of an acute coronary event or of angina is more likely to be crushing or squeezing than sharp and is not relieved by sitting forward.
   B. See A.
   C. Costochondritis may present with sharp pain associated with movement but has no associated ECG changes.
   D. This presentation is classic for acute pericarditis following a viral infection, which is the most common cause of in-flammatory pericarditis.

269. The answer is **C** [Cardiology, Surgery, Geriatrics].
   A. Acute myocardial infarction presents with chest pain with or without dyspnea, nausea, or vomiting. The pain typically radiates to the jaw or left arm.
   B. Acute pulmonary embolus presents with sudden dyspnea and chest pain which is sensitive to inspiration.
   C. A classic triad of hypotension, pulsatile abdominal mass, and flank or back pain has been described but is not present in every patient with dissecting abdominal aortic aneurysm. The vast majority of abdominal aortic aneurysms are asymp-tomatic until expansion or rupture. The presence of unex-plained syncope in a male patient over the age of 60 should raise the possibility.
   D. Wolff–Parkinson–White syndrome is an arrhythmia char-acterized by a wide QRS and delta wave (slur) on ECG. Clinical manifestations include palpitations, SVT, and syncope.

270. The answer is **D** [Nephrology and Urology].
   A. Bran significantly lowers urinary calcium, reducing the risk for stone recurrence.
   B. Carbohydrates and fat do not have any impact on urinary stone disease.
   C. Increased fluids throughout the day and night are impor-tant in reducing stone recurrence.
   D. Sodium intake increases sodium and calcium excretion and increases monosodium urate saturation. Protein also increases calcium, oxalate, and uric acid excretion. All these factors can lead to stone formation.

271. The answer is **A** [Nephrology and Urology, Infectious Disease].
   A. Ceftriaxone or cefpodoxime is the drug of choice for the treatment of *Neisseria gonorrhoeae*.
   B. See A.
   C. Tetracyclines, such as doxycycline, are drugs of first choice for *Chlamydia* which is often present along with gonorrhea.
   D. See A.

272. The answer is **B** [Gastroenterology].
   A. A body mass index (BMI) of 14.5 to 18.4 is considered underweight.
   B. BMI is the body weight in kilograms divided by the height in meters squared. An ideal BMI is between 18.5 and 24.9.
   C. A BMI of 25 to 29.9 is considered overweight.
   D. A BMI of 30 to 34.9 is considered class I obesity.

273. The answer is **B** [Gastroenterology].
   A. Alcoholic fatty liver produces right upper quadrant pain, tender hepatomegaly, and elevated transaminase levels.
   B. Alcoholic hepatitis presents with nausea, jaundice, hep-atomegaly, leukocytosis, and elevated transaminase levels. Patients may also have anorexia, vomiting, weight loss, abdominal pain, and splenomegaly.
   C. Cirrhosis is associated with jaundice, bruising, a nonpal-pable liver, and hypoalbuminemia.
   D. Acute pancreatitis presents with nausea and vomiting, continuous epigastric pain, and elevated serum amylase levels.

274. The answer is **A** [Cardiology].
   A. Patients with mitral valve prolapse and no regurgitation routinely have no sequelae.
   B. Infective endocarditis may occur in mitral valve prolapse, but primarily in patients with evidence of regurgitation. Prophylaxis is not recommended for patients with isolated prolapse.
   C. Mitral valve prolapse is a common condition (up to 10% of all females); there is nothing emergent about her presentation.
   D. Only routine health care is recommended; close monitor-ing is not warranted.

275. The answer is **D** [Cardiology].
   A. Cardiogenic syncope typically has no prodrome and is found in persons with preexisting cardiac problems.
   B. Orthostatic hypotension as a cause of syncope most often occurs in the elderly, persons with blood loss, autonomic neuropathy, or who are taking certain medications.
   C. PSVT, while common in young people, is more often experienced as mild chest pain or breathlessness; it usually occurs more often than once.
   D. Vasomotor syncope has premonitory symptoms as desc-ribed and is most common in young women in stressful, painful, or claustrophobic situations.

276. The answer is **B** [Gastroenterology, Surgery].
  A. Atrophic gastritis, a nonerosive gastritis, results in achlorhydria, which causes impaired release of B$_{12}$ from food. Achlorhydria may lead to gastrin levels greater than 1,000 pg/mL.
  B. Peptic ulcers develop in 90% of patients with Zollinger–Ellison syndrome which is caused by gastrinomas, which are gastrin-secreting tumors. When ulcers are refractory to standard therapies, are larger than 2 cm, or are located distal to the duodenal bulb, screening for Zollinger–Ellison syndrome is appropriate. A serum gastrin level over 1,000 pg/mL and acid hypersecretion establish the diagnosis of Zollinger–Ellison syndrome. With lower levels of serum gastrin (150 to 1,000 pg/mL) and acid hypersecretion, a secretin stimulation test is conducted to rule out other causes of increased gastrin levels.
  C. Gastric outlet obstruction is due to narrowing of the duodenal bulb or pyloris of the stomach. This can be caused by peptic ulcer disease or neoplasm as well as other etiologies. Symptoms are early satiety, weight loss, and vomiting.
  D. Insulinomas, adenomas in the islets of Langerhans of the pancreas, are insulin-secreting tumors that cause hypoglycemia typically after exercise, in the early morning, or after missing a meal.

277. The answer is **C** [Endocrinology, Cardiology].
  A. Familial hypercholesteremia is associated with thickening of the Achilles' tendon, not pes planus (flat feet).
  B. Eye findings in hypercholesterolemia include premature arcus cornea, not senile cataracts. Lipema retinalis occurs with extremely high triglycerides.
  C. Tendinous xanthomas occur in approximately 75% of patients with familial hypercholesterolemia. Common areas include the Achilles' tendons or extensor tendons of the hands.
  D. Tophi are associated with gout.

278. The answer is **D** [Cardiology].
  A. Aspirin does not adequately maintain the recommended INR for DVT prophylaxis. It may be used if warfarin is contraindicated.
  B. Lifelong anticoagulation is recommended after two or more DVTs.
  C. Vena cava filter implantation is recommended for chronic, recurrent DVTs.
  D. Warfarin for at least 6 months is the treatment of choice after an acute DVT.

279. The answer is **C** [Obstetrics/Gynecology].
  A. Laparoscopy is used for ectopic pregnancy, not molar pregnancy.
  B. Methotrexate can be used as a follow-up treatment after suction curettage but not as an initial treatment for molar pregnancy
  C. The scenario describes a hydatidiform mole or molar pregnancy. The initial treatment of choice is suction curettage.
  D. Watchful waiting is never a choice with molar pregnancies.

280. The answer is **C** [Pulmonology, Infectious Disease].
  A. Betamethasone may be helpful in later stages involving paroxysmal coughing.
  B. Ciprofloxacin is not indicated in pertussis.
  C. The patient is in the early phase of infection with *Bortadella pertussis* and would benefit from antibiotic treatment. Erythromycin is the drug of choice; however, it is not effective once the patient is in the paroxysmal stage of the disease. Macrolides are also recommended prophylactically for all susceptible close contacts.
  D. Antihistamines and cough suppressants are contraindicated in pertussis, as they can induce paroxysmal cough.

281. The answer is **A** [Ophthalmology and Otolaryngology, Infectious Disease].
  A. The thick, white coating from *Candida* infection can be scraped off revealing a raw, reddened surface underneath. *Candida* infections are commonly seen in patients who are immunocompromised.
  B. Cancer of the tongue is more common in men over age 50, especially in patients who abuse tobacco and alcohol. Cancers occur most often on the side of the tongue and any persistent nodule or ulcer must be suspect. Lesions can be red or white.
  C. Physical examination of a patient infected with *Corynebacterium diphtheria* reveals a dull, red throat with a gray exudate present on the uvula, pharynx, and tongue.
  D. HIV-positive patients are vulnerable to the whitish raised, feathery coating seen in hairy leukoplakia. In contrast to candidiasis, these areas cannot be scraped off.

282. The answer is **C** [Nephrology and Urology, Surgery].
  A. Initial management of renal calculi up to 6 mm in diameter involves at least 6 weeks of conservative management. Invasive procedures such as pyelolithotomy are reserved until spontaneous stone passage has failed.
  B. Increasing fluid intake and analgesia are important in the management of a stone that is passing down the ureter, but is not adequate for a stone that is in the pelvis with a rising BUN.
  C. Lithotripsy is the procedure of choice for a renal calculus that is obstructing renal output as evidenced by a rising BUN.
  D. Allopurinol is utilized when uric acid stones are confirmed and if hyperuricemia is present.

283. The answer is **B** [Obstetrics/Gynecology].
  A. Breast cysts may be single or multiple and may appear bilaterally. Cysts are filled with fluid, tend to fluctuate in size, and are associated with cyclic breast pain. Increase in size and pain typically occurs premenstrually and resolves postmenstrually.
  B. Fibroadenoma is the most common benign tumor of the female breast. It most commonly presents as a single nodule that is sharply circumscribed, freely mobile, and ranges in size from 2 to 4 cm. It is most common before the age of 30 years.
  C. Galactoceles are cystic dilatations of the ducts that are filled with thick milky fluid. They are associated with lactation.
  D. Intraductal papillomas are neoplastic growths that occur within the ducts of the breast. They are most common just before or after menopause. Intraductal papillomas are most commonly associated with a bloody, serous, or turbid nipple discharge. They are rarely palpable.

284. The answer is **A** [Gastroenterology].
  A. Oral rehydration is appropriate in diarrhea; aggressive replacement is particularly important for those who are elderly, children, immunocompromised, or frail. In otherwise healthy persons, supportive care is all that is warranted.
  B. The stool tests are appropriate for diarrhea that is more severe, longer standing, or with a fever, or in patients who are immunocompromised or elderly.
  C. Starting empiric antibiotic therapy is not appropriate for a mild acute diarrhea in an otherwise healthy individual even if it is inflammatory (bloody), as the symptoms often resolve in a few days. Empiric antibiotic treatment is more appropriate for those with positive fecal white blood cell, dehydration, who are immunocompromised, or those requiring hospitalization.
  D. Antidiarrheal treatment may be appropriate for mild to moderate diarrhea that is noninflammatory (nonbloody). However, these agents may cause over-slowing of peristalsis leading to constipation.

285. The answer is **C** [Neurology].
  A. IVIG is not beneficial in this typically self-limiting disease.
  B. Low-salt diet is beneficial in Meniere's disease.
  C. This patient has developed Bell's palsy. Lubricating drops are needed to prevent corneal abrasions or keratitis.
  D. Prednisone is beneficial but only if started within the first 5 days of symptoms.

286. The answer is **B** [Ophthalmology and Otolaryngology, Surgery].
  A. If pterygia become inflamed, artificial tears can be helpful.
  B. Excision is recommended if growth of the pterygium approaches the visual axis or causes significant astigmatism or eye irritation.
  C. Iridotomy is the definitive treatment for acute-angle closure glaucoma.
  D. Topical NSAIDs or corticosteroids may be required for inflamed pterygia or pingueculae.

287. The answer is **A** [Cardiology].
  A. Dobutamine is a β-agonist that is the first-line therapy for cardiogenic shock.
  B. Epinephrine is an α- and β-blocker that is used during resuscitation efforts.
  C. Milrinone has a longer duration of action and its effects are difficult to reverse.
  D. Norepinephrine is a last choice option in this case, as it does not increase coronary perfusion.

288. The answer is **D** [Gastroenterology].
  A. Anal fissures that are off the midline should prompt a workup for infection (HIV/AIDS, syphilis, tuberculosis), inflammatory bowel disease (Crohn's disease, ulcerative colitis), or carcinoma.
  B. See A.
  C. See A.
  D. Anal fissures most commonly occur in the posterior midline and are attributed to straining, high internal sphincter tone, or constipation.

289. The answer is **A** [Psychiatry].
  A. Serotonin is involved in antidepressant action.
  B. Adrenergic transmitters are involved in antihypertensive action.
  C. Cholinergic transmitters are involved in antiparkinsonian action.
  D. Adrenergic and cholinergic transmitters are involved in the regulation of cardiac function.

290. The answer is **C** [Cardiology].
  A. Calf tenderness develops with deep vein thrombosis.
  B. Erythema, dermatitis, and ulcers are seen in venous insufficiency.
  C. Pallor, acute focal pain, pulselessness, and paresthesia develop rapidly with an acute arterial occlusion.
  D. Paralysis develops later in the process as ischemia worsens.

291. The answer is **B** [Rheumatology and Orthopaedics, Infectious Disease].
  A. Imaging tests are not helpful in diagnosing septic arthritis.
  B. Classic signs of inflammation (rubor, calor, dolor, tumor; erythema, heat, pain, swelling) along with fever and chills indicate septic arthritis. Evaluation of synovial fluid for cell count, Gram stain, and culture and sensitivity will guide antibiotic therapy.
  C. ESR is a nonspecific marker of inflammation.
  D. See A.

292. The answer is **B** [Pulmonary, Ophthalmology and Otolaryngology].
  A. Adenocarcinoma of the lung presents as peripheral nodules or masses. It is not associated with asthma or nasal polyps.
  B. Aspirin may precipitate bronchospasm in patients with polyps and asthma (Samter's triad).
  C. Cystic fibrosis typically results in recurrent lung infections; nasal polyps and asthma are not common.
  D. Rhinitis medicamentosa occurs with overuse of nasal decongestants (Afrin, others).

293. The answer is **A** [Cardiology, Rheumatology and Orthopaedics].
  A. This is the classic description of amyloidosis, which is the most common cause of restrictive cardiomyopathy.
  B. Chronic untreated hypertension would typically produce a dilated cardiomyopathy.
  C. Ethanol abuse typically causes a dilated cardiomyopathy.
  D. Sarcoidosis can cause heart disease, although rarely. Biopsy would reveal noncaseating granulomatous disease.

294. The answer is **C** [Pulmonology].
  A. A chest x-ray is not indicated in asthma exacerbations unless a diagnosis of pneumonia is suspect.
  B. A methacholine challenge test is indicated in patients whose diagnosis of asthma is uncertain.
  C. Peak expiratory flow rate is reduced during acute exacerbations and should improve with treatment. It is easy to do and reliable for monitoring disease status.
  D. Pulse oximetry will be abnormal in severe exacerbations. Retention of CO_2 is more likely than loss of O_2 during asthma exacerbations.

295. The answer is **D** [Ophthalmology and Otolaryngology, Infectious Disease, Pediatrics].
  A. Epiglottitis should be suspected when a patient presents with a rapidly developing sore throat or when pain with swallowing is out of proportion to minimal findings on physical exam. It is less common today in children secondary to Hib (*Haemophilus influenzae* type b) vaccination programs.
  B. Mononucleosis is suggested by prominent adenopathy and a shaggy, white-gray tonsillar exudate, which may extend into the nasopharynx, especially in young adults.
  C. Peritonsillar abscess presents with severe sore throat, pain on swallowing, trismus ("lockjaw"), medial deviation of the soft palate, and a muffled ("hot potato") voice.
  D. These clinical features (fever, tender anterior cervical adenopathy, lack of cough, and pharyngotonsillar exudate) strongly suggest group A β-hemolytic streptococcus.

296. The answer is **C** [Rheumatology and Orthopaedics].
  A. See C.
  B. See C.
  C. The mechanism of injury in acromioclavicular separation is usually a direct blow caused by a fall onto the shoulder. Presentation involves pain, swelling, and direct tenderness over the joint. Plain radiographs will not reveal the extent of the injury or separation unless performed as weight-bearing views on both shoulders for comparison.
  D. See C.

297. The answer is **C** [Ophthalmology and Otolaryngology].
  A. Treatment of corneal abrasion does include antibiotic ophthalmic ointment (i.e., polymyxin–bacitracin), mydriatics, and analgesics. However, the next initial step would be to instill fluoroscein to visualize the suspected abrasion.
  B. After diagnosis and treatment, the patient should have follow-up within 48 hours to make sure the cornea has healed.
  C. See A.
  D. With corneal abrasions, patching or padding of the eye does not help and may, in fact, retard healing.

298. The answer is **D** [Hematology].
  A. See D.
  B. See D.
  C. See D.
  D. Hemophilia A is an X-linked recessive disorder which leads to affected males and carrier females. The gene would therefore be passed to all daughters.

299. The answer is **A** [Psychiatry, Gastroenterology].
  A. The GGTP is generally elevated in alcohol abuse and is one of the best early indicators of alcohol abuse.
  B. Although high-density lipoproteins tend to be elevated in alcohol abuse, this finding is not specific to alcohol abuse and may indicate healthy lipid status.
  C. With alcohol abuse, the CBC more often reveals macrocytosis. The enlarged mean corpuscular volume (MCV) results from the toxic effect of alcohol on erythrocyte development and nutritional deficiencies.
  D. Liver transaminases (ALT, AST) are often elevated, but may be normal or low in advanced liver disease and are not supportive in this case.

300. The answer is **A** [Neurology].
  A. Migraine headaches are commonly precipitated by menses, stress, red wine, chocolates, or other factors. They are more commonly throbbing and unilateral, although they may be bilateral and constant. The underlying mechanism is believed to be activation of the trigeminal nerve.
  B. Abnormality in acetylcholine function is implicated in myasthenia gravis, although this is not an autoimmune disease.
  C. The surge of estrogen occurs just prior to ovulation, not menses.
  D. Serotonin deficiency is implicated in depression.

301. The answer is **A** [Psychiatry, Gastroenterology].
  A. Elevated cholesterol, liver enzymes, and BUN and creatinine are common in patients with anorexia nervosa.
  B. In anorexia nervosa, T_4 is mildly decreased due to depression of thyroid function.
  C. FSH and LH are typically decreased in anorexia nervosa.
  D. Bradycardia and hypotension are common in anorexia nervosa.

302. The answer is **A** [Rheumatology and Orthopaedics, Surgery].
  A. Avascular necrosis (AVN) usually presents with groin pain that radiates to the knee; decreased ROM on internal rotation and normal x-ray findings are common in early AVN.
  B. Herniated lumbar disc can present with pain radiating down the leg, but it generally does not cause decreased ROM in the hip.
  C. Osteoarthritis of the hip usually presents in older patients with groin pain that may radiate to the knee and decreased ROM. It would show decreased joint space, osteophytes, and sclerosis on x-ray.
  D. Rheumatoid arthritis usually affects the smaller joints of the hands and wrist and is symmetrical. Systemic symptoms are usually present.

303. The answer is **D** [Dermatology, Infectious Disease].
  A. Griseofulvin therapy is not effective for onychomycosis.
  B. Pulse oral itraconazole is inferior to oral terbinafine therapy for onychomycosis. It is an acceptable alternative for those who cannot tolerate terbinafine.
  C. Ketoconazole is not recommended for the treatment of onychomycosis due to the risk of hepatotoxicity.
  D. Terbinafine is FDA approved for the treatment of onychomycosis. Monthly liver enzymes and CBC with platelets should be performed.

304. The answer is **B** [Obstetrics/Gynecology, Infectious Disease].
   A. Atrophic vaginitis is due to decreased levels of estrogen and is the most common cause of vaginitis in the climacteric female. It is characterized by vulvar irritation and a clear or yellowish discharge. It may also be associated with symptoms of frequency, urgency, and stress incontinence. Vaginal epithelium is usually pale.
   B. Bacterial vaginosis is due to overgrowth of *Gardnerella vaginalis* and other anaerobes. It is associated with a malodorous, grayish, nonadherent discharge which demonstrates an amine "fishy" odor after alkalization with KOH. On wet mount, the epithelial cell borders are studded with bacteria (clue cells).
   C. Trichomoniasis is a sexually transmitted infection associated with pruritus and a malodorous, frothy, yellow to greenish discharge. Red maculopapular lesions may be visible on the cervix. Wet mount demonstrates motile flagellate protozoans.
   D. Vulvovaginal candidiasis is associated with pruritus, erythema of the vulva and vagina, and a white, curd-like, nonodorous discharge. Risk factors include pregnancy, diabetes, recent antibiotic use, and occlusive clothing. Wet prep demonstrates budding yeast cells, filaments, and spores.

305. The answer is **A** [Obstetrics/Gynecology].
   A. External fetal monitoring (EFM) is commonly used to assess fetal status during labor. A good, reassuring EFM is a heart rate of 110 to 160 with variability and accelerations but no decelerations. Bradycardia and late decelerations often indicate fetal hypoxia, which can lead to fetal morbidity and mortality.
   B. This EFM is within normal limits and would be considered reassuring.
   C. This EFM is within normal limits and would be considered reassuring.
   D. This heart rate is borderline high but still normal. Early decelerations are an indication of head compression when a woman is fully dilated and delivery is near. Generally, early decelerations are considered benign.

306. The answer is **D** [Psychiatry, Endocrinology, Pediatrics].
   A. See D.
   B. See D.
   C. See D.
   D. This patient is at high risk for anorexia nervosa. Her initial workup includes a complete chemistry panel, CBC, ESR, urinalysis, ECG, and thyroid function tests.

Ophthalmology and Otolaryngology

1

Nancy E. Orr

I. DISORDERS OF THE EYES

A. Disorders of the globe

1. Trauma

    a. General characteristics

    (1) Traumatic disorders affecting the globe include blunt or penetrating trauma, foreign bodies, and chemical burns.

    (2) All management steps should be taken as soon as possible, especially with penetrating trauma and foreign bodies. The first step of the history is to find out when and how the accident, trauma, or burn occurred.

    b. Physical examination

    (1) Observe: inspect, noticing any abnormalities.

       (a) Orbit: for edema or hematoma.

       (b) Lids: for laceration, hematomas, edema, and foreign bodies.

       (c) Pupils: for irregularity.

       (d) Extraocular muscles: for unequal, limited, or decreased movement, which may indicate laceration or entrapment of eye muscles.

       (e) Anterior chamber: for hyphema.

       (f) Interior of eye with funduscope: for ruptured retinal vessels, which may indicate physical abuse, such as shaken baby syndrome.

    (2) Palpate orbital rim: for irregularity, which may indicate a fracture. If rupture of the globe is suspected, do not palpate.

    c. Measurements

    (1) Visual acuity is tested using the Snellen chart. This is important to establish a baseline; any decrease indicates serious trauma.

    (2) Pupillary reactions should be checked. Unequal reactions might indicate severe trauma to the globe, head trauma, or nerve palsies.

    (3) Check for intraocular pressure. After appropriate topical anesthesia, carefully use the Schiötz tonometer.

    d. Treatment

    (1) Penetrating trauma

       (a) The object should not be removed.

       (b) The patient should be transported to the emergency room for consult with an ophthalmologist.

    (2) Foreign body

       (a) The eyelids should be carefully everted, stained with fluorescein, and observed with a Wood's lamp.

       (b) Gently attempt to remove the foreign body using a moistened, cotton-tipped swab.

       (c) Patching may be beneficial if a large corneal abrasion occurs. Patching should be limited to 24 hours. Reexamine the next day.

       (d) A rust ring on the cornea indicates metallic foreign bodies. These may be removed with a rotating burr, or the patient may be referred to an ophthalmologist.

    (3) Chemical burns (acid or alkali)

       (a) The eye should be irrigated with water or normal saline for at least 30 minutes. Use sterile solution if available. A chemical burn can continue to cause damage even after flushing.

       (b) An eye shield should be placed on the eye.

       (c) Because an acid or alkali burn is severe, transport the patient to the emergency room and refer to an ophthalmologist.

1

2. Blow-out fracture
    a. General characteristics
        (1) The orbital floor is composed of maxillary, palatine, and zygomatic bones. These bones are very thin.
        (2) Blunt trauma, such as that from a fist or a ball, causes the floor to fracture, trapping the orbital structures.
    b. Clinical features
        (1) Patients present with swelling and misalignment. Movement of the globe is restricted, specifically an inability to look up due to entrapment of the infraorbital nerve and the musculature.
        (2) Double vision is common.
        (3) Subcutaneous emphysema and exophthalmos are present.
    c. Treatment
        (1) Prompt referral to an ophthalmologist is important.
        (2) Patients should be kept calm and avoid sneezing or anything that would increase pressure.
        (3) Nasal decongestants, ice packs or cold compresses, and antibiotics are started during transport.
3. Corneal abrasion
    a. General characteristics: It usually is caused by minor trauma, such as that from a fingernail, contact lens, eyelash, or small foreign body.
    b. Clinical features
        (1) Pain and sensation of a foreign body can be accompanied by photophobia, tearing, injection, and blepharospasm.
        (2) Record visual acuity before examining or treating.
        (3) A slit-lamp examination or fluorescein staining will reveal an epithelial defect but a clear cornea. A search for foreign bodies is required.
    c. Treatment
        (1) Topical anesthetic will provide immediate relief; however, it should be used only to assist in confirming the diagnosis and should not be prescribed.
        (2) Antibiotic ointment, such as polymyxin/bacitracin, should be applied. Acetaminophen is given for analgesia.
        (3) Patching for no longer than 24 hours is recommended only for large abrasions (>5 to 10 mm) to promote healing. Patching for longer than 24 hours may retard healing.
        (4) Follow-up of all abrasions within 1 to 2 days is essential.
4. Retinal disorders
    a. Retinal detachment
        (1) General characteristics
            (a) The underlying pathogenesis is a separation of the retina from the pigmented epithelial layer, causing the detached tissue to appear as flapping in the vitreous humor.
            (b) The tear usually begins at the superior temporal retinal area.
            (c) The tear can happen spontaneously or be secondary to trauma or extreme myopia.
        (2) Clinical features
            (a) The patient may report acute onset of blurred or blackened vision that occurs over several hours and progresses to complete or partial monocular blindness.
            (b) It is classically described as a curtain being drawn over the eye from top to bottom.
            (c) The patient may sense floaters or flashing lights at the initiation of symptoms.
        (3) There will be a relative afferent pupillary defect. Funduscopic examination may reveal the rugous retina flapping in the vitreous humor.
        (4) Treatment
            (a) An emergency consult with an ophthalmologist regarding possible laser surgery or cryosurgery is needed.
            (b) Patients with retinal detachment should remain supine, with the head turned to the side of the retinal detachment.
            (c) Prognosis is good: 80% will recover without recurrence, 15% will require retreatment, and 5% will never reattach.

   b. Macular degeneration

     (1) This disorder may be age related or secondary to the toxic effects of drugs, such as chloroquine or phenothiazine. It is the leading cause of irreversible central visual loss.

     (2) Drusen deposits are found in Bruch's membrane, leading to degenerative changes, loss of nutritional supply, atrophy, and neovascularization.

     (3) It usually has an insidious onset, and its chief clinical feature is gradual loss of vision. Metamorphopsia is the phenomenon of wavy or distorted vision and can be measured with an Amsler grid.

     (4) Mottling, serous leaks, and hemorrhages commonly develop on the retina.

     (5) There is no effective treatment. If detected early, laser therapy or intravitreal injections of monoclonal antibody drugs (anti-VEGF [vascular endothelial growth factor]) may slow the progression of macular degeneration. Vitamins and antioxidants may also reduce the progression of age-related macular degeneration.

   c. Central retinal artery occlusion

     (1) General characteristics

       (a) This disorder is considered to be an ophthalmic emergency; prognosis is poor, even with immediate treatment.

       (b) Common causes are emboli, thrombotic phenomenon, and vasculitides.

     (2) Clinical features

       (a) It is characterized by sudden, painless, and marked unilateral loss of vision.

       (b) Funduscopy reveals arteriolar narrowing, separation of arterial flow (box-carring), retinal edema, and perifoveal atrophy (cherry red spot). Ganglionic death leads to optic atrophy and a pale retina.

     (3) Treatment

       (a) Emergency referral to an ophthalmologist is necessary. Vessel dilation and paracentesis are attempted to save the eye.

       (b) Workup and management of atherosclerotic disease is warranted to reduce the risk of recurrence.

   d. Central retinal vein occlusion

     (1) This usually occurs secondary to a thrombotic event.

     (2) Patients present with sudden, unilateral, painless blurred vision or complete visual loss.

     (3) Examination reveals an afferent pupillary defect and a "blood and thunder" retina (dilated veins, hemorrhages, edema, and exudates).

     (4) Vision typically is resolved with time, at least partially. A workup for further thrombosis is warranted.

   e. Retinopathy

     (1) Systemic disorders, including diabetes, hypertension, preeclampsia–eclampsia, blood dyscrasias, and HIV disease, may affect the retina.

     (2) Diabetic retinopathy

       (a) This is the leading cause of blindness in adults in the United States. Patients with diabetes should have yearly dilated ophthalmoscopic examinations.

       (b) Nonproliferative: venous dilation, microaneurysms, retinal hemorrhages, retinal edema, hard exudates.

       (c) Proliferative: neovascularization, vitreous hemorrhage.

     (3) Treatment includes optimized glucose control, regulation of blood pressure, laser photocoagulation, and vitrectomy. Severe disease is permanent.

5. Cataract

   a. General characteristics

     (1) A cataract is any opacity of the natural lens of the eye. It may involve a small part of the lens or the entire lens. The degree of opacification also is variable.

     (2) Cataracts may develop secondary to the natural aging process, trauma, congenital causes, or medication use (e.g., corticosteroids, lovastatin).

     (3) Excess sun exposure predisposes to cataract development.

b. Clinical features

(1) The insidious onset of decreased vision is the main clinical feature.

(2) A gradual diminution of vision is characteristic. Patients also may complain of double vision, fixed spots, or reduced color perception.

(3) On examination, there is a translucent, yellow discoloration in the lens. On funduscopy, the cataract appears black on a red background.

c. Treatment

(1) Treatment is warranted to improve activities of daily living, prevent secondary glaucoma, and permit visualization of the fundus.

(2) Treatment involves intracapsular or extracapsular extractions of the cataract with lens replacement.

(3) Prognosis is excellent; postoperative bleeding occurs in less than 0.1%.

6. Glaucoma

a. General characteristics

(1) This condition is defined as increased intraocular pressure with optic nerve damage. Any impediment to the flow of aqueous humor through the trabecular meshwork and canal of Schlemm will increase pressure in the anterior chamber.

(2) Glaucoma may be acute or chronic. Types include angle-closure glaucoma and open-angle glaucoma.

(3) Open-angle glaucoma affects people older than 40 years and is more common in African Americans and in patients with a family history of glaucoma.

b. Clinical features

(1) Angle-closure glaucoma is an ophthalmic emergency.

(a) Painful eye and loss of vision are important clinical features.

(b) Physical examination reveals circumlimbal injection, steamy cornea, fixed mid-dilated pupil, and decreased visual acuity.

(c) The anterior chamber is narrowed; intraocular pressure is acutely elevated.

(d) Nausea, vomiting, and diaphoresis are common.

(2) Open-angle glaucoma

(a) This is a chronic, asymptomatic, and potentially blinding disease defined as increased intraocular pressure, defects in the peripheral visual field, and increased cup-to-disc ratios.

c. Treatment

(1) Angle-closure glaucoma

(a) These patients must be referred immediately to an ophthalmologist. Start intravenous (IV) carbonic anhydrase inhibitor, topical β-blocker, and osmotic diuresis.

(b) Mydriatics should not be administered to these patients.

(c) Treatment is via laser or surgical iridotomy.

(2) Open-angle glaucoma

(a) Patients need to be referred to an ophthalmologist.

(b) Treatment consists of topical and/or systemic medications to decrease the intraocular pressure by decreasing aqueous production and increasing outflow.

7. Orbital cellulitis

a. General characteristics

(1) Orbital cellulitis is more common in children than in adults. Median age is 7 to 12 years.

(2) Orbital cellulitis has several possible causes, including sinusitis, dental infections, facial infections, infection of the globe or eyelids, and infections of the lacrimal system. Less often, it results from trauma.

(3) Causative agents in children include *Streptococcus pneumoniae, Staphylococcus aureus, Haemophilus influenzae,* and Gram-negative bacteria. In adults it occurs secondary to acute or chronic sinusitis and has many possible causative agents. An increase in methicillin-resistant *Staphylococcus aureus* (MRSA) has been noted.

    b. Clinical features

        (1) Orbital cellulitis presents with ptosis, eyelid edema, exophthalmos, purulent discharge, and conjunctivitis.

        (2) Examination will reveal fever, decreased range of motion in the eye muscles, and a sluggish pupillary response.

    c. Laboratory studies

        (1) Workup includes complete blood count (CBC), blood cultures, and cultures of any drainage.

        (2) Sinus radiography and computed tomography (CT) may help to determine the cause and extent of the disease. CT will show broad infiltration of the orbital soft tissue.

    d. Treatment

        (1) Orbital cellulitis constitutes a medical emergency requiring hospitalization and IV antibiotics.

        (2) Antibiotics should be broad spectrum until the causative agent is identified.

B. Disorders of the adnexa

  1. Disorders of the lacrimal system

    a. Dacryostenosis is common in the newborn after the first month of life and occurs when the duct does not open.

        (1) The obstruction usually resolves by 9 months of age.

        (2) Treatment includes warm compresses and massage; if no resolution, surgical probe is indicated.

    b. Dacryocystitis is an inflammation of the lacrimal gland caused by obstruction. Common pathogens include *Staphylococcus aureus*, β-hemolytic streptococci, *Staphylococcus epidermidis*, and *Candida* sp.

        (1) Pain, swelling, tenderness, redness, and purulent discharge are characteristic.

        (2) Treatment is warm compresses and antibiotics.

  2. Eyelids

    a. Blepharitis is chronic inflammation of the lid margins.

        (1) Causes include seborrhea, staphylococcal or streptococcal infection, or dysfunction of the meibomian glands.

        (2) Clinical features

            (a) Rims are red, and eyelashes adhere.

            (b) Dandruff-like deposits (scurf) and fibrous scales (collarettes) may be seen.

            (c) The conjunctiva is clear or slightly erythematous.

        (3) Treatment

            (a) Lid scrubs using diluted baby shampoo on cotton-tipped swabs are helpful.

            (b) Topical antibiotics can be used if infection is suspected. Systemic antibiotics are reserved for recalcitrant cases.

    b. Hordeolum

        (1) General characteristics

            (a) A hordeolum is an acute development of a small, painful nodule or pustule within a gland in the upper or lower eyelid.

            (b) Types

                (i) Internal hordeola: caused by the inflammation and infection of a meibomian gland, with pustular formation in that gland. They are situated deep from the palpebral margin.

                (ii) External hordeola (commonly referred to as a sty): caused by the inflammation and infection of the glands of Moll or Zeis, with pustular formation in those glands. They are situated immediately adjacent to the edge of the palpebral margin.

            (c) Causal pathogen for either type of hordeolum is typically *Staphylococcus aureus*.

            (d) Hordeolum is not contagious.

        (2) Clinical features

            (a) Hordeolum is characterized by acute onset of pain and edema of the involved eyelid.

            (b) There is a palpable, indurated area in the involved eyelid, which has a central area of purulence with surrounding erythema.

(3) Treatment

    (a) Warm compresses should be applied several times per day for 48 hours.

    (b) Topical antibiotics should be used if secondary infection develops.

    (c) Incision and drainage may be indicated if it does not resolve.

c. Chalazion

  (1) General characteristics

    (a) This is a relatively painless, indurated lesion deep from the palpebral margin.

    (b) It often is secondary to a chronic inflammation of an internal hordeolum of the meibomian gland.

  (2) Clinical features

    (a) The chalazion is characterized by insidious onset with minimal irritation.

    (b) It can become pruritic and cause erythema of the involved lid.

  (3) Treatment involves warm compresses and referral to an ophthalmologist for an elective excision if not resolved.

d. Entropion and ectropion

  (1) Entropion: The lid and lashes are turned in secondary to scar tissue or a spasm of the orbicularis oculi muscles.

  (2) Ectropion: The edge of the eyelid everts secondary to advanced age, trauma, infection, or palsy of the facial nerve.

  (3) Treatment: Involves surgical repair if the condition causes trauma, excessive tearing, exposure keratitis, or cosmetic distress.

C. Disorders of the conjunctiva

1. Viral conjunctivitis

a. General characteristics

  (1) Viral infection in the conjunctiva usually is caused by adenovirus type 3, 8, or 19.

  (2) Viral conjunctivitis is highly contagious. Transmission is by direct contact, usually via the fingers, with the contralateral eye or with other persons.

  (3) Viral conjunctivitis can be transmitted in swimming pools (epidemic keratoconjunctivitis), and it is most common in midsummer to early fall.

b. Clinical features: Viral conjunctivitis is characterized by the acute onset of unilateral or bilateral erythema of the conjunctiva, copious watery discharge, and ipsilateral tender preauricular lymphadenopathy.

c. Treatment

  (1) Therapy includes eye lavage with normal saline twice a day for 7 to 14 days; vasoconstrictor–antihistamine drops also may have beneficial effects.

  (2) Warm to cool compresses reduce discomfort.

  (3) Ophthalmic sulfonamide drops may prevent secondary bacterial infection but are not routinely prescribed.

2. Bacterial conjunctivitis

a. General characteristics: Bacterial infection in the conjunctiva may occur with common or rare pathogens.

  (1) Common pathogens include *Streptococcus pneumoniae, Staphylococcus aureus, Haemophilus aegyptius*, and *Moraxella* sp.

    (a) Transmission is via direct contact or via fomites. Autoinoculation, from one eye to the other, usually via the fingers, is typical.

    (b) The natural history of an infection caused by these common pathogens usually is self-limiting, but a secondary keratitis can develop.

  (2) Rare pathogens include *Chlamydia trachomatis* and *Neisseria gonorrhoeae*.

    (a) Transmission is by direct contact or fomites, including nonchlorinated swimming sources. It also can be transmitted via sexual contact or to a neonate via vaginal delivery.

    (b) The natural history of an infection caused by these rare pathogens is a severe conjunctivitis and keratitis with development of permanent visual impairment.

b. Clinical features

  (1) Bacterial conjunctivitis is characterized by the acute onset of copious, purulent discharge from both eyes.

  (2) Patients may have a mild decrease in visual acuity and mild discomfort. The eyes may be "glued" shut on awakening.

    c. Laboratory studies

        (1) Common pathogens: Gram stain should show the presence of polymorphonuclear cells (PMNs) and a predominant organism.

        (2) Rare pathogens: Gram stain and Giemsa stain should show PMNs.

            (a) When *Chlamydia trachomatis* is the pathogen, no organisms will be seen.

            (b) When *Neisseria gonorrhoeae* is the pathogen, intracellular Gram-negative diplococci will be present.

    d. Treatment

        (1) Specific therapy includes application of topical antibiotics.

        (2) For the rare pathogens, treatment also may require concurrent systemic antibiotics.

3. Pinguecula

    a. General characteristics: It is caused by chronic actinic exposure, repeated trauma, and dry and windy conditions.

    b. Clinical features

        (1) Elevated, yellowish, fleshy conjunctival mass found on the sclera adjacent to the cornea.

        (2) Painless inflammation may occur.

    c. Treatment

        (1) No treatment is necessary.

        (2) If it is cosmetically undesirable or chronically inflamed, it can be resected.

4. Pterygium

    a. General characteristics

        (1) Slowly growing thickening of the bulbar conjunctiva.

        (2) It can be unilateral or bilateral.

    b. Clinical features

        (1) A highly vascular, triangular mass grows from the nasal side toward the cornea.

        (2) It occasionally encroaches on the cornea and interferes with vision.

    c. Treatment

        (1) Excision is warranted if it interferes with vision.

        (2) Recurrence is common.

D. Optic nerve and visual pathways

  1. Papilledema

    a. This condition is defined as an increase in intracranial pressure.

    b. Causes are numerous but may include malignant hypertension, hemorrhagic strokes, acute subdural hematoma, and pseudotumor cerebri.

    c. The disc appears swollen, and the margins are blurred, with an obliteration of the vessels.

    d. The patient may be asymptomatic or may complain of transient visual alterations that last for seconds.

    e. Treatment consists of therapy for the underlying cause.

  2. Blurred vision and decreased visual acuity

    a. The location of the lesion determines the effect on vision (Fig. 1-1).

        (1) Lesions anterior to the optic chiasm will affect only one eye.

        (2) Lesions at the optic chiasm will affect both eyes partially.

        (3) Lesions posterior to the chiasm will yield corresponding defects in both visual fields.

    b. The quality of visual loss helps to determine the diagnosis.

        (1) Transient visual loss may be secondary to a transient ischemic attack, an emboli (amaurosis fugax), or temporal (giant cell) arteritis.

            (a) Temporal arteritis (giant cell arteritis) is one of the more common causes and is characterized by a tender temporal artery, fever, malaise, and a strikingly increased erythrocyte sedimentation rate.

            (b) Prompt treatment with systemic corticosteroids is necessary to prevent permanent blindness.

        (2) Sudden visual loss may be secondary to central retinal vein or branch vein occlusion, optic neuropathy, papillitis, and retrobulbar neuritis.

        (3) Gradual visual loss may be secondary to macular degeneration, tumors, cataracts, or glaucoma.

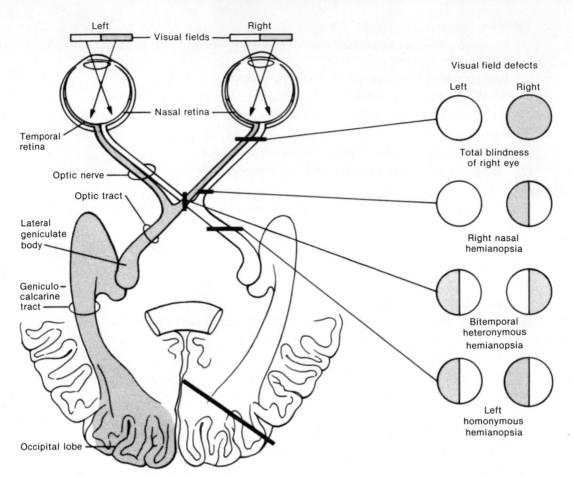

FIGURE 1-1 Optic pathways. (From Harwood-Nuss A, Wolfson AB, Linden CH, et al. *The Clinical Practice of Emergency Medicine*. 3rd ed. Philadelphia: Lippincott Williams & Wilkins; 2001.)

3. Strabismus

   a. Strabismus is a condition in which binocular fixation is not present.

   b. Strabismus may occur in one eye or both. A corneal light reflex test will reveal misalignment (manifest or heterotropia strabismus). A cover–uncover test may reveal latent (heterophoria) strabismus which may not be readily apparent otherwise.

   c. Inward misalignment is termed *esotropia;* outward misalignment is termed *exotropia.*

   d. Strabismus may be corrected with eye exercises (patch therapy) or, in severe cases, with surgery. If left untreated after the age of 2, amblyopia will result.

4. Amblyopia

   a. Amblyopia is reduced visual acuity not correctable by refractive means.

   b. It may be caused by strabismus (most commonly), uremia, or toxins, such as alcohol, tobacco, lead, and other toxic substances.

5. Icterus or jaundice, which is a yellowing of the sclera, is caused by the retention of bilirubin.

6. Blue or cyanotic sclera may be normal or seen in infants with osteogenesis imperfecta.

II. DISORDERS OF THE EARS

   A. Hearing impairment (hearing loss) may be of acute or gradual onset.

     1. General characteristics

       a. Hearing loss may result from either conductive or sensorineural physiologic causes.

       b. The Weber and Rinne tests are used to help differentiate conductive from sensorineural hearing loss.

        (1) Lateralization to the affected ear on the Weber test indicates conductive hearing loss. Conductive loss also will result in bone conduction greater than air conduction on the affected side (Rinne sign).

      (2) Sensorineural defects will have impairment of both air conduction and bone conduction, but air conduction will remain greater than bone conduction.

  2. Conductive hearing loss is caused by impaired transmission of sound along the external canal, across the ossicles, and through the oval window. It is often temporary.

    a. There is an increased threshold for perceived sound intensity.

    b. Possible causes of conductive hearing loss

      (1) Cerumen impaction may require removal either by irrigation or by use of a wire loop or cerumen spoon.

      (2) Acute otitis externa also may cause a conductive hearing loss because of the exudate in the external canal.

      (3) Otosclerosis, which is caused by abnormal new bone formation in the oval window, causes conductive hearing loss and is amenable to surgery.

      (4) Otitis media also may cause conductive hearing loss.

  3. Sensorineural hearing loss is any hearing loss secondary to a disruption in the nerves or the mechanics of hearing. It has many causes (e.g., neural degeneration, decreased cilia, problems in the ossicles).

    a. Presbycusis

      (1) General characteristics

        (a) Presbycusis is the most common cause of sensorineural hearing loss.

        (b) It occurs with age in most people; men are affected more often than women.

        (c) There is probably a genetic predisposition; it may be caused or exacerbated by noise exposure.

      (2) Clinical features

        (a) It usually involves the higher frequencies and may be associated with tinnitus.

        (b) The patient or family members may complain that there is difficulty in sound discrimination.

      (3) Treatment: This type of loss may or may not be helped by hearing aids.

    b. Ménière's disease

      (1) General characteristics

        (a) This is a recurrent and usually progressive group of symptoms, including acquired chronic hearing loss, tinnitus, and dizziness or vertigo.

        (b) The cause is unknown; symptoms result from distention of the endolymphatic compartment of the inner ear.

      (2) Clinical features

        (a) Hearing loss is accompanied by episodes of tinnitus, vertigo, and nausea and vomiting. The attacks may last from minutes to hours, but unsteadiness may last longer.

        (b) The hearing loss may abate with each attack, but hearing rarely returns to the pre-attack level.

      (3) Treatment

        (a) Most cases can be managed with diuretics and salt restriction.

        (b) Surgical intervention may be indicated if symptoms progress.

    c. Acoustic trauma (e.g., an explosion, a shotgun blast) or chronic noise exposure can cause sensorineural hearing loss.

    d. Acoustic neuroma (vestibular schwannoma) is a neoplastic cause of hearing loss.

      (1) It is more predominant in females and usually is unilateral.

      (2) The patient may present with insidious hearing loss; with progressive growth, a patient may develop tinnitus, vertigo, ataxia, and brain stem dysfunction.

      (3) It is diagnosed via CT or magnetic resonance imaging (MRI), and the treatment is surgical.

  4. Drug-induced hearing loss

    a. It may be caused by streptomycin, kanamycin, neomycin, ethacrynic acid, chloramphenicol, and other drugs.

    b. The onset is insidious, and tinnitus may be the first symptom.

    c. Hearing loss usually is high frequency.

    d. It may or may not be reversible with cessation of the drug.

5. Infancy and childhood hearing loss
   a. Congenital causes include asphyxia, erythroblastosis, and maternal rubella.
   b. Acquired causes include measles, mumps, pertussis, meningitis, influenza, and labyrinthitis.
   c. Clinical features include inattentiveness to human voices or lack of reaction to noise.
   d. Treatment: Involves correction of underlying causes.

B. Otitis media (infection of the middle ear)
   1. General characteristics
      a. The pathophysiology involves underlying poor drainage from the eustachian tubes because of age (i.e., the tubes are usually straighter in children), inflammation and edema, or a congenital deformity (e.g., Down syndrome, cleft palate, adenoidal hypertrophy).
      b. Otitis media is most common in children 4 to 24 months of age, but can occur at any age.
      c. It is caused by bacteria in 70% to 90% of cases; the most common organisms are *Streptococcus pneumoniae*, *Haemophilus influenzae*, *Moraxella catarrhalis*, *Streptococcus pyogenes*, and *Staphylococcus aureus*.
      d. Recurrent cases often are associated with allergies or exposure to secondhand smoke.
   2. Clinical features
      a. The patient may present with fever, pressure, pain, and hearing loss.
      b. The eardrum will be immobile and may appear erythematous and bulging. Bullae suggest mycoplasmal infection.
      c. Rupture of the tympanic membrane results in otorrhea and decreased pain; typically, chronic otitis media ensues.
      d. Inadequate treatment of otitis media may cause mastoiditis. Patients will exhibit spiking fevers, postauricular pain, and erythema.
   3. Treatment
      a. First-line antibiotics include amoxicillin, erythromycin/sulfonamide, clavulanic acid/amoxicillin, trimethoprim/sulfamethoxazole, and cefaclor. If the patient is allergic to penicillin, erythromycin or clarithromycin is indicated. In uncomplicated cases, antibiotics may not be necessary.
      b. When medication fails to heal the otitis media, the patient may need myringotomy, tympanostomy, adenoidectomy, or a combination of these procedures.
      c. Mastoiditis is treated with IV antibiotics; if medication fails, mastoidectomy is indicated.

C. Otitis externa
   1. General characteristics
      a. Otitis externa, generally known as swimmer's ear, is common in children and adolescents.
      b. The cause is a combination of mechanical obstruction that inhibits drainage of water from the external ear canal and the presence of an infectious agent.
      c. Certain conditions may predispose to otitis externa (e.g., eczema, seborrheic dermatitis, psoriasis). The causative organisms include *Pseudomonas* sp., Enterobacteriaceae, *Proteus* sp., and, rarely, fungi.
   2. Clinical features
      a. Physical signs include pain in the ear and tenderness with manipulation of the tragus or the auricle.
      b. Otoscopic examination reveals a canal that is edematous and obscured with purulent debris.
   3. Treatment
      a. Using otic antibacterial drops and keeping the canal dry usually are effective.
      b. In diabetic or immunocompromised patients, malignant otitis externa may develop, which is a necrotizing infection extending to the blood vessels, bone, and cartilage; this requires hospitalization and parenteral antibiotics.

D. Vertigo
   1. General characteristics
      a. True vertigo is the sensation of movement (spinning, tumbling, or falling) or a person's sensation of objects spinning around him or her.
      b. Peripheral vertigo is caused by labyrinthitis, Meniere's disease, positional (or positioning) vertigo, vestibular neuronitis, migrainous vertigo, and obstructing anatomic abnormalities.
      c. Central vertigo is caused by brain stem vascular disease, arteriovenous malformations, tumors of the brain stem or cerebellum, multiple sclerosis, or vertebrobasilar migraine syndrome.

2. Clinical features

a. Vertigo usually is accelerated with movement.

b. It may be accompanied by nystagmus.

(1) Peripheral vertigo is characterized by sudden onset, nausea and vomiting, tinnitus, and decreased hearing. Nystagmus is horizontal with a rotary component, fast-phase beats away from the diseased side, and fixation inhibition.

(2) Central vertigo is characterized by a slower-onset, nonfatigable nystagmus, vertical greater than horizontal plane, and no latency or suppression by fixation. There usually are accompanying motor, sensory, or cerebellar deficits.

c. The condition may last from days to weeks.

3. Laboratory studies

a. The Hallpike or Nylen–Barany maneuver (i.e., quickly turning the patient's head 90 degrees while the patient is in the supine position) is used to reproduce the vertigo. This test is more likely to be positive with peripheral causes.

b. Audiometry, caloric stimulation, electronystagmography, CT, MRI, and evoked potentials are performed as indicated by history and physical examination findings.

4. Treatment is per underlying cause.

a. Acute attacks can be treated with diazepam; injection or per rectum is advised.

b. Mild vertigo may respond to meclizine, cyclizine, or dimenhydrinate.

c. Severe vertigo may be treated with scopolamine.

d. Bed rest may be necessary during acute attacks; however, patients with chronic vertigo should be encouraged to move about.

e. Interventional and surgical therapies are available for recalcitrant cases.

E. **Labyrinthitis** is a phenomenon of severe acute vertigo, hearing loss, and tinnitus. The cause is unknown, but it may occur after an otitis or viremia. It may be treated with meclizine, promethazine, or dimenhydrinate.

F. **Barotrauma** is the inability to equalize barometric stress on the middle ear, resulting in pain.

1. Barotrauma is caused by auditory tube dysfunction. This can result from congenital narrowing or acquired mucosal edema.

2. Symptoms are most likely to occur during airplane descent, rapid altitude change, or underwater diving.

3. Patients should be instructed to swallow or yawn to autoinflate the tube. Systemic or topical decongestants also may help. If the pressure is not equalized, the tympanic membrane may rupture. A middle ear infection often follows this trauma.

4. If symptoms persist after removal of the offending agent, then decongestants, autoinflation, or myringotomy can be tried.

G. **Tympanic membrane rupture**

1. Small ruptures in the tympanic membrane usually will close on their own in time.

2. Larger ruptures may require a tympanoplasty for closure.

3. It is important not to allow any water into the ear until the rupture is closed.

III. DISORDERS OF THE NOSE, SINUS, AND THROAT

A. **Sinusitis**

1. General characteristics

a. Sinusitis refers to any inflammation of the sinus cavities.

b. It usually follows an upper respiratory tract infection (URI).

c. Causative agents include viruses (most commonly) or bacteria (the less common acute sinusitis). Bacterial pathogens are the same as for otitis media (see II.B, Otitis media).

d. Specific risk factors for the development of acute sinusitis include a recent URI, chronic rhinitis, cigarette smoking, history of trauma or presence of a foreign body, any of which can obstruct drainage and increase the risk of infection.

2. Clinical features

a. Patients complain of headache and pain in the face that worsens when leaning forward, purulent drainage, fever, and malaise.

    b. Physical examination reveals tenderness to palpation over the sinuses or opacification of the sinus with transillumination. Unilateral or severe localized symptoms support a diagnosis of acute sinusitis.

    c. Osteomyelitis, cavernous sinus thrombosis, or an orbital cellulitis are among the complications of sinusitis.

  3. Laboratory studies

    a. Diagnosis is clinical.

    b. CT scan is indicated in chronic sinusitis resistant to treatment or other complications or if the host is immunocompromised.

    c. Waters view radiograph may reveal opacification but is less sensitive than CT.

    d. MRI is more sensitive than CT in determining malignancy.

  4. Treatment

    a. Treatment of sinusitis includes saline nasal spray, decongestants, and hot packs or steam.

    b. Antibiotics are recommended in cases of acute sinusitis and should be used appropriately.

    c. Treatment should last for 10 to 14 days; patients should be carefully monitored for any signs of complications.

B. Rhinitis

  1. General characteristics

    a. Rhinitis refers to any inflammation of the nasal mucosa.

    b. There are three basic types: allergic rhinitis, vasomotor rhinitis, and rhinitis medicamentosa.

      (1) Allergic rhinitis is an immunoglobulin E–mediated reactivity to airborne antigens (e.g., pollen, molds, danders, dust). It commonly occurs in people who have other atopic diseases (e.g., asthma, eczema, atopic dermatitis) and who have a family history.

      (2) Vasomotor rhinitis is rhinorrhea caused by increased secretion of mucus from the nasal mucosa. It may be precipitated by changes in temperature or humidity, odors, alcohol, or result from a neurovascular imbalance.

      (3) Rhinitis medicamentosa is caused by the overzealous use of decongestant drops or sprays containing oxymetazoline or phenylephrine. This causes a rebound congestion, which prompts increased use of the agent, creating a vicious cycle.

  2. Clinical features

    a. Allergic rhinitis

      (1) Symptoms may be confused with those of a common cold.

      (2) Signs may include allergic shiners (bluish discoloration below the eyes), rhinorrhea, itchy or watery eyes, sneezing, nasal congestion, dry cough, and pale, boggy, or bluish mucosa. Children may develop a horizontal nasal crease (the allergic salute) from habitual rubbing of the nose.

      (3) The discharge usually is clear and watery.

    b. Vasomotor rhinitis

      (1) In its purest form, vasomotor rhinitis consists of bogginess of the nasal mucosa associated with a complaint of stuffiness and rhinorrhea.

      (2) The symptoms are labile and can clear quickly.

    c. Rhinitis medicamentosa

      (1) Patients experience severe congestion and pain.

      (2) Discharge is typically minimal.

  3. Treatment

    a. Allergic rhinitis: Avoid any known allergens and use antihistamines, cromolyn sodium, nasal or systemic corticosteroids, nasal saline drops, and immunotherapy.

    b. Vasomotor rhinitis: Avoid the irritant.

    c. Rhinitis medicamentosa: Discontinue the irritant. It may be quite uncomfortable for the patient; sometimes the use of topical corticosteroids is warranted through the withdrawal period.

C. Pharyngitis/Tonsillitis

  1. General characteristics

    a. Sore throat is one of the most common reasons for outpatient visits.

    b. The causes of pharyngitis are bacterial and viral; differentiation between the two types of causes is important to direct treatment. Viral cases are much more common than bacterial.

    2. Clinical features

        a. The overall manifestations of pharyngitis include sore throat, difficulty swallowing, fever, erythema of the tonsils and posterior pharynx, lymph node enlargement, rhinitis, and cough, all in varying degrees.

        b. Infection that penetrates the tonsillar capsule leads to cellulitis and peritonsillar abscess, a medical emergency.

        c. The Centor criteria were developed to help guide proper diagnosis and treatment.

            (1) Criteria include fever greater than $38°C$ ($100.4°F$), tender anterior cervical adenopathy, lack of a cough, and pharyngotonsillar exudates.

            (2) Presence of three out of four criteria is highly suggestive of group A β-hemolytic strep (GABHS).

            (3) With only one criteria, GABHS is highly unlikely.

            (4) Presence of two criteria indicates the need for culture.

    3. Common types of pharyngitis and their management

        a. Streptococcal pharyngitis

            (1) Clinical features

                (a) Acute onset, fever, exudate in posterior pharynx or on tonsils, and cervical adenopathy suggest GABHS as the cause. In children, it may present as abdominal pain secondary to adenopathy in the abdomen.

                (b) Rapid strep screening is indicated; if negative and the diagnosis is still suspicious, throat culture should be obtained to confirm.

            (2) Treatment

                (a) Treat with penicillin or erythromycin.

                (b) Complications of improper or incomplete treatment include rheumatic fever, Ludwig's angina, and tonsillar abscess.

        b. Viral pharyngitis

            (1) Clinical features

                (a) Insidious onset, often with coryza, and usually lacking exudate. Fever is low grade; lymphadenopathy may or may not be present.

                (b) Obtain a rapid strep screen or throat culture to rule out streptococcal infection.

            (2) Treatment: Treatment is supportive in nature.

        c. Peritonsillar cellulitis and abscess (quinsy)

            (1) Clinical features include severe sore throat, pain on swallowing or opening the mouth wide, deviation of the soft palate and uvula, and a muffled voice.

            (2) Treatment requires either aspiration or incision and drainage followed by a course of antibiotics. Tonsillectomy may be indicated in about 10% of cases.

            (3) Indications for tonsillectomy include air way obstruction causing sleep apnea or persistent marked asymmetry of tonsils. Relative indications include recurrent streptococcal infection causing loss of work or school, recurrent abscess or chronic tonsillitis.

D. Laryngitis

    1. General characteristics: It typically is viral and follows a URI.

    2. Clinical features: Hoarseness is the hallmark; there is little to no pain with loss of voice.

    3. Treatment is supportive; to prevent the formation of vocal nodules, patients should not overuse their voice (e.g., shouting, singing).

E. Aphthous ulcers (canker sores) and other oral lesions

    1. General characteristics: Canker sores can be idiopathic or associated with herpes virus.

    2. Clinical features: They are found on the buccal mucosa, can be single or multiple, and manifest as painful, round ulcers with red halos. Typically, they are recurrent.

    3. Treatment is nonspecific; symptomatic treatment includes topical steroids or anesthetics and anti-inflammatories.

    4. Candidiasis causes burning pain in areas of the tongue, inside the cheek, or in the throat. It can be scraped off, which leaves the underlying area raw, erythematous, and friable. It often is seen in immunocompromised patients and in the use of broad-spectrum antibiotics. It is treated with antifungals in the form of a liquid, with which the patient performs a "swish and swallow" technique, or in a troche that is allowed to dissolve in the mouth.

    5. Leukoplakia is a painless white area on the tongue, inside the cheek, on the lower lip, or on the floor of the mouth. It usually is seen in patients who use chewing tobacco, smokers, those with AIDS, and with ethanol

(ETOH) abuse. Unlike candidiasis, it cannot be scraped off. The area should be biopsied to rule out cancer; however, less than 5% of these areas have been shown to be malignant. Malignancies are more likely in an erythroplastic lesion.

F. Epiglottitis

   1. General characteristics

      a. Epiglottitis is a life-threatening infection of the epiglottis and surrounding tissues that leads to obstructive respiratory disease.

      b. It is most commonly caused by group A streptococci, pneumococci, staphylococci, or *Haemophilus influenzae*.

      c. It was once more common in children, but can occur at any age. It is more common in adults since the onset of the vaccine against *Haemophilus influenzae*.

      d. Diabetics are at higher risk.

   2. Clinical features: Onset is abrupt, with high fever, difficulty swallowing, sore throat, drooling, and in children, sitting in the tripod or sniffing position.

   3. Laboratory studies

      a. A lateral soft-tissue neck radiograph reveals a thumb-like projection (the classic thumb sign).

      b. Controlled intubation should be performed, and the patient should not be left alone until intubation has occurred.

      c. Examination should be limited, causing no undue distress until the airway is maintained.

   4. Treatment

      a. Patients need IV fluids and antibiotics for 24 to 72 hours, followed by oral antibiotics to complete a 10-day course.

      b. All unimmunized close contacts should be given prophylaxis with rifampin.

G. Epistaxis (nosebleed)

   1. Kiesselbach's plexus on the anterior aspect of the nose is the most common site of epistaxis.

   2. Epistaxis may be caused by minor trauma, dry mucosa, nasal trauma, or an acquired or genetic coagulopathy.

   3. Treatment

      a. Begin with the patient sitting or standing upright, apply firm pressure to the nares for 10 to 15 minutes, and then identify the bleeding site. Visualization is aided by use of a light source and a nasal speculum.

      b. If a bleeding site can be identified, anesthetize with cocaine or lidocaine, and cauterize with a silver nitrate stick.

      c. Recauterize and pack if necessary. The packing is left in place for 24 hours.

      d. The patient should be told to return if bleeding recurs.

   4. Posterior bleed (Woodruff's plexus) is uncommon and significant, requiring emergency evaluation and treatment.

      a. It usually is caused by acute trauma, and the bleeding generally is arterial. Often, blood is seen in the posterior pharynx.

      b. The bleeding may compromise the airway, and a posterior pack must be placed. This usually requires an ear, nose, and throat consult.

      c. The patient is at risk for toxic shock syndrome secondary to retained packing.

H. Polyps

   1. Polyps are pedunculated tumors found on the nasal mucosa.

   2. They often are seen in patients with allergic rhinitis, and they often are easily visualized. There is a somewhat common triad of asthma, nasal polyps, and aspirin sensitivity.

   3. Patients may have nasal phonations and complain of feeling congested all the time.

   4. In most cases, polyps are benign. They should be removed if corticosteroid treatment fails to diminish their size.

Pulmonology

Matthew A. McQuillan

I. INFECTIOUS DISORDERS

A. Pneumonia

1. Pneumonia denotes inflammation in the alveoli or interstitium of the lung caused by microorganisms.

2. Pneumonia ranks as the primary cause of mortality from infectious diseases.

3. Classic community-acquired pneumonia (CAP)

   a. General characteristics

      (1) Acquired in the home or nonhospital environment.

      (2) In most cases of CAP, the causative agent is not identified. However, in those cases where an agent is identified, bacteria are more commonly found.

      (3) Causative agents include *Streptococcus pneumoniae, Haemophilus influenzae, Moraxella catarrhalis, Staphylococcus aureus, Klebsiella pneumoniae*, and other Gram-negative bacilli. Viral causes include influenza virus, respiratory syncytial virus (RSV), adenovirus, and parainfluenza.

   b. Clinical features

      (1) Typical presentation is a 1- to 10-day history of increasing cough, purulent sputum, shortness of breath, tachycardia, pleuritic chest pain, fever or hypothermia, sweats, and rigors.

      (2) Physical examination may reveal altered breath sounds and crackles, dullness to percussion if an effusion is present, and bronchial breath sounds over an area of consolidation. *Note:* The chest exam alone is not sufficient to confirm or exclude the diagnosis.

      (3) Table 2-1 provides classic descriptions of pneumonias caused by specific organisms. Although these characteristics may help in attempting to identify specific pathogens, exceptions and less typical presentations are common.

      (4) Table 2-2 lists the pathogens more likely to occur in certain patient groups. *Streptococcus pneumoniae* remains the most common cause of bacterial pneumonia in all groups.

   c. Laboratory findings

      (1) Organisms may be detected with conventional stain or sputum culture, although typically this is not done before starting treatment. The most common bacterial pathogen identified is *Streptococcus pneumoniae*.

      (2) Chest radiography (CXR) shows lobar or segmental infiltrates, air bronchograms, and pleural effusions. There is no pathognomonic radiographic presentation.

   d. Treatment

      (1) The patient who is otherwise healthy and free of respiratory distress or complications may be treated as an outpatient with oral antibiotics and appropriate supportive care.

      (2) Doxycycline, erythromycin, macrolides (clarithromycin, azithromycin), or fluoroquinolones are appropriate choices for outpatient treatment.

      (3) Neutropenia, involvement of more than one lobe, or poor host resistance indicates a need for hospitalization. Also, consider hospitalization for patients older than 50 years with comorbidities, altered mental status, or hemodynamic instability.

      (4) If inpatient treatment is necessary, consider coverage of *Streptococcus pneumoniae* and *Legionella* sp. with ceftriaxone or cefotaxime plus azithromycin or a fluoroquinolone.

      (5) The polyvalent pneumococcal vaccine (Pneumovax) contains antigens of 23 common strains of the pneumococcus. Studies have shown efficacy ranging from 51% to 86% in reducing serious pneumococcal disease. The pneumococcal conjugate vaccine (PCV) is recommended as a series of 4 doses for children aged 6 weeks to 15 months. The pneumococcal polysaccharide vaccine (PPV) is recommended for children aged 2 to 5 years who have not been previously immunized, persons ≥65 years of age or any person with a chronic illness that increases the risk of CAP including cardiopulmonary diseases, sickle cell disease, splenectomy, and liver disease. Booster shots are needed about every 6 years. Some sources recommend PPV for any person requesting vaccination.

TABLE 2-1	Typical Manifestations of Pneumonia per Pathogen
Organism	**Typical Manifestations**
Mycoplasma pneumoniae	Low-grade fever
	Cough
	Bullous myringitis
	Cold agglutinins
Pneumocystis jiroveci (nee carinii)	Slower onset, immunosuppression
	Increased lactate dehydrogenase
	More hypoxemic than appears on chest radiography
	Interstitial infiltrates
Legionella pneumoniae	Chronic cardiac or respiratory disease
	Hyponatremia
	Diarrhea, other systemic symptoms
Chlamydia pneumoniae	Longer prodrome
	Sore throat, hoarseness
Streptococcus pneumoniae	Single rigor
	Rust-colored sputum
Klebsiella pneumoniae	Currant jelly sputum
	Chronic illness, including alcohol abuse

TABLE 2-2	Pathogens More Likely to Cause Pneumonia in Certain Patient Groups
Patient Characteristic	**Pathogen More Likely Seen in this Group**
Alcohol abuse	Klebsiella pneumoniae
COPD	Haemophilus pneumoniae
Cystic fibrosis	Pseudomonas sp.
Young adults, college settings	Mycoplasma pneumoniae
	Chlamydia pneumoniae
Air conditioning/aerosolized water	Legionella pneumoniae
Postsplenectomy	Encapsulated organisms
	Streptococcus pneumoniae
	Haemophilus pneumoniae
Leukemia, lymphoma	Fungus
Children, <1 year	Respiratory syncytial virus
Children, <2 year	Parainfluenza virus

COPD, chronic obstructive pulmonary disease.

4. Atypical CAP
   a. General characteristics
      (1) As the term *atypical* implies, this form of pneumonia has a clinical presentation different from that of classic CAP.
      (2) *Mycoplasma pneumoniae* is the most common cause of atypical pneumonias. Other causes include viruses (influenza types A and B and adenoviruses), *Chlamydia pneumoniae*, *Legionella* sp., and *Moraxella* sp.
   b. Clinical features
      (1) The typical presentation of atypical pneumonia is a low-grade fever with relatively mild pulmonary symptoms, which are self-limited, occurring in young, otherwise healthy adults. A nonproductive cough, myalgia, and fatigue are common.

(2) *Legionella* infection is associated with exposure to contaminated water droplets from cooling and ventilation systems. Acute development of high fever, dry cough, dyspnea, and systemic symptoms is common.

(3) Viral pneumonias are variable in presentation but often are associated with epidemics and upper respiratory symptoms.

c. Laboratory findings

(1) Organisms usually are not detected with conventional stain or culture of sputum.

(2) The white blood cell (WBC) count is normal or only slightly elevated.

(3) Radiography shows segmental unilateral lower lung zone infiltrates or diffuse infiltrates.

d. Treatment

(1) Antibiotic treatment is started empirically based on the clinical features. Regimens include erythromycin (for suspected *Mycoplasma pneumoniae* and *Legionella* infection) and tetracycline (for suspected *Chlamydia* infection).

(2) Viral pneumonias are treated with supportive measures (analgesics, fluids, cough suppressants) unless influenza is suspected. Amantadine and rimantadine are no longer recommended in the treatment of influenza because of increasing resistance. Neuraminidase inhibitors (inhaled zanamivir or oral oseltamivir) may be used if antiviral therapy is indicated. Influenza type A resistance to oseltamivir is a developing issue; Centers for Disease Control and Prevention (CDC) recommendations call for use of confirmatory tests and, if positive for influenza A, combination treatment with oseltamivir and rimantadine.

5. Hospital-acquired (nosocomial) pneumonia

a. General characteristics

(1) Hospital-acquired pneumonia is caused by organisms that colonize ill patients, staff, and equipment, producing clinical infection more than 48 hours after admission to the hospital. Those at highest risk are intensive care unit (ICU) patients on mechanical ventilation.

(2) Pneumonia is the second most common cause of hospital-acquired infection.

(3) The causative organisms are unique and the mortality rate is 20% to 50%.

(a) The usual organisms are *Staphylococcus aureus* and Gram-negative bacilli, which are easy to recover from respiratory secretions.

(b) *Pseudomonas aeruginosa* is the most likely pathogen in ICUs and carries the worst prognosis. Others include *Staphylococcus aureus*, *Klebsiella* sp., *Escherichia coli*, and *Enterobacter* sp.

b. Clinical features are similar to those with CAP.

c. Laboratory findings: Diagnosis is clinical and supported with Gram's stain and culture of sputum and blood. The CXR may help to support the diagnosis.

d. Treatment includes use of appropriate empiric antibiotics such as cefepime, ticarcillin/clavulanic acid, piperacillin/tazobactam, meropenem. If an organism is isolated, therapy can be based on the culture results. Patients may need aggressive supportive measures including mechanical ventilation as appropriate.

6. Pneumonia: HIV related

a. General characteristics

(1) *Pneumocystis jiroveci* (formerly *P. carinii*) is the most common opportunistic infection in patients with HIV disease, typically with CD4 counts of less than 200 cells/μL.

(2) *Pneumocystis* infection also occurs in patients with cancer, malnourished states, and immunosuppression.

(3) Other pathogens common in patients with HIV and pneumonia include *Streptococcus*, *Haemophilus*, *Pseudomonas*, and *Mycobacterium* sp.

b. Clinical features

(1) Pneumocystis pneumonia typically presents with fever, tachypnea, dyspnea, and nonproductive cough.

(2) Nonpneumocystis pneumonia typically follows a more fulminant course than in non–HIV-infected persons.

c. Laboratory findings

(1) CXR is the cornerstone of diagnosis. The radiograph typically shows diffuse or perihilar infiltrates; no effusions are seen.

(2) Lymphopenia and a low CD4 count are typical.

(3) Sputum staining, via either induced sputum or bronchoalveolar lavage, will establish the diagnosis in more than 90% of patients.

d. Treatment

(1) Trimethoprim/sulfamethoxazole (Bactrim) is the treatment of choice.

(2) There is an extremely high mortality rate (near 100%) if not treated.

(3) Prophylaxis is recommended in all patients with a CD4 count of less than 200 cells/μL or with a history of *Pneumocystis* infection. Trimethoprim/sulfamethoxazole is the antibiotic of choice.

B. Tuberculosis (TB)

1. General characteristics

   a. *Mycobacterium tuberculosis* infection is acquired by inhaling organisms within aerosol droplets expelled during coughing by people with active disease.

   b. Most exposed people mount an immune response sufficient to prevent progression from primary infection to clinical illness. Overall, 10% of persons infected with TB will develop the disease. This is called primary TB.

   c. Approximately 5% of exposed people fail to contain the primary infection and progress to active TB within 2 years; this is known as progressive primary TB.

   d. Approximately 95% of infected persons will contain the bacterium without becoming symptomatic. This is known as latent TB infection (LTBI). These patients are not considered to be infectious, nor can they spread the disease. They are asymptomatic but have inactive TB in their body, most commonly in the apices of the lungs. Reactivation TB develops from LTBI in the setting of immune compromise.

   e. Outbreaks since the mid-1990s have seen an emergence of organisms resistant to multiple antituberculous drugs.

2. Clinical features

   a. Cough is the most common symptom. It begins as a dry cough and progresses to a productive cough, with or without hemoptysis, typically over 3 weeks or longer.

   b. The classic symptom complex includes fever, drenching night sweats, anorexia, and weight loss. Other common pulmonary symptoms are cough, pleuritic chest pain, dyspnea, and hemoptysis. Posttussive rales are classic.

   c. On examination, the patient may appear chronically ill and malnourished.

3. Laboratory findings

   a. Radiography

      (1) Primary TB: Homogeneous infiltrates, hilar/paratracheal lymph node enlargement, segmental atelectasis, cavitations with progressive disease.

      (2) Reactivation TB: Fibrocavitary apical disease, nodules, infiltrates, posterior and apical segments of the right upper lobe, apical–posterior segments of the left upper lobe, superior segments of the lower lobes.

      (3) Ghon complexes (calcified primary focus) and Ranke complexes (calcified primary focus and calcified hilar lymph node) represent healed primary infection.

   b. The tuberculin skin test (TST) identifies individuals who have been infected, but it does not differentiate between active and latent infection. Tuberculin skin testing (such as the PPD [purified protein derivative]) is reported according to the diameter of induration, not erythema (Table 2-3).

   c. Definitive diagnosis requires the identification of *Mycobacterium tuberculosis* from cultures or by DNA or RNA amplification techniques. Demonstration of acid-fast bacilli on sputum supports, but does not confirm, a diagnosis of TB.

   d. Biopsy revealing caseating granulomas (also known as necrotizing granulomas) is the histologic hallmark.

4. Treatment

   a. Antituberculous drugs, including isoniazid (INH), rifampin (RIF), pyrazinamide (PZA), and ethambutol (EMB), are the cornerstone of therapy. CDC recommends multiple drug regimens such as:

      (1) LTBI: INH for 9 months *or* RIF for 4 months *or* RIF and PZA for 2 months (only if in contact with TB-resistant persons). *Note*: Treat for LTBI only after active TB is ruled out as active TB is treated with a multidrug regimen.

      (2) Active TB: INH/RIF/PZA/EMB for 2 months, followed by INH/RIF for 4 months. This regimen is only recommended if the isolate is INH sensitive.

      (3) Drug-resistant TB: Other regimens are recommended for patients who are drug resistant. Expert advice should be sought if the clinician is unfamiliar with drug-resistant TB.

      (4) For more information and alternative treatment regimens, see www.cdc.gov

   b. Antituberculous class-specific side effects

      (1) INH: hepatitis, peripheral neuropathy; coadminister vitamin B$_6$ (pyridoxine) to reduce the risk.

      (2) RIF: hepatitis, flu syndrome, orange body fluid (e.g., orange urine).

      (3) EMB: optic neuritis (red–green vision loss).

TABLE 2-3	**Classification of Positive Tuberculin Skin Test Reactions**
Reaction Size	**Group**
≥5 mm	HIV-positive persons
	Recent contacts of those with active tuberculosis
	Persons with evidence of tuberculosis on chest radiography
	Immunosuppressed patients on steroids
≥10 mm	Recent immigrants from countries with high rate of tuberculosis
	HIV-negative injection drug users
	Mycobacteriology laboratory personnel
	Residents/employees of high-risk congregate settings
	Persons with certain medical conditions: diabetes mellitus, silicosis, chronic renal failure, etc.
	Children younger than 4 years, or infants, children and adolescents exposed to adults at high risk
	Infants, children, adolescents exposed to adults at high risk
≥15 mm	Persons with no risk factors for tuberculosis

    c. Patients with active disease require combination chemotherapy for 6 to 9 months; patients infected with HIV require therapy for at least 1 year.

    d. INH for 6 to 12 months is indicated for prophylaxis in patients who have tested negative in the past but are now positive with known or unknown exposure (converters).

    e. Persons exposed to active TB should be screened with TST. Indurations greater than 5 mm should be treated aggressively.

    f. The bacille Calmette–Guérin (BCG) vaccine can be administered to a tuberculin-negative person in cases with a high risk for intense, prolonged exposure to untreated or ineffectively treated cases of infectious TB. This practice is not recommended in the United States, but it is common in areas with endemic TB.

    g. Children, adolescents, and the immunocompromised who have been in close contact with a person with active TB should be offered treatment until a TST is negative 12 weeks after exposure. Treatment of other cases should be dictated by TST status.

C. Acute bronchitis

  1. General characteristics

    a. More than 90% of cases are caused by viruses including rhinovirus, coronavirus, and RSV.

    b. Bronchitis is defined as inflammation of the airways (trachea, bronchi, bronchioles) characterized by cough.

    c. In patients with chronic lung disease, causes also include *Haemophilus influenzae*, *Streptococcus pneumoniae*, and *Moraxella catarrhalis*.

  2. Clinical features

    a. Signs and symptoms include cough (with or without sputum), dyspnea, fever, sore throat, headache, myalgias, substernal discomfort, and expiratory rhonchi or wheezes. *Note*: Sputum color is not predictive of bacterial involvement.

    b. Bronchitis can be difficult to distinguish from pneumonia, so the examination should be conducted to identify comorbid conditions that may influence the treatment.

  3. Laboratory findings: Generally, no laboratory evaluation is required unless there is a strong need to differentiate bronchitis from pneumonia. The CXR will be negative in acute bronchitis.

  4. Treatment

    a. Supportive measures include hydration, expectorants, analgesics, β_2-agonists, and cough suppressants.

    b. For acute exacerbations of chronic bronchitis, in which bacterial causes are more likely, empiric first-line treatment is a second-generation cephalosporin; second-line treatment is a second-generation macrolide or trimethoprim/sulfamethoxazole.

    c. Antibiotics are indicated for the following: Elderly patients, those with underlying cardiopulmonary diseases and a cough for more than 7 to 10 days, and any patient who is immunocompromised.

    d. For acute exacerbations in otherwise healthy adults, no empiric treatment is needed.

D. Acute bronchiolitis

1. General characteristics

   a. Bronchiolitis refers to inflammation of the bronchioles (airways smaller than 2 mm in diameter). It is primarily an illness of young children and infants.

   b. RSV is the most common cause; other agents include parainfluenza, adenovirus, and rhinovirus.

2. Clinical features

   a. Signs and symptoms include rhinorrhea, sneezing, wheezing, and low-grade fever.

   b. Nasal flaring, tachypnea, and retractions indicate respiratory distress.

3. Laboratory findings

   a. The CBC usually is normal. Nasal washings for RSV culture and antigen assay often are done in infants.

   b. CXR is normal but can show air trapping and peribronchial thickening.

4. Treatment

   a. If RSV is present, consider hospitalization and administration of ribavirin. This is especially important for infants born premature or who are severely ill.

   b. Supportive measures, such as nebulized albuterol, intravenous (IV) fluids, antipyretics, chest physiotherapy, and humidified oxygen, are important.

E. Acute epiglottitis

1. General characteristics

   a. This is a severe, life-threatening infection of the epiglottis.

   b. It may be of viral or bacterial origin.

   c. It may occur at any age; in children, it is most common between ages 2 and 7 years. In adults, most cases occur in the 45 to 65 age group.

   d. The widespread administration of the *H. influenzae* type B (Hib) vaccine has decreased the incidence of epiglottitis in children. Most adults, however, have not been immunized; therefore, the incidence of Hib-induced epiglottitis has increased in this population. The most common etiologies in adults include group A *Streptococcus*, *Streptococcus pneumoniae*, *Haemophilus parainfluenzae*, and *Staphylococcus aureus*.

2. Clinical findings

   a. Signs and symptoms include sudden onset of high fever, respiratory distress, severe dysphagia, drooling, and muffled voice.

   b. Examination may reveal mild stridor with little or no coughing; patients usually sit upright with their necks extended.

3. Laboratory findings

   a. Direct visualization of the epiglottis is diagnostic, but manipulation may initiate sudden, fatal airway obstruction in children. This is less common in adults.

   b. Once the airway is secured, obtain a complete blood count (CBC) and blood and epiglottic cultures.

   c. A lateral neck radiograph shows swollen epiglottis (thumbprint sign).

4. Treatment

   a. Secure airway: Do not move or upset the child unless ready to manage the airway.

   b. Administer broad-spectrum second- or third-generation cephalosporin such as cefotaxime or ceftriaxone for 7 to 10 days.

F. Croup

1. General characteristics

   a. Also known as acute viral laryngotracheobronchitis, which more commonly affects children 6 months to 5 years.

   b. Most common cause is the parainfluenza virus types 1 and 2. RSV, adenovirus, influenza, and rhinovirus are also implicated.

2. Clinical findings

   a. Harsh barking seal–like cough, inspiratory stridor, hoarseness, aphonia, low-grade fever, and rhinorrhea.

   b. The diagnosis is usually clinical.

3. Laboratory findings

   a. Posteroanterior (PA) neck film may show steeple sign due to subglottic narrowing. Lateral neck film will differentiate croup from epiglottitis.

4. Treatment
   a. Mild croup does not usually require treatment.
   b. Corticosteroids, humidified air or oxygen, and nebulized epinephrine may also be recommended.
   c. Hospitalization may be required for patients with severe symptoms.

II. NEOPLASTIC DISEASE

A. Bronchogenic carcinoma
   1. General
      a. Bronchogenic carcinoma is the leading cause of cancer deaths in men and women. There are more deaths from lung cancer than from colon, breast, and prostate combined.
      b. The overall 5-year survival rate is 15%.
      c. Smoking is the number one risk factor.
      d. Bronchogenic carcinoma is divided into two major categories based on staging and treatment options: small cell lung cancer (SCLC), and non-SCLC (NSCLC).
         (1) SCLC (oat cell) accounts for 25% to 35% of cases; it is more likely to spread early and rarely is amenable to surgery (mean survival is 6 to 18 weeks). SCLC tends to originate in the central bronchi and to metastasize to regional lymph nodes. It is prone to early metastasis and an aggressive clinical course; assume micrometastases at presentation.
         (2) NSCLC grows more slowly and is more amenable to surgery. NSCLC includes squamous cell carcinoma, adenocarcinoma, and large cell carcinoma.
            (a) Squamous cell carcinoma: Represents 25% to 35% of cases; bronchial in origin and a centrally located mass; more likely to present with hemoptysis and therefore more likely to be diagnosed via sputum cytology.
            (b) Adenocarcinoma: The most common type of bronchogenic carcinoma, accounting for 35% to 40% of cases; typically metastatic to distant organs; this tumor arises from mucous glands, usually appears in the periphery of the lung, and is not amenable to early detection through sputum examination. Bronchoalveolar cell carcinoma, a subtype of adenocarcinoma, is a low-grade carcinoma.
            (c) Large cell carcinoma: A heterogeneous group of undifferentiated types that do not fit elsewhere; cytology typically shows large cells; doubling time is rapid, and metastasis is early; there may be central or peripheral masses.
   2. Clinical features
      a. Symptoms include cough, hemoptysis, pain, anorexia, weight loss, or asthenia.
      b. Patients may also exhibit lymphadenopathy, hepatomegaly, and clubbing.
      c. Paraneoplastic syndromes occur in 10% to 20% of patients with lung cancer (Table 2-4).
   3. Laboratory findings
      a. CXR and CT scans usually demonstrate abnormalities.
      b. Cytologic examination of sputum, if adequate cells are obtained, permits definitive diagnosis of a specific cell type in many cases.
      c. Bronchoscopy, examination of pleural fluid, and biopsy also are used to establish a diagnosis by looking at specific cell types through direct visualization.
      d. Positron emission tomography (PET) scans may also aid in diagnosis and prevent unnecessary surgery.
   4. Treatment
      a. For NSCLC, surgery remains the treatment of choice. The 5-year survival rate after resection is 35% to 40%.
      b. For SCLC, combination chemotherapy is the treatment of choice and results in improved median survival, although patients rarely live for more than 5 years after the diagnosis is established.
   5. Complications common to all types of bronchogenic carcinoma are listed in Table 2-5.

B. Solitary pulmonary nodule
   1. General characteristics
      a. Pulmonary nodules also are known as coin lesions. If the lesion measures greater than 3 cm, it is referred to as a mass.
      b. Most solitary nodules are infectious granulomas from old or active TB, fungal infection, or foreign body reaction. Approximately 40% are malignant and represent carcinoma, hamartoma, or metastasis (but these are usually multiple) as well as bronchial adenoma (95% are carcinoid tumors).

TABLE 2-4 **Paraneoplastic Syndromes**

Classification	Syndrome	Histological Type
Endocrine/metabolic	Cushing's syndrome	Small cell
	SIADH	Small cell
	Hypercalcemia	Squamous cell
	Gynecomastia	Large cell
Neuromuscular	Peripheral neuropathy	Small cell
	Myesthenia (Eaton–Lambert)	Small cell
	Cerebellar degeneration	Small cell
Cardiovascular	Thrombophlebitis	Adenocarcinoma
Hematologic	Anemia	All
	DIC	All
	Eosinophilia	All
	Thrombocytosis	All
Cutaneous	*Acanthosis nigricans*	All

SIADH, syndrome of inappropriate antidiuretic hormone; *DIC*, disseminated intravascular coagulation.

TABLE 2-5 **Sphere of Lung Cancer Complications**

SVC syndrome	Compression of SVC: plethora, headache, mental status changes
Pancoast's tumor	Tumor of the lung apex
	Causes Horner's syndrome and shoulder pain
	Affects brachial plexus and cervical sympathetic nerve
Horner's syndrome	Unilateral facial anhidrosis, ptosis, miosis
Endocrine	Carcinoid syndrome: flushing, diarrhea, telangiectasias
Recurrent laryngeal nerve	Hoarseness
Effusions	Exudative

SVC, superior vena cava.

   c. Malignancy is rare in patients younger than 30 years. Smokers have an increased risk of malignancy; this increased risk rises with the number of pack-years smoked.

  2. Clinical features: Most pulmonary nodules are found unexpectedly at radiography and are asymptomatic.

  3. Laboratory findings

   a. A solitary pulmonary nodule (coin lesion) is a round or oval, sharply circumscribed pulmonary lesion/mass (up to 5 cm in diameter) surrounded by normal lung tissue.

   b. Central cavitation, calcification, or surrounding (satellite) lesions may occur.

   c. A lesion that has not enlarged in more than 2 years suggests a benign cause. Most are infectious granulomas.

   d. Malignant lesions occasionally are symptomatic, tend to occur in patients older than 45 years, usually are greater than 2 cm in diameter, often have indistinct margins, exhibit rapid progression in size, and rarely are calcified.

  4. Treatment

   a. Lesions with a low probability of malignancy can be watched. Patients should undergo CT every 3 months for a year; if stable, frequency of CT can be reduced to every 6 months for the next 2 years.

   b. Lesions with a high probability of malignancy should be resected as soon as possible. An interim biopsy is not recommended.

   c. Lesions with intermediate probability of malignancy should be biopsied; use transthoracic needle biopsy or bronchoscopy if the lesion is peripheral. False-positive rates can be as high as 25%. High-resolution CT or PET may aid in establishing the diagnosis. High-resolution CT is best to delineate the mass and detect adenopathy or the presence of multiple nodules.

 C. Carcinoid tumors

  1. General characteristics

    a. Also known as carcinoid adenomas or bronchial gland tumors, these are well-differentiated neuroendocrine tumors that affect men and women equally. Patients usually are younger than 60 years.

    b. Carcinoid tumors are low-grade malignant neoplasms. They grow slowly and rarely metastasize.

  2. Clinical features

    a. Hemoptysis, cough, focal wheezing, and recurrent pneumonia. Bleeding and obstruction are common.

    b. Carcinoid syndrome (flushing, diarrhea, wheezing, hypotension) is rare.

  3. Laboratory findings

    a. Bronchoscopy reveals a pink or purple central lesion that is well vascularized. The lesion can be pedunculated or sessile.

    b. CT and octreotide scintigraphy localize the disease. CT will localize the lesion as well as monitor for growth.

  4. Treatment: Surgical excision carries a good prognosis. The lesions are resistant to radiation therapy and chemotherapy.

III. OBSTRUCTIVE PULMONARY DISEASE

  A. Asthma

    1. General characteristics

      a. Asthma is characterized by three components: obstruction of airflow, bronchial hyperreactivity, and inflammation of the airway. It is a disease of chronic inflammation leading to airway narrowing and increased mucus production.

      b. Asthma affects 5% of the population. Prevalence, hospitalization, and mortality have risen during the past 20 years.

      c. Many asthma syndromes have been identified: extrinsic allergic, allergic bronchopulmonary aspergillosis, intrinsic asthma, extrinsic nonallergic, aspirin sensitivity, exercise induced, and asthma associated with chronic obstructive pulmonary disease (COPD).

      d. The strongest predisposing factor to asthma is atopy. The atopic triad consists of wheeze, eczema, and seasonal rhinitis.

      e. Exacerbations often are correlated with common precipitants: allergens (especially dust and dust mites, dander, cockroaches, and pollen), exercise, upper respiratory tract infections, postnasal drip, gastroesophageal reflux disease, drugs (β-blockers, angiotensin-converting enzyme inhibitors, aspirin, nonsteroidal anti-inflammatory drugs [NSAIDs]), stress, cold air or change in the weather, environmental irritants, and others.

    2. Clinical features

      a. Patients have an intermittent occurrence of cough, chest tightness, breathlessness, and wheezing. One-third of children have no wheeze.

      b. Patients undergo asymptomatic periods between these attacks.

      c. Asthma is classified according to the frequency of symptoms and pulmonary function testing. In children, especially those under the age of 5, the classification of asthma severity is more aggressive (Table 2-6).

    3. Laboratory findings

      a. Airflow obstruction is indicated by decreased ratio of forced expiratory volume in 1 second to forced vital capacity (FEV_1/FVC: <75%). A greater than 10% increase in FEV_1 after bronchodilator therapy is supportive of the diagnosis.

      b. Arterial blood gas (ABG) measurements may be normal in mild cases, but in severe cases, they can reveal hypoxemia and hypercapnia, with a PaO_2 of less than 60 mm Hg and a $PaCO_2$ of more than 40 mm Hg. ABGs are rarely indicated or obtained unless the patient is severely ill or nonresponsive to treatment.

      c. CXR may show hyperinflation. Radiography is only indicated if pneumonia is suspected, the asthma is complicated, or another disorder is suspected.

      d. Handheld peak expiratory flow meters estimate variability and quantify severity of attacks. Use of this objective device should be encouraged in patients with chronic disease.

      e. A histamine or methacholine challenge test (bronchial provocation test) may help to establish the diagnosis of asthma when spirometry is nondiagnostic. An FEV_1 decrease of more than 20% is diagnostic.

    4. Treatment

      a. The goals of treatment are to minimize chronic symptoms; prevent recurrent exacerbations and, thus, minimize the need for urgent care visits; and maintain near-normal pulmonary function.

      b. Asthma medications can be divided into long-term control (corticosteroids, cromolyn, nedocromil, long-acting bronchodilators, leukotriene modifiers, and theophylline) and quick-relief medications (short-acting inhaled β_2-agonists, ipratropium bromide, and systemic corticosteroids).

TABLE 2-6	Classification of Severity of Chronic Stable Asthma			
Severity	Symptoms	Nighttime Symptoms	Use of Rescue Medication	Lung Function
Intermittent	Symptoms ≤2 days per week	≤2 times per month	<2 days per week	FEV_1 >80% predicted
	No interference with daily activities			FEV_1/FVC normal
Mild persistent	>2 days per week but not daily	3–4 times per month	>2 days per week but not daily, and not more than once on any day	FEV_1 >80% predicted
	Minor limitation			FEV_1/FVC normal
Moderate persistent	Daily symptoms	>1 time per week but not nightly	Daily	FEV_1 >60% but <80% predicted
	Some limitation in daily activity			FEV_1/FVC reduced 5%
Severe persistent	Continual symptoms	Often 7 times per week	Several times per day	FEV_1 <60% predicted
	Extremely limited physical activities			FEV_1/FVC reduced >5%

FEV_1, forced expiratory volume in 1 second; FVC, forced vital capacity.

From the National Asthma Education and Prevention Program Expert Panel Report 3: *Guidelines for the Diagnosis and Management of Asthma.* Bethesda, MD: National Institutes of Health; 2007. Publication 08-4051.

c. Treatment algorithms are based on both the severity of the patient's baseline asthma and the severity of asthma exacerbations. In children, especially those under the age of 5, the stepwise approach to treatment is more aggressive (Fig. 2-1).

d. β-adrenergic agonists should be available to induce bronchodilation during acute symptoms (rescue medication).

e. Inhaled corticosteroids are the most effective anti-inflammatory medications for management of chronic asthma.

f. Patients should be educated about their disease and the use of peak flow monitoring. Daily evaluation of pulmonary function with a peak flow meter is an important component of optimal asthma management. This type of monitoring warns of changes in disease status and allows for adjustments on a daily basis if needed. Changes in peak flow will occur prior to clinical symptoms.

B. Bronchiectasis

1. General characteristics

a. Bronchiectasis is defined as an abnormal, permanent dilatation of the bronchi and destruction of bronchial walls. It can be congenital (cystic fibrosis) or acquired from recurrent infections (TB, fungal infection, lung abscess) or obstruction (tumor).

b. Bronchiectasis results from bronchial injury subsequent to severe infection and/or inflammation.

c. Cystic fibrosis causes half of all cases.

2. Clinical features

a. Symptoms include chronic purulent sputum (often foul smelling), hemoptysis, chronic cough, and recurrent pneumonia.

b. Physical examination may reveal localized chest crackles and clubbing.

3. Laboratory findings

a. High-resolution chest CT is the imaging modality of choice; it reveals dilated, tortuous airways.

b. CXR in patients with clinically significant bronchiectasis is abnormal. The degree of abnormality depends on the extent and severity of the disease. Crowded bronchial markings and basal cystic spaces are characteristic. CXR may reveal tram-track lung markings, honeycombing, and atelectasis.

c. Bronchoscopy is warranted to evaluate hemoptysis, remove secretions, and rule out obstructing lesions.

4. Treatment

a. A productive cough should be managed with the appropriate antibiotic, bronchodilators, and chest physiotherapy.

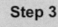

Intermittent Asthma	**Persistent Asthma: Daily Medication** Consult with asthma specialist if step 4 care or higher is required. Consider consultation at step 3.

Step 1

Preferred:

SABA PRN

Step 2

Preferred:

Low-dose ICS

Alternative:

Cromolyn, LTRA, Nedocromil, or Theophylline

Step 3

Preferred:

Low-dose ICS + LABA OR Medium-dose ICS

Alternative:

Low-dose ICS + either LTRA, Theophylline, or Zileuton

Step 4

Preferred:

Medium-dose ICS + LABA

Alternative:

Medium-dose ICS + either LTRA, Theophylline, or Zileuton

Step 5

Preferred:

High-dose ICS + LABA

AND

Consider Omalizumab for patients who have allergies

Step 6

Preferred:

High-dose ICS + LABA + oral corticosteroid

AND

Consider Omalizumab for patients who have allergies

Step up if needed

(first, check adherence, environmental control, and comorbid conditions)

Assess control

Step down if possible

(and asthma is well controlled at least 3 months)

Each step: Patient education, environmental control, and management of comorbidities.

Steps 2–4: Consider subcutaneous allergen immunotherapy for patients who have allergic asthma (see notes).

Quick-Relief Medication for All Patients

- SABA as needed for symptoms. Intensity of treatment depends on severity of symptoms: up to 3 treatments at 20-minute intervals as needed. Short course of oral systemic corticosteroids may be needed.
- Use of SABA >2 days a week for symptom relief (not prevention of EIB) generally indicates inadequate control and the need to step up treatment.

Key: **Alphabetical order is used when more than one treatment option is listed within either preferred or alternative therapy.** ICS, inhaled corticosteroid; LABA, long-acting inhaled beta$_2$-agonist; LTRA, leukotriene receptor antagonist; SABA, inhaled short-acting beta$_2$-agonist

Notes:

- The stepwise approach is meant to assist, not replace, the clinical decisionmaking required to meet individual patient needs.
- If alternative treatment is used and response is inadequate, discontinue it and use the preferred treatment before stepping up.
- Zileuton is a less desirable alternative due to limited studies as adjunctive therapy and the need to monitor liver function. Theophylline requires monitoring of serum concentration levels.
- In step 6, before oral corticosteroids are introduced, a trial of high-dose ICS + LABA + either LTRA, theophylline, or zileuton may be considered, although this approach has not been studied in clinical trials.
- Step 1, 2, and 3 preferred therapies are based on Evidence A; step 3 alternative therapy is based on Evidence A for LTRA, Evidence B for theophylline, and Evidence D for zileuton. Step 4 preferred therapy is based on Evidence B, and alternative therapy is based on Evidence B for LTRA and theophylline and Evidence D zileuton. Step 5 preferred therapy is based on Evidence B. Step 6 preferred therapy is based on (EPR—2 1997) and Evidence B for omalizumab.
- Immunotherapy for steps 2–4 is based on Evidence B for house-dust mites, animal danders, and pollens; evidence is weak or lacking for molds and cockroaches. Evidence is strongest for immunotherapy with single allergens. The role of allergy in asthma is greater in children than in adults.
- Clinicians who administer immunotherapy or omalizumab should be prepared and equipped to identify and treat anaphylaxis that may occur.

FIGURE 2-1   Stepwise approach for managing asthma. (From the National Asthma Education and Prevention Program Expert Panel Report 3: *Guidelines for the Diagnosis and Management of Asthma.* Bethesda, MD: National Institutes of Health, U.S. Department of Health and Human Services; 2007. Available at: http://www.nhlbi.nih.gov/guidelines/asthma/asthsumm.pdf.)

   b. Antibiotics are prescribed for 10 to 14 days for acute symptoms; suppressive therapy may be helpful in severe disease or in patients with rapid recurrence. Amoxicillin, amoxicillin/clavulanate, trimethoprim/sulfamethoxazole, and tetracyclines are effective choices.

   c. Bronchodilators are helpful for maintenance and for treating acute exacerbations.

   d. Patients with disabling symptoms or progressive bronchiectasis can be considered for surgery; however, surgery has little long-term benefit.

TABLE 2-7	COPD Comparisons	
	Emphysema Predominant	**Bronchitis Predominant**
Patient type	"Pink puffers"	"Blue bloaters"
Clinical findings	Exertional dyspnea	Mild dyspnea
	Cough is rare	Chronic productive cough
	Quiet lungs	Noisy lungs: rhonchi and wheeze
	No peripheral edema	Peripheral edema
	Thin; recent weight loss	Overweight and cyanotic
	Barrel chest	Pursed-lip breathing
	Hyperventilation	
Chest radiography	Decreased lung markings at apices	Increased interstitial markings at bases
	Flattened diaphragms	Diaphragms not flattened
	Hyperinflation	Parenchymal bullae and blebs
	Small, thin-appearing heart	

COPD, chronic obstructive pulmonary disease.

C. Chronic obstructive pulmonary disease (COPD)

1. General characteristics

a. COPD is a clinical and pathophysiologic syndrome that includes emphysema and chronic bronchitis. These disorders have overlapping features, and because patients often have characteristics of more than one disorder, both are classified together as COPD (Table 2-7).

(1) Emphysema is a condition in which the air spaces are enlarged as a consequence of destruction of alveolar septae.

(2) Chronic bronchitis is a disease characterized by a chronic cough that is productive of phlegm occurring on most days for 3 months of the year for 2 or more consecutive years without an otherwise-defined acute cause.

b. Smoking is the most important cause of COPD. Other causes include environmental pollutants, recurrent upper respiratory infections, eosinophilia, bronchial hyperresponsiveness, and α_1-antitrypsin deficiency.

2. Clinical features

a. Patients present with a history of progressive shortness of breath, excessive cough, and sputum production. Patients with predominantly emphysematous COPD may have dry cough and weight loss.

b. The physical examination of a patient with advanced COPD may reveal asthenia, dyspnea, pursed-lip breathing, and grunting expirations.

c. Chest examination

(1) Signs of hyperinflation with increase in the anteroposterior dimension are noted.

(2) Percussion yields increased resonance.

(3) Auscultation reveals decreased breath sounds and early inspiratory crackles.

(4) Wheezing may not be present at rest but can be evoked with forced expiration or exertion.

(5) The duration of expiration is prolonged.

d. In patients with chronic bronchitis, rhonchi reflect secretions in the airways, and breathing typically is raspy and loud.

3. Laboratory findings

a. Chest radiography

(1) CXR may show hyperinflation of the lungs and flat diaphragms; however, a CXR is not sensitive or specific enough to serve as a diagnostic or screening tool.

(2) If emphysema is the main clinical feature, parenchymal bullae or subpleural blebs are pathognomonic.

(3) In chronic bronchitis, nonspecific peribronchial and perivascular markings may be present.

b. Pulmonary function testing

(1) Airflow obstruction demonstrated on forced expiratory spirometry is suggestive.

(2) The FEV_1/FVC ratio is decreased.

c. The CBC may show polycythemia caused by chronic hypoxemia.

4. Treatment

    a. In symptomatic patients, the goal of treatment is to improve functional state and relieve symptoms.

    b. Smoking cessation is the single most important intervention.

    c. Anticholinergic inhalers (ipratropium or tiotropium) are superior to β-adrenergic agonists in achieving bronchodilation.

    d. Short-acting bronchodilators should be prescribed for acute exacerbations of dyspnea.

    e. These patients are at high risk for acute infections; therefore, oral antibiotics frequently are necessary.

    f. Supplemental oxygen is the only therapy that may alter the course of COPD in patients with resting hypoxemia ($PaO_2 < 55$mm Hg or $SaO_2 < 88\%$).

    g. Graded aerobic physical exercise should be encouraged.

    h. Steroids are effective but should be used with caution.

    i. Human α_1-antitrypsin replacement may be recommended for patients who are deficient.

    j. Patients should receive the pneumococcal vaccine and yearly influenza vaccine.

D. Cystic fibrosis

  1. General characteristics

    a. Cystic fibrosis is an autosomal recessive disorder that results in the abnormal production of mucus by almost all exocrine glands, causing obstruction of those glands and ducts.

    b. Patients are at increased risk of malignancies of the gastrointestinal (GI) tract, osteopenia, and arthropathies.

    c. Median survival is about 31 years of age.

  2. Clinical features

    a. The diagnosis should be suspected in any young patient who presents with a history of chronic lung disease, pancreatitis, or infertility.

    b. Symptoms include cough, excess sputum, decreased exercise tolerance, sinus pain, purulent nasal discharge, steatorrhea, diarrhea, and abdominal pain.

    c. Signs include clubbing, increased anteroposterior chest diameter, and apical crackles.

  3. Laboratory findings

    a. ABG studies reveal hypoxemia and, in advanced disease, a chronic, compensated respiratory acidosis.

    b. Pulmonary function tests reveal a mixed obstructive and restrictive pattern.

    c. CXR may reveal hyperinflation; peribronchial cuffing; mucous plugging; bronchiectasis; increased interstitial markings; small, round peripheral opacities; focal atelectasis; or pneumothorax.

    d. Thin-section CT may confirm the presence of bronchiectasis.

    e. An elevated quantitative sweat chloride test (>60 mEq/L) performed on two different days can be diagnostic; however, a normal result does not exclude the diagnosis. If the diagnosis is strongly suspected, DNA testing can provide definitive evidence of cystic fibrosis.

  4. Treatment

    a. Comprehensive multidisciplinary therapy improves the control of symptoms and the chances of survival.

    b. Therapies focus on the following areas: clearance of airway secretions, reversal of bronchoconstriction, treatment of respiratory infections, replacement of pancreatic enzymes, and nutritional and psychosocial support.

IV. PLEURAL DISEASES

A. Pleural effusion

  1. General characteristics

    a. Pleural effusions (the accumulation of significant volumes of pleural fluid) may result from inflammation of structures adjacent to the pleural space or lesions within the chest.

    b. Small effusions may not cause symptoms and may be first discovered on routine radiography.

    c. About 25% of effusions are associated with malignancy.

    d. There are four types of effusions.

      (1) Exudates are associated with "leaky capillaries"; examples include infection, malignancy, and trauma.

      (2) Transudates ("intact capillaries") are associated with increased hydrostatic or decreased oncotic pressure; examples include congestive heart failure, atelectasis, and renal or liver disease (cirrhosis).

(3) An empyema is an infection within the pleural space.

(4) A hemothorax indicates bleeding into the pleural space, commonly as a result of trauma or malignancy.

2. Clinical features

   a. With a small inflammatory effusion, patients are often asymptomatic.

   b. Large or bilateral pleural effusions may lead to dyspnea, but orthopnea is uncommon in the absence of congestive heart failure.

   c. A dull to flat percussion note over the area of fluid may be heard with reduced or absent breath sounds.

   d. The mediastinum usually is shifted away from the side of the large effusion.

3. Laboratory findings

   a. Radiographic findings include blunting of the costophrenic angle, loss of sharp demarcation of the diaphragm and heart, and mediastinal shift to the uninvolved side.

   b. Lateral decubitus radiographs can help to identify small effusions and differentiate free-flowing versus loculated fluid.

   c. CT may be useful if plain-film radiography cannot separate parenchymal and pleural densities.

   d. Thoracentesis is the gold standard; the fluid is sent for protein, lactate dehydrogenase (LDH), pH, total WBC and differential cell counts, glucose, cytology, and Gram stain with culture and sensitivity.

   e. Transudates versus exudates (Light's criteria): Fluid is considered to be an exudate if it meets any *one* of the following:

      (1) Pleural fluid protein to serum protein ratio of greater than 0.5.

      (2) Pleural fluid LDH to serum LDH ratio of greater than 0.6.

      (3) Pleural fluid LDH greater than two-thirds the upper limit of normal for serum LDH.

4. Treatment

   a. Unless the cause has been clearly established, the presence of fluid is an indication for thoracocentesis. Removal of fluid via thoracocentesis allows fluid examination, radiographic visualization of the lung parenchyma, and relief of symptoms.

   b. Transudate pleural effusions resolve when underlying causes are treated.

   c. Malignant effusions may require drainage and pleurodesis. The most commonly used irritants are doxycycline and talc.

   d. Empyema requires drainage and antibiotic therapy.

B. Pneumothorax

1. General characteristics

   a. Pneumothorax is the accumulation of air in the pleural space.

   b. The cause may be spontaneous (primary pneumothorax), traumatic, or iatrogenic.

   c. Tall, thin males between 10 and 30 years of age are at greatest risk of primary pneumothorax.

   d. Tension pneumothorax is secondary to a sucking chest wound or a pulmonary laceration that allows air to enter the chest with inspiration but does not allow it to leave on expiration.

2. Clinical features

   a. Pneumothorax is characterized by the acute onset of ipsilateral chest pain and dyspnea. Physical findings depend on the size of the pneumothorax and may include unilateral chest expansion, decreased tactile fremitus, hyperresonance, and diminished breath sounds.

   b. Tension pneumothorax is associated with a mediastinal shift to the contralateral side and impaired ventilation, leading to cardiovascular compromise.

3. Laboratory findings

   a. Expiratory CXR reveals the presence of pleural air. A visceral pleural line may be the only evidence of a small pneumothorax.

   b. ABG analysis, if done, reveals hypoxemia.

4. Treatment depends on the severity.

   a. Small pneumothoraces resolve spontaneously.

   b. For severely symptomatic or large pneumothoraces, chest tube placement is performed.

   c. Tension pneumothorax is a medical emergency. If it is suspected, a large-bore needle should be inserted to allow air to move out of the chest. Placement of chest tube follows the decompression.

   d. Patients should be followed with serial CXR every 24 hours until resolved.

V. PULMONARY CIRCULATION

A. Pulmonary embolism (PE)

1. General characteristics

   a. PE arises from thrombi in the systemic venous circulation or the right side of the heart, from tumors that have invaded the venous circulation, and from other sources. More than 90% of pulmonary emboli originate as clots in the deep veins of the lower extremities; others include air emboli from central lines, amniotic fluid from active labor, and fat from long bone (femur) fracture.

   b. Risk factors revolve around Virchow's triad: hypercoagulable state, venous stasis, and vascular intimal inflammation or injury. Specific risks include surgical procedures (orthopaedic, pelvic, abdominal), cancer, oral contraceptives, and pregnancy.

   c. Approximately 50% to 60% of patients with deep vein thrombosis will experience a PE; half of these will be asymptomatic, often the PE is found only on autopsy. Symptomatic PE is a serious and potentially fatal condition.

   d. PE is the third leading cause of death in hospitalized patients.

2. Clinical features

   a. Symptoms include pleuritic chest pain, dyspnea, apprehension, cough, hemoptysis, and diaphoresis.

   b. Signs include tachycardia, tachypnea, crackles, accentuation of the pulmonary component of the second heart sound, and a low-grade fever. Homans' sign lacks sensitivity and specificity.

3. Laboratory findings

   a. ABG measurements show acute respiratory alkalosis secondary to hyperventilation.

   b. Electrocardiography shows tachycardia and nonspecific ST–T wave changes. The classic $S_1Q_3T_3$ pattern, indicating cor pulmonale, is seen in fewer than 20% of patients with symptomatic PE.

   c. CXR may show nonspecific abnormalities such as basilar atelectasis. The main purpose of obtaining CXR is to rule out other abnormalities and aid in interpreting a ventilation–perfusion scan.

   d. A ventilation–perfusion lung scan shows perfusion defects with normal ventilation. A normal scan rules out clinically significant thromboembolism. Nondiagnostic scans warrant further testing.

   e. Pulmonary angiography remains the definitive test for diagnosis but is reserved for cases in which the diagnosis is uncertain after noninvasive testing.

   f. Measuring plasma D-dimer may be useful especially to rule out PE if clinical suspicion is low and D-dimer is negative.

   g. Spiral CT has now replaced ventilation-perfusion scans as the initial method of identifying pulmonary embolus.

4. Treatment

   a. Anticoagulation therapy is initiated; heparin is the anticoagulant of choice. Low-molecular-weight heparin or warfarin is continued after the acute phase.

   b. Duration of therapy depends on the clinical situation. A minimum of 3 months is advised.

   c. Vena cava interruption (filter) is helpful in patients at high risk of recurrence who are unable to tolerate anticoagulants.

   d. Prevention is the key. For high-risk patients, consider the following: early ambulation; intermittent pneumatic compression stockings; low-dose heparin and low-molecular-weight heparin; or a combination of mechanical and pharmacologic measures.

B. Pulmonary hypertension

1. General characteristics

   a. Pulmonary hypertension is present when the pulmonary arterial pressure rises to a level inappropriate for a given cardiac output. Once present, it is self-perpetuating.

   b. Primary (idiopathic) pulmonary hypertension is rare and has a fatal outcome.

   c. Secondary pulmonary hypertension has many causes that develop as a result of obliteration and obstruction of the pulmonary arterial tree.

   d. Hypoxia is the most important and potent stimulus of pulmonary arterial vasoconstriction. Other causes include acidosis and veno-occlusive conditions.

2. Clinical features

   a. Clinical manifestations may include dyspnea, angina-like retrosternal chest pain, weakness, fatigue, edema, ascites, cyanosis, and syncope.

   b. Signs may include narrow splitting and accentuation of the second heart sound and a systolic ejection click.

3. Laboratory findings

   a. CXR may show enlarged pulmonary arteries, and electrocardiography may show right ventricular hypertrophy, atrial hypertrophy, and right ventricular strain.

   b. Echocardiography may be useful in estimating pulmonary arterial pressure, but right heart catheterization offers more precise hemodynamic monitoring.

4. Treatment

   a. Treatment of primary pulmonary hypertension may include chronic oral anticoagulants, calcium channel blockers to lower systemic arterial pressure, and prostacyclin (a potent pulmonary vasodilator). Despite these measures, heart–lung transplantation usually is needed.

   b. Treatment of secondary pulmonary hypertension consists of treating the underlying disorder in addition to those mentioned earlier.

VI. RESTRICTIVE PULMONARY DISEASE

A. Idiopathic fibrosing interstitial pneumonia (formerly idiopathic pulmonary fibrosis)

1. General characteristics

   a. This is the most common diagnosis among patients with interstitial lung disease.

   b. There are three histopathologic patterns with different natural histories and treatments: usual interstitial pneumonia; respiratory bronchiolitis–associated interstitial lung disease; and acute interstitial pneumonitis.

2. Clinical features

   a. Symptoms include an insidious dry cough, exertional dyspnea, and constitutional symptoms (fatigue, malaise, etc.).

   b. Examination may reveal clubbing and inspiratory crackles.

3. Laboratory findings

   a. CXR demonstrates evidence of progressive fibrosis over several years.

   b. CT shows diffuse, patchy fibrosis with pleural-based honeycombing.

   c. Pulmonary function tests may show a restrictive pattern (decreased lung volume with a normal to increased FEV_1/FVC ratio).

4. Treatment remains controversial, because none has been shown to improve survival or quality of life compared to no treatment.

B. Pneumoconioses

1. General characteristics

   a. Pneumoconioses are chronic fibrotic lung diseases caused by the inhalation of coal dust or various inert, inorganic, or silicate dusts.

   b. Clinically important pneumoconioses include coal workers' pneumoconiosis, silicosis, and asbestosis.

TABLE 2-8	**Comparison of Pneumoconioses**		
Disease	**Occupation**	**Diagnosis**	**Complications**
Asbestosis	Insulation, demolition, construction	Bx: asbestos bodies	Increased risk of lung cancer and mesothelioma, especially if a smoker
		CXR: linear opacities at bases and pleural plaques	
Coal workers' pneumoconiosis	Coal mining	CXR: nodular opacities at upper lung fields	Progressive massive fibrosis
Silicosis	Mining, sand blasting, quarry work, stone work	CXR: nodular opacities at upper lung fields	Increased risk of tuberculosis; progressive massive fibrosis
Berryliosis	High-technology fields: aerospace, nuclear power, ceramics, foundries, tool and die manufacturing	CXR: diffuse infiltrates and hilar adenopathy	Requires chronic steroids

Bx, biopsy; CXR, chest radiography.

2. Clinical features
   a. In simple cases, pneumoconioses usually are asymptomatic.
   b. In complicated cases, patients have dyspnea, inspiratory crackles, clubbing, and cyanosis.
   c. Table 2-8 provides a comparison of the most common pneumoconioses.
3. Laboratory findings
   a. Pulmonary function tests show restrictive dysfunction and reduced diffusing capacity.
   b. Chest radiography
      (1) Coal workers' pneumoconiosis: Small opacities are prominent in the upper lung fields.
      (2) Silicosis: Small rounded opacities are seen throughout the lung, and hilar lymph nodes may be calcified.
      (3) Asbestosis: Interstitial fibrosis, thickened pleura, and calcified plaques appear on the diaphragms or lateral chest wall.
4. Treatment
   a. Treatment is primarily supportive as no effective treatment is available. Supportive therapy includes oxygen, vaccinations (pneumovax, influenza vaccine), and rehabilitation.
   b. Corticosteroids may relieve the chronic alveolitis in silicosis.
   c. Smoking cessation is especially important for patients with asbestosis, because smoking interferes with short asbestos fiber clearance from the lung. Smoking and asbestos are synergistically linked to lung cancer.

C. Sarcoidosis
1. General characteristics
   a. Sarcoidosis is a multiorgan disease of idiopathic cause. It is characterized by noncaseating granulomatous inflammation in affected organs (e.g., lungs, lymph nodes, eyes, skin, liver, spleen, salivary glands, heart, nervous system).
   b. Approximately 90% of patients have lung involvement.
   c. The incidence is highest in North American blacks (especially women) and northern European whites.
2. Clinical features
   a. Common respiratory symptoms include cough, dyspnea of insidious onset, and chest discomfort.
   b. Patients may present with malaise, fever, and symptoms consistent with the involvement of various organs.
   c. Extrapulmonary findings are common and include erythema nodosum or enlargement of parotid glands, lymph nodes, liver, or spleen.
3. Laboratory findings
   a. Serum blood tests may show leukopenia, eosinophilia, elevated erythrocyte sedimentation rate, hypercalcemia, and hypercalciuria.
   b. Angiotensin-converting enzyme levels are elevated in 40% to 80% of patients.
   c. Radiographic findings demonstrate symmetric bilateral hilar and right paratracheal adenopathy and bilateral diffuse reticular infiltrates.
   d. Transbronchial biopsy of the lung or fine-needle node biopsy confirms the diagnosis. Biopsy shows noncaseating granulomas.
4. Treatment: Approximately 90% of cases are responsive to corticosteroids and can be controlled with modest maintenance doses.

VII. OTHER PULMONARY DISEASES

A. Acute (adult) respiratory distress syndrome (ARDS)
1. General characteristics
   a. Three clinical settings account for 75% of ARDS cases: sepsis syndrome (the single most important), severe multiple trauma, and aspiration of gastric contents. Other causes include shock, toxic inhalation, near-drowning, and multiple transfusions.
   b. The underlying abnormality in ARDS is increased permeability of the alveolar capillary membranes, which leads to development of protein-rich pulmonary edema.
2. Clinical features
   a. Rapid onset of profound dyspnea occurring 12 to 24 hours after the precipitating event.
   b. Physical examination shows tachypnea, frothy pink or red sputum, and diffuse crackles.
   c. Many patients are cyanotic with increasingly severe hypoxemia that is refractory to administered oxygen.

3. Laboratory findings
   a. CXR may be normal at first. Infiltrates tend to be peripheral (spares the costophrenic angles) with air bronchograms in 80% of patients. The heart is normal in size. Upper lung venous engorgement is uncommon. Pleural effusions are small to absent.
   b. Pulmonary capillary wedge pressure is normal.
   c. Multiple organ failure is common.
4. Treatment
   a. Treatment includes identification and specific treatment of the underlying precipitating and secondary conditions.
   b. Supportive care also is required to compensate for the severe respiratory dysfunction. Oxygen should be delivered via endotracheal intubation with positive pressure ventilation and low levels of positive end-expiratory pressure (PEEP). Hypoxia often is refractory to treatment.
   c. The mortality rate associated with ARDS is high, which reflects the severity of the predisposing conditions.
   d. One-third of deaths occur within 3 days of the onset of symptoms. The remaining deaths occur within 2 weeks of diagnosis and are caused by infection and multiple organ failure.

B. Aspiration of foreign bodies
1. General characteristics
   a. Knowledge of the Heimlich maneuver is lifesaving.
   b. Aspiration may be of gastric contents, inert material, toxic material, or poorly chewed food. The degree of injury depends on the substance aspirated.
2. Clinical features
   a. An episode of choking and coughing or unexplained wheezing or hemoptysis should raise the suspicion of foreign body aspiration.
   b. Asphyxia may result from the aspiration of obstructing material.
   c. Pneumonia may develop secondary to aspiration of toxic materials.
   d. Acute gastric aspiration is one of the most common causes of ARDS.
3. Laboratory studies: Expiratory radiography may reveal regional hyperinflation caused by a check valve effect.
4. Treatment
   a. Bronchoscopy may help to establish the diagnosis but also can be the treatment of choice for removal of the object.
   b. Cultures should be obtained if postobstructive pneumonia is suspected.

C. Hyaline membrane disease
1. General characteristics
   a. Hyaline membrane disease is the most common cause of respiratory disease in the preterm infant.
   b. It is caused by a deficiency of surfactant.
2. Clinical features: The infant will demonstrate typical signs of respiratory distress.
3. Laboratory findings: CXR demonstrates air bronchograms, diffuse bilateral atelectasis causing a ground glass appearance, and doming of the diaphragm.
4. Treatment
   a. Synchronized intermittent mandatory ventilation should be used.
   b. Administration of exogenous surfactants can be used in the delivery room as prophylaxis or as rescue in established hyaline membrane disease.

Cardiology

Rebecca Lovell Scott

I. MAJOR PRINCIPLES OF CARDIAC CARE

A. Three factors are needed to maintain adequate pressure in the cardiovascular system.

   1. A functioning pump

   2. Sufficient fluid volume

   3. Resistance

B. All cardiac pathologies result from abnormalities of electrical or contractile functions of the heart muscle, fluid load, or vascular resistance.

C. Quantification and monitoring of severity of symptoms is important to management (Table 3-1).

II. SHOCK

A. General characteristics

   1. Shock is severe cardiovascular failure caused by poor blood flow or inadequate distribution of flow.

   2. Inadequate oxygen delivery to body tissues results in shock, which may lead to organ failure and death.

   3. The physical responses to shock are mediated by catecholamines, renin, antidiuretic hormone, glucagon, cortisol, and growth hormone.

   4. Shock may result from multiple causes.

      a. Hypovolemic shock is caused by hemorrhage, loss of plasma, or loss of fluid and electrolytes, resulting in decreased intravascular volume. This may be caused by obvious loss or by "third-space" sequestration.

      b. Cardiogenic shock may arise from myocardial infarction (MI), dysrhythmias, heart failure, defects in the valves or septum, hypertension, myocarditis, cardiac contusion, rupture of the ventricular septum, or myocardiopathies.

      c. Causes of obstructive shock include tension pneumothorax, pericardial tamponade, obstructive valvular disease, and pulmonary problems, including massive pulmonary embolism.

      d. Shock caused by poorly regulated distribution of blood volume ("distributive shock") includes septic shock, systemic inflammatory response syndrome (signs of systemic inflammation without end-organ damage), anaphylaxis, and neurogenic shock.

         (1) Septic shock is the most common cause, has a mortality rate of 30% to 87%, and is most often associated with Gram-negative sepsis in persons at the extremes of age, persons with diabetes or immunosuppression, or those who have recently had an invasive procedure.

         (2) Causes of neurogenic shock include spinal cord injury or adverse effects of spinal or epidural anesthetic.

B. Clinical features

   1. Signs and symptoms of shock include low blood pressure, orthostatic changes, tachycardia, peripheral hypoperfusion, altered mental status, oliguria or anuria, insulin resistance, and metabolic acidosis.

   2. The actual blood pressure reading in shock is not as important as the decrease in blood pressure compared to the usual blood pressure for the individual patient.

   3. End-organ hypoperfusion usually results in cool or mottled extremities and weak ("thready") or absent peripheral pulses.

   4. Mental status may remain normal, or the patient may be agitated, restless, confused, obtunded, or comatose.

C. Laboratory studies

   1. All patients require a complete blood count (CBC), blood type and cross-match, and coagulation parameters.

   2. Electrolytes, glucose, urinalysis, and serum creatinine will aid in determining the cause of shock.

   3. Pulse oximetry or serial arterial blood gases are needed to monitor oxygenation.

D. Treatment must address both the specific cause and the manifestations of shock.

   1. The first step in treatment is attention to basic life support (airway, breathing, circulation).

   2. Specific treatments depend on the cause of shock.

   3. The Trendelenburg or supine position with legs elevated maximizes blood flow to the brain.

TABLE 3-1	New York Heart Association Functional Classification of Heart Disease
Class	**Definition**
I	No limitation of physical activity; ordinary physical activity does not cause undue fatigue, dyspnea, or anginal pain
II	Slight limitation of physical activity; ordinary physical activity results in symptoms
III	Marked limitation of physical activity; comfortable at rest, but less than ordinary activity causes symptoms
IV	Unable to engage in any physical activity without discomfort; symptoms may be present even at rest

From Criteria Committee of the New York Heart Association. *Nomenclature and Criteria for Diagnosis of Diseases of the Heart and Great Vessels.* 9th ed. Boston: Little, Brown & Co.; 1994.

4. Oxygen and intravenous (IV) fluids are essential.

5. Urine flow should be monitored via indwelling catheter and sustained at 0.5 mL/kg/hr or more.

6. Continuous cardiac monitoring is preferable to intermittent cardiac monitoring. Central venous pressure monitoring or capillary wedge pressure is helpful.

7. Pressors (dopamine, others) will increase glomerular filtration rate, contractility, and heart rate.

III. ORTHOSTASIS/POSTURAL HYPOTENSION

A. General characteristics

1. Postural hypotension may be related to reduced cardiac output, paroxysmal cardiac dysrhythmias, low blood volume, medications, and various endocrine and metabolic disorders.

2. Postural hypotension is a reversible cause of syncope and a major cause of falls in the elderly.

B. Clinical features

1. Postural hypotension is a greater than 20 mm Hg drop in systolic blood pressure between supine and sitting and/or standing measurements.

2. If accompanied by a rise in pulse of more than 15 bpm, depleted blood volume is the probable cause.

3. If no change in pulse occurs, medications, central nervous system (CNS) disease (Parkinsons, Shy–Drager), or peripheral neuropathies should be considered.

C. Laboratory studies are directed at the suspected cause.

D. Treatment is directed at the suspected cause.

IV. HYPERTENSION

A. General characteristics

1. Primary (essential) hypertension causes 95% of cases of elevated blood pressure. It has no specific identifiable cause; pathogenesis is multifactorial.

a. Genetic predisposition is an important factor; it is more prevalent with increased age and in blacks.

b. Environmental factors also are important and include excessive or increased salt intake and obesity.

c. Other hypothesized factors are related to sympathetic nervous system hyperactivity, abnormal cardiovascular or renal development, imbalance in the renin–angiotensin system, defects in sodium excretion, and abnormalities in sodium and potassium exchange at the cellular level.

d. Exacerbating factors include excessive use of alcohol, cigarette smoking, lack of exercise, polycythemia, use of nonsteroidal anti-inflammatory drugs (NSAIDs), and low potassium intake.

e. The metabolic syndrome (truncal obesity, hyperinsulinemia and insulin resistance, hypertriglyceridemia, and hypertension) is associated with development of diabetes and increased risk of cardiovascular complications.

2. Secondary causes of hypertension (5%) include sleep apnea, estrogen use, pheochromocytoma, coarctation of the aorta, pseudotumor cerebri, parenchymal renal disease, renal artery stenosis, chronic steroid therapy, Cushing's syndrome, thyroid and parathyroid disease, primary hyperaldosteronism, and pregnancy.

3. Essential hypertension is exacerbated in males, blacks, sedentary individuals, and smokers.

TABLE 3-2	**Classification of Blood Pressure for Adults 18 Years of Age and Older**	
Category	**Systolic Pressure (mm Hg)**	**Diastolic Pressure (mm Hg)**
Normal	<120	<80
Prehypertension	120–139	80–99
Hypertension		
Stage 1	140–159	90–99
Stage 2	≥160	≥100

From Chobanian AV, Bakris GL, Black HR, et al. The Seventh Report of the Joint National Committee on Prevention, Detection, Evaluation, and Treatment of High Blood Pressure: The JNC7 Report. *JAMA.* 2003;289:2560–2572.

4. Hypertension plays a major role in the genesis and exacerbation of other forms of cardiovascular disease and causes numerous secondary disorders.

5. Hypertensive urgencies reflect blood pressures that must be reduced within hours.

6. Hypertensive emergencies reflect blood pressure that must be reduced within 1 hour to prevent progression of end-organ damage or death.

7. Malignant hypertension is defined as elevated blood pressure associated with papilledema and either encephalopathy or nephropathy; if untreated, progressive renal failure occurs.

8. Complications of untreated hypertension include cardiovascular disease, cerebrovascular disease, dementia, renal disease, aortic dissection, and atherosclerotic complications.

B. Clinical features (Table 3-2)

1. The essential diagnostic criterion is a systolic pressure of greater than 140 mm Hg or a diastolic pressure of greater than 90 mm Hg measured on three separate occasions.

2. Most patients with mild to moderate hypertension are asymptomatic; the most commonly voiced symptom is nonspecific headache.

3. End-organ damage in untreated hypertension includes heart failure, renal failure, stroke, dementia, aortic dissection, atherosclerosis, and retinal hemorrhage.

4. In hypertensive urgencies, the systolic pressure usually is greater than 220 mm Hg, or the diastolic pressure is greater than 125 mm Hg.

5. In hypertensive emergencies, the diastolic pressure usually is greater than 130 mm Hg. Optic disc edema (papilledema) indicates the presence of end-organ damage. Complications include hypertensive encephalopathy, nephropathy, intracranial hemorrhage, aortic dissection, preeclampsia or eclampsia, pulmonary edema, unstable angina, or MI.

C. Laboratory studies

1. Electrocardiography (ECG) may reveal left ventricular hypertrophy or heart failure (Fig. 3-1). A strain pattern is associated with advanced disease and a poorer prognosis.

2. Chest radiography may show ventricular hypertrophy (Fig. 3-2); however, chest radiography is not considered to be necessary in the evaluation of uncomplicated hypertension.

3. Decreased hemoglobin or hematocrit or elevations in blood urea nitrogen (BUN), creatinine, and glucose (serum or urine) may indicate related renal disease or diabetes. Other parameters that should be measured include serum uric acid, plasma aldosterone concentration, plasma renin activity, calculation of plasma aldosterone to renin ratio, and serum electrolytes.

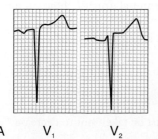
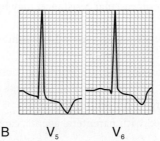

A   V₁   V₂   B   V₅   V₆

FIGURE 3-1 Electrocardiographic findings in left ventricular hypertrophy. **A:** Deep S waves in V₁ and V₂. **B:** Tall R waves in V₅ and V₆. (From Stein E. *Rapid Analysis of Electrocardiograms: A Self-study Program.* 3rd ed. Philadelphia: Lippincott Williams & Wilkins; 2000.)

FIGURE 3-2 Hypertensive cardiovascular disease, frontal view. Note the left ventricular prominence and a slight increase in the tortuosity of the aorta at its arch. There is calcification in the descending aorta *(arrow)*. (From Daffner RH. *Clinical Radiology: The Essentials.* 2nd ed. Baltimore: Williams & Wilkins; 1999.)

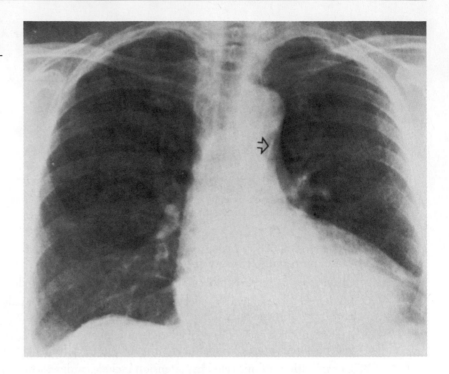

4. A lipid profile is important for ascertaining the associated risk of atherosclerosis.

5. In hypertensive urgencies and emergencies, diagnostic testing targets end-organ function.

D. Treatment

1. Nonpharmacologic therapies of essential hypertension should be stressed and include following the DASH (**D**ietary **A**pproaches to **S**top **H**ypertension) diet (low saturated fat, cholesterol, and total fat; increased fruits, vegetables; fat-free or low-fat milk or milk products; and increased fiber), weight loss, exercise, cessation of smoking, limitation of alcohol, and in some cases, limitation of sodium.

2. Therapy may be initiated with a number of agents.

   a. Diuretics initially reduce plasma volume and chronically reduce peripheral resistance. They are recommended as initial therapy for essential hypertension. Potassium supplements may be needed for some patients. Thiazide diuretics are most consistently effective; loop diuretics should be used only in those with renal dysfunction and when close electrolyte monitoring is assured.

   b. β-Adrenergic antagonists are used to decrease heart rate and cardiac output. They tend to be more effective in younger white patients.

   c. Angiotensin-converting enzyme (ACE) inhibitors, which also inhibit bradykinin degradation and stimulate synthesis of vasodilating prostaglandins, are the initial drug of choice for hypertensive patients with diabetes and are increasingly the treatment of choice for mild or moderate hypertension, especially in younger white patients, or when diuretics are insufficient. The major side effect of ACE inhibitors is cough.

   d. Angiotensin II receptor–blocking agents block the interaction of angiotensin II on receptors. They do not increase bradykinins and, therefore, do not cause cough.

   e. Calcium channel blockers for peripheral vasodilation may be preferable in blacks and elderly patients.

   f. Aliskiren, a renin inhibitor, was recently approved for mono- or combination therapy.

3. Other agents are available for use in refractory cases or special situations.

   a. α-Adrenergic antagonists, which lower peripheral vascular resistance, may be the initial drug of choice in men with symptomatic prostatic hyperplasia.

   b. Central sympatholytics, arteriolar dilators, and peripheral sympathetic inhibitors also may play a role in treatment of refractory hypertension.

   c. Aldosterone receptor antagonists, such as spironolactone, are increasingly used in refractory hypertension as additions to other antihypertensives.

4. Treatment of secondary causes of hypertension targets the underlying cause.

5. Hypertensive urgencies and emergencies are treated with parenteral agents; care must be taken not to decrease the blood pressure too rapidly.

    a. Preferred agents include sodium nitroprusside and, if myocardial ischemia is present, nitroglycerin or a β-blocker. Aortic dissection calls for nitroprusside and a β-blocker, usually labetalol or esmolol, and urgent surgery.

    b. Other acceptable agents include nicardipine, enalaprilat, diazoxide, hydralazine, trimethaphan, fenoldopam, and loop diuretics.

    c. Oral agents for less severe emergencies include clonidine, captopril, and nifedipine.

V. CONGESTIVE HEART FAILURE

A. General characteristics

  1. Congestive heart failure (CHF) is a clinical syndrome characterized by dyspnea and abnormal retention of water and sodium.

  2. CHF results from changes in one or more of the following: contractile ability of the heart muscle, preload and afterload of the ventricle, and heart rate.

  3. Alterations may result from multiple causes, including myocardial and pericardial disorders as well as valvular and congenital abnormalities. High-output failure has noncardiac causes (e.g., thyrotoxicosis, severe anemia).

  4. CHF adversely affects left atrial pressure and cardiac output.

  5. CHF is increasing in incidence and prevalence as the population ages; it occurs in 10% of persons over 80 years of age.

B. Clinical features

  1. Left-sided failure causes exertional dyspnea plus nonproductive cough, fatigue, orthopnea, paroxysmal nocturnal dyspnea, basilar rales, gallops, and exercise intolerance.

  2. Right-sided failure is characterized by distended neck veins, tender or nontender hepatic congestion, nausea, and dependent pitting edema; it often is caused by left-sided failure. Predominant features are edema and hepatomegaly.

  3. Cardiac signs include parasternal lift, enlarged apical impulse, diminished first heart sound, and an S_3 gallop. An S_4 gallop may be heard in diastolic failure.

  4. Sympathetic activity produces pallor and cold, clammy skin.

  5. Nocturia is a common symptom.

  6. Hypotension and a narrow pulse pressure are typical.

C. Laboratory studies

  1. Patients may have anemia, renal insufficiency, hyperkalemia, hyponatremia, and elevated liver enzymes; those on diuretics may develop hypokalemia.

  2. Chest radiography may show cardiomegaly and bilateral or right-sided pulmonary effusions, perivascular or interstitial edema (Kerley B lines), venous dilation, and alveolar fluid (Fig. 3-3).

  3. ECG may show nonspecific changes (e.g., low voltage), underlying arrhythmia, intraventricular conduction defects, left ventricular hypertrophy, nonspecific repolarization changes, or new or old MI.

  4. Echocardiography is useful to determine size and function of the chambers, valve abnormalities, pericardial effusion, shunting, and segmental wall abnormalities.

  5. Serum B-type natriuretic peptide (BNP) or N-terminal pro-BNP may be elevated.

  6. Stress imaging, radionuclide angiography, and cardiac catheterization may be indicated to assess cause or severity of disease.

  7. Older patients should have thyroid function testing; iron studies are indicated in suspected cases of CHF due to hemochromatosis.

D. Treatment

  1. Correction of reversible causes is key to management.

  2. Preventive and rehabilitative nonpharmacologic measures include progressive aerobic exercise, low-sodium diet, and stress reduction.

  3. Diuretic therapy reduces fluid volume and produces relief of symptoms.

  4. Initial therapy in most patients is a thiazide or loop diuretic and an ACE inhibitor. Other drugs include potassium-sparing diuretics, angiotensin II receptor blockers, β-blockers, direct inotropic agents (digitalis), and arterial and venous vasodilators.

  5. Calcium channel blockers, preferably amlodipine, are used only to treat associated angina or hypertension.

FIGURE 3-3 Congestive heart failure, frontal view. Note the mild pulmonary edema and pulmonary venous engorgement. (From Daffner RH. *Clinical Radiology: The Essentials.* 2nd ed. Baltimore: Williams & Wilkins; 1999.)

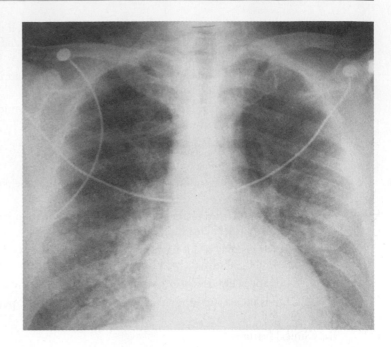

6. Patients may require anticoagulants or antiarrhythmics, as dictated by the underlying disease.

7. Increasingly, implantable cardioverter-defibrillators and biventricular pacing are being used.

8. Coronary revascularization or cardiac transplantation may be indicated.

VI. ATHEROSCLEROTIC OCCLUSIVE DISEASE

A. General characteristics

1. Atherosclerosis is characterized by lipid deposition, fibrosis, calcification, and plaque formation in the intima of large and medium vessels.

2. Atherosclerosis is associated with premature coronary and peripheral vascular morbidity and mortality.

a. Atherosclerotic heart disease is the most common cause of cardiac-related death and disability.

b. Men are affected fourfold more often than women; however, by the age of 70 years, the ratio is 1:1.

3. The cause is closely related to smoking and elevated cholesterol levels (>200 mg/dL) due to diet or familial dyslipidemias. C-reactive protein is an important marker.

4. Management of both blood glucose and blood pressure is essential to the control of vascular disease.

5. Obesity, sedentary lifestyle, and homocystinuria must be addressed.

B. Clinical features: These depend on the location of the vessels involved (e.g., cerebral occlusions lead to cognitive disorders, renal artery blockage leads to kidney failure).

C. Treatment

1. Smoking cessation is essential.

2. Exercise, dietary modifications, and treatment of dyslipidemias are important.

3. Areas under investigation include the use of macrolide antibiotics, anti-inflammatory agents, and various forms of gene therapy.

VII. ISCHEMIC HEART DISEASE

A. General characteristics

1. Ischemic heart disease is characterized by insufficient oxygen supply to cardiac muscle, most commonly caused by atherosclerotic narrowing and less often by constriction of coronary arteries. Rare causes include congenital anomalies, emboli, arteritis, and dissection.

2. Risk factors include male gender, increased age, low-estrogen state, cigarette smoking, family history, hypertension, diabetes mellitus, abdominal obesity, inactivity, dyslipidemias, increased alcohol intake, and low intake of fruits and vegetables.

3. Metabolic syndrome is a major contributor to coronary heart disease and includes three or more of the following: abdominal obesity, triglycerides greater than 150 mg/dL, HDL less than 40 for men and less than 50 for women, fasting glucose greater than 110 mg/dL, and hypertension.

4. Cocaine use is an important cause of myocardial ischemia and infarction.

B. Clinical features

1. Ischemia causes angina pectoris. Angina is characterized by paroxysmal chest "squeezing" or pressure, often accompanied by a sensation of smothering and a fear of impending death.

   a. Stable angina is exacerbated by physical activity and is relieved by rest.

   b. Prinzmetal's, or variant angina, is caused by vasospasm at rest, with preservation of exercise capacity.

   c. Unstable angina is an increasing pattern of pain in previously stable patients. It is less responsive to medication, lasts longer, and occurs at rest or with less exertion.

2. Levine's sign, which is a clenched fist over the sternum and clenched teeth when describing chest pain, may be seen in patients with ischemia.

3. Angina pectoris usually is midsternal but may radiate to the jaw, shoulders, arms, wrists, back of the neck, or some combination of these, usually on the left.

4. Angina pectoris usually lasts for less than 3 minutes. Angina pectoris lasting for more than 30 minutes suggests unstable angina, MI, or another diagnosis.

5. Angina is relieved by sublingual nitroglycerin.

C. Laboratory studies

1. Horizontal or downsloping ST-segment depression on ECG during an anginal attack is among the most sensitive clinical signs, although the ECG will be normal in 25% of those with angina. T waves may flatten or invert.

2. Exercise testing is the most useful and cost-effective noninvasive test. An ST-segment depression of 1 mm (0.1 mV) is considered to be a positive test.

3. Myocardial stress imaging includes myocardial perfusion scintigraphy, radionuclide angiography, and stress echocardiography; these may follow exercise testing.

4. Echocardiography is used to evaluate left ventricular function, an important prognostic indicator.

5. Positron emission tomography (PET), single-photon emission computed tomography (SPECT) cameras, computed tomography (CT) angiography, electron beam CT (EBCT), cardiac magnetic resonance imaging (MRI), and ambulatory ECG monitoring may be indicated.

6. Coronary angiography is the definitive diagnostic procedure but should be used selectively because of cost and invasiveness.

D. Treatment

1. Preventive and rehabilitative treatment includes exercise, weight reduction, diet low in fat and cholesterol, smoking cessation, and aggressive control of diabetes, hypertension, and hyperlipidemias.

2. Aggravating factors (e.g., hypertension) must be identified and treated.

3. Sublingual or translingual spray nitroglycerin or sublingual isosorbide dinitrate is the primary pharmacotherapy for acute anginal attacks.

4. Long-acting nitrate (oral, ointment, or transdermal patches) therapy should include a daily 8- to 10-hour treatment-free interval to prevent drug tolerance. Major adverse effects of nitrates include headache, nausea, light-headedness, and hypotension.

5. β-Blockers prolong life in patients with coronary disease and are first-line therapy for chronic angina.

6. Ranolazine prolongs exercise duration and time to angina.

7. Calcium channel blockers decrease cardiac muscle oxygen demand but are considered third-line therapy.

8. Platelet-inhibiting agents (e.g., aspirin, clopidogrel) reduce the possibility of infarction secondary to emboli.

9. Revascularization provides long-term relief of ischemia in suitable patients.

VIII. ACUTE CORONARY SYNDROMES

A. General characteristics

1. Acute coronary syndromes (ACS) include a spectrum of problems ranging from unstable angina to MI.

2. These conditions are classified simply as ST-elevated or non–ST-elevated events rather than as unstable angina, Q-wave infarction, or non–Q-wave infarction.

   a. Based on initial findings, patients can be triaged to acute reperfusion therapy if indicated.

   b. Determination of the occurrence of acute MI is based on evolution of cardiac markers.

(1) MI is a result of prolonged myocardial ischemia, usually as a result of thrombus formation on a preexisting atherosclerotic plaque. Other causes include prolonged vasospasm, reduced myocardial blood flow, excessive metabolic demand, embolic occlusion, vasculitis, aortitis, coronary artery dissection, and cocaine use.

(2) Signs and symptoms, prognosis, and complications depend on the size and location of the infarct.

3. One-fifth of patients with acute MI will die, usually of ventricular fibrillation, before reaching a hospital.

4. About one-third of acute MIs are "silent" or accompanied by minor pain only. Older people, women, and those with diabetes mellitus are more likely to present atypically.

B. Clinical features

1. Chest pain is the most common presenting factor in ACS.

2. The patient with MI usually develops increasingly severe, prolonged (>30 minutes) anterior chest pain at rest, most often during the early morning hours, which can lead to arrhythmias, hypotension, shock, and heart failure.

3. Diaphoresis, weakness, anxiety, restlessness, light-headedness, syncope, cough, dyspnea, orthopnea, nausea, vomiting, and abdominal bloating often are present in patients with MI.

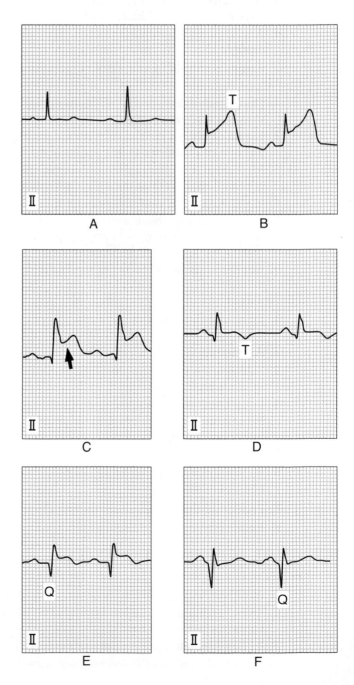

FIGURE 3-4 Evolutionary changes of a Q-wave infarction as seen from lead II. Examples are not necessarily from the same patient. **A:** Normal. **B** and **D:** T wave becomes tall, then inverts symmetrically. **C:** ST segment elevates *(arrow)*. **E:** Significant Q waves develop. **F:** Healed infarction. Q waves persist, but ST segment and T wave return to normal. (From Mulholland GC, Brewer BB. *Improving Your Skills in 12-Lead ECG Interpretation.* Baltimore: Williams & Wilkins; 1990.)

TABLE 3-3	Determining Location of Cardiac Damage by Examining ECG Changes
ECG Location	**ECG Leads Most Likely to Exhibit Changes**
Inferior	II, III, aVF
Posterior	V_1, V_2
Anteroseptal	V_1, V_2
Anterior	V_1, V_2, V_3
Anterolateral	V_4, V_5, V_6

ECG, electrocardiogram.

4. Patients may be bradycardic or tachycardic as well as hypotensive or hypertensive.

5. Low-grade fever may develop after 12 hours and last for several days.

6. Lung fields may be clear, or rales and wheezing may be present.

7. The cardiovascular examination may be quite normal, or it may reveal jugular venous distention, soft heart sounds, murmur of mitral regurgitation, and an S_4 gallop.

8. Pericardial friction rubs may appear after 24 hours.

9. Dressler's syndrome (post-MI syndrome) includes pericarditis, fever, leukocytosis, and pericardial or pleural effusion, usually 1 to 2 weeks post-MI.

C. Laboratory studies

1. ECG changes form the basis of an initial and ongoing evaluation of ACS.

   a. In acute MI, progression from peaked T waves to ST-segment elevations (or depressions) to Q waves to T-wave inversions classically occurs over hours to days, but is not present in all cases (Fig. 3-4).

   b. The location of cardiac damage may be determined by examining changes on the ECG (Table 3-3).

2. Serial cardiac enzymes—isoenzyme of creatine kinase containing M and B subunits (CK-MB), troponin T, and troponin I—demonstrate characteristic elevations (Table 3-4).

3. Echocardiography may show abnormalities of cardiac wall motion; Doppler studies may show postinfarction ventricular septal defect or mitral regurgitation.

4. Chest radiography may indicate congestive failure or signs of aortic dissection.

5. MRI with gadolinium contrast is one of the most sensitive tests to quantify the extent of an infarction.

6. Scintigraphy and radionuclide angiography may be helpful in establishing the diagnosis; hemodynamic studies may be useful in the management of cases with cardiogenic shock.

D. Treatment

1. All patients with suspected ACS should receive IV fluids, oxygen, nitroglycerin, and pain management. Serial ECG and pulse oximetry are important components of monitoring. Some patients may require sedation with a benzodiazepine.

TABLE 3-4	Cardiac Markers in Acute Myocardial Infarction			
Marker	**Timing of Initial Elevation (hr)**	**Peak Elevation (hr)**	**Return to Normal**	**Sampling Schedule**
Myoglobin	1–4	6–7	24 hr	Often beginning 1–2 hr after onset of chest pain
Cardiac troponin I	3–12	24	5–10 days	12 hr after onset of chest pain
Cardiac troponin T	3–12	12–48	5–14 days	12 hr after onset of chest pain
Total CK	3–5	24	28–72 hr	May not be drawn owing to many false positives; CK-MB more sensitive
CK-MB	3–12	24	48–72 hr	Three times, 12 hr apart
LDH	10	24–48	10–14 days	Once, at least 24 hr after onset of chest pain

CK, creatine kinase; CK-MB, isoenzyme of CK containing M and B subunits; LDH, lactate dehydrogenase.

2. ACS patients without ST-segment elevations should receive antiplatelet (aspirin, clopidogrel) and anticoagulant (unfractionated heparin, enoxaparin, fondoparinux, or bivalirudin) therapy.

3. β-Blockers should be initiated in the absence of contraindications (heart failure, bradycardia, heart block).

4. Calcium channel blockers are used only in patients who cannot take nitrates and β-blockers or in those with contraindications to these drugs.

5. Patients with ACS (including non–ST-segment elevation) must undergo risk stratification. Rating systems aid in deciding which patients should undergo aggressive treatment. Several scoring systems are available based on the risk of reinfarction or death.

   a. The TIMI (**T**hrombolysis **I**n **M**yocardial **I**nfarction) system is the quickest and easiest scoring system and can be completed easily at the bedside. One point is given for each of the following factors: age 65 years or more, three or more risk factors for coronary artery disease, use of aspirin within the last 7 days, known coronary artery disease with stenosis 50% or greater, more than one episode of rest angina within the last 24 hours, ST-segment deviation, and elevated cardiac markers. Scores of 3 or more are considered to be high risk.

   b. GRACE (**G**lobal **R**egistry of **A**cute **C**oronary **E**vents) is a somewhat more complex scoring method. Age, gender, vital signs, ST-segment changes, and historical factors are included to predict risk.

   c. It is essential to carefully monitor patients with non–ST-segment elevation and to intervene in cases of patients likely to progress to infarction.

6. Patients with ACS and an acute ST-segment elevation MI (STEMI) should undergo immediate interventions to promote reperfusion.

   a. Aspirin and clopidogrel should be given at once.

   b. Immediate (within 90 minutes) coronary angiography and primary percutaneous coronary intervention are superior to thrombolysis in high-volume centers with experienced operators.

   c. Thrombolytic therapy within the first 3 hours of the onset of pain reduces mortality and limits the size of infarction. Some benefit may occur if therapy is initiated within the first 12 hours. In the United States, alteplase, reteplase, and tenecteplase are the most commonly used agents. Absolute contraindications include previous hemorrhagic stroke, any stroke within past one year, known intracranial neoplasm, active internal bleeding, or suspected aortic dissection. Known bleeding diasthesis, trauma within past 2–4 weeks, major surgery within past 3 weeks, prolonged or traumatic cardiopulmonary resuscitation, recent internal bleeding, noncompressible vascular puncture, active diabetic retinopathy, pregnancy, active peptic ulcer disease, current use of anticoagulatants, and blood pressure >180/>110 are relative contraindications.

7. Statin therapy should be started in most patients in the days following ACS.

IX. CONGENITAL HEART ANOMALIES

A. General characteristics

1. Congenital heart anomalies are the most common congenital structural malformations.

2. Congenital heart anomalies are classified as either cyanotic or noncyanotic.

   a. Cyanotic types all involve right-to-left shunts.

      (1) Tetralogy of Fallot consists of a subaortic septal defect, right ventricular outflow obstruction, overriding aorta, and right ventricular hypertrophy.

      (2) Pulmonary atresia most often occurs with an intact ventricular septum. The pulmonary valve is closed; an atrial septal opening and patent ductus arteriosus are present.

      (3) Hypoplastic left heart syndrome actually is a group of defects with a small left ventricle and normally placed great vessels.

      (4) Transposition of the great vessels most commonly is a complete transposition of the aorta and pulmonary artery.

   b. Noncyanotic types

      (1) Atrial septal defect is an opening between the right and left atria. Of the four types, ostium secundum is the most common.

      (2) Ventricular septal defects may be muscular, perimembranous, or outlet openings between the ventricles.

      (3) Atrioventricular (AV) septal defect (canal) is due to incomplete fusion of the endocardial cushions. It is common in Down syndrome.

      (4) Patent (persistent) ductus arteriosus is a failure to close or a delay in closure of the channel bypassing the lungs, which allows placental gas exchange during the fetal state.

      (5) Coarctation of the aorta involves narrowing in the proximal thoracic aorta.

B. Clinical features: See Table 3-5.

TABLE 3-5   **Comparison of Findings in Various Congenital Defects**

Anomaly	Frequency	Murmur	Other Physical Findings	Important Clinical Information
CYANOTIC DEFECTS				
Tetralogy of Fallot	6–10% of significant congenital heart defects	Crescendo–decrescendo holosystolic at LSB, radiating to back	Cyanosis; clubbing; increased RV impulse at LLSB; loud S_2	Polycythemia usually present; TET (hypercyanotic) spells include extreme cyanosis, hyperpnea, and agitation—a medical emergency
Pulmonary atresia	1–3% of congenital heart disease	Depends on presence of tricuspid regurgitation	Cyanosis with tachypnea at birth; tachypnea without dyspnea; hyperdynamic apical impulse; single S_1 and S_2	Sudden onset of severe cyanosis and acidosis requires emergency treatment
Hypoplastic left heart syndrome	7–9% of significant congenital heart defects	Variable; not diagnostic	Shock; early heart failure; respiratory distress; single S_2; presentation varies with specific syndrome	Occurs more often in males; accounts for 25% of cardiac deaths before age 7 days
Transposition of the great vessels	5–7% of all congenital heart defects	Systolic murmur if associated VSD; systolic ejection murmur if pulmonary stenosis	Cyanosis in newborn is most common sign; tachypnea without respiratory distress; if large VSD, symptoms of CHF and poor feeding; single loud S_2; absent LE pulses if aortic arch obstruction	
NONCYANOTIC DEFECTS				
Atrial septal defect	7% of congenital heart disease; second most common	Systolic ejection murmur second LICS; early to middle systolic rumble	Failure to thrive; fatigability; RV heave; wide fixed split S_2	
VSD	Most common of all congenital heart defects	Systolic murmur at LLSB; others depend on severity of defect	Depends on size of defect—from asymptomatic to signs of CHF	Outlet VSDs more common in Japanese and Chinese
PDA	12–15% of significant congenital heart disease; higher in premature infants	Continuous (machinery) murmur in patients with isolated PDA	Wide pulse pressure, hyperdynamic apical pulse	
Coarctation of the aorta		Systolic, LUSB and left interscapular area; may be continuous	Infants may present with CHF; older children may have systolic hypertension or murmur	Differences between arterial pulses and blood pressure in UE and LE pathognomonic
VARIABLE				
Atrioventricular canal defect (endocardial cushion defect, AV septal defect)	5% of all defects; more common in infants with Down syndrome (15–20% of Down syndrome patients)	Depends on the degree of the defect	Cyanosis may be present; infants present with CHF if defect is large enough; first diagnosis may occur in adulthood with partial defects	As this refers to a constellation of defects, presentation is variable depending on whether the defect is complete, partial, or transitional

LSB, left sternal border; RV, right ventricle; LLSB, left lower sternal border; VSD, ventricular septal defect; CHF, congestive heart failure; LE, lower extremity; LICS, left intercostal space; PDA, patent ductus arteriosus; LUSB, left upper sternal border; UE, upper extremity.

C. Laboratory studies to evaluate cardiac anomalies may include ECG, echocardiography, Doppler ultrasound, MRI, chest radiography, radionuclide flow studies, cardiac catheterization, and angiography.

D. Treatment of most congenital heart anomalies is surgical.

X. VALVULAR DISORDERS

A. Aortic and mitral valve disorders

1. General characteristics

a. Aortic stenosis narrows the valve opening, impeding the ejection function of the left side of the heart.

b. Aortic insufficiency (regurgitation) results in volume overloading of the left ventricle.

c. Mitral stenosis impedes blood flow between the left atrium and ventricle.

d. Mitral insufficiency causes backflow and volume overload of the left atrium.

e. Mitral valve prolapse usually is asymptomatic, but it may cause mitral regurgitation.

f. Valve-related progressive heart failure leads to pulmonary hypertension and congestion.

g. The most frequent causes of mitral and aortic valve disorders are congenital defects; others include rheumatic heart disease, connective tissue disorders, infection, and senile degeneration.

h. Most patients present as adults after extended periods of asymptomatic conditions.

2. Clinical features (Table 3-6)

a. The most common presenting symptoms include dyspnea, fatigue, and decreased exercise tolerance.

b. Patients also may have cough, rales, paroxysmal nocturnal dyspnea or hemoptysis, and hoarseness.

c. Carotid pulses typically are thready in aortic stenosis; aortic insufficiency produces widened pulse pressures.

d. Most patients with mitral valve prolapse are thin females with minor chest wall deformities, midsystolic clicks, and late systolic murmur.

3. Laboratory studies

a. ECG is not useful in establishing the diagnosis.

TABLE 3-6 Comparison of Findings in Aortic and Mitral Valve Disorders

Valve Disorder	Murmur Location	Radiation	Intensity	Pitch/Quality	Aids to Hearing	Associated Findings	Timing
Aortic stenosis	2nd RICS	To neck and LSB	Often loud with a thrill	Medium pitch; harsh	Patient sitting and leaning forward		Midsystolic
Aortic regurgitation	2nd–4th LICS	To apex and RSB	Grade 1–3	High pitch; blowing	Patient sitting and leaning forward; full exhalation	Midsystolic or Austin Flint murmur suggests large flow; arterial pulses large and bounding	Systolic (soft) and diastolic decrescendo
Mitral stenosis	Apex	Little or none	Grade 1–4	Low pitch	Patient in left lateral position; full exhalation	S_1 accentuated; opening snap follows S_2	Middiastolic
Mitral regurgitation	Apex	To left axilla	Soft to loud	Medium to high pitch; blowing		S_2 often decreased; apical impulse prolonged	Pansystolic

RICS, right intercostal space; LSB, left sternal border; LICS, left intercostal space; RSB, right sternal border.

   b. Chest radiography
   (1) With aortic valve disorders, chest radiography may show left-sided atrial enlargement and ventricular hypertrophy.
   (2) With mitral valve disorders, chest radiography may show atrial enlargement alone.
   c. Echocardiography, particularly transesophageal, and cardiac catheterization are the only definitive methods of identifying structural and functional abnormalities. Doppler ultrasound is particularly useful for pressure gradient assessment.

4. Treatment
   a. The only effective long-term treatments are surgical repair, replacement of the defective valve, and balloon valvuloplasty.
   b. Patients with good exercise tolerance may be treated medically with diuretics and vasodilators for pulmonary congestion and with digoxin or β-blockers for dysrhythmias.
   c. Anticoagulant therapy is recommended for the prevention of thromboemboli, particularly if atrial fibrillation occurs.
   d. Antibiotics may be indicated for prevention of endocarditis and recurrent rheumatic fever, especially in the presence of regurgitation.

B. Tricuspid and pulmonic valve disorders
1. General characteristics
   a. Patients with congenital anomalies of these valves usually present during infancy or childhood; adults may present with stenosis resulting from rheumatic scarring or connective tissue disease.
   b. Tricuspid regurgitation may be intrinsic or functional.
   c. In all cases, right-sided pressure overload leads to right-sided cardiomegaly, systemic venous congestion, and right-sided heart failure.

2. Clinical features (Table 3-7)
   a. Patients usually present with exercise intolerance.
   b. Jugular venous distention, peripheral edema, and hepatomegaly reflect systemic venous congestion.

3. Laboratory studies
   a. Chest radiography may show a prominent right heart border with dilation of the superior vena cava.
   b. ECG findings may show right-axis deviation, P-wave abnormalities associated with right atrial enlargement, or the prominent R and deep S waves of right ventricular hypertrophy.
   c. Echocardiography or cardiac catheterization is the only definitive method of identifying structural or functional abnormalities.

4. Treatment
   a. Sodium restriction and diuretic therapy decrease fluid volume and right atrial filling pressure.
   b. Underlying conditions causing pulmonary hypertension are treated with arterial vasodilators or positive inotropic agents.
   c. Definitive treatment includes surgical repair, valvuloplasty, or replacement with porcine or synthetic prostheses.

TABLE 3-7	**Comparison of Findings in Tricuspid Regurgitation and Pulmonic Stenosis**						
Valve Disorder	Murmur Location	Radiation	Intensity	Pitch/Quality	Aids to Hearing	Associated Findings	Timing
Tricuspid regurgitation	LLSB; holosystolic	To right sternum and xiphoid area	Variable	Medium; blowing	Increases slightly with inspiration	JVP often elevated	Pansystolic
Pulmonic stenosis	2nd–3rd LICS; midsystolic crescendo–decrescendo	To left shoulder and neck	Soft to loud, possibly associated with thrill	Medium; harsh	—	Early pulmonic ejection sound common	Systolic

LLSB, left lower sternal border; JVP, jugular venous pressure; LICS, left intercostal space.

XI. RATE AND RHYTHM DISORDERS

A. Overview of arrhythmias

1. General characteristics

a. How dangerous an arrhythmia is depends on how much it impairs cardiac output or how likely it is to deteriorate into a more serious disturbance.

b. Susceptibility is based on genetic abnormalities and acquired structural heart disease.

c. Electrolyte abnormalities, hormonal imbalances, hypoxia, drug effects, and myocardial ischemia increase susceptibility.

d. Classification of arrhythmias includes those caused by disorders of impulse formation or automaticity, abnormalities of conduction, reentry, and triggered activity.

2. Clinical features

a. Presentation ranges from asymptomatic to symptomatic to lethal.

b. Specific features depend on the individual arrhythmia (see the following text).

3. Laboratory studies include ECG monitoring, measurements of heart rate variability, signal-averaged ECG, electrophysiologic testing, and autonomic testing.

4. Treatment: Antiarrhythmic drugs are divided into four classes based on the mechanism of action (Table 3-8).

B. Supraventricular arrhythmias

1. General characteristics

a. Sinus bradycardia (heart rate <60 bpm) may be normal in athletes; in others, it usually represents sinus node pathology, with increased risk for ectopic rhythms.

b. Sinus tachycardia (heart rate >100 bpm) occurs with fever, exercise, pain, emotion, shock, thyrotoxicosis, anemia, heart failure, and use of many drugs.

c. Atrial premature beats frequently are found in normal hearts and do not alone constitute heart disease.

d. Paroxysmal supraventricular tachycardia (PSVT) is the most common paroxysmal tachycardia and usually occurs in persons without structural problems.

TABLE 3-8	**Antiarrhythmic Drugs**		
Class	**Action**	**Indications**	**Examples**
Ia	Sodium channel blockers; depress phase 0 depolarization; slow conduction; prolong repolarization	Supraventricular tachycardia; V tach; prevention of V fib; symptomatic ventricular premature beats	Quinidine, procainamide, disopyramide, moricizine
Ib	Shorten repolarization	V tach; prevention of V fib; symptomatic ventricular premature beats	Lidocaine, mexiletine
Ic	Depress phase 0 repolarization; slow conduction	Life-threatening V tach or fibrillation; refractory supraventricular tachycardia	Flecainide, propafenone
II	β-Blockers; slow AV conduction	Supraventricular tachycardia; may prevent ventricular fibrillation	Esmolol, propranolol, metoprolol
III	Prolong action potential	Refractory V tach; supraventricular tachycardia; individual agents have specific indications	Amiodarone, sotalol, dofetilide, ibutilide
IV	Slow calcium channel blockers	Supraventricular tachycardia	Verapamil, diltiazem
V	Adenosine: slows conduction time through AVnode, interrupts reentry pathways; digoxin: direct action on cardiac muscle and indirect action on cardiovascular system via ANS	Supraventricular tachycardia	Adenosine, digoxin

V tach, ventricular tachycardia; V fib, ventricular fibrillation; AV, atrioventricular; ANS, autonomic nervous system.

e. Atrial fibrillation is the most common chronic arrhythmia, and both incidence and prevalence increase with age. It is called "holiday heart" when caused by excessive alcohol use or withdrawal.

f. Atrial flutter usually occurs in patients with chronic obstructive pulmonary disease, CHF, atrial septal defect, or coronary artery disease.

g. Junctional rhythms occur in patients with normal hearts or those with myocarditis, coronary artery disease, or digitalis toxicity.

2. Clinical features

   a. Patients may present with palpitations, angina, fatigue, and other symptoms of heart failure.

   b. Patients may be completely asymptomatic.

3. Laboratory studies: Characteristic ECG findings assist in the diagnosis of supraventricular arrhythmias (Fig. 3-5).

4. Treatment depends on the specific arrhythmia.

   a. Mechanical measures to interrupt acute PSVT include Valsalva maneuver, coughing, breath holding, stretching, putting the head between the knees, applying cold water to the face, and unilateral carotid sinus massage.

   b. Nonpharmacologic interventions may include surgical or radiofrequency ablation of abnormal sites, cardioversion, and electrical pacing. Synchronized cardioversion nearly always is successful, but it should not be used in cases of suspected digitalis toxicity.

   c. Pharmacotherapy may be used to terminate or prevent supraventricular arrhythmias.

      (1) IV administration of adenosine or IV or oral administration of verapamil terminates most episodes of PSVT. Other possibilities include esmolol, diltiazem, metoprolol, and digoxin.

      (2) Prevention usually is initiated with diltiazem and/or verapamil or a β-blocker.

   d. Treatment of acute atrial fibrillation depends on the presentation and includes electric cardioversion, treatment of underlying disease, and control of rate. Treatment of chronic atrial fibrillation includes control of rate and prevention of thromboembolism.

   e. Chemical conversion with ibutilide or electric cardioversion usually is successful in the treatment of atrial flutter. Amiodarone or dofetilide is the treatment of choice for chronic atrial flutter. Radiofrequency ablation is recommended for refractory or recurrent conditions.

C. Ventricular arrhythmias

1. General characteristics

   a. Ventricular premature beats may be benign or may lead to sudden death in persons with underlying heart disease.

   b. Ventricular tachycardia (V tach)

      (1) V tach is defined as three or more consecutive ventricular premature beats.

      (2) It may be sustained or unsustained.

      (3) It is a frequent complication of acute MI and dilated cardiomyopathy.

   c. Torsades de pointes is a V tach in which the QRS complex twists around the baseline. The ECG exhibits a continuously changing axis ("turning of the points"). It may occur spontaneously or when the patient has hypokalemia or hypomagnesemia, or following administration of drugs that prolong the QT.

   d. Long QT syndrome may be congenital or acquired and causes recurrent syncope, a QT interval usually 0.5 to 0.7 seconds long, ventricular arrhythmias, and sudden death.

   e. Brugada's syndrome is a genetic disorder, more common in Asians and in men, that causes syncope, ventricular fibrillation, and sudden death.

   f. In ventricular fibrillation, no effective pumping action exists; without intervention, death ensues.

2. Clinical features

   a. Patients with ventricular premature beats may be asymptomatic or aware of skipped beats.

   b. Patients with V tach may be asymptomatic or experience dizziness and syncope.

   c. Ventricular fibrillation is associated with sudden death, most often occurring in the early morning.

3. Laboratory studies: Characteristic ECG findings assist in diagnosing ventricular arrhythmias (Fig. 3-6).

4. Treatment is based on hemodynamic compromise and duration of the dysrhythmia.

   a. Ventricular premature beats may be treated with β-blockers only if the patient is symptomatic; class I and III agents may be used with caution only in symptomatic individuals.

   b. In V tach with severe hypotension or loss of consciousness, synchronized cardioversion may be necessary; ventricular overdrive pacing may help.

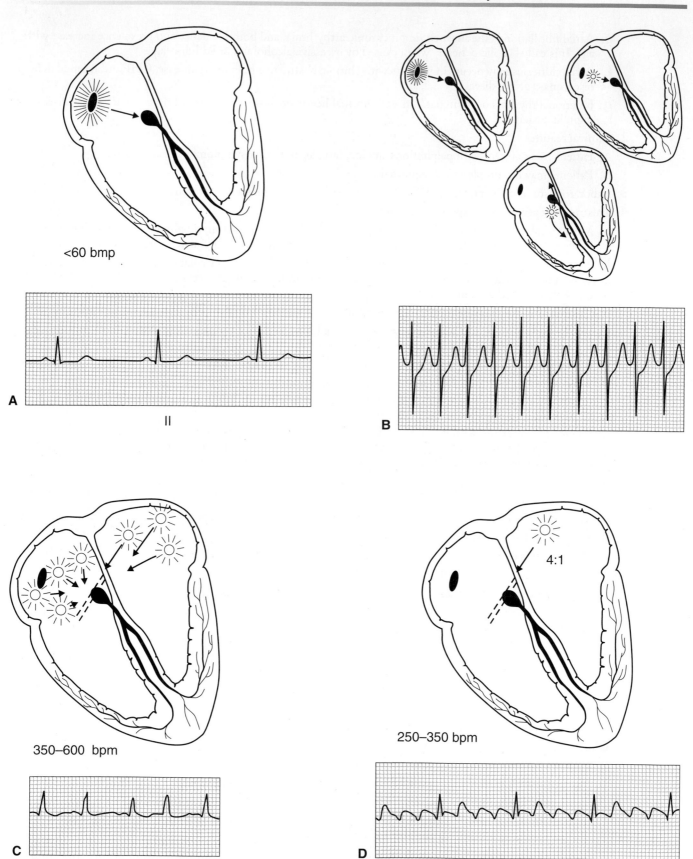

FIGURE 3-5 Electrocardiographic findings in supraventricular arrhythmias. **A:** Sinus bradycardia. **B:** Supraventricular tachycardia. **C:** Atrial fibrillation. **D:** Atrial flutter. **E:** Junctional rhythm, P waves. (From Stein E. *Rapid Analysis of Electrocardiograms: A Self-study Program.* 3rd ed. Philadelphia: Lippincott Williams & Wilkins; 2000.)

FIGURE 3-5 *Continued.*

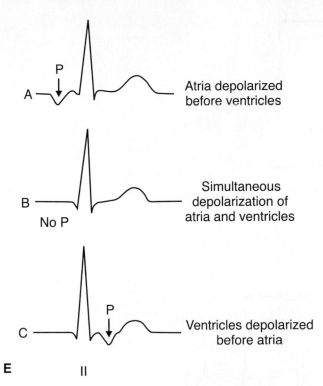

A — P↓ — Atria depolarized before ventricles

B — No P — Simultaneous depolarization of atria and ventricles

C — P↓ — Ventricles depolarized before atria

E — II

   c. The preferred pharmacologic interventions for acute V tach include lidocaine, procainamide, and amiodarone (Table 3-8). Empiric magnesium may help.

   d. In many types of ventricular arrhythmias, patients with an identifiable site of arrhythmic origin benefit from radiofrequency ablation.

   e. For chronic recurrent sustained V tach without a reversible cause, for congenital long QT syndrome, and for Brugada's syndrome, an implantable defibrillator is indicated.

   f. For acquired long QT syndrome, treatment includes discontinuation of drugs that prolong the QT interval.

   g. Torsades de pointes is treated with β-blockers, magnesium, and temporary atrial or ventricular pacing.

XII. CONDUCTION DISTURBANCES

  A. General characteristics

    1. Sick sinus syndrome

      a. Sick sinus syndrome most often is found in the elderly, but it may occur even in infants.

      b. It may be caused or exacerbated by digitalis, calcium channel blockers, β-blockers, sympatholytic agents, and antiarrhythmic drugs. It may result from underlying collagen vascular or metastatic disease, surgical injury, or, rarely, coronary disease.

      c. It is reversible if caused by digitalis, quinidine, β-blockers, or aerosols.

    2. AV block is characterized by refractory conduction of impulses from the atria to the ventricles through the AV node and/or bundle of His and is divided into first-degree, second-degree (subdivided into Mobitz type I [Wenckebach] and Mobitz type II), and complete or third-degree block.

  B. Clinical features

    1. Most patients with sick sinus syndrome are asymptomatic, but patients may have syncope, dizziness, confusion, heart failure, palpitations, or angina.

    2. AV conduction block may produce weakness, fatigue, light-headedness, and syncope.

  C. Laboratory studies: ECG changes associated with conduction disturbances are shown in Figure 3-7.

  D. Treatment

    1. Most symptomatic patients with sick sinus syndrome require permanent pacing.

    2. The only effective long-term treatment for AV conduction disorders is cardiac pacing.

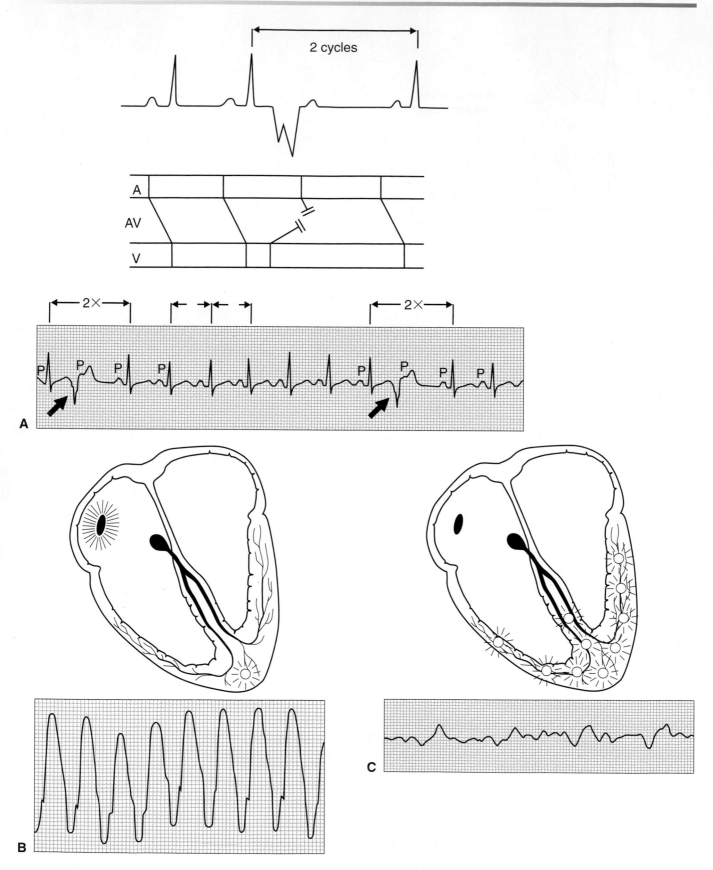

FIGURE 3-6 Electrocardiographic findings in ventricular arrhythmias. **A:** Premature ventricular contractions *(arrows)* frequently are identified by the accompanying compensatory pause. **B:** Ventricular tachycardia showing sustained tachycardia (it can also be intermittent). **C:** Ventricular fibrillation. (From Stein E. *Rapid Analysis of Electrocardiograms: A Self-study Program.* 3rd ed. Philadelphia: Lippincott Williams & Wilkins; 2000.)

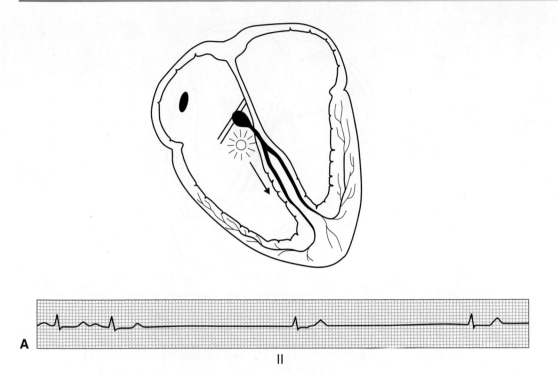

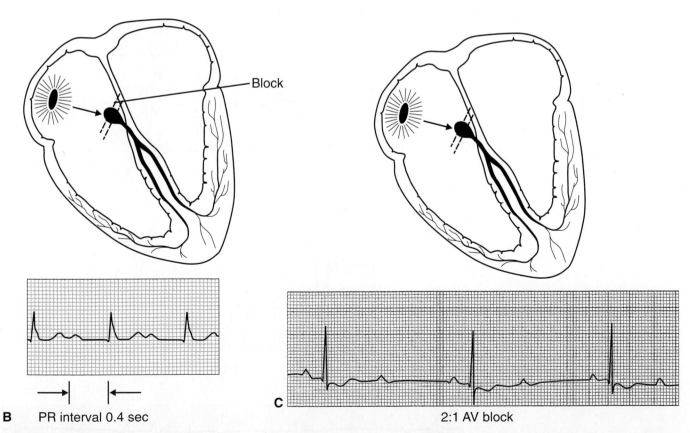

A

II

Block

B PR interval 0.4 sec

C 2:1 AV block

FIGURE 3-7 Electrocardiographic findings in conduction disturbances. **A:** Sinus arrest. **B:** First-degree atrioventricular (AV) block. **C:** Second-degree AV block. **D:** Second-degree AV block (Mobitz I block). **E:** Second-degree AV block. **F:** Third-degree (complete) AV block. SA, sinoatrial. (From Stein E. *Rapid Analysis of Electrocardiograms: A Self-study Program*. 3rd ed. Philadelphia: Lippincott Williams & Wilkins; 2000.)

FIGURE 3-7 *Continued.*

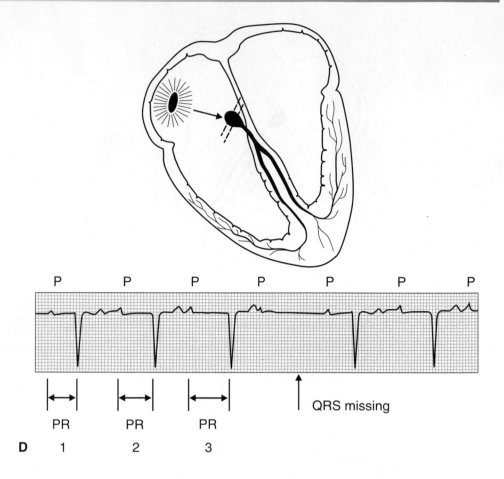

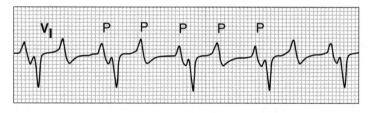

2:1

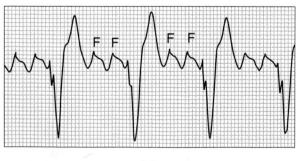

4:1

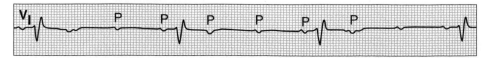

E   3:1

FIGURE 3-7 *Continued.*

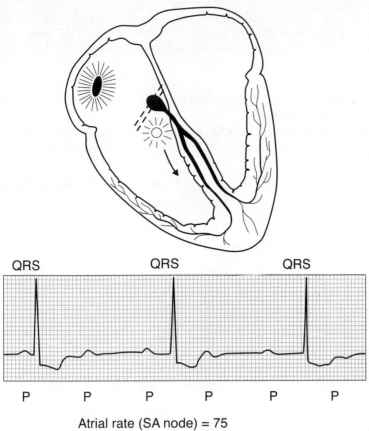

QRS   QRS   QRS

P   P   P   P   P   P

Atrial rate (SA node) = 75
F   Ventricular rate (AV junction) = 33

XIII. CARDIOMYOPATHIES

A. General characteristics

1. Cardiomyopathies are categorized by their presentation and pathophysiology.

2. Dilated cardiomyopathy

a. Dilated cardiomyopathies are the most common type (95%) and are associated with reduced strength of ventricular contraction, resulting in dilation of the left ventricle.

b. Causes include genetic abnormalities (25% to 30%), excessive alcohol consumption, postpartum state, chemotherapy toxicity, endocrinopathies, and myocarditis; it may be idiopathic.

c. It is more common in men (especially black men).

d. Takotsubo cardiomyopathy occurs after a major catecholamine discharge and is an apical left ventricular ballooning with symptoms indistinguishable from acute MI.

3. Hypertrophic cardiomyopathy

a. This cardiomyopathy (4%) has massive hypertrophy, particularly of the septum, small left ventricle, systolic anterior mitral motion, and diastolic dysfunction.

b. It is almost exclusively transmitted genetically. The apical variety is more common in persons of Asian descent; hypertrophic cardiomyopathy in the elderly is a distinct form.

c. Sudden cardiac death occurs in patients younger than 30 years at a rate of 2% to 3% yearly.

4. Restrictive cardiomyopathy

a. Restrictive cardiomyopathy (1%) results from fibrosis or infiltration of the ventricular wall because of collagen-defect diseases, most commonly amyloidosis, radiation, postoperative changes, diabetes, and endomyocardial fibrosis.

b. The left ventricle is small or normal, with mildly reduced function.

B. Clinical features

1. Dilated cardiomyopathies result in signs and symptoms of left or biventricular congestive failure; the most common presentation is dyspnea. Patients may have an S_3 gallop, rales, and increased jugular venous pressure.

2. Hypertrophic cardiomyopathy

    a. Patients most commonly present with dyspnea and angina. Syncope and arrhythmias are common. It may be asymptomatic. Sudden death may be the initial presentation.

    b. Physical examination may show sustained point of maximal impulse or triple apical impulse, loud S_4 gallop, variable systolic murmur, a bisferiens carotid pulse, and jugular venous pulsations with a prominent "a" wave.

3. Restrictive cardiomyopathy

    a. Patients present with decreased exercise tolerance; in advanced disease, patients develop right-sided congestive failure.

    b. Pulmonary hypertension usually is present.

C. Laboratory studies

1. Dilated cardiomyopathies

    a. ECG may show nonspecific ST- and T-wave changes, conduction abnormalities, and ventricular ectopy.

    b. Chest radiography in long-standing disease shows cardiomegaly and pulmonary congestion.

    c. Echocardiography, nuclear studies, and cardiac catheterization show left ventricular dilation and dysfunction, with high diastolic pressures and low cardiac output.

2. Hypertrophic obstructive cardiomyopathy

    a. Chest radiography often is not remarkable.

    b. ECG abnormalities include nonspecific ST- and T-wave changes, exaggerated septal Q waves, and left ventricular hypertrophy.

    c. Echocardiography, Doppler ultrasound, myocardial perfusion studies, cardiac MRI, and cardiac catheterization show left ventricular hypertrophy, asymmetric septal hypertrophy, small left ventricle, and diastolic dysfunction.

3. Restrictive cardiomyopathy

    a. Chest radiography may show a mildly to moderately enlarged cardiac silhouette.

    b. Echocardiography is the key to diagnosis; other low-voltage changes on ECG are typical. Cardiac MRI is distinctive, and cardiac catheterization may demonstrate normal or mildly reduced left ventricular function.

    c. Endomyocardial biopsy may be necessary to differentiate restrictive disease from other forms of cardiomyopathy or pericarditis.

D. Treatment

1. Dilated cardiomyopathies

    a. Abstinence from alcohol is essential.

    b. Underlying disease should be treated.

    c. CHF requires supportive treatment.

2. Hypertrophic cardiomyopathies

    a. Initial treatment employs β-blockers or calcium channel blockers; disopyramide is used for its negative inotropic effects.

    b. Surgical or nonsurgical ablation of the hypertrophic septum may be required.

    c. Dual-chamber pacing, implantable defibrillators, or mitral valve replacement may be indicated.

3. Diuretics may help patients with restrictive cardiomyopathies.

4. Cardiac transplantation may be indicated for severe disease.

XIV. PERICARDIAL DISORDERS

A. General characteristics

1. Pericarditis most often occurs as the result of infection (viral or bacterial), autoimmune or connective tissue disease, neoplasms, radiation therapy, chemotherapy or other drug toxicity, cardiac surgery, or myxedema; tuberculous pericarditis is common outside of developed nations. Pericarditis is more common in men and those under 50 years of age.

2. Pericardial effusion (secondary to pericarditis, uremia, or cardiac trauma) produces restrictive pressure on the heart.

3. Cardiac tamponade occurs when fluid compromises cardiac filling and impairs cardiac output.

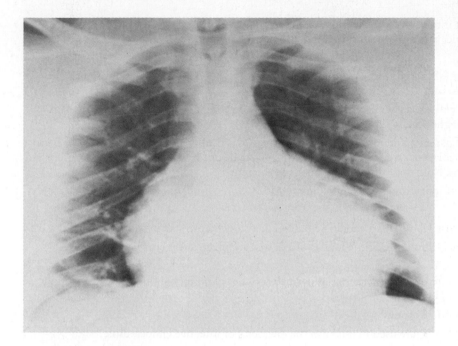

FIGURE 3-8 Pericardial effusion, frontal view. Note the massive enlargement of the patient's cardiac silhouette (water bottle heart). (From Daffner RH. *Clinical Radiology: The Essentials.* 2nd ed. Baltimore: Williams & Wilkins; 1999.)

B. Clinical features

1. The primary presenting symptom of acute pericarditis is pleuritic substernal radiating chest pain relieved by sitting upright and leaning forward; a friction rub is characteristic.

2. Constrictive pericarditis presents with slowly progressive dyspnea, fatigue, and weakness, accompanied by edema, hepatomegaly, and ascites.

3. Pericardial effusions may be painful or painless, often accompanied by cough and dyspnea.

4. In infectious conditions, patients may be febrile.

5. Cardiac tamponade typically presents with tachycardia, tachypnea, narrow pulse pressure, and pulsus paradoxus.

C. Laboratory studies

1. Elevated white blood cell (WBC) indicates infection, necessitating blood and pericardial fluid cultures.

2. Chest radiography or echocardiography is useful to determine the extent of cardiac effusion (Fig. 3-8) and calcification.

3. ECG changes include nonspecific T-wave changes and low QRS voltage. Electrical alternans is pathognomonic of effusion.

4. Echocardiography, Doppler ultrasonography, CT, and MRI may be helpful for more accurate diagnosis or before invasive procedures.

D. Treatment

1. In the presence of hemodynamic compromise, pericardiocentesis is necessary to relieve fluid accumulation.

2. Strictly inflammatory conditions may be treated with steroids or NSAIDs.

3. Infectious conditions require antibiotic therapy only if bacterial infection is suspected.

XV. INFECTIVE ENDOCARDITIS

A. General characteristics

1. Most cases of infective endocarditis are caused by *Staphylococcus aureus*, group D streptococci, enterococci, and HACEK organisms.

2. In IV drug users, *Staphylococcus aureus* is the most common cause, and the tricuspid valve frequently is involved.

3. Prosthetic valve endocarditis most often is caused by staphylococci, Gram-negative organisms, and fungi during the first 2 months after implantation. Later disease is typically due to strep or staph.

4. Most patients with endocarditis have an underlying regurgitant cardiac defect that provides a nidus for development of vegetation.

     5. Infection may result from direct intravascular contamination or from bacteremia, which is common during dental, upper respiratory, urologic, and lower gastrointestinal (GI) procedures.

B. Clinical features

     1. Most patients present with fever (although this may be absent in the elderly) and nonspecific symptoms (e.g., cough, dyspnea, arthralgias, back or flank pain, GI complaints).

     2. Approximately 90% of patients will have a stable murmur, but this may be absent in right-sided infections. A changing murmur is rare, but diagnostically significant.

     3. Classic features occur in 25% of patients and include palatal, conjunctival, or subungual petechiae; splinter hemorrhages; Osler nodes (painful, violaceous, raised lesions of the fingers, toes, or feet); Janeway lesions (painless red lesions of the palms or soles); and Roth spots (exudative lesions in the retina).

     4. Pallor and splenomegaly are common; strokes and emboli may occur.

C. Laboratory studies

     1. Three sets of blood cultures at least 1 hour apart should be obtained, ideally before starting antibiotics.

     2. Echocardiography is useful to identify the specific valves involved; transesophageal echocardiography is particularly useful.

     3. Chest radiography may demonstrate underlying cardiac abnormality or reveal pulmonary infiltrates if the right side of the heart is involved.

     4. The ECG has no specific diagnostic features.

     5. The modified Duke criteria (Table 3-9) are used to establish the diagnosis of infective endocarditis.

D. Treatment

     1. Empiric antibiotic treatment should include coverage of staphylococci, streptococci, and enterococci pending blood culture results. Vancomycin plus ceftriaxone is appropriate.

     2. Antibiotic prophylaxis to prevent endocarditis is recommended before invasive dental work or surgical procedures in patients with prosthetic valves, previous infective endocarditis, some congenital heart disease, some acquired valve disorders, hypertrophic cardiomyopathy, and cardiac transplant recipients with valvulopathy. Amoxicillin is the main drug of choice.

     3. Valve replacement, especially of the aortic valve, may be necessary if the condition does not resolve with antibiotic therapy, if an abscess develops, or if a fungal infection is the cause.

     4. Anticoagulants are not beneficial in patients with native valve infection and are controversial in patients with prosthetic valves.

XVI. RHEUMATIC HEART DISEASE

A. General characteristics

     1. Rheumatic fever is a systemic immune response occurring usually 2 to 3 weeks following a β-hemolytic streptococcal pharyngitis.

TABLE 3-9 | **Clinical Criteria for Infective Endocarditis**

Patient must have (1) two major, (2) one major and one minor, or (3) three minor criteria for the diagnosis to be made on clinical grounds

Major Criteria

- Two positive blood cultures of a typically causative microorganism
- Evidence of endocardial involvement on echocardiography
- Development of a new regurgitant murmur

Minor Criteria

- Predisposing factor
- Fever higher than 100.48°F (38.8°C)
- Vascular phenomena (e.g., embolic disease or pulmonary infarction)
- Immunologic phenomena (e.g., glomerulonephritis, Osler nodes, Roth spots)
- Positive blood culture not meeting major criteria

For details, see Bayer AS, Bolger AF, Taubert KA, et al. Diagnosis and management of infective endocarditis and its complications. *Circulation.* 1998;98:2936–2948.

2. It is most common in recent immigrants, but new U.S. outbreaks have occurred. Children from 5 to 15 years of age most often are affected.

3. Rheumatic valve disease may be self-limited or lead to progressive deformity of the valve; the typical lesion is a perivascular granuloma with vasculitis.

4. The mitral valve most often is involved (75% to 80%), followed by the aortic valve (30%). Aortic or tricuspid involvement rarely occurs in isolation.

B. Clinical features

1. Two major or one major and two minor Jones criteria are required to establish the diagnosis of rheumatic fever.

   a. Major criteria: carditis, erythema marginatum, subcutaneous nodules, chorea, and polyarthritis.

   b. Minor criteria: fever, polyarthralgias, reversible prolongation of the PR interval, rapid erythrocyte sedimentation rate, or C-reactive protein.

2. Supportive evidence includes positive throat culture or rapid strep test and elevated or rising streptococcal antibody titer.

C. Treatment

1. Strict bed rest is essential until the patient is stable.

2. Salicylates reduce fever and relieve joint problems; corticosteroid use relieves joint symptoms but does not seem to prevent cardiac disease.

3. Intramuscular (IM) penicillin is used for documented streptococcal infection; in patients who are allergic to penicillin, erythromycin is used.

4. Prevention includes early treatment of streptococcal pharyngitis. Prevention of recurrence is essential to prevent heart damage; benzathine penicillin every 4 weeks is adequate.

XVII. PERIPHERAL VASCULAR DISORDERS

A. Peripheral arterial disease

1. General characteristics

   a. Peripheral arterial disease usually is a result of atherosclerosis and is a significant independent risk factor for cardiovascular morbidity and mortality.

   b. Lower extremity disease results in ischemia and pain, causing significant limitation of activity or disability.

   c. Acute arterial occlusion may be caused by thrombosis or embolism.

   d. Thrombotic disease also may be a result of trauma, hypovolemia, inflammatory arteritis, polycythemia, dehydration, repeated arterial punctures, and hypercoagulable states.

   e. Three patterns of disease exist.

      (1) Type 1: 15% to 20% of patients, limited to the aorta and common iliac artery, most commonly found in men and women 40 to 55 years of age who smoke heavily or have hyperlipidemia.

      (2) Type 2: 25% of patients; involves the aorta, common iliac artery, and external iliac artery.

      (3) Type 3: most common, 60% to 70% of patients; multilevel disease affecting the aorta and the iliac, femoral, popliteal, and tibial arteries.

   f. Patients with type 2 and 3 peripheral arterial disease have typical risk factors for atherosclerotic disease and, usually, a high incidence of cerebrovascular and coronary artery disease.

2. Clinical features

   a. Lower leg pain with exercise, which is relieved by rest (intermittent claudication), usually is the first symptom of peripheral disease. Later, pain at rest occurs.

   b. Femoral and distal pulses will be weak or absent; an aortic, iliac, or femoral bruit may be present.

   c. Erectile dysfunction occurs with iliac artery disease (Leriche's syndrome).

   d. Severe, chronic disease results in numbness, tingling, and ischemic ulcerations, which may lead to gangrene.

   e. Symptoms of occlusion depend on the artery, the area it supplies, and the collateral circulation.

   f. Extremity occlusion usually results in pain, pallor, pulselessness, paresthesias, poikilothermia, and paralysis.

3. Laboratory studies

   a. Doppler flow studies are used to determine systolic pressures in the posterior tibial and dorsalis pedis arteries.

   b. An ankle–brachial index of less than 0.9 indicates significant disease.

    c. CT or magnetic resonance angiography is used for locating stenotic sites and for accurate diagnosis of thrombosis or embolism.

  4. Treatment

    a. Cigarette smoking is contraindicated. Progressive exercise is recommended. Lipid-lowering medications reduce the risk for new-onset or worsening claudication.

    b. Cilostazol is the main drug treatment. Antiplatelet therapy should be used routinely in all patients without a contraindication.

    c. Erectile dysfunction may require revascularization or treatment with a phosphodiesterase, such as sildenafil.

    d. Lower extremity revascularization must be preceded by a thorough cardiac and carotid evaluation.

    e. Thromboendarterectomy, embolectomy, thrombolytic therapy, and endovascular surgery may be indicated.

B. Varicose veins

  1. General characteristics

    a. Approximately 15% of adults, particularly women who have been pregnant, develop varicosities. Other risk factors include family history, prolonged sitting or standing, and history of phlebitis.

    b. The main mechanisms are superficial venous insufficiency and valvular incompetence; inherited defects in vein walls or valves also play a role.

  2. Clinical features

    a. Dilated, tortuous veins develop superficially in the lower extremities, particularly in the distribution of the long saphenous vein. Smaller blue-green, flat reticular veins, telangiectasias, and spider veins are further evidence of venous dysfunction.

    b. Varicosities may be asymptomatic or associated with aching and fatigue.

    c. Chronic distal edema, abnormal pigmentation, fibrosis, atrophy, and skin ulceration may develop in severe or prolonged disease.

    d. The Brodie–Trendelenburg test differentiates saphenofemoral valve incompetence from perforator vein incompetence.

  3. Laboratory studies are not necessary; however, Doppler sonography locates incompetent valves before surgery and identifies those due to congenital malformation.

  4. Treatment

    a. Graduated elastic stockings give external support.

    b. Leg elevation and regular exercise provide symptomatic relief.

    c. Small venous ulcers heal with leg elevation and compression bandages; larger ulcers may require compression boot dressing or skin grafts.

    d. Interventional techniques include endovenous radiofrequency or laser ablation, compression sclerotherapy, and sometimes surgical stripping of the saphenous tree.

C. Thrombophlebitis and deep venous thrombosis (DVT)

  1. General characteristics

    a. Thrombophlebitis involves partial or complete occlusion of a vein and inflammatory changes. Virchow's triad of stasis, vascular injury, and hypercoagulability predispose a vein to development of thrombophlebitis.

    b. Superficial thrombophlebitis may occur spontaneously or following trauma and occurs frequently at the site of intravenous or peripherally inserted central catheter (PICC) lines.

    c. DVT most often occurs in the lower extremities and pelvis.

    d. DVT is associated with major surgical procedures (especially total hip replacement), prolonged bed rest, use of oral contraceptives and hormone replacement therapy, and inherited (e.g., factor V Leiden) and cancer-associated hypercoagulable states. Increasingly, air travel is being recognized as a cause.

    e. Other risk factors include advanced age, type A blood, obesity, multiparity, inflammatory bowel disease, and lupus erythematosus.

  2. Clinical features

    a. Superficial thrombophlebitis may present with dull pain, erythema, tenderness, and induration of the involved vein or with no symptoms. It is most common in the long saphenous vein. A cord may be palpable following resolution of acute symptoms.

    b. Half of patients with DVT have no early signs or symptoms. Classic findings of DVT include swelling of the involved area with heat and redness over the site; Homan's sign in unreliable.

3. Diagnostic studies
   a. Duplex ultrasonography is the preferred study for DVT. Negative results in a patient with a high suspicion for DVT indicate the need for further study.
   b. Venography is the most accurate method for definitive diagnosis of DVT, but it is associated with increased risk and rarely is needed.
   c. D-Dimer is a fibrin degradation product that is elevated in the presence of thrombus. An elevated D-dimer does not sufficiently diagnose thrombophlebitis; most hospitalized patients will have an elevated level. A negative D-dimer test (<500 ng/dL), however, suggests that ultrasonography may be omitted.
4. Treatment
   a. Superficial disease is usually treated with bed rest, local heat, elevation of the extremity, and NSAIDs. More serious disease may require surgical intervention.
   b. Prevention of DVT in bedridden patients is accomplished by elevation of the foot of the bed, leg exercises, and compression hose; in high-risk patients, anticoagulation may be appropriate.
   c. Prevention of perioperative and travel-associated DVT includes early or frequent ambulation, leg exercises, and compression hose.
   d. Preferred treatment is anticoagulation with low-molecular-weight heparin; heparin followed by warfarin may be used.

D. Chronic venous insufficiency
   1. General characteristics
      a. Chronic venous insufficiency is characterized by loss of wall tension in veins, which results in stasis of venous blood and often is associated with a history of DVT, leg injury, or varicose veins.
      b. Prevention is accomplished by early aggressive treatment of venous reflux states, such as acute thrombophlebitis or varicose veins, use of compression hose, and weight reduction.
   2. Clinical features
      a. Progressive edema starting at the ankle is followed by skin and subcutaneous changes.
      b. Itching, dull pain with standing and pain with ulceration is common.
      c. Skin is shiny, thin, and atrophic with dark pigmentary changes and subcutaneous induration.
      d. Ulcers most commonly occur just above the ankle (stasis ulcer).
   3. Treatment
      a. General therapeutic measures include elevation of the legs, avoidance of extended sitting or standing, and compression hose.
      b. Stasis dermatitis should be treated with wet compresses and hydrocortisone cream; chronic dermatitis may require addition of zinc oxide with ichthammol and an antifungal cream.
      c. Ulcerations may be treated with wet compresses, compression boots or stockings, and, occasionally, skin grafting.

XVIII. GIANT CELL ARTERITIS

A. General characteristics
   1. Giant cell arteritis is a systemic inflammatory condition of medium and large vessels. It primarily affects those older than 50 years and frequently coexists with polymyalgia rheumatica.
   2. It most frequently involves the temporal artery and other extracranial branches of the carotid artery.
   3. If not treated aggressively, it can cause blindness.
   4. Large vessel problems (e.g., thoracic aortic aneurysm) occur in 15% of patients within 7 years.
B. Clinical features
   1. Patients have headache, scalp tenderness, jaw claudication, throat pain, and visual abnormalities.
   2. Symptoms of polymyalgia rheumatica (pain and stiffness mainly of shoulder and pelvic girdle) are present in 50% of patients.
   3. Nonclassic symptoms include respiratory tract problems, mononeuritis multiplex, fever of unknown origin, or unexplained neck and head pain.
   4. The temporal artery examination is usually normal, but may be nodular, enlarged, tender, or pulseless.
C. Laboratory studies
   1. Erythrocyte sedimentation rate and C-reactive protein are markedly elevated.

FIGURE 3-9 A CT scan through the abdomen showing a large abdominal aortic aneurysm *(arrows)*. Note the central enlarged lumen (L), the more peripheral hematoma (H), and the calcification of the wall on the left side. (From Daffner RH. *Clinical Radiology: The Essentials.* 2nd ed. Baltimore: Williams & Wilkins; 1999.)

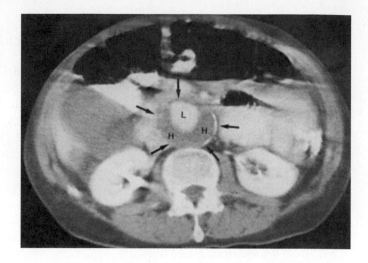

2. Most patients have a normochromic normocytic anemia and thrombocytosis; some have elevated alkaline phosphatase.

3. Temporal artery biopsy should be performed promptly for definitive diagnosis.

D. Treatment is high-dose prednisone (1 to 2 months before tapering) and low-dose aspirin.

XIX. AORTIC ANEURYSMS

A. General characteristics

1. An aortic aneurysm is a weakness and subsequent dilation of the vessel wall, usually caused by genetic defect or atherosclerotic damage to the intima.

2. Atherosclerosis is the most common cause, although some exist as congenital defects or as a result of syphilis, giant cell arteritis, vasculitis, trauma, Marfan's syndrome, or Ehlers–Danlos syndrome.

3. Males are eight times more likely to have an aneurysm; the classic picture is an elderly male smoker with coronary artery disease, emphysema, and renal impairment.

4. Aneurysms may occur in the abdominal (90%) or thoracic (10%) aorta.

5. Rupture (dissection) leads to rapid death in 90% of patients.

B. Clinical features

1. Abdominal aortic aneurysm may be asymptomatic or present as a pulsating abdominal mass, sometimes accompanied by abdominal or back pain.

2. Renal or lower extremity occlusive disease is present in 25% of patients.

3. Thoracic aortic aneurysms may be asymptomatic or cause substernal, back, or neck pain; dyspnea, stridor, and cough; dysphagia; hoarseness; or symptoms of superior vena cava syndrome.

4. Symptoms often indicate dissection.

5. Rupture causes severe back, abdominal, or flank pain and hypotension and shock.

C. Laboratory studies

1. Abdominal ultrasonography is the study of choice for abdominal aneurysms; this may be followed by contrast-enhanced CT (Fig. 3-9).

2. Thoracic aneurysms may require aortography for diagnosis; CT and MRI are preferred over ultrasonography.

D. Treatment

1. The only effective treatment is endovascular or open surgical repair.

2. Five-year survival after repair is greater than 60%.

Hematology

Rebecca Lovell Scott

4

I. ANEMIAS

A. General characteristics

1. Anemias are conditions involving hemoglobin concentrations or packed red blood cell (RBC) concentrations at levels below normal (Table 4-1).

2. Anemias may be caused by increased red cell destruction, decreased red cell production, or bleeding, or they may be secondary to a systemic disease.

3. Congenital anemia may be suggested by personal or family history.

4. Anemias present in many forms, including hypochromic microcytic anemias (iron deficiency anemia, thalassemia, sickle cell anemia, and long-standing anemia of chronic disease), normochromic normocytic anemias, and macrocytic anemias (Fig. 4-1). Macrocytic anemias may develop from megaloblastic or nonmegaloblastic causes.

   a. In microcytic anemias with mean corpuscular volume (MCV) of less than 80 fL, the cause is iron deficiency or thalassemia.

   b. Macrocytic anemia is defined as MCV greater than 100 fL; anemias with MCV of greater than 125 fL almost always are megaloblastic, except for those associated with myelodysplastic syndromes.

5. Anemias also may be classified on a pathophysiologic basis: diminished production or increased rate of loss of RBCs (Table 4-2).

B. Clinical features

1. Many patients have few signs or symptoms. The most common are fatigue, headache, and exertional dyspnea.

2. Acute anemia of rapid onset may cause tachycardia, orthostatic hypotension, faintness, and pale, cold extremities.

3. Chronic anemia may cause findings associated with hyperkinetic circulation (e.g., large pulse volume, tachycardia).

4. Pronounced anemia may cause pallor, cheilosis, jaundice, beefy red tongue, and koilonychia.

5. Smooth tongue and other mucosal changes suggest nutritional deficiencies (iron, folate, vitamin B_{12}).

6. Signs of primary hematologic disease (lymphadenopathy, hepatosplenomegaly, bone tenderness) may be present.

C. Laboratory studies (Table 4-3)

1. Hemoglobin (Hgb), hematocrit (Hct), red cell indices, and red cell distribution width (RDW) will help distinguish the type of anemia.

2. Peripheral smear will provide shape, color, size, and cell structure.

3. Corrected reticulocyte count assesses whether the bone marrow is responding by releasing immature red cells in response to low counts. It will distinguish whether the anemia is due to loss of cells (reticulocyte count high) or inadequate production (reticulocyte count low).

D. Hypochromic microcytic anemias (MCV <80 fL)

1. Iron deficiency anemias

   a. General characteristics

      (1) Iron deficiency anemias result from an inadequate supply of iron for synthesis of hemoglobin. Iron deficiency is the most common cause of anemia in the world.

      (2) In adults, blood loss, particularly from the gastrointestinal (GI) tract, almost universally is the cause of the iron deficiency. Chronic aspirin or nonsteroidal anti-inflammatory drug (NSAID) use also may be contributory.

      (3) Although menstrual blood loss plays a major role, menstruation should not automatically be assumed to cause a woman's iron deficiency.

      (4) Low dietary intake of iron may occur in children and pregnant women.

      (5) Other causes include decreased absorption of iron, increased requirements, hemoglobinuria, blood donation, iron sequestration, trauma, and intravascular hemolysis.

TABLE 4-1	Values for Normal Adult Blood	
Parameter	**Males**	**Females**
Hemoglobin	13.6–17.5 g/dL	12.0–15.5 g/dL
Hematocrit	39–49%	35–45%
Red blood cells	4.6–6.3 million/mL	4.2–5.4 million/mL

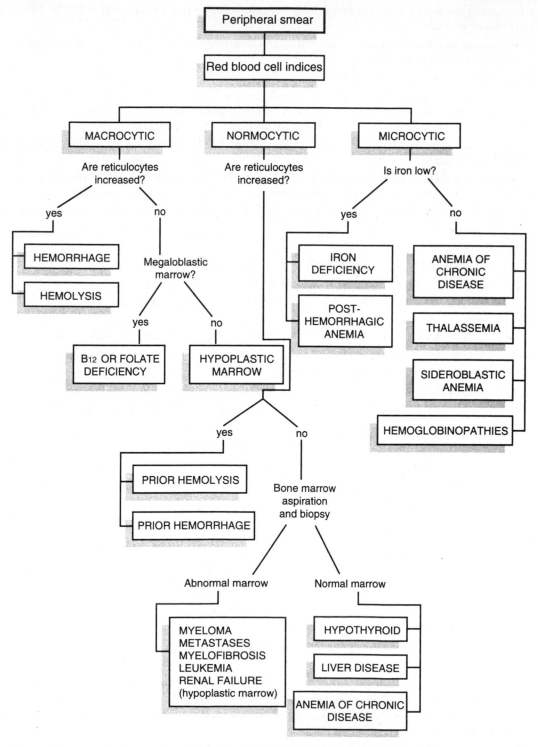

FIGURE 4-1 Diagnostic approach to anemias. (From Nirula R. *High-Yield Internal Medicine.* Baltimore: Lippincott Williams & Wilkins; 2003.)

TABLE 4-2	Pathophysiologic Classification of Anemias	
Decreased Production		**Increased Production**
Hemoglobin synthesis		Blood loss
Iron deficiency		Intrinsic hemolysis
Thalassemia		Hereditary spherocytosis
Anemia of chronic disease		Elliptocytosis
DNA synthesis		Sickle cell
Megaloblastic anemia		Unstable hemoglobin
Stem cell		G6PD deficiency
Aplastic anemia		Extrinsic hemolysis
Myeloproliferative leukemia		Warm and cold antibody
Bone marrow infiltration		TTP–HUS
Carcinoma		Mechanical cardiac valve
Lymphoma		Clostridial infection
Pure red cell aplasia		Hypersplenism

G6PD, glucose-6-phosphate dehydrogenase; TTP–HUS, thrombotic thrombocytopenic purpura–hemolytic uremic syndrome.

TABLE 4-3	Red Blood Cell Studies
Parameter	**Normal Range**
Mean corpuscular hemoglobin	26–34 pg
Mean corpuscular volume	80–100 fL
Mean corpuscular hemoglobin concentration	31–36 g/dL
Red cell distribution width	11.5–14.5%
Corrected reticulocyte count	0.5–2.5%

b. Clinical features
  (1) Lack of iron causes few specific complaints. General complaints in moderate to severe iron deficiency include pallor, easy fatigability, irritability, anorexia, tachycardia, tachypnea on exertion, and poor weight gain in infants.
  (2) Pica is a hallmark of iron deficiency.
  (3) Severe deficiency (Hct <25%) may cause brittle nails, cheilosis, smooth tongue, and formation of esophageal webs (Plummer–Vinson syndrome).
  (4) Iron deficiency anemia responds promptly to iron therapy.
c. Laboratory findings
  (1) Hemoglobin and hematocrit are decreased.
  (2) Peripheral smear
    (a) Initially, there are no changes in red cell size.
    (b) Later, the peripheral smear shows hypochromic microcytic red cells. Smear shows anisocytosis and poikilocytosis.
    (c) Severe anemia causes severely hypochromic cells, target cells, and nucleated red cells.
  (3) A plasma ferritin level of less than 30 µg/L reliably indicates iron deficiency anemia.
  (4) Serum iron is decreased to less than 30 µg/dL, and total iron-binding capacity is elevated. Transferrin saturation decreases to less than 15%.
  (5) MCV is normal early on but falls later in the course of the disease.
  (6) Platelet count is elevated in severe anemia.

d. Treatment

(1) Ferrous sulfate, 325 mg three times per day, should be given in a slowly escalating dose. It is best absorbed on an empty stomach but is frequently given with meals due to intolerability. Orange juice may enhance absorption.

(2) Although hematocrit will be within the normal range in 2 months, therapy should be continued for up to 6 months or longer to replenish tissue stores.

(3) Supplementation during pregnancy and lactation is essential.

(4) Parenteral iron is appropriate for patients with intolerance to oral iron, GI disease, and continuing blood loss. Sodium ferric gluconate is less likely than iron dextran to cause anaphylaxis.

(5) Identification of sources of occult blood loss is imperative.

(6) Treatment failures may be caused by nonadherence, poor absorption, incorrect diagnosis, or ongoing blood loss.

2. Thalassemia syndromes

a. General characteristics

(1) Thalassemia syndromes are hereditary anemias in which synthesis of α- or β-globin chains is reduced, resulting in defective hemoglobinization of RBCs.

(a) α-Thalassemia results from gene deletion; β-thalassemia results from point mutations.

(b) α-Thalassemia is more common in people of Southeast Asian or Chinese origin; β-thalassemia is more common in Mediterranean populations.

(2) The most prominent feature is microcytosis out of proportion to the degree of anemia.

(3) Thalassemia should be suspected in a person with a positive family history or a personal history of life-long microcytic anemia, especially if unresponsive to iron therapy.

(4) Thalassemias also may be classified as hypoproliferative anemias, hemolytic anemias, or anemias related to abnormal hemoglobin.

b. Clinical features

(1) Deficits range from silent carrier status to profound anemia.

(2) α-Thalassemia

(a) Patients may have mild symptoms or none (thalassemia trait; carriers). Patients often are diagnosed after a nonresponse to treatment for a prescribed iron deficiency.

(b) Patients with one α-globin chain have hemoglobin H disease, which is variably symptomatic; when all four chains are deleted, stillbirth occurs from hydrops fetalis.

(3) β-Thalassemia major (Cooley anemia)

(a) Problems begin at 4 to 6 months, when the switch from fetal hemoglobin (Hgb F) to adult hemoglobin (Hgb A) occurs. These problems include severe anemia, growth retardation, abnormal facial structure, pathologic fractures, osteopenia, bone deformities, hepatosplenomegaly, and jaundice.

(b) Before effective iron chelation and allogeneic stem cell transplantation, patients usually died from cardiac failure by age 30.

c. Laboratory findings

(1) Table 4-4 differentiates the thalassemias per typical hematocrit, hemoglobin electrophoresis, reticulocyte count, and peripheral smear.

(2) Serum iron and ferritin levels characteristically are normal or elevated.

(3) Hemoglobin level usually is between 3 and 6 g/dL.

(4) Thalassemia produces more marked microcytosis for degree of anemia than iron deficiency does; red cell morphologic changes occur earlier.

(5) Diagnosis is confirmed by hemoglobin electrophoresis.

d. Treatment

(1) Patients with mild disease should not receive iron because of the risk of iron overload.

(2) Persons with hemoglobin H disease need folic acid supplements and should avoid iron supplements and oxidative drugs (e.g., dapsone, primaquine, quinidine, sulfonamides, nitrofurantoin).

(3) Treatment for β-thalassemia major consists of transfusions to keep hemoglobin concentrations at least 12 g/dL; however, iron overload may result in hemosiderosis, heart failure, cirrhosis, and endocrinopathies. Deferoxamine is used to avoid or postpone hemosiderosis.

		Hemoglobin	Peripheral	Reticulocyte
TABLE 4-4	**Differentiation of Thalassemias per Laboratory Parameters**			
Type	**Hematocrit**	**Hemoglobin Electrophoresis**	**Peripheral Smear**	**Reticulocyte Count**
α-Thalassemia minor (trait)	28–40%	Normal	Target cells Acanthocytes	Normal
α-Thalassemia H	22–32%	Hemoglobin H	Target cells Poikilocytes	Increased
β-Thalassemia minor	28–40%	Hemoglobin A_2 Hemoglobin F	Target cells Basophilic stippling	Normal or increased
β-Thalassemia major	As low as 10%	Hemoglobin F Hemoglobin A_2	Target cells Poikilocytes Basophilic stippling Nucleated RBCs	Increased

RBCs, red blood cells.

(4) Allogeneic bone marrow transplantation also is used with increasing success; splenectomy may also be required.

(5) Genetic counseling, testing, and prenatal diagnosis for severe forms are essential.

3. Other hypochromic microcytic anemias

a. Sideroblastic anemias are acquired disorders with reduced hemoglobin synthesis causing iron accumulation, especially in the mitochondria.

(1) Prussian blue staining of bone marrow cells shows ringed sideroblasts.

(2) Causes include myelodysplasia, chronic alcoholism, and lead poisoning.

(3) Laboratory findings

(a) Hematocrit usually is 20% to 30%.

(b) MCV varies.

(c) Peripheral smear shows normal and hypochromic cells.

(d) In lead poisoning, basophilic stippling of red cells is present.

(e) Bone marrow evaluation is necessary to establish the diagnosis.

(4) Treatment

(a) Treat the underlying cause.

(b) Transfusion may be required.

(c) Patients do not respond to erythropoietin.

b. Hypochromic microcytic anemia may be associated with systemic or chronic disease or with copper deficiency.

E. Normochromic normocytic anemias (MCV = 80 to 100 fL)

1. General characteristics: These anemias are caused by organ failure or impaired marrow function resulting from systemic disease. Upregulation of hepcidin in response to inflammatory mediators is an important cause.

a. The organ failure causing these anemias may be associated with kidney, endocrine, thyroid, or liver disease; anemia of renal disease usually is more severe due to reduced production of erythropoietin.

b. Significant anemia in patients with chronic disease usually indicates coexisting iron or folate deficiency.

c. The impaired marrow function causing these anemias may be associated with chronic infection, aplastic anemia, infiltrative marrow disease (myelophthisic syndromes), and pure red cell aplasia.

d. Aplastic anemia arises from injury or abnormal expression of the pluripotent hematopoietic stem cell.

e. T cell–mediated autoimmune suppression of hematopoiesis is the most common cause; other causes are radiation, chemotherapy, toxins, pharmaceuticals, and systemic lupus erythematosus.

2. Clinical features

a. Anemia associated with chronic disease usually is mild and remits with treatment of the disease.

b. Clinical features are consistent with the underlying disease.

    c. Patients with aplastic anemia have weakness, fatigue, vulnerability to infection, pallor, purpura, and petechiae. Hepatosplenomegaly, lymphadenopathy, and bone tenderness suggest an alternative diagnosis.

3. Laboratory studies are ordered according to the underlying disease.

    a. Anemia of chronic disease usually is normochromic normocytic or mildly hypochromic microcytic.

    b. Anemia of chronic disease has normal or increased bone marrow iron stores and serum ferritin and normal or low total iron-binding capacity.

    c. Red cell morphology and reticulocyte count are unremarkable or mildly abnormal.

    d. Serum iron and transferrin saturation may be extremely low, but serum ferritin should be normal or elevated, except in cases of coexisting iron deficiency.

    e. Pancytopenia is the hallmark of aplastic anemia; bone marrow is hypocellular.

4. Treatment

    a. In anemia of chronic disease, the underlying disease must be treated.

    b. Erythropoietin is effective in treating anemia of renal failure, cancer, and inflammatory disorders.

    c. Mild aplastic anemia is treated supportively with transfusions of red cells and platelets; severe disease is treated with bone marrow transplantation or immunosuppression.

F. Macrocytic anemias (MCV >100 fL)

1. General characteristics

    a. These include anemias caused by acute hemorrhage and hemolysis.

    b. Macrocytic anemias also include deficiencies leading to megaloblastic states.

2. Folic acid deficiency anemia

    a. General characteristics

        (1) Folic acid deficiency most often is caused by poor dietary intake; other causes include defective absorption, pregnancy, hemolytic anemias, alcohol abuse, and consumption of folic acid antagonists (i.e., phenytoin, trimethoprim–sulfamethoxazole, sulfasalazine).

        (2) Inadequate intake is the most common cause in alcoholics, persons with anorexia, and those whose diet is low in fruits and vegetables.

        (3) Malabsorption is a rare cause as folic acid is absorbed throughout the GI tract.

        (4) The daily requirement of folic acid is 50 to 100 mg/dL and usually is met by the diet.

        (5) Pregnancy, hemolytic anemias, and exfoliative skin disease increase requirements.

    b. Clinical features

        (1) Sore tongue (glossitis)

        (2) Vague GI symptoms

        (3) No neurologic symptoms (in contrast to vitamin B_{12} deficiency)

    c. Laboratory findings

        (1) Macro-ovalocytes and hypersegmented polymorphonuclear cells are pathognomonic.

        (2) Howell–Jolly bodies (nuclear DNA remnants) are typical.

        (3) RBC folate level of less than 150 ng/mL is diagnostic.

        (4) Serum vitamin B_{12} level is normal.

    d. Treatment

        (1) Oral replacement (1 mg/day) with folic acid is the first line of treatment.

        (2) Avoid alcohol and folic acid metabolism antagonists (trimethoprim, seizure medications, others).

3. Vitamin B_{12} (cobalamin) deficiency

    a. General characteristics

        (1) Pernicious anemia is the most common cause and leads to atrophic gastritis and increased risk of gastric carcinoma. Other autoimmune diseases may be present.

        (2) Other causes include strict vegan diet, gastric surgery, blind loop syndrome, pancreatic insufficiency, and Crohn's disease.

        (3) Irreversible neurologic damage can be caused by uncorrected deficiency. Folate administration can mask the deficiency but does not correct it.

        (4) Foods of animal origin supply vitamin B_{12}.

        (5) Absorption occurs in the terminal ileum and storage in the liver.

    b. Clinical features

        (1) The physical examination will be unremarkable in most patients; glossitis, pale icterus, and vague GI symptoms may be present.

        (2) Neurologic findings include stocking–glove paresthesias, loss of position, fine touch and vibratory sensation, clumsiness, dementia, and ataxia.

    c. Laboratory studies

        (1) Anemia may be severe, and MCV usually is markedly elevated but may be normal.

        (2) Anisocytosis, poikilocytosis, macro-ovalocytosis, and hypersegmented neutrophils are seen.

        (3) Reticulocyte count is reduced.

        (4) Serum lactate dehydrogenase (LDH) and indirect bilirubin are elevated.

        (5) Serum vitamin B_{12} is abnormally low.

        (6) Schilling test (a 24-hour urine collection of radioactive vitamin B_{12}) is rarely used today.

    d. Treatment

        (1) Lifelong supplemental vitamin B_{12} usually is given intramuscularly (IM) for pernicious anemia.

        (2) Daily oral cobalamin may be used but must be given in high doses. A nasal spray or gel is also available.

        (3) Reversible causes of malabsorption should be treated.

        (4) Strict vegans, persons who have undergone gastrectomy or resection of the ileum, and those with blind loop syndrome require supplementation to prevent anemia.

        (5) Neurologic signs and symptoms are reversible if treated within 6 months.

  4. Hemolytic anemias

    a. General characteristics

        (1) Hemolytic anemias are those characterized by episodic or continuous RBC destruction.

        (2) Classification usually is based on intrinsic red cell defects or extracellular causes.

            (a) Intrinsic causes include hereditary spherocytosis and elliptocytosis, paroxysmal nocturnal hemoglobinuria, glucose-6-phosphate dehydrogenase (G6PD) deficiency, methemoglobinemia, and sickle cell syndromes.

            (b) Causes external to the erythrocyte include autoimmune and lymphoproliferative diseases, drug toxicity, thrombotic thrombocytopenic purpura (TTP), hemolytic uremic syndrome (HUS), disseminated intravascular coagulation (DIC), valvular hemolysis, metastatic adenocarcinoma, vasculitides, infections, hypersplenism, and burns.

    b. Clinical features

        (1) Anemia from both causes may present with jaundice, gallstones, pallor, and symptoms related to decreased oxygen delivery to the tissues.

        (2) Infection with parvovirus B19 can lead to a transient aplastic crisis. Risk for infection with *Salmonella* and *Pneumococcus* sp. is increased.

    c. Laboratory findings

        (1) An elevated reticulocyte count in the presence of a falling or stable hematocrit is the hallmark of hemolytic anemia.

        (2) Peripheral smear may reveal immature red cells, nucleated red cells, or morphologic changes.

        (3) Transient hemoglobinemia indicates intravascular hemolysis and may be accompanied by hemoglobinuria.

        (4) Unconjugated (indirect) bilirubin is elevated; total bilirubin may rise to 4 mg/dL.

        (5) Serum LDH indicates microangiopathic hemolysis.

    d. Treatment depends on the underlying disorder.

  5. Sickle cell anemia

    a. General characteristics

        (1) Sickle cell anemia is an autosomal recessive hemolytic anemia.

        (2) RBCs containing primarily hemoglobin S sickle under deoxygenated conditions.

        (3) In the United States, this disease most often is seen in blacks (1 in 400 births); 8% carry the hemoglobin S gene as the sickle cell trait.

    b. Clinical features

      (1) Problems begin in infancy, when hemoglobin F levels fall.

      (2) By childhood or adolescence, vascular occlusions produce painful crises, lasting for hours to days, with organ swelling and dysfunction and infarction.

      (3) Sickling is increased by red cell dehydration, acidosis, and hypoxemia. Patients with sickle cell disease should avoid high altitudes due to the risk of precipitating a crisis.

      (4) Patients with sickle cell anemia are at increased risk for cholelithiasis, splenomegaly, poorly healing ulcers, infection with encapsulated organisms (e.g., *Streptococcus pneumoniae*), strokes, priapism, retinopathies leading to blindness, and osteomyelitis.

      (5) Hemolytic or aplastic crises may be life threatening.

      (6) Avascular necrosis of the femoral head is common.

      (7) Life expectancy is 40 to 50 years.

      (8) Sickle cell trait may result in difficulty concentrating urine.

    c. Laboratory findings

      (1) Electrophoresis demonstrates hemoglobin S in red cells.

      (2) Peripheral smear reveals sickled cells (5% to 50%) and target cells, nucleated RBCs, and Howell–Jolly bodies.

      (3) Reticulocyte count is elevated.

      (4) White blood cell (WBC) count is elevated; thrombocytosis may be present.

      (5) Indirect bilirubin may be elevated.

    d. Treatment

      (1) Symptomatic treatment includes administration of analgesics, fluids, and oxygen.

      (2) Vaso-occlusive crises may require exchange transfusion.

      (3) Patients should receive pneumococcal vaccine (booster vaccine every 10 years) and folate supplementation.

      (4) Genetic counseling for patients with either the disease or trait is recommended. Prenatal testing is available.

  6. G6PD deficiency

    a. General characteristics

      (1) G6PD deficiency is an X-linked recessive disorder commonly seen in American black males (10% to 15%) and some Mediterranean populations.

      (2) G6PD activity declines as erythrocytes age beyond 40 days.

      (3) Oxidative drugs (e.g., aspirin, dapsone, primaquine, quinidine, sulfonamides, nitrofurantoin) and infection cause episodic hemolysis.

      (4) Severe deficiency may cause chronic hemolysis.

    b. Clinical features

      (1) Patients with episodic hemolysis usually are healthy and have no splenomegaly.

      (2) Female carriers rarely are affected.

    c. Laboratory findings

      (1) During hemolytic episodes, reticulocytes and serum indirect bilirubin increase.

      (2) Peripheral smear reveals bite cells and Heinz bodies (denatured hemoglobin).

      (3) G6PD levels will be low between hemolytic episodes; in severe cases, G6PD levels will always be low.

    d. Treatment

      (1) In most cases, hemolytic episodes are self-limited as red cells are replaced.

      (2) Oxidative drugs should be avoided.

II. POLYCYTHEMIA VERA

  A. General characteristics

    1. Polycythemia vera is a slowly progressive bone marrow disorder characterized by increased numbers of RBCs and increased total blood volume. The presence of the JAK2 mutation is diagnostic.

    2. Unregulated expansion of red cell mass causes hyperviscosity, which leads to decreased cerebral blood flow.

3. Secondary causes of erythrocytosis include chronic hypoxia, often caused by cigarette smoking, and renal tumors.

4. Morbidity and mortality most commonly result from thrombosis; other complications include bleeding, peptic ulcer disease, and GI bleeding.

5. Median age at presentation is 60 years, and 60% of patients are male. Median survival time for patients with polycythemia vera is 11 to 15 years.

6. Polycythemia vera may convert to myelofibrosis or chronic myeloid leukemia and, rarely, to acute myeloid leukemia.

B. Clinical features

1. Diagnostic criteria include splenomegaly, normal arterial oxygen saturation, and an elevated red cell mass.

2. Patients may present with symptoms of increased blood viscosity and volume (i.e., headache, dizziness, fullness in the head and face, weakness, fatigue, tinnitus, blurred vision); burning, pain, and redness of the extremities; and, rarely, stroke.

3. Generalized pruritus after bathing is characteristic.

4. Epistaxis may be the presenting complaint.

5. Incidence of peptic ulcer disease is high.

6. Plethora, systolic hypertension, engorged retinal veins, and splenomegaly may be found on physical examination.

7. Thrombosis is the most common complication and the cause of most morbidity and mortality; increased bleeding also occurs.

8. Absence of splenomegaly suggests secondary polycythemia.

C. Laboratory findings

1. At sea level, hematocrit levels in polycythemia vera are typically greater than 54% in males and greater than 51% in females.

2. Patients without splenomegaly must have two of the following to establish the diagnosis: thrombocytosis, leukocytosis, elevated leukocyte alkaline phosphatase, elevated serum vitamin B_{12}, or elevated vitamin B_{12}–binding capacity.

3. Peripheral smear shows neutrophilic leukocytosis, increased basophils and eosinophils, and increased numbers of large, bizarre platelets.

4. Red cell morphology usually is normal; erythropoietin levels generally are low.

5. The bone marrow is hypercellular in all cell lines; iron stores usually are absent.

6. Hyperuricemia also develops.

D. Treatment

1. Phlebotomy is the treatment of choice.

2. Myelosuppressive therapy with hydroxyurea may be indicated; anagrelide may be added or substituted.

3. Low-dose aspirin reduces the risk of thrombosis without increasing the risk of bleeding.

III. **MALIGNANCIES**

A. Leukemias

1. General characteristics

a. Leukemias are diseases characterized by unrestrained growth of leukocytes and leukocyte precursors in the tissues.

b. Leukemias are classified according to cell type and may be myeloid or lymphoid.

c. They also are classified as either acute or chronic.

d. Risk factors include a positive family history and exposures to ionizing radiation, benzene, and certain alkylating agents.

2. Acute leukemias

a. General characteristics

(1) There are two types of acute leukemias: acute lymphocytic leukemia (ALL), and acute myelogenous leukemia (AML).

(2) The incidence increases with age. In children, ALL (80%) is more common than AML. Most diagnoses are made in children between 3 and 7 years of age.

(3) AML primarily is a disease of adulthood (median age at onset is 60 years).

b. Clinical features

(1) Most clinical findings are related to replacement of normal bone marrow with malignant cells.

(2) Gingival bleeding, epistaxis, and menorrhagia may be the presenting complaint; DIC is less common.

(3) Infections from neutropenia commonly are caused by Gram-negative bacteria or fungi; common presentations include cellulitis, pneumonia, and perirectal infection. Death may occur if treatment is delayed.

(4) Children and young adults present with fatigue, abrupt onset of fever, lethargy, headache, and bone and/or joint pain, especially in the sternum, tibia, and femur.

(5) Older adults have a slow, progressive onset, with lethargy, anorexia, and dyspnea.

(6) Symptoms of anemia, thrombocytopenia, gingival hyperplasia, rashes, or cranial nerve palsies occur in most patients.

(7) Lymphadenopathy and hepatosplenomegaly are more common with ALL than in AML.

c. Laboratory findings

(1) The hallmark of acute leukemia is pancytopenia with circulating blasts; blasts make up at least 20% of nucleated cells in the bone marrow.

(2) Hyperuricemia is present.

(3) Different leukemias express specific antigens.

(4) Auer rods (rod-shaped structures in cell cytoplasm) signify myeloid leukemia.

(5) WBC counts usually are high.

(6) Bone marrow biopsy confirms the diagnosis.

(7) In ALL, a mediastinal mass may be seen on chest radiography.

(8) Terminal deoxynucleotidyl transferase is present in 95% of ALL cases.

(9) Cytogenetic studies are the most powerful prognostic factors; presence of the Philadelphia chromosome is unfavorable in ALL.

d. Treatment

(1) Induction (remission-inducing) chemotherapy is targeted toward eradication of most of the leukemic cells.

(2) Consolidation therapy destroys the remainder of the leukemic cells.

(3) Increased serum urate levels may be caused by the treatment. Allopurinol and diuretics may be needed to prevent uric acid stones.

(4) Allogeneic bone marrow transplantation is used in patients with adverse cytogenetics or poor response to treatment.

(5) Greater than 50% of children with ALL can be cured with chemotherapy (induction plus consolidation therapy). Prognosis is related to age and WBC count at diagnosis.

(6) Greater than 70% of adults younger than 60 years achieve complete remission with treatment for AML; further chemotherapy leads to cure in 30% to 40% of patients.

3. Chronic leukemias

a. General characteristics

(1) Chronic lymphocytic leukemia (CLL) is a clonal malignancy of B lymphocytes.

(2) CLL is the most prevalent of all leukemias. It is twice as common in men as in women. Incidence increases with advancing age; median age at presentation is 65 years.

(3) The B cell form accounts for 95% of CLL cases.

(4) Prognostic staging uses the Rai system.

(5) Chronic myelocytic leukemia (CML) is a myeloproliferative disorder.

b. Clinical features

(1) CML

(a) CML presents in young to middle-aged adults (median age at presentation is 55 years). Greater than 80% are alive 6 years later.

(b) It occurs in three phases: chronic, accelerated, and acute (blast crisis, defined as >30% blast cells in the blood or bone marrow).

(c) It inevitably transforms into acute disease.

    (d) Symptoms

        (i) Fatigue, anorexia, weight loss, low-grade fever, and excessive sweating are common.

        (ii) Most patients also have abdominal fullness caused by splenomegaly.

        (iii) Rare presentations include blurred vision, respiratory distress, and priapism.

    (e) The symptoms of CML develop gradually. CML generally runs a mild course until the blast-crisis phase, which indicates accelerated disease and short survival.

  (2) CLL

    (a) CLL usually has an indolent course, with a median survival time of 6 years. Patients with stage 0 or I have a median survival of 10 to 15 years. It often is harmless but is resistant to cure. A variant, polylymphocytic leukemia, is more aggressive.

    (b) Clinical manifestations of CLL include peripheral lymphocytosis and lymphocytic invasion of bone marrow, liver, spleen, and lymph nodes.

    (c) Patients may have recurrent infections, splenomegaly, and lymphadenopathy.

    (d) Richter's syndrome occurs in 5% of cases; an isolated node transforms into aggressive, large-cell lymphoma.

c. Laboratory findings

  (1) The hallmark of CLL is isolated lymphocytosis, with a leukocytosis of greater than 20,000 cells/mL.

  (2) The hallmark of CML is leukocytosis, with a median WBC count of 150,000 cells/mL. The Philadelphia chromosome is identified in 95% of cases.

  (3) Identification of the BCR-ABL gene by polymerase chain reaction has replaced the search for the Philadelphia chromosome to establish the diagnosis.

  (4) Peripheral smear

    (a) CML may show anemia and thrombocytosis.

    (b) CLL shows increased mature small lymphocytes; smudge cells are pathognomonic.

  (5) Bone marrow is hypercellular with a left shift.

d. Treatment

  (1) CML

    (a) STI571 (imatinib mesylate; Gleevec) has replaced the former standard therapy. It is very effective during the chronic phase.

    (b) Dasatinib or nilotinib is used in cases of imatinib intolerance.

    (c) Allogeneic bone marrow transplantation may be the initial treatment and is the only therapy proven to be curative. A cure rate of 80% is achieved in those under 40 years with transplantation from HLA-matched siblings. Bone marrow transplantation is reserved for patients with disease, which progresses after initial treatment.

  (2) CLL: Treatment of CLL usually is palliative once the disease is advanced.

B. Hodgkin's disease

  1. General characteristics

    a. Hodgkin's disease refers to a group of cancers characterized by enlargement of lymphoid tissue, spleen, and liver and the presence of Reed–Sternberg cells.

    b. The Epstein–Barr virus also appears to be an important factor; it can be found in 40% to 50% of cases.

    c. Hodgkin's disease usually arises in a single area and spreads to contiguous nodes.

    d. It is most common between the ages of 15 and 45 years, peaking in the 20s, and again after age 50. It is rare in children under the age of 5.

    e. Among adults 15 to 45 years of age, it is more common in men.

  2. Clinical features

    a. Patients usually present with painless cervical, supraclavicular, and mediastinal lymphadenopathy. Pain in the affected node after ingestion of alcohol may occur.

    b. The nodular sclerosis subtype commonly is seen in young women; other subtypes are lymphocyte predominant, mixed cellularity, and lymphocyte depletion.

TABLE 4-5	Staging for Hodgkin's Disease: The Ann Arbor Criteria
Stage	**Criteria**
I	Single LNR (I) or a single ELS (IE)
II	Two or more LNRs on the same side of the diaphragm (II) or one solitary ELS and one or more LNRs on the same side of the diaphragm (IIE)
III	LNR on both sides of the diaphragm (III) With spleen involvement (IIIS) or solitary involvement of an ELS (IIIE) or both (IIIES) III_1 = upper abdomen; III_2 = lower abdomen
IV	Diffuse involvement of ELS with or without node involvement
A, B	Constitutional symptoms (fever, night sweats, loss of 10% of body weight); presence = B; absence = A

LNR, lymph node region; ELS, extralymphatic site.

    c. Stage A designation indicates a lack of constitutional symptoms. One-third of patients present with constitutional (stage B) symptoms (fever, night sweats, weight loss, pruritus, and fatigue), which are associated with a poorer prognosis.

3. Laboratory studies

    a. The Ann Arbor system is used to stage Hodgkin's and non-Hodgkin's lymphoma (Table 4-5).

    b. Basic staging includes CT of neck, chest, abdomen, and pelvis as well as biopsy of the bone marrow; laparotomy is no longer routine.

    c. Reed–Sternberg cells confirm the diagnosis.

4. Treatment

    a. Combination chemotherapy cures more than 50% of patients, even those with advanced-stage disease.

    b. Radiation therapy is the initial treatment of choice for patients with low-risk stage IA and IIA disease; the 10-year survival rate exceeds 80%.

    c. Most other patients receive adriamycin, bleomycin, vinblastine, and dacarbazine (ABVD) chemotherapy; shorter, intensive treatments are under study.

C. Non-Hodgkin's lymphoma

  1. General characteristics

    a. Lymphomas are a group of malignancies that arise from lymphocytes; pathogenesis is related to cytogenetic abnormalities.

    b. About 90% of cases are derived from B lymphocytes.

    c. The incidence of B cell lymphomas is higher in patients with HIV disease and other immunodeficiencies.

    d. Peak incidence occurs between 20 and 40 years of age.

    e. These lymphomas are divided into clinically indolent and aggressive groups.

      (1) Indolent lymphomas tend to convert to aggressive disease.

      (2) One-third of aggressive lymphomas are curable with chemotherapy.

  2. Clinical features

    a. Diffuse or isolated, painless, persistent lymphadenopathy is the most common presentation; bone marrow involvement is frequent.

    b. Common extralymphatic sites are the GI tract, skin, bone, and bone marrow. Burkitt's lymphoma is likely to present with abdominal fullness.

    c. Fever, night sweats, weight loss, pruritus, and fatigue are less likely than with Hodgkin's disease but do occur in intermediate- and high-grade disease.

  3. Laboratory studies

    a. Persistent, unexplained, enlarged nodes should be biopsied.

    b. Staging is accomplished by chest radiography, CT of the abdomen and pelvis, bone marrow biopsy, and possibly lumbar puncture.

c. Serum LDH is a useful prognostic marker.

d. Molecular profiling is under study.

4. Treatment is based on the stage of disease and the patient's clinical status.

a. No clear consensus exists regarding treatment because of multiple new modalities. In some cases, spontaneous remission may occur.

b. Patients with a single involved node may be treated with radiation.

c. Low-grade lymphoma may be treated with rituximab with or without chemotherapy or radioimmune conjugates.

d. Patients with aggressive low-grade lymphoma may be suitable for allogeneic transplant.

e. Intermediate- or high-grade lymphomas are treated with chemotherapy and autologous stem cell transplantation.

D. Multiple myeloma

1. General characteristics

a. Multiple myeloma is a malignancy of plasma cells, possibly caused by a herpes virus.

b. Replacement of bone marrow leads to failure; bone destruction leads to pain, osteoporosis, lytic lesions, hypercalcemia, and pathologic fractures. Plasmacytomas may cause spinal cord compression.

c. Patients are prone to recurrent infections, particularly with encapsulated organisms, because of neutropenia and failure of antibody production in response to antigen challenge.

d. Paraprotein levels are increased (IgG or IgA may cause hyperviscosity; light-chain components may lead to renal failure).

2. Clinical features

a. Median age at diagnosis is 65 years.

b. The most common presenting complaints include anemia, bone pain (particularly in the low back or ribs), and infection. Less common presenting complaints include renal failure, spinal cord compression, and hyperviscosity syndrome.

c. Some cases are found simply through abnormal laboratory studies, including hypercalcemia, proteinuria, and elevated erythrocyte sedimentation rate; follow-up electrophoresis will be abnormal.

3. Laboratory studies

a. Patients will be anemic, with normal cell morphology; rouleaux formation is common (RBCs stack like coins).

b. The hallmark of myeloma is a monoclonal spike on serum protein electrophoresis.

c. Lytic lesions are present on radiography of the axial skeleton; generalized osteoporosis may be the only finding.

d. Positron-emission tomography (PET) scanning, while showing more disease than radiography, is not yet standardized.

e. Bone scans are not helpful, because multiple myeloma does not have an osteoblastic component.

f. Prognosis is evaluated based on bone marrow cytogenetic characteristics.

4. Treatment options are changing rapidly and include lenalidomide (a thalidomide derivative), dexamethasone, and doxorubicin. Bisphosphonates are important adjuncts.

IV. BLEEDING DISORDERS

A. General characteristics

1. Bleeding disorders involve excessive or repetitive bleeding or bleeding at unusual sites.

a. If the bleeding is caused by problems with platelets, the mucosa and skin usually are involved (e.g., epistaxis, gum bleeding, menorrhagia). Petechiae are seen almost exclusively in thrombocytopenia rather than in platelet dysfunction.

b. If the bleeding is caused by coagulation problems, the skin and muscles are involved; spontaneous hemarthroses are found only in severe hemophilia.

c. Bleeding disorders may be classified as either congenital or acquired.

B. Clinical features vary with the cause of the bleeding.

1. Congenital disorders usually involve single defects related to vascular integrity, platelet function, coagulation, or fibrinolytic systems.

2. Acquired disorders involve more than one system (liver, kidneys, collagen vascular system, or immune system).

   a. Abnormal bleeding is seen with neoplasia, infection, malabsorption, shock, and obstetric complications.

   b. Drugs associated with bleeding include NSAIDs, aspirin, certain antibiotics, anticoagulants, thiazides, gold, and heparin.

   c. Systemic lupus erythematosus and CLL are common causes of secondary thrombocytopenic purpura.

C. Laboratory studies

   1. Initial assessment

      a. Platelet count, peripheral smear, and bleeding time should be analyzed in patients with suspected coagulation disorders.

      b. Prothrombin time (PT), partial thromboplastin time (PTT), and/or activated PTT are helpful in differentiating cause.

      c. Thrombin clotting time measures the rate of conversion of fibrinogen to fibrin in the presence of thrombin.

   2. Special studies should be done as indicated.

D. Thrombocytopenia

   1. General characteristics

      a. Thrombocytopenia is an abnormal decrease in the number of platelets in the blood. It is the most common cause of abnormal bleeding.

      b. It may be caused by impaired production, increased destruction, splenic sequestration, or dilution.

         (1) Acute immune (idiopathic) thrombocytopenic purpura (ITP) is a self-limited, autoimmune (IgG) disorder found most commonly in children of both sexes and is associated with a preceding viral upper respiratory infection.

         (2) Chronic ITP may occur at any age (peak incidence is from 20 to 50 years) and is more common in women; it often coexists with other autoimmune diseases.

   2. Clinical features

      a. Acute ITP is characterized by the abrupt appearance of petechiae, purpura, and hemorrhagic bullae on the skin and mucous membranes.

      b. Chronic ITP patients develop petechiae on the skin and mucous membranes.

      c. Patients are otherwise well and rarely febrile; other common presenting complaints are epistaxis, oral bleeding, and menorrhagia.

      d. Splenomegaly usually is not present.

      e. Heparin is the drug that most commonly causes an ITP-like reaction in hospitalized patients (HIT: heparin-induced thrombocytopenia). Others include sulfonamides, quinine, thiazides, cimetidine, and gold. Other causes of secondary thrombocytopenia are systemic lupus erythematosus and CLL.

   3. Laboratory findings

      a. Acute ITP shows decreased platelets (10,000 to 20,000/mcL), eosinophilia, and mild lymphocytosis.

      b. Chronic ITP shows a platelet count of 25,000 to 75,000/mcL.

      c. Mild anemia may be present, unless autoimmune hemolytic anemia coexists (10%).

      d. Peripheral smear shows megathrombocytes; coagulation studies are normal.

   4. Treatment

      a. Acute ITP usually resolves spontaneously; some patients require corticosteroids or splenectomy.

      b. Chronic ITP rarely resolves spontaneously; initial treatment is high-dose prednisone. For treatment failures, intravenous (IV) immunoglobulin, danazol, immunosuppressive therapy, and stem cell transplantation are used. Splenectomy is definitive and often required. Platelet transfusions may be used for life-threatening bleeding.

      c. Platelet antagonists (e.g., aspirin) should be avoided.

E. Platelet consumption syndromes

   1. General characteristics: There are three major types of platelet consumption syndromes.

      a. Thrombocytopenic purpura (TTP) is rare but often fatal. It is found in previously healthy people, most commonly between the ages of 20 and 50. It occurs more often in women than in men and in patients with HIV disease. TTP may be precipitated by estrogen use, pregnancy, and drugs, such as quinine and ticlopidine.

      b. Hemolytic uremia syndrome (HUS) is similar to TTP but is found primarily in children. Pregnancy and estrogen use may precipitate HUS in adults.

c. Disseminated intravascular coagulopathy (DIC) causes generalized hemorrhage in patients with severe underlying systemic illness such as sepsis, tissue injury, obstetric complications, cancer and in severe transfusion reactions.

2. Clinical features

a. TTP is characterized by severe thrombocytopenia with purpura, petechiae, pallor, abdominal pain, microangiopathic hemolytic anemia, fever, abnormal neurologic signs, renal failure, and, possibly, pancreatitis. Neurologic symptoms may wax and wane over minutes.

b. HUS is similar to TTP but does not have associated neurologic findings. It has more renal problems than TTP. It affects primarily children younger than 10 years, particularly after infection with *Escherichia coli* 0157:H7, *Shigella* sp., *Salmonella* sp., and various viruses.

c. In DIC, skin and mucous membrane bleeding (particularly at puncture/wound sites) and shock are more common; thrombosis (commonly digital ischemia and gangrene) less often predominates.

3. Laboratory findings

a. TTP and HUS

(1) Anemia, red cell fragmentation (schistocytes), normal leukocytes, polychromatophilia, reticulocytosis, and thrombocytopenia (less severe in HUS than in TTP) are found; Coombs' test is negative. ADAMTS 13 (a metalloprotease enzyme) is low.

(2) LDH is markedly elevated; indirect bilirubin increases.

(3) Coagulation tests are normal.

(4) Renal insufficiency may be found.

b. DIC

(1) Evidence of coagulopathy includes hypofibrinogenemia, elevated fibrin degradation products (D-dimer is most sensitive), thrombocytopenia, and prolonged PT. ADAMTS 13 usually is absent.

(2) Microangiopathic hemolytic anemia with fragmented red cells (schistocytes) is present in 25% of cases.

4. Treatment

a. TTP

(1) TTP requires emergency large-volume plasmapheresis.

(2) Prednisone and antiplatelet agents have also been used.

b. HUS

(1) In children, conservative management usually is all that is required. Fluids and management of electrolyte imbalance are important.

(2) Treatment of adults is plasmapheresis.

c. DIC

(1) Treatment primarily is prompt and aggressive therapy for the underlying cause.

(2) Component blood transfusions are important, particularly the replacement of fibrinogen through the administration of cryoprecipitate. The role of heparin is controversial.

F. Disorders of platelet function

1. General characteristics

a. Congenital abnormalities are varied; most result in normal counts and morphology but prolonged bleeding time.

b. Acquired platelet dysfunction is more common than congenital.

(1) The most common causes of acquired platelet dysfunction are aspirin and other NSAIDs.

(2) Acquired platelet dysfunction also is seen with the use of certain other drugs, uremia, alcoholism, myeloproliferative diseases, hypothermia, various vitamin deficiencies, and other conditions.

2. Clinical features are prolonged bleeding time and skin and mucosal bleeding.

3. Laboratory findings indicate a normal number of platelets, but platelet function study results are abnormal.

4. Treatment

a. In drug-related cases, the drug should be discontinued.

b. Dialysis may help patients with uremia.

c. Transfusion with platelets is necessary for serious bleeding.

G. Disorders associated with coagulation protein defects

1. Von Willebrand disease
   a. General characteristics
      (1) Von Willebrand disease is an autosomal dominant, congenital bleeding disorder. It is the most common congenital coagulopathy. Most cases are mild.
      (2) It is characterized by reduced levels of factor VIII antigen or ristocetin cofactor.
      (3) Both men and women may be affected.
      (4) It occurs in six major types, all characterized by deficient or defective von Willebrand factor (vWF). Type I accounts for 75% to 80% of cases.
   b. Clinical features
      (1) Bleeding occurs in nasal, sinus, vaginal, and GI mucous membranes.
      (2) Spontaneous hemarthrosis and soft-tissue bleeds are less common than in hemophilia A.
      (3) Bleeding is exacerbated by aspirin and decreases with use of estrogen or pregnancy.
   c. Laboratory findings
      (1) PT and PTT are generally normal. Bleeding time is usually prolonged, particularly following aspirin use.
      (2) vWF is low.
   d. Treatment varies according to the type of disease.
      (1) Desmopressin acetate is useful in type I.
      (2) Factor VIII concentrates are preferred if factor replacement is necessary.

2. Hemophilia A (factor VIII deficiency or classic hemophilia)
   a. General characteristics
      (1) Hemophilia A is a hereditary disease characterized by excessively prolonged coagulation time.
      (2) It is the most severe bleeding disorder and the most common congenital coagulopathy after von Willebrand disease.
      (3) It is X-linked recessive and occurs in about 1/7,500 male births.
      (4) Recent genetic mutation causes one-third of all cases of hemophilia A.
      (5) Many older patients are seropositive for HIV because of infected factor VIII transfusions given before widespread blood product testing for HIV.
   b. Clinical features
      (1) Severely affected patients have repeated spontaneous hemorrhagic episodes with hemarthroses, epistaxis, intracranial bleeding, hematemesis, melena, microscopic hematuria, and bleeding into the soft tissue and gingiva.
      (2) Less severely affected patients may experience excessive bleeding following trauma or surgery.
   c. Laboratory findings
      (1) PTT is prolonged.
      (2) PT, bleeding time, fibrinogen level, and platelet count are normal.
      (3) Factor assay shows reduced factor VIII:C levels; vWF is normal.
      (4) Low platelet count suggests HIV-related immune thrombocytopenia.
      (5) Female carriers will have low or normal factor VIII:C and normal factor VIII antigen.
   d. Treatment
      (1) Infusion of heat-treated or recombinant factor VIII concentrates is standard treatment.
      (2) Desmopressin may elevate factor VIII levels in patients with mild to moderate disease.
      (3) Patients should avoid aspirin; celecoxib or opioids may be used to control pain.

3. Hemophilia B, also known as factor IX deficiency or Christmas disease, is a heterogeneous group of disorders similar to hemophilia A but occurring less frequently. It is an X-linked recessive disorder affecting males (1/25,000).

4. Factor XI deficiency is a usually mild, autosomal recessive disorder seen primarily in Ashkenazi Jews. It is treated with fresh frozen plasma.

5. Vitamin K–dependent factor deficiencies
   a. General characteristics
      (1) These are the most common acquired coagulopathies.
      (2) Deficiencies may be secondary to poor diet, liver failure, malabsorption, malnutrition, and use of some drugs, especially broad-spectrum antibiotics.
   b. Clinical features
      (1) The typical patient is postoperative, not eating well, and receiving broad-spectrum antibiotics that suppress colonic bacteria.
      (2) Features of the underlying cause are evident.
      (3) Soft-tissue bleeding may occur.
   c. Laboratory findings
      (1) PT is prolonged and PTT may be prolonged.
      (2) Fibrinogen, thrombin time, and platelet count are normal.
      (3) Liver enzymes may be elevated.
      (4) Levels of vitamin K and factors II, VII, IX, and X are decreased.
   d. Treatment
      (1) Treatment is directed at the underlying cause.
      (2) Oral or parenteral vitamin K (phytonadione) rapidly restores factor production.
      (3) Treat hemorrhage with fresh frozen plasma.
      (4) Prevention includes a diet high in leafy vegetables and treatment of malabsorption.

V. THROMBOTIC DISORDERS AND HYPERCOAGULABLE CONDITIONS

A. General characteristics
   1. Predisposing factors in patients who present with thrombus include the following:
      a. Age older than 40 years
      b. Venous thrombosis in the neck, arms, abdomen, or central nervous system; arterial thrombosis may result in large vessel or microvascular events.
      c. Recurrent thrombosis
      d. Family history of thrombosis
      e. Repeated thrombosis despite adequate anticoagulation, which suggests a neoplasm
   2. Congenital disorders associated with thrombotic states typically are autosomal dominant.
   3. Acquired hypercoagulable states are associated with malignancy (Trousseau's syndrome), pregnancy, nephrotic syndrome, ingestion of certain medications (especially oral contraceptive agents and pure estrogen compounds), immobilization, myeloproliferative disease, ulcerative colitis and Crohn's disease, Behçet's syndrome, intravascular devices, DIC, hyperlipidemia (particularly familial type II hyperbetalipoproteinemia), paroxysmal nocturnal hemoglobinuria, TTP–HUS, hyperviscosity syndrome, anticardiolipin antibodies, HIT, and antiphospholipid syndrome.
   4. Heparin use is a rare but important cause and is not dose dependent. Thrombocytopenia also is associated with heparin-induced thrombosis.
   5. Congenital causes include antithrombin III deficiency, factor V Leiden, protein C deficiency, protein S deficiency, dysfibrogenemia, abnormal plasminogen, and activated protein C resistance.
   6. Lupus anticoagulant
      a. An IgM or IgG immunoglobulin is seen in 5% to 10% of patients with systemic lupus erythematosus but is more common in persons without lupus or in those taking phenothiazines.
      b. It causes bleeding in conjunction with an additional bleeding disorder and is associated with risk of thrombosis and spontaneous abortion.
B. Clinical features include typical signs and symptoms of arterial or venous thrombus formation.
C. Laboratory findings: PTT is prolonged; Russell's viper venom time is specific to detect lupus anticoagulant.

D. Treatment
1. Prednisone usually eliminates lupus anticoagulant.
2. Treatment for thrombosis is standard anticoagulation; low-molecular-weight heparin may be preferred.
3. If caused by heparin, all heparin must be withheld from the patient.
4. No prophylaxis is indicated in an at-risk person who has not had a previous thrombotic event.
5. At-risk persons with previous thrombotic events should be anticoagulated for prolonged periods.

Gastroenterology

Susan LeLacheur

5

I. DISEASES OF THE ESOPHAGUS

A. Gastroesophageal reflux disease (GERD; reflux esophagitis)

1. General characteristics

   a. Reflux esophagitis is the recurrent reflux of gastric contents into the distal esophagus because of mechanical or functional abnormality of the lower esophageal sphincter.

   b. GERD is present in an estimated 10% of the population; up to 60% of the population experiences heartburn at some point in their lives. In infants, about 50% have reflux, but less than 10% have evidence of esophagitis.

   c. Factors that protect the esophagus include gravity, lower esophageal sphincter tone, esophageal motility, salivary flow, gastric emptying, and tissue resistance.

   d. In a minority of patients, reflux causes erosion of the esophagus that leads to Barrett's esophagitis (replacement of normal squamous epithelium with metaplastic columnar epithelium), which can predispose to malignancy.

2. Clinical features

   a. Heartburn is the most common presenting feature; it generally is worse after meals and when lying down, and often is relieved with antacids. Regurgitation or dysphagia may occur.

   b. Hoarseness, halitosis, cough, hiccupping, and atypical chest pain are less common symptoms of reflux.

   c. More severe disease, generally caused by a severe impairment of lower esophageal sphincter tone, occurs spontaneously when supine, while less severe disease is associated with a pattern of heartburn following meals but not associated with nighttime symptoms.

3. Laboratory studies

   a. Most often a clinical diagnosis is made based on a history of heartburn and regurgitation of gastric contents, especially if relieved by antacids. More severe disease warrants endoscopy to confirm the diagnosis and to assess for epithelial damage.

   b. Endoscopy is also warranted in patients older than 45 years with a new onset of symptoms, long-standing or frequently recurring symptoms, and failure to respond to therapy or symptoms, indicating more severe conditions such as anemia, dysphagia, or recurrent vomiting.

   c. Be sure to consider the possibility that symptoms are caused by myocardial ischemia; an electrocardiography (ECG) and appropriate cardiac workup should be considered.

   d. Barium swallow, esophageal manometry, and ambulatory 24-hour pH monitoring may be indicated in more severe or refractory cases.

4. Treatment

   a. Lifestyle modifications should be implemented on presumptive diagnosis, with further workup if symptoms persist. Appropriate lifestyle modifications include cessation of smoking, avoidance of eating at bedtime, avoidance of large meals, avoidance of alcohol and foods that cause irritation, and raising the head of the bed.

   b. Pharmacotherapy

      (1) Antacids or alginic acid may be used for mild symptoms.

      (2) Histamine (H_2) blockers may be used, but generally in larger doses than for peptic ulcer disease (PUD). H_2-blockers are first-line treatment for mild GERD.

      (3) An acid-suppressant proton pump inhibitor (PPI) is the most powerful anti-GERD medication. PPIs are first-line treatment in moderate to severe disease or in patients who are unresponsive to H_2-blockers or have evidence of erosive gastritis.

      (4) A combination of an H_2-blocker at bedtime and a PPI in the daytime may be helpful in patients with significant nighttime symptoms.

      (5) β-Agonists, α-adrenergic antagonists, nitrates, calcium channel blockers, anticholinergics, theophylline, morphine, meperidine, diazepam, and barbiturate agents decrease lower esophageal sphincter pressure and, therefore, should be avoided.

   c. Surgical and endoscopic techniques are available for refractory cases but have not been shown to prevent complications of the disease.

B. Infectious esophagitis
  1. General characteristics
    a. Infectious esophagitis is rare, except in immunocompromised persons.
    b. Causes
      (1) Fungal: *Candida* sp. should be considered, especially if oral thrush is present.
      (2) Viral: Cytomegalovirus (CMV) and herpes simplex virus (HSV) are common causes.
      (3) HIV, *Mycobacterium tuberculosis*, Epstein–Barr virus (EBV), and *Mycobacterium avium intracellulare* are additional but uncommon causes of infectious esophagitis.
  2. Clinical features: The main clinical feature is odynophagia (painful swallowing) or dysphagia (difficult swallowing) in an immunocompromised patient.
  3. Laboratory findings
    a. Endoscopy in patients with CMV or HIV reveals large, deep ulcers. Infection with HSV is characterized by multiple shallow ulcers. Candidal infection shows white plaques.
    b. Cytology or culture from endoscopic brushings is needed for definitive diagnosis.
  4. Treatment
    a. Treatment is specific to the type of infection.
    b. Fluconazole or ketoconazole for *Candida* sp.
    c. Acyclovir for HSV.
    d. Ganciclovir for CMV.
C. Esophageal dysmotility
  1. General characteristics
    a. Disorders of esophageal motility include neurogenic dysphagia, Zenker's diverticulum, esophageal stenosis, achalasia, diffuse esophageal spasm, and scleroderma.
    b. Dysmotility can be caused by neurologic factors, intrinsic or external blockage, or malfunction of esophageal peristalsis.
  2. Clinical features
    a. Dysphagia is the most common presenting symptom for all motility disorders. Its presentation can help to determine the underlying cause.
    b. Neurogenic dysphagia causes difficulty with both liquids and solids and is caused by injury or disease of the brain stem or the cranial nerves involved in swallowing.
    c. Zenker's diverticulum is an outpouching of the posterior hypopharynx that can cause regurgitation of undigested food and liquid into the pharynx several hours after eating.
    d. Esophageal stenosis causes dysphagia for solid foods. Slow progression of solid food dysphagia indicates a more benign process (e.g., webs or rings), and rapid progression indicates malignancy.
    e. Achalasia is a global esophageal motor disorder in which peristalsis is decreased and lower esophageal sphincter tone is increased, causing slowly progressive dysphagia with episodic regurgitation and chest pain.
    f. Diffuse esophageal spasm is characterized by dysphagia or intermittent chest pain that may or may not be associated with eating.
    g. Scleroderma eventually progresses to involve the esophagus in most patients with the disease, causing decreased esophageal sphincter tone and peristalsis, predisposing the patient to the symptoms and complications of reflux esophagitis.
  3. Laboratory findings
    a. Barium swallow can reveal both structural and motor abnormalities of the esophagus that may cause dysphagia. Achalasia typically has a "parrot-beaked" appearance (i.e., a dilated esophagus tapering to the distal obstruction) on barium swallow.
    b. Pharyngoscopy or esophagoscopy must be done (generally by an otolaryngologist) to clarify the nature of a structural lesion.
    c. Esophageal manometry can be used to assess the strength and coordination of peristalsis.
  4. Treatment
    a. Neurogenic dysphagia must be managed by treating the underlying disease.
    b. Strictures

(1) Most benign strictures can be managed by dilation.

(2) Malignant strictures must be resected.

   c. Diverticula, achalasia, and stenosis may be managed medically (calcium channel blockers, nitrates, botulinum) or surgically (endoscopic dilatation, resection) if the condition is severe enough to warrant intervention.

D. Esophageal neoplasms

  1. General characteristics

    a. Squamous cell carcinomas and adenocarcinomas are the most common types.

    b. Barrett's esophagitis is associated with adenocarcinomas in the distal third of the esophagus, while squamous cell lesions tend to occur in the proximal two-thirds.

    c. Local spread to the mediastinum is common, because the esophagus has no serosa.

    d. Esophageal cancers are frequently related to cigarette smoking and chronic alcohol use. Contributing factors include exposure to other caustic agents (e.g., nitrosamines, fungal toxins, other carcinogens), hot foods, mucosal abnormalities, poor oral hygiene, and human papilloma virus (HPV).

  2. Clinical features: The main clinical feature of esophageal cancer is progressive dysphagia for solid food associated with marked weight loss. Heartburn, vomiting, and hoarseness may occur.

  3. Laboratory findings

    a. Biphasic barium esophagram is the best initial test to visualize the lesion.

    b. Endoscopy with brushings is used for diagnosis.

    c. Endoscopic sonography and CT may be used for staging.

  4. Treatment

    a. Treatment of esophageal cancer is generally surgical. Radiotherapy and adjunctive chemotherapy have been used in various combinations with or without surgery, but a survival benefit has not yet been demonstrated.

    b. Prognosis depends on stage of disease at diagnosis ranging from 4% to 60% 5-year survival.

E. Mallory–Weiss tear

  1. A Mallory–Weiss tear is a linear mucosal tear in the esophagus, generally at the gastroesophageal junction, that occurs with forceful vomiting or retching, causing hematemesis.

  2. A Mallory–Weiss tear often is associated with alcohol use, but it should be considered in all cases of upper gastrointestinal (GI) bleed.

  3. Diagnosis is established by endoscopy.

  4. Most episodes resolve without treatment, but endoscopic injection of epinephrine or thermal coagulation may be required.

F. Esophageal varices

  1. General characteristics

    a. Esophageal varices are dilations of the veins of the esophagus, generally at the distal end.

    b. The underlying cause in adults is portal hypertension, most commonly caused by cirrhosis either from alcohol abuse or from chronic viral hepatitis. Use of nonsteroidal anti-inflammatory drugs (NSAIDs) can exacerbate bleeding (hepatic vein obstruction).

    c. Budd–Chiari syndrome may cause thrombosis of the portal vein, leading to esophageal varices.

  2. Diagnosis

    a. Diagnosis generally is established clinically when a patient with signs of cirrhosis presents with hematemesis.

    b. Varices generally are asymptomatic until they bleed, at which point they frequently are life threatening.

  3. Treatment

    a. Hemodynamic support with high-volume fluid replacement and vasopressors and immediate control of bleeding are necessary, because bleeding varices have high mortality (~30% with first bleed and 50% within 6 weeks).

    b. Endoscopic therapy and pharmacologic vasoconstriction (e.g., octreotide) are the preferred therapies.

II.   DISEASES OF THE STOMACH

A. Gastritis and duodenitis

  1. General characteristics

    a. Gastritis and duodenitis can be defined as inflammation of the stomach or duodenum.

    b. Protective factors include mucus, bicarbonate, mucosal blood flow, prostaglandins, alkaline state, hydrophobic layer, and epithelial renewal. Any imbalance in protective factors can lead to inflammation.

c. Causes

(1) Autoimmune disorders (e.g., pernicious anemia) and other noninfectious factors cause type A gastritis, which involves the body of the stomach.

(2) *Helicobacter pylori* (HP) is a Gram-negative, spiral-shaped bacillus. It is implicated in almost all non-NSAID–induced GI mucosal inflammation.

(a) HP causes type B gastritis, which involves the antrum and body of the stomach.

(b) HP tolerates well the acidity of a normal stomach and also is associated with peptic ulcer, gastric adenocarcinoma, and gastric lymphoma.

(3) NSAIDs can cause gastric injury by diminishing local prostaglandin production in the stomach or duodenum.

(4) Stress from central nervous system injury, burns, sepsis, or surgery can lead to erosion of the stomach or duodenum.

(5) Alcohol use is another leading cause of gastritis.

2. Clinical features

a. The clinical features of gastritis generally reflect the underlying syndrome rather than the gastric injury itself.

b. Dyspepsia and abdominal pain are common indicators of gastritis.

3. Laboratory studies

a. Endoscopy with biopsy reveals the location and extent of gastritis as well as the presence of HP.

b. A urea breath test can be used to detect HP, because urea is a product of the bacterial metabolism. Fecal antigen testing or serology for HP also is helpful.

c. Specific tests for underlying conditions (e.g., vitamin B_{12} level, complete blood count [CBC] for pernicious anemia) should be used as indicated by history.

4. Treatment

a. Remove the causative factor (e.g., NSAIDs alcohol).

b. Treat the underlying cause.

B. Delayed gastric emptying

1. General characteristics

a. Delayed gastric emptying can be defined as an alteration in gastric motility.

b. Causes include myopathic diseases of the smooth muscles and neurologic dysfunction.

2. Clinical features include nausea and a feeling of excessive fullness after meals.

3. Treatment: Prokinetic medications (e.g., cisapride, metoclopramide) can sometimes help to speed the movement of food through the stomach.

C. Peptic ulcer disease

1. General characteristics

a. PUD describes any ulcer of the upper digestive system (e.g., gastric ulcer, duodenal ulcer).

b. Causes: Any discreet break in mucosa caused by injury, NSAIDs, stress, alcohol, or other irritants will lead to an ulcer.

(1) HP is the most common cause of PUD.

(2) When HP is the cause, the ulcer disease can be eradicated with treatment.

c. The lifetime risk of ulcer disease is 5% to 10%.

d. Men and women are equally affected.

e. Both gastric ulcers and HP are highly associated with gastric malignancy. Although most patients with HP or a gastric ulcer will not get gastric cancer, almost all patients with gastric cancer have had HP or a gastric ulcer.

2. Differential diagnosis: Dyspepsia, abdominal pain, discomfort, or nausea often is associated with gastric or duodenal ulcers but also can occur in a variety of other conditions including gastritis, malignancy, and ischemic heart disease.

3. Clinical features

a. Abdominal pain or discomfort is the primary clinical feature.

(1) The pain may be described as burning or gnawing and often radiates to the back.

(2) The pain of a duodenal ulcer often improves with food, whereas the pain of a gastric ulcer typically worsens, which leads to anorexia and associated weight loss.

b. Dyspepsia (belching, bloating, distention, heartburn) or nausea also is reported.

c. Complications include bleeding, perforation, and penetration.

  (1) Bleeding typically manifests as melena.

  (2) PUD is the most common cause of nonhemorrhagic GI bleeds.

4. Laboratory studies

  a. Endoscopy is best for detecting small or healing ulcers. It differentiates gastritis from ulcer disease and allows immediate biopsy of gastric or suspicious ulcers to rule out malignancy.

  b. Barium radiography was once widely used and cheaper, but it is less sensitive, with a 30% false-negative rate. Endoscopy is more sensitive and definitive.

  c. Urea breath test may be helpful for detecting HP, as will stool or blood antibody tests.

5. Treatment

  a. Irritating factors (smoking, NSAIDs, alcohol) should be avoided.

  b. Combination therapy for HP regimen should be taken for 14 days. Options include the following:

  (1) PPI with clarithromycin and amoxicillin (sometimes with the addition of metronidazole)

  (2) Bismuth subsalicylate plus tetracycline, metronidazole, and PPI

  c. Prophylactic treatment with misoprostol or a PPI should be considered in patients with a history of ulcer who require daily NSAID use; a history of complications, such as a bleed; a need for chronic steroids or anticoagulants; or significant other comorbidities.

D. Gastric neoplasm

  1. Zollinger–Ellison syndrome (ZES)

  a. General characteristics

  (1) In ZES, a gastrin-secreting tumor (gastrinoma) causes hypergastrinemia, which results in refractory PUD.

  (2) Only 1% of cases of PUD are caused by ZES.

  (3) Most gastrinomas are found in the pancreas or duodenum, but they may be found anywhere or may metastasize.

  (4) About one-third of gastrinomas are part of a syndrome known as multiple endocrine neoplasia, type I (MEN1), an autosomal dominant condition.

  b. Clinical features

  (1) Most commonly, the clinical presentation is indistinguishable from that of PUD, although ZES usually is more advanced or refractory to treatment.

  (2) Abdominal pain may be accompanied by a secretory diarrhea that improves with H_2-blockers (ranitidine, cimetidine) or PPIs (omeprazole, lansoprazole).

  (3) Occult or frank bleeding, causing anemia, may be present.

  c. Laboratory findings

  (1) A fasting gastrin level greater than 150 pg/mL indicates hypergastrinemia.

  (2) A secretin test is needed to confirm the presence of ZES.

  (a) Patients are given secretin, 2 U/kg intravenous (IV).

  (b) In most patients with ZES, the gastrin levels will increase by more than 200 pg/mL.

  (3) Endoscopy, computed tomography (CT), or magnetic resonance imaging (MRI) may help to localize the tumor.

  d. Treatment

  (1) Use of PPIs controls gastrin secretion.

  (2) Surgical resection of the gastrinoma should be attempted when possible.

  2. Gastric adenocarcinoma

  a. General characteristics

  (1) Gastric adenocarcinoma is among the most common types of cancer worldwide but is less common in the United States.

  (2) Gastric adenocarcinoma is almost twice as common in men than in women.

  (3) It almost never occurs in a patient younger than 40 years.

    (4) With early diagnosis, an 80% cure rate can be accomplished. If the muscularis propria is involved, the cure rate is 50%, but if there is lymphatic spread, the cure rate is 10%.

    (5) There is a strong association of gastric adenocarcinoma with HP, although genetic factors are involved in some types.

b. Clinical features

    (1) Dyspepsia and weight loss associated with anemia and occult GI bleeding in a patient older than 40 years are the common presenting complaints.

    (2) Progressive dysphagia may be caused by a neoplasm impinging on the esophagus.

    (3) Postprandial vomiting may be caused by a neoplasm near the pylorus.

    (4) Signs of metastatic spread include left supraclavicular lymphadenopathy (Virchow's node) and an umbilical nodule (Sister Mary Joseph nodule).

c. Laboratory studies

    (1) Iron deficiency anemia is the most common finding.

    (2) Liver enzymes may be elevated with hepatic metastases.

    (3) Endoscopy with cytology should be done on any patient older than 40 years with dyspepsia who is unresponsive to therapy.

    (4) After the diagnosis has been established, abdominal CT is used to determine the extent of disease.

d. Treatment

    (1) Treatment is either curative or palliative resection of the tumor.

    (2) Chemotherapy or radiation may provide some palliative benefit.

3. Carcinoid tumors of the stomach rarely occur in response to hypergastrinemia and generally are benign and self-limited.

4. Gastric lymphoma

a. General characteristics

    (1) Gastric lymphomas account for less than 2% of gastric malignancies, but the stomach is the most common extranodal site for non-Hodgkin's lymphoma.

    (2) The risk of gastric lymphoma is greater by sixfold if HP infection is present.

b. Clinical features: Clinical features are the same as those for gastric adenocarcinoma.

c. Laboratory findings: Findings differ from those of gastric adenocarcinoma only in the pathology of the lesion.

d. Treatment: Treatment is resection with or without radiation or chemotherapy.

III. DISEASES OF THE SMALL INTESTINE AND COLON

A. Diarrhea

1. Diarrhea is increased frequency or volume of stool (e.g., three or more liquid or semisolid stools daily for at least 2 to 3 consecutive days).

2. Causes of diarrhea may be infectious (Table 5-1), toxic, dietary (e.g., laxative use), or other GI disease.

3. Patient history: The history should include all current medications as well as illnesses among others who have shared meals with the patient.

4. Clinical features

a. Secretory diarrhea (large volume without inflammation) indicates pancreatic insufficiency, ingestion of preformed bacterial toxins, or laxative use.

b. Inflammatory diarrhea (bloody diarrhea with fever) indicates invasive organisms or inflammatory bowel disease.

c. Antibiotic-associated diarrhea is almost always caused by *Clostridium difficile* colitis, which in the most severe cases causes the classic pseudomembranous colitis.

5. Laboratory findings

a. White blood cells (WBCs) in stool denote an inflammatory process.

b. Cultures for bacterial agents, microscopy for parasites, or toxin identification (if enterotoxic *Escherichia coli* or *Clostridium difficile* is suspected) can identify infectious agents in stool.

6. Treatment

a. Supportive therapy is sufficient for most patients with viral or bacterial diarrhea.

TABLE 5-1	**Foodborne and Waterborne Causes of Diarrhea**						
Agent	**Source**	**Onset**	**Nausea and Vomiting**	**Diarrhea**	**Fever**	**Duration**	**Therapy**
Norovirus	Food, water, person to person	1–3 days	Yes	Watery	Low grade	1–2 days	Hydration (Prevention: hand-washing)
Rotavirus	Person to person	1–3 days	Yes	Watery	Low grade	5–8 days	Hydration (Prevention: hand-washing)
Staphylococcus aureus (toxin)	Food, after cooking	1–7 hr	Yes, rapid onset	Cramping, some diarrhea	Uncommon	Acute (4–6 hr); total (1–2 days)	Supportive
Clostridium perfringens (toxin)	Food, before cooking	8–14 hr	Uncommon	Cramping, watery	Rare	24 hr	Supportive
Vibrio spp. (cholera)	Water	2–3 days	Some	Profuse, watery	Rare	Days	Hydration
Enterotoxic *Escherichia coli*	Food	5–15 days	Some	Cramping, watery	Low grade	1–5 days	Hydration, bismuth/loperamide
Giardia lamblia	Water, person to person	5–25 days	Nausea	Diarrhea, bloating	None possible	Until treated	Metronidazole, 250 mg twice a day for 10 days
Cryptosporidia	Water, outbreaks	2–10 days	Yes	Watery	Possible	30 days (unless HIV)	Supportive, HIV treatment
Cyclospora	Imported, uncooked foods	7 days	Nausea, anorexia	Watery	Low grade	Weeks	Trimethoprim/sulfamethox-azole twice a day for 7 days
Salmonella (invasive)	Poultry	6–72 hr	Nausea, some vomiting	Purulent	Yes, septicemia common	4–7 days	Hydration
Enterohemorrhagic *Escherichia coli* (invasive)	Undercooked ground beef	12–60 hr	No	Purulent, bloody, cramping	Yes	5–10 days	Supportive unless severe
Shigella (invasive)	Fecal–oral	1–6 days	No	Purulent, bloody, cramping	Yes	1–7 days	Supportive
Campylobacter (invasive)	Undercooked poultry	2–5 days	Some	Purulent, bloody, cramping	Yes	2–5 days	Supportive

> **b.** Antibiotics may be indicated for patients with severe diarrhea and systemic symptoms (e.g., *Shigella* sp., *Campylobacter* sp., severe cases of *Clostridium difficile*).
>
> **c.** Treatment of the underlying cause is required for noninfectious diarrhea.

B. Constipation

    1. General characteristics

        a. Normal bowel function ranges from three stools per day to three stools per week. Constipation is a decrease in stool volume and an increase in stool firmness accompanied by straining.

        b. Patients older than 50 years with new-onset constipation should be evaluated for colon cancer.

2. Treatment

   a. In most cases, an increase in fiber (to 10–20 g/day) and fluid intake (up to 1.5 to 2 L/day) and increased exercise will resolve the problem.

   b. A patient with constipation lasting for more than 2 weeks or with constipation refractory to modifications in diet, exercise, and fluid intake should undergo further investigation to detect the underlying cause. If a treatable underlying cause is found, constipation will resolve with treatment of the disease process.

C. Bowel obstruction

   1. General characteristics

      a. Most small bowel obstructions are due to adhesions or hernias; other causes include neoplasm, inflammatory bowel disease, and volvulus.

      b. Large bowel obstructions are more likely due to neoplasm; other causes include strictures, hernias, volvulus, intussusception, and fecal impaction.

      c. Complete strangulation of bowel tissue leads to infarction, necrosis, peritonitis, and death.

   2. Clinical features

      a. Small bowel obstruction presents with abdominal pain, distention, vomiting of partially digested food, and obstipation.

      b. Bowel sounds are high pitched and come in rushes. Later in the process the bowel becomes silent.

      c. Large bowel obstruction presents with distention and pain.

      d. Patients may be febrile and tachycardic. Shock may ensue.

   3. Laboratory findings

      a. Dehydration and electrolyte imbalance is common.

      b. Upright radiographs may illustrate air–fluid levels.

      c. Treatment includes nothing by mouth (NPO), nasogastric suctioning, IV fluids, and monitoring. Surgery is very likely, especially with large bowel obstruction.

D. Volvulus

   1. Volvulus is twisting of any portion of the bowel on itself, most commonly in the sigmoid or cecal area of the bowel, requiring emergent decompression to avoid ischemic injury.

   2. Clinical features

      a. Patients present with cramping abdominal pain and distention, nausea, vomiting, and obstipation.

      b. Ischemia caused by volvulus can lead to gangrene, peritonitis, and sepsis.

      c. Abdominal tympany will be found on exam, along with tachycardia, fever, and severe pain if ischemia is present.

   3. Diagnosis is generally confirmed by abdominal plain film, which will show colonic distension.

   4. Treatment

      a. Endoscopic decompression is possible in many cases.

      b. Surgical evaluation and treatment is required urgently if volvulus fails to quickly resolve by nonsurgical means.

E. Malabsorption

   1. General characteristics

      a. Malabsorption may involve a single nutrient, as with pernicious anemia (vitamin B_{12}) or lactase deficiency (lactose), or it may be global, as with celiac disease or AIDS.

      b. Malabsorption may be caused by problems in digestion, absorption, or impaired blood and lymph flow.

   2. Clinical features

      a. Diarrhea usually is the primary complaint and may be accompanied by bloating and abdominal discomfort.

      b. Weight loss and edema also may be present.

      c. Steatorrhea may occur.

      d. Specific deficiencies may cause bone demineralization, tetany, bleeding, or anemia.

   3. Laboratory findings

      a. If a 72-hour fecal fat test is normal, specific defects, such as pancreatic insufficiency and abnormal bile salt metabolism, should be considered.

      b. A D-xylose test will distinguish maldigestion (e.g., pancreatic insufficiency, bile salt deficiency) from malabsorption.

      c. Specific tests may be used to detect vitamin B_{12}, calcium, or albumin deficiency.

4. Therapeutic trials of the following can help in both diagnosis and treatment:

    a. Lactose-free diet for lactase deficiency

    b. Gluten-free diet for celiac disease

    c. Pancreatic enzyme replacement for pancreatic insufficiency

    d. Antibiotics may be indicated for specific bacterial infections if the agent is known.

F. Celiac disease (celiac sprue)

  1. General characteristics

    a. It is among the most common genetic conditions in Europe and the United States (multifactorial inheritance).

    b. It is characterized by inflammation of the small bowel, with the ingestion of gluten-containing foods such as wheat, rye, and barley leading to malabsorption.

    c. Clinical presentation is highly variable, often leading to a delay in diagnosis in milder cases.

  2. Clinical presentation

    a. Diarrhea, steatorrhea, flatulence, weight loss, weakness, and abdominal distension are common.

    b. Infants and children may present with failure to thrive.

    c. Older patients may present with iron deficiency, coagulopathy, and hypocalcemia.

  3. Diagnosis

    a. IgA antiendomysial and antitissue transglutaminase antibodies are the serologic screening tests.

    b. Small bowel biopsy is needed to confirm the diagnosis.

  4. Treatment

    a. Treatment involves a gluten-free diet. Patients should be referred to a nutritionist for assistance because of the pervasive nature of gluten in the North American diet. A lactose-free diet may also be needed initially until the intestinal inflammation resolves.

    b. Supplementation may be needed to correct nutritional deficiencies in iron, B_{12} and folic acid, calcium and vitamin D.

    c. Prednisone may be required in refractory cases.

G. Crohn's disease (regional enteritis)

  1. General characteristics

    a. Crohn's disease is an inflammatory bowel disease for which there is some genetic predisposition, although the cause is unknown. Crohn's disease must be differentiated from ulcerative colitis (UC) (Table 5-2).

    b. Crohn's disease may involve both the small and large bowels as well as the mouth, esophagus, and stomach. Most commonly, the terminal ileum and right colon are involved, but the rectum frequently is spared. Skip areas are characteristic.

    c. Complications include fistulas, abscesses, aphthous ulcers, renal stones, and predisposition to colonic cancer.

    d. The success or failure of treatment is variable. The disease usually waxes and wanes throughout life.

  2. Clinical features

    a. Abdominal cramps and diarrhea in a patient younger than 40 years are the most common presenting complaints.

    b. Low-grade fever, polyarthralgia, anemia, and fatigue frequently are encountered.

    c. Blood is often present in stool.

TABLE 5-2	**Differentiation of Crohn's Disease and Ulcerative Colitis**	
Characteristic	**Crohn's Disease**	**Ulcerative Colitis**
Onset	Gradual	Sudden or gradual
Distribution	Mouth to anus, predominantly, right sided; skip areas	Distal to proximal, continuous
Depth of lesions	Transmural	Mucosal surface
Symptoms	Diarrhea and pain	Bloody, pus-filled diarrhea, tenesmus
Complications	Fistulas (common), toxic megacolon, colon cancer	Toxic megacolon, colon cancer

3. Laboratory findings

   a. Colonoscopy is the most valuable tool for establishing the diagnosis, determining the extent and severity of disease, and guiding the treatment.

   b. Contrast studies and endoscopic procedures should be avoided in patients with fulminant disease because of the possibility of inducing toxic megacolon or perforation.

   c. Biopsy will reveal involvement of the entire bowel wall in Crohn's disease. Granulomas are frequent.

   d. Blood tests may include increased sedimentation rate, anemia, and nutritional and electrolyte imbalances during exacerbations.

4. Treatment

   a. For acute attacks, oral corticosteroids (prednisone) are used with or without aminosalicylates. Metronidazole or ciprofloxacin is added in perianal disease, fissures, or fistulae. Infliximab may be used in refractory cases.

   b. Elemental diet is nearly as effective as corticosteroids, but relapse is more likely.

   c. Mesalamine is generally the best option for maintenance therapy.

   d. For patients with malabsorption, supplementation may be needed especially for vitamin B_{12}, folic acid, and vitamin D.

   e. Smoking cessation is critical for reducing the frequency and severity of attacks.

   f. Surgery is not curative in Crohn's disease and is reserved for treatment of complications. Segmental resection is the approach of choice.

H. Ulcerative colitis

1. General characteristics

   a. UC must be differentiated from inflammatory infectious conditions (Table 5-1) and Crohn's disease (Table 5-2).

   b. The disease generally starts distally, at the rectum, and progresses proximally. Disease is continuous, and skip areas are not seen.

   c. Onset generally is gradual but also can be abrupt.

2. Clinical features

   a. Tenesmus and bloody, pus-filled diarrhea are the most common symptoms.

   b. Pain is less common but may occur, typically in the lower left quadrant.

   c. Weight loss, malaise, and fever may occur in more severe disease.

   d. Toxic megacolon and malignancy are more likely in UC than in Crohn's disease.

   e. Other complications include scleritis and episcleritis, arthritides, sclerosing cholangitis, and skin manifestations (erythema nodosum and pyoderma gangrenosum).

   f. As opposed to Crohn's disease, where smoking increases disease, ironically smoking seems protective in UC. Smokers who have recently quit will often have a disease flare.

3. Laboratory findings

   a. Anemia, increased sedimentation rate, and decreased serum albumin are common.

   b. Abdominal plain-film radiography may show colonic dilatation. Sigmoidoscopy or colonoscopy is the best method of establishing the diagnosis.

   c. Colonoscopy and barium enema should be avoided in acute disease because of the risks of perforation and toxic megacolon.

4. Treatment

   a. Topical or oral aminosalicylates and corticosteroids are the mainstays of medical treatment. Immunomodulators are indicated for refractory disease.

   b. Surgery can be curative in UC. Segmental resection is possible, but total proctocolectomy is the most common surgical cure.

I. Irritable bowel syndrome (IBS)

1. General characteristics

   a. IBS is a functional disorder without a known pathology. It is thought to be a combination of altered motility, hypersensitivity to intestinal distention, and psychological distress.

   b. IBS is the most common cause of chronic or recurrent abdominal pain in the United States.

   c. IBS generally remains an intermittent, lifelong problem. Symptoms typically begin during early to mid adulthood.

    d. IBS is more common in women than in men. Exacerbations may be associated with menses or stress.

    e. IBS is a diagnosis of exclusion. The differential diagnosis includes lactose intolerance, cholecystitis, chronic pancreatitis, intestinal obstruction, chronic peritonitis, and carcinoma of the pancreas or stomach.

2. Clinical features

    a. Abdominal pain may occur anywhere or may be localized to the hypogastrium or left lower quadrant.

        (1) Pain may be worsened by food intake and typically is relieved with defecation.

        (2) Pain may be associated with bowel distention from accumulation of gas and associated spasm of the smooth muscle; postprandial urgency is common.

    b. Physical examination generally is normal but may include a tender, palpable sigmoid colon and hyperresonance on percussion over the abdomen.

    c. IBS is strongly identified with changes in stool frequency and character. Constipation, diarrhea, or alternating constipation and diarrhea may occur.

    d. Dyspepsia is common.

    e. Urinary frequency and urgency are common in women.

3. Laboratory findings generally are normal.

    a. The stool should be tested for blood, bacteria, parasites, and lactose intolerance.

    b. Colonoscopy, barium enema, ultrasonography, or CT should be performed to rule out other pathology.

    c. Endoscopic studies are indicated in patients with persistent symptoms, weight loss or anorexia, bleeding, or history of other GI pathology.

4. Treatment

    a. Reassurance and a strong provider–patient relationship are key. Avoidance of any known triggers is important.

    b. A high-fiber diet and bulking agents, such as psyllium hydrophilic mucilloid, are the mainstays of treatment.

    c. Antispasmodics, antidiarrheals, prokinetics, or antidepressants can be used if indicated by the patient's symptoms or course of illness.

J. Intussusception

1. General characteristics

    a. Intussusception is the invagination of a proximal segment of the bowel into the portion just distal to it.

    b. It occurs most commonly in children (95% of cases), generally following a viral infection.

    c. In adults, intussusception almost always is caused by a neoplasm.

2. Clinical features

    a. Children will exhibit signs of severe colicky pain. Stool, if passed, will contain mucus and blood (currant jelly stools). A sausage-like mass may be felt on abdominal examination.

    b. Adults may present with a more indolent course of crampy abdominal pain. Bloody stool and abdominal mass are rare.

3. Laboratory findings

    a. For children, barium or air enema may be both diagnostic and therapeutic.

    b. For adults, barium enema should not be used, and abdominal plain-film radiography shows nonspecific obstruction. CT is the best means of establishing the diagnosis, but many cases are diagnosed only at surgery.

4. Treatment

    a. All patients with suspected intussusception should be hospitalized.

    b. Air or barium enema may be curative for children; if not, surgery is needed.

    c. Adults generally require surgery.

K. Diverticular disease

1. General characteristics

    a. Diverticulosis can be described as large outpouchings of the mucosa in the colon.

    b. Diverticulitis is defined as inflammation of the diverticula caused by obstructing matter.

    c. Approximately 60% of people older than 60 years have diverticula; of these, 20% become symptomatic.

    d. Approximately 20% of patients with acute diverticulitis are younger than 40 years.

    e. In patients with diverticulosis, diverticulitis and its complications can be prevented with a high-fiber diet and avoidance of obstructing or constipating foods.

2. Clinical features
    a. Diverticulitis
        (1) It generally presents with sudden-onset abdominal pain, usually in the left lower quadrant or suprapubic region, with or without fever.
        (2) Symptoms may range from mild disease to severe infection with peritonitis.
        (3) Altered bowel movement as well as nausea and vomiting are common.
    b. Diverticular bleeding generally presents as sudden-onset, large-volume hematochezia. It resolves spontaneously, although continuous or recurrent bleeding are indications for surgery.
3. Laboratory findings
    a. Occult blood in the stool and mild to moderate leukocytosis may occur with diverticulitis.
    b. Plain-film radiography should be done to rule out free air.
    c. CT is warranted if patients do not respond to therapy.
    d. Barium enema should be avoided during an acute episode, because it may lead to perforation and peritonitis.
4. Treatment
    a. Low-residue diet and broad-spectrum antibiotics are appropriate for patients with mild diverticulitis.
    b. Hospitalization for IV administration of antibiotics, bowel rest, and analgesics often is required. A nasogastric tube is inserted if ileus develops.
    c. Surgical management may be necessary in severe cases including peritonitis, large abscesses, fistulae or obstruction.
    d. Patients with diverticulosis should maintain a high-fiber diet to prevent diverticulits. Recent studies have negated the need to recommend avoidance of nuts, seeds, and popcorn.
L. Ischemic bowel disease
    1. General characteristics
        a. Mesenteric ischemia (MI) can be acute (AMI) or chronic (CMI). In chronic ischemia, the blood supply is present but insufficient to meet the needs of the intestine.
        b. For both AMI and CMI, patients generally will be older than 50 years and have other signs of cardiovascular or collagen vascular disease.
        c. AMI
            (1) AMI may be caused by arterial embolus, arterial thrombosis, or venous thrombosis, with differing risk factors and prognosis for each.
            (2) AMI represents an emergency. Mortality remains high despite advances in treatment.
        d. Intestinal infarction is more common in the small bowel than in the large bowel. Shock is common.
    2. Clinical features
        a. CMI presents as abdominal angina, with pain occurring 10 to 30 minutes after eating, which is relieved somewhat by squatting or lying down.
        b. AMI presents with sudden onset of severe abdominal pain out of proportion to examination findings. Later in the process involuntary guarding, rebound, and heme-positive stool may develop.
    3. Laboratory findings
        a. Plain-film radiography and CT are performed to rule out other causes of abdominal pain or to show areas of edema or dilatation.
        b. Colonoscopy is the optimal test to evaluate for ischemia of the colon.
        c. Angiography may be helpful if the diagnosis is in question.
    4. Treatment for AMI or CMI is surgical revascularization. Hydration is also a critical factor.
M. Toxic megacolon
    1. General characteristics
        a. Toxic megacolon is extreme dilatation and immobility of the colon and represents a true emergency.
        b. Hirschsprung's disease is a congenital aganglionosis of the colon, leading to functional obstruction in the newborn.
        c. In adults, toxic megacolon occurs as a complication of UC, Crohn's colitis, pseudomembranous colitis, and specific infectious causes (particularly amebiasis, *Shigella* sp., *Campylobacter* sp., and *Clostridium difficile*).

2. Clinical features

   a. Symptoms include fever, prostration, severe cramps, and abdominal distention.

   b. A rigid abdomen and localized, diffuse, or rebound abdominal tenderness are found on physical examination.

3. Laboratory findings: Abdominal plain-film radiography will show colonic dilatation.

4. Treatment

   a. Decompression of the colon is required. In some cases, colostomy or even complete colonic resection may be required.

   b. Careful attention must be paid to fluid and electrolyte balance.

N. Colonic polyps

1. General characteristics

   a. Colonic polyps are common in the industrialized world and can be either benign or malignant.

   b. Removal of polyps can reduce the occurrence of colon cancer.

   c. Familial polyposis syndrome is a genetic predisposition to multiple colonic polyps with a near-100% risk of developing colonic cancer.

2. Clinical features

   a. Polyps generally are asymptomatic, although constipation, flatulence, and rectal bleeding may occur.

   b. Bleeding polyps may cause iron deficiency anemia.

3. Laboratory findings

   a. Heme-positive stool is common.

   b. Barium enema, flexible sigmoidoscopy, and colonoscopy can detect polyps.

   c. Histologic evaluation is needed to determine dysplasia.

   d. Family members of those with familial polyposis syndrome should be evaluated every 1 to 2 years beginning at 10 to 12 years of age.

4. Treatment depends on the size and histology of polyps. Larger and dysplastic polyps should be removed and frequent follow-up arranged.

O. Colorectal cancer

1. General characteristics

   a. Colorectal cancer is the third leading cause of cancer death in the United States after lung cancer and skin cancers.

   b. Approximately 90% of cases occur in people older than 50 years.

   c. Hereditary nonpolyposis colorectal cancer also leads to an extremely high risk of colon cancer, and those with familial polyposis have a virtually 100% risk of developing the disease.

   d. Prognosis

     (1) Prognosis is good in early disease.

     (2) When the cancer involves only the mucosa (Dukes A), the 5-year survival rate is greater than 90%.

     (3) Penetration through the wall or involvement of regional lymph nodes (Dukes B) has a 5-year survival rate of 70% to 80%.

     (4) When there is metastasis (Dukes C [lymph node positive] and D [distant metastases]), the 5-year survival rate drops to 5%.

2. Clinical features

   a. Colorectal cancer is slow growing, and symptoms often appear late in the disease. Abdominal pain, change in bowel habits, occult bleeding, and intestinal obstruction are common presentations.

   b. Fatigue and weakness may occur if chronic blood loss has led to anemia.

   c. Changes in stool size and shape may be noted, as may frank blood in the stool.

3. Laboratory findings

   a. Occult blood in the stool can be an early marker and is used for screening adults older than 40 years. Flexible colonoscopy is recommended in those older than 40 or 50 years. Debate continues regarding specific screening schedules, but overall the data support regular screening for the general population after age 50 (every 5 to 10 years depending on the method).

   b. Carcinoembryonic antigen may be used to monitor, although not to detect, colorectal cancer.

    c. Sigmoidoscopy, colonoscopy, or barium enema may all be used to visualize suspected colonic masses, whereas chest radiography and CT are used to detect metastases.

  4. Treatment

    a. Treatment is by surgical resection, which is accompanied by chemotherapy in patients stage III (Dukes C or higher) or higher (and sometimes in stage II [Dukes B] lesions).

    b. Radiation may be used for rectal tumors.

IV. DISEASES OF THE RECTUM AND ANUS

A. Anorectal abscess/fistula

  1. General characteristics

    a. Anorectal abscess is a result of infection, whereas fistula is a chronic complication of abscess.

    b. Fistula is an open tract between two epithelium-lined areas and most commonly is associated with deeper anorectal abscesses.

  2. Clinical features

    a. Perirectal and perianal abscesses are most common and produce painful swelling at the anus as well as painful defecation. Examination reveals localized tenderness, erythema, swelling, and fluctuance; fever is uncommon.

    b. Deeper abscesses may produce buttock or coccyx pain and rectal fullness; fever is more likely.

    c. Fistula will produce anal discharge and pain when the tract becomes occluded. The tract should not be explored on examination, because this may open new tracts.

  3. Treatment

    a. Treatment of abscess requires surgical drainage, followed by warm-water cleansing, analgesics, stool softeners, and high-fiber diet (WASH regimen).

    b. Fistulae must be treated surgically.

B. Anal fissure

  1. Anal fissures are linear lesions in the rectal wall, most commonly found on the posterior midline.

  2. Patients describe severe tearing pain on defecation, often accompanied by hematochezia; bright red blood often is noted on the stool or tissue paper.

  3. Treatment includes bulking agents and increased fluids to avoid straining. Sitz baths will relieve acute pain. Topical nitroglycerin ointment or topical styptic, such as silver nitrate (1% to 2%) or gentian violet solution (1%), may help with healing.

C. Hemorrhoids

  1. General characteristic: Hemorrhoids are varices of the hemorrhoidal plexus.

  2. Clinical features

    a. External hemorrhoids are visible perianally.

    b. Stage I internal hemorrhoids are confined to the anal canal and may bleed with defecation.

    c. Stage II internal hemorrhoids protrude from the anal opening but reduce spontaneously. Bleeding and mucoid discharge may occur.

    d. Stage III internal hemorrhoids require manual reduction after bowel movements. Patients may develop pain and discomfort.

    e. Stage IV internal hemorrhoids are chronically protruding and risk strangulation.

  3. Treatment

    a. Stage I and II disease can be managed with a high-fiber diet and increased fluids. Bulk laxatives are helpful.

    b. Higher-stage hemorrhoidal disease may benefit from suppositories with anesthetic and astringent properties.

    c. Surgical treatment is indicated for those unresponsive to conservative treatment and all stage IV hemorrhoids. Choices include injection, rubber band ligation, or sclerotherapy.

D. Pilonidal disease

  1. General characteristics

    a. Pilonidal cyst is an abscess in the sacrococcygeal cleft associated with subsequent sinus tract development.

    b. Pilonidal cysts are four times more likely in males than in females, are more common in hirsute and obese individuals, and are rare in those older than 40 years.

2. Clinical presentation is a painful, fluctuant area at the sacrococcygeal cleft.

3. Treatment

   a. Treatment is surgical drainage, which may be supplemented with antibiotics.

   b. Follicle removal may be required, with unroofing of sinus tracts.

E. Fecal impaction

1. General characteristics

   a. Fecal impaction is a large mass of hard, retained stool. It generally occurs in the rectum but also may occur higher in the colon.

   b. Complications

      (1) Complications include urinary tract obstruction and infection, spontaneous perforation of the colon, and stercoral ulcer where the mass has pressed on the colon.

      (2) Fecaliths may develop and cause appendicitis.

   c. More proximal impaction generally indicates neoplasm.

2. Clinical features

   a. Abdominal pain, rectal discomfort, anorexia, nausea, and vomiting are common but nonspecific.

   b. Headache and a general sense of illness are common, and acute confusional states may appear.

   c. Incontinence of small amounts of water and semiformed stool may occur as leakage passes by a large impaction.

   d. Rock-hard stool in the rectal vault on examination is diagnostic. Abdominal mass also may be palpated, and sigmoidoscopy or barium enema may be needed to confirm a more proximal impaction.

3. Treatment

   a. Treatment involves breaking up the impaction digitally, followed by a saline or tepid-water enema.

   b. More proximal impaction can be broken up by sigmoidoscopic water irrigation and suction.

   c. Subsequent attention must be paid to bowel habits and hydration.

V. APPENDICITIS

A. General characteristics

1. Appendicitis occurs when obstruction of the appendix leads to inflammation and infection.

   a. The most common cause is a fecalith.

   b. Less common causes include infection (CMV, adenovirus, histoplasma, other), collagen vascular disease, and inflammatory bowel disease.

2. Patients usually are between 10 and 30 years of age.

3. Appendicitis affects 10% of the U.S. population, making it the most common abdominal surgical emergency.

4. Perforation and peritonitis occur in about 20% of patients with appendicitis, causing high-grade fever, generalized abdominal pain, and increased leukocytosis.

B. Clinical features

1. The initial symptom is intermittent periumbilical or epigastric pain.

2. In about 12 hours, pain typically localizes to the right lower quadrant (McBurney's point), becomes constant, and is worsened by movement, leading to rebound tenderness on examination.

3. Nausea and anorexia are common. Vomiting may occur, but generally is isolated and begins subsequent to the onset of pain.

4. Diarrhea may occur but is not common.

5. A low-grade fever is common; a high-grade fever is unlikely.

6. Psoas sign (patient is supine and attempts to raise the leg against resistance) and obturator sign (patient is supine and attempts to flex and internally rotate the right hip with the knee bent) generally are positive, indicating inflammation adjacent to those muscles.

7. Variability in anatomy can cause unusual presentations of appendicitis, with symptoms reflecting the location of the appendix.

C. Laboratory findings

1. Leukocytosis (usually 10,000 to 20,000 cells/mL) is characteristic. Higher levels suggest perforation and peritonitis.

2. Some microscopic hematuria and pyuria may be seen.

3. Abdominal CT may be used in some cases to confirm the diagnosis and to locate an abnormally placed appendix.

D. Treatment

1. Treatment is appendectomy.

2. If there is any reason to suspect perforation, broad-spectrum antibiotics are administered before and after surgery.

VI. DISEASES OF THE PANCREAS

A. Acute pancreatitis

1. General characteristics

a. Causes

(1) The most common causes are cholelithiasis or alcohol abuse, but hyperlipidemia, trauma, drugs, hypercalcemia, and penetrating PUD also may cause pancreatitis.

(2) Pancreatitis also is associated with medications, especially many of the antiretroviral medications used to treat HIV.

b. The range of presentation is wide, ranging from mild episodes of deep epigastric pain with nausea and vomiting to the sudden onset of severe pain with shock.

2. Clinical features

a. The classic presentation is epigastric pain radiating to the back. The pain typically lessens when the patient leans forward or lies in a fetal position.

b. Nausea and vomiting are common.

c. Fever, leukocytosis, and sterile peritonitis may occur.

d. Severe hypovolemia, adult respiratory distress syndrome, and tachycardia of greater than 130 bpm indicate a grave prognosis.

3. Laboratory studies

a. Elevation of serum amylase occurs but may be transient and can return to normal after 48 to 72 hours.

b. Serum lipase is more sensitive and specific than amylase for acute pancreatitis, but only with elevations of threefold or greater.

c. WBC count generally is elevated, and hemoconcentration may occur with third spacing of fluid.

d. Liver enzymes may increase as a result of biliary obstruction.

e. Mild hyperbilirubinemia and bilirubinuria, hyperglycemia, and hypocalcemia may occur.

f. Poor prognosis is indicated by Ranson's criteria (Table 5-3). Risk of mortality rises with each additional factor.

4. Treatment

a. Oral intake must be stopped to prevent continued secretion of pancreatic juices.

b. Fluid volume must be restored and maintained. Parenteral hyperalimentation should be started early to prevent nutritional depletion.

TABLE 5-3	Ranson's Criteria for Poor Prognosis for Pancreatitis
Leukocyte count	>16,000 cells/mL
Blood glucose level	>200 mg/dL
Lactate dehydrogenase	>350 IU/dL (normal, <20–50 IU/dL)
AST	>250 IU/dL (normal, <120 IU/dL)
Arterial PO$_2$	<60 mm Hg
Base deficit	>4 mEq/L
Calcium	Falling
BUN	Rising

AST, aspartate aminotransferase; BUN, blood urea nitrogen.

     c. Pain is managed with meperidine. Antibiotics should be considered.

     d. The patient must be monitored closely for complications, including pancreatic pseudocyst, renal failure, pleural effusion, hypocalcemia, and pancreatic abscess.

B. Chronic pancreatitis

  1. General characteristics

     a. Almost 90% of cases of chronic pancreatitis in the United States are caused by alcohol abuse; other causes include cholelithiasis, PUD, hyperparathyroidism, and hyperlipidemia.

     b. Some chronic cases can resolve if alcohol consumption is decreased.

     c. The classic triad of pancreatic calcification, steatorrhea, and diabetes mellitus occurs in only 20% of patients.

  2. Clinical features are the same as those of acute pancreatitis, with the addition of fat malabsorption and steatorrhea late in the disease. Fecal fat will be elevated if malabsorption is present.

  3. Laboratory studies

     a. The amylase level may be elevated early but will decrease with each episode of pancreatitis and cease to be a useful marker.

     b. Abdominal plain-film radiography reveals calcification in 20% to 30% of patients.

  4. Treatment

     a. Treatment is as for acute pancreatitis. A low-fat diet should be recommended at discharge.

     b. Surgical removal of part of the pancreas can control pain.

     c. The only definitive treatment for chronic pancreatitis is to address the underlying cause, which most commonly is alcohol.

C. Pancreatic neoplasm

  1. General characteristics

     a. Pancreatic cancer is the fifth leading cause of cancer death in the United States.

     b. Risk factors include increased age, obesity, tobacco, chronic pancreatitis, previous abdominal radiation, and family history.

  2. Clinical presentation

     a. Abdominal pain occurs in most patients and, depending on the location of the tumor, can radiate.

     b. Jaundice and a palpable gallbladder (Courvoisier's sign) may be seen in patients with cancer of the pancreatic head.

  3. Diagnostic studies include CT to delineate disease and search for metastases and angiography to look for vascular invasion.

  4. Treatment

     a. Treatment is surgical resection (modified Whipple's procedure) in those without metastases.

     b. Subsequent radiation and chemotherapy are controversial.

     c. Prognosis is poor.

VII. DISEASES OF THE BILIARY TRACT

A. Choledocholithiasis

  1. General characteristics

     a. By age 75, 35% of women and 20% of men have gallstones.

     b. Only 30% of people with gallstones develop symptomatic disease.

  2. Treatment

     a. Generally, only the complications of choledocholithiasis should be treated, because most people with gallstones will never develop the disease.

     b. Complications include cholecystitis, pancreatitis, and acute cholangitis.

B. Acute cholecystitis

  1. Acute cholecystitis is caused by obstruction of the bile duct, generally by a stone, leading to chronic inflammation.

  2. Clinical presentation

     a. Colicky epigastric or right upper quadrant (RUQ) pain becomes steady and increases in intensity. It often occurs after a high-fat meal.

b. Right shoulder or subscapular pain may occur.

c. Nausea, vomiting, and low-grade fever are common.

d. Constipation and mild paralytic ileus may occur.

3. Laboratory findings

a. After 24 hours, bilirubin levels increase in blood and urine.

b. Leukocytosis is common.

c. Gallstones are found in 95% of patients with cholecystitis. Although only 20% are radiopaque, the remainder generally are visible by sonography.

d. Hepatobiliary imaging (hepatoiminodiacetic acid [HIDA] scan or others) can be used for confirmation of the diagnosis.

e. Endoscopic retrograde cholangiopancreatography (ERCP) can identify cause, location, and extent of biliary obstruction.

4. Treatment is surgical.

C. Acute cholangitis

1. General characteristics

a. It is a potentially deadly condition of common bile duct obstruction combined with ascending infection, most commonly caused by *Escherichia coli, Enterococcus, Klebsiella,* and *Enterobacter,* that can lead to sepsis and death.

b. It is most often caused by choledocholelithiasis, although neoplasms, postoperative strictures, or other causes of obstruction may be involved.

2. Clinical presentation

a. Presentation varies from mild to fulminant.

b. RUQ tenderness, jaundice, and fever (Charcot's triad) is present in 50% to 70% of cases.

c. In additional to Charcot's triad, altered mental status and hypotension may also be present (Reynold's pentad) and indicate sepsis. If present, the disease can become rapidly fatal.

d. Elderly patients may present with confusion, falls, and incontinence.

3. Laboratory findings

a. RUQ ultrasonography will generally show biliary dilation or stones and is a good initial test.

b. Leukocytosis with left shift along with increased bilirubin and mildly increased transaminase levels support the diagnosis.

c. ECRP is the optimal procedure both for diagnosis and for treatment but, unless urgent decompression is necessary, should not be done until the patient is stable.

4. Treatment

a. Antibiotics (generally fluoroquinolone, ampicillin, and gentamycin with or without metronidazole), fluid and electrolyte replacement, and analgesia are the initial treatment.

b. ECRP for drainage, sphincterotomy, and stone removal and stent placement can be done when the patient is stable. Percutaneous transhepatic biliary drainage or surgical biliary drainage may be required.

c. Cholecystectomy should be performed after the acute syndrome is resolved when choledocholilithiasis is present.

D. Primary sclerosing cholangitis (PSC)

1. General characteristics

a. PSC is a chronic thickening of the bile duct walls of unknown etiology, although 80% of cases are associated with inflammatory bowel disease, generally UC (although only 10% of patients with UC will develop PSC).

b. PSC is strongly associated with cholangiocarcinoma (10% to 30% of patients) as well as with an increased risk of pancreatic and colorectal carcinoma.

c. Male to female ratio is 7:3, and the age at diagnosis is between 21 and 67 years (mean 39).

2. Clinical presentation

a. Jaundice and pruritis are the most common presenting features, with fatigue, malaise, and weight loss seen in many patients.

b. Hepatomegaly and/or splenomegaly may be found on exam.

3. Labs are the same as for acute cholangitis.
4. Treatment
   a. Ursodiol is used, as is endoscopic management of stricture, although the effect of these interventions on quality of life and survival is unknown.
   b. Liver transplant is the only treatment with a known survival benefit.

VIII. DISEASES OF THE LIVER

A. Hepatitis
   1. General characteristics
      a. Hepatitis can describe acute or chronic hepatocellular damage.
      b. The most common cause of acute hepatitis is viral; toxins (e.g., alcohol) are the second most common cause.
      c. Chronic hepatitis most often results from viral infection (hepatitis B, C, D) but often is caused by inherited disorders (e.g., Wilson's disease, α_1-antitrypsin deficiency), autoimmune disease of the liver, or hepatic effects of systemic disease.
   2. Viral hepatitis
      a. General characteristics
         (1) The severity of the disease is highly variable, ranging from asymptomatic to fulminant, generally fatal, infection.
         (2) Hepatitis A and E are transmitted by fecal–oral contamination and can be prevented by maintaining a sanitary water supply and hand washing.
         (3) Hepatitis B, C, and D are transmitted parenterally or by mucous membrane contact.
         (4) Of those with chronic hepatitis C, only 20% to 30% will progress to serious liver disease, which occurs most often when alcohol is involved or the patient is coinfected with hepatitis B or HIV.
      b. Clinical features
         (1) Fatigue, malaise, anorexia, nausea, tea-colored urine, and vague abdominal discomfort are common presenting complaints.
         (2) Hepatitis A and E are self-limited and mild, without long-term sequelae.
         (3) Hepatitis B and C can have a highly variable presentation, ranging from asymptomatic to fulminant. Chronic hepatitis B or C causing liver damage may require treatment.
         (4) Hepatitis D is seen only in conjunction with hepatitis B and is associated with a more severe course.
         (5) Hepatitis C and HIV are frequent coinfections, as are hepatitis B and HIV, necessitating specialist care if treatment of the hepatitis is indicated.
      c. Laboratory findings
         (1) Aminotransferase elevations are seen in all types of acute hepatitis, indicating hepatocellular damage.
         (2) Bilirubin of greater than 3.0 mg/dL will be associated with scleral icterus, if not frank jaundice.
         (3) Immunoglobulin M antibody to hepatitis A virus (anti-HAV) can be detected with the onset of clinical disease (after a 15- to 40-day incubation period), but it disappears after several months. HAV IgG indicates resolved hepatitis A.
         (4) Hepatitis B surface antigen (HBsAg) indicates ongoing infection of any duration; antibody against hepatitis B surface antigen (anti-HBs) indicates immunity by past infection or vaccination (Fig. 5-1).
         (5) Hepatitis B core antibody (anti-HBc) is present between the disappearance of HBsAg and the appearance of anti-HBs, indicating acute hepatitis.
         (6) Hepatitis B envelope antigen (HBeAg) indicates active infection that is highly contagious, whereas anti-HBe indicates a lower viral titer.
         (7) Hepatitis C or D generally is detected by its antibody, which for hepatitis C generally indicates ongoing infection, as it does for hepatitis D if hepatitis B infection is ongoing.
         (8) Hepatitis B may exist in a carrier state or a chronic infection. Both exhibit positive HBsAg, but in chronic infection, liver damage is demonstrated by elevated aspartate aminotransferase (AST) and alanine aminotransferase (ALT) and by hepatocellular damage on biopsy. In chronic infection, the viral DNA load will be greater than 10^5 copies. HBeAg seroconversion (to negative) tends to occur with a reduction in viral DNA.

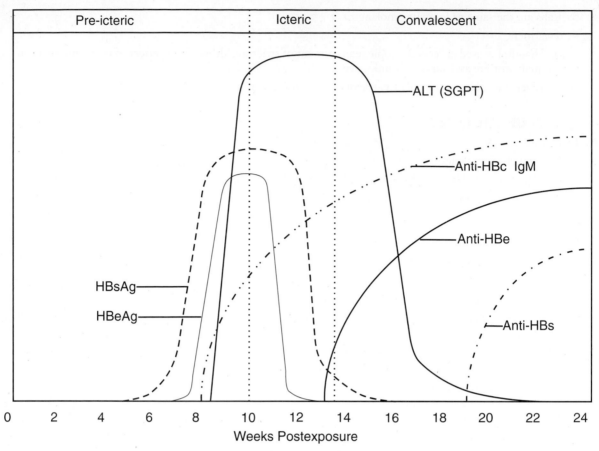

FIGURE 5-1 Relationship of clinical and laboratory features of hepatitis B. ALT, alanine aminotransferase; anti-HBc, hepatitis B core antibody; anti-HBe, hepatitis B envelope antigen; anti-HBs, hepatitis B surface antigen antibody; HBsAg, hepatitis B surface antigen; SGPT, serum glutamate pyruvate transaminase.

(9) Hepatitis C antibody–positive patients should be evaluated for genotype and viral load. Types 2 and 3 have a better treatment prognosis than type 1, as does a lower HCV viral load. Liver biopsy is currently the preferred method for evaluating the level of fibrosis and the need for treatment.

d. Treatment

(1) Treatment of acute viral hepatitis is supportive. Patients with hepatitis A must be cautious about transmission to others by not sharing food or dishes and by frequent hand washing.

(2) All patients with acute or chronic hepatitis should avoid alcohol and other hepatotoxins.

(3) All HIV-positive patients with chronic hepatitis B should be treated for HIV, regardless of CD4 count, with therapies that cover both infections. Tenofovir with either emtricitabine or lamivudine will cover the hepatitis B and the addition of either efavirenz or a boosted protease inhibitor will cover the HIV infection.

(4) Patients with hepatitis C should be vaccinated against hepatitis A and B.

(5) Patients with hepatitis C should be evaluated for the level of fibrosis. Therapy, when indicated, involves pegylated interferon α-2a or α-2b given with ribavirin. Newer therapies are evolving. The goal of therapy is reduction of viral RNA to undetectable at 6 months post therapy.

3. Toxic hepatitis

a. Toxic hepatitis may be caused by numerous agents, including alcohol, acetaminophen, carbon tetrachloride, isoniazid, halothane, phenytoin, and many others.

b. Both diagnosis and treatment are accomplished by discontinuing the suspected agent. Acetylcysteine can be used for acetaminophen toxicity.

c. Toxic hepatitis may be reversible, depending on the amount of the toxin. If the patient survives the acute episode, the prognosis is good.

B. Cirrhosis
1. General characteristics
   a. Cirrhosis is irreversible fibrosis and nodular regeneration throughout the liver.
   b. In the United States, more than 45% of cases are alcohol related, with the remainder associated with hepatitis B or C or with congenital disorders.
2. Clinical presentation
   a. Weakness, fatigue, and weight loss are common.
   b. Nausea, vomiting, and anorexia usually are present.
   c. Menstrual changes (generally amenorrhea), impotence, loss of libido, and gynecomastia occur.
   d. Abdominal pain and hepatomegaly generally are present.
   e. Late-stage disease includes ascites, pleural effusions, peripheral edema, ecchymoses, esophageal varices, and signs of hepatic encephalopathy (e.g., asterixis, tremor, dysarthria, delirium, and, eventually, coma).
3. Laboratory findings
   a. Laboratory values often are minimally abnormal until late in the disease.
   b. Anemia is common, as are mild elevations of AST and alkaline phosphatase, increased γ-globulin, and decreased albumin.
   c. Ultrasonography, CT, or MRI can confirm the size and number of nodules and is helpful in guiding biopsy.
4. Treatment
   a. Abstinence from alcohol is the key feature of treatment.
   b. Salt restriction and bed rest may be sufficient treatment for ascites, although spironolactone, 100 mg daily, may be added as a diuretic.
   c. Liver transplant is indicated in selected patients.

C. Liver abscess generally is caused by *Entamoeba histolytica* or the coliform bacteria. It may occur either after travel or secondary to an intra-abdominal infection and presents with fever and abdominal pain. Treatment includes antibiotics and percutaneous drainage or surgical excision.

D. Liver neoplasm
1. General characteristics
   a. Liver neoplasms may be malignant or benign, and malignant neoplasms may be primary or metastatic.
   b. Benign liver neoplasms include cavernous hemangioma, hepatocellular adenoma, and infantile hemangioendothelioma.
   c. The liver is a common site of metastasis for other primary cancers, especially lung and breast cancers. If the primary tumor is silent, liver manifestations may be the presenting complaints.
   d. Primary hepatocellular carcinoma is associated with hepatitis B, hepatitis C, aflatoxin B1 exposure (produced by *Aspergillus* species and found in contaminated vegetation and contaminated food), and cirrhosis.
2. Clinical characteristics
   a. Presenting complaints include malaise, weight loss, abdominal swelling, weakness, jaundice, and upper abdominal pain.
   b. Hepatomegaly, splenomegaly, hepatic bruit, ascites, jaundice, wasting, and fever may be detected on examination.
3. Laboratory findings
   a. α-Fetoprotein may be elevated in hepatic carcinoma.
   b. Imaging with sonography, CT, MRI, or hepatic angiography can show the lesion.
   c. Needle biopsy generally should not be used if the tumor is resectable.
4. Treatment
   a. Benign neoplasms should be treated if the tumor size indicates a danger of rupturing the hepatic capsule.
   b. Treatment of metastatic disease involves treatment of the primary lesion.
   c. Surgical resection of hepatic carcinoma may be attempted if the cancer is confined to one lobe and there is no concurrent cirrhosis. Liver transplant also can be considered. The overall prognosis is poor.

IX. HERNIAS

A. General characteristics
   1. A hernia is a protrusion of an organ or structure through the wall that normally contains it.
   2. Hernias of various types can entrap the intestines and cause intestinal blockage.
B. Types
   1. Umbilical hernia generally is congenital and appears at birth. Many umbilical hernias resolve on their own, but surgery may be indicated.
   2. Diaphragmatic or hiatal hernia involves protrusion of the stomach through the diaphragm via the esophageal hiatus. It can cause GERD. Acid reduction may suffice, and surgical repair can be used for more serious cases.
   3. Incisional hernias are associated more commonly with vertical incisions, especially in patients with concurrent obesity or wound infection.
   4. Inguinal hernias can be indirect (most common; passage of intestine through the internal inguinal ring down the inguinal canal, may pass into the scrotum), direct (passage of intestine through external inguinal ring at Hesselbach's triangle, rarely enters the scrotum), or femoral (least common; passage through femoral ring).
   5. Ventral hernia occurs when there is a weakening in the anterior abdominal wall and may be either incisional or umbilical.
C. Treatment of hernias is surgical.

X. CONGENITAL ABNORMALITIES

A. Esophageal atresia commonly is associated with tracheoesophageal fistulae.
   1. Atresia presents in newborns as excessive saliva and choking or coughing with attempts to feed.
   2. Inability to pass a nasogastric tube will establish the diagnosis.
   3. Treatment is surgical, but pulmonary aspiration should be prevented in the interim by suction and withholding of oral feedings.
B. Diaphragmatic hernia causes immediate respiratory distress in the newborn, because the affected lung is compressed by pressure from abdominal contents.
   1. Immediate intubation and ventilation is required, along with suction of the stomach by nasogastric tube.
   2. Diagnosis can be made if bowel sounds are heard in the chest.
   3. Radiography shows loops of bowel in the involved hemithorax, with displacement of the heart and mediastinal structures.
   4. Treatment is surgical.
C. Pyloric stenosis
   1. General characteristics
      a. The gastric outlet is obstructed by pyloric hypertrophy.
      b. Males are affected about five times more often than females.
   2. Clinical features
      a. Progressive, nonbilious, often projectile vomiting occurs in a child who remains hungry, generally presenting between 4 and 6 weeks of age.
      b. Weight loss and dehydration are common.
      c. An olive-shaped mass may be felt to the right of the umbilicus in most cases, especially shortly after vomiting.
   3. Laboratory findings
      a. Ultrasonography will generally demonstrate the lesion, although barium swallow, showing delayed emptying and "string sign," may be required in some cases.
   4. Treatment is surgical.
D. Bowel atresia can occur in the ileum (most common), duodenum, jejunum, or colon and presents with signs of obstruction within the first few days of life.
E. Hirschsprung's disease (congenital megacolon) is caused by congenital absence of Meissner's and Auerbach's autonomic plexuses enervating the bowel wall.
   1. Symptoms may include constipation or obstipation, vomiting, and failure to thrive.
   2. Treatment is surgical resection of the affected bowel.

XI. NUTRITIONAL DEFICIENCIES

Vitamin	Sources	Function(s)	At-risk Groups	Deficiency	Toxicity
Vitamin A	Liver, fish oils, fortified milk, eggs	Vision, epithelial cell maturity, resistance to infection, antioxidant	Elderly, alcoholics, liver disease	Night blindness, dry skin	Skin disorders, hair loss, teratogenicity
Vitamin D	Fortified milk	Calcium regulation, cell differentiation	Elderly, shut-ins with low sun exposure	Rickets, osteomalacia	Hypercalcemia, kidney stones, soft-tissue deposits
Vitamin E	Plant oils, wheat germ, asparagus, peanuts, margarine	Retard cell aging, vascular and red cell wall integrity, antioxidant	Rare	Hemolytic anemia, degenerative nerve changes	Inhibition of vitamin K, myalgia, headache, weakness
Vitamin K	Liver, green leafy vegetables, broccoli, peas, green beans	Clotting	Rare	Bleeding	Anemia, jaundice
Thiamin	Pork, grains, dried beans, peas, brewer's yeast	Carbohydrate metabolism, nerve function	Alcoholism, poverty	Beriberi (nervous tingling, poor coordination, edema, weakness, cardiac dysfunction)	N/A
Riboflavin	Milk, spinach, liver, grains	Energy	N/A	Oral inflammation, eye disorders	N/A
Niacin	Bran, tuna, salmon, chicken, beef, liver, peanuts, grains	Energy, fat metabolism	Poverty, alcoholism	Flushing	N/A
Pantothenic acid	Liver, broccoli, eggs	Energy, fat metabolism	Alcoholism	Tingling, fatigue, headache	N/A
Biotin	Cheese, eggs, cauliflower, peanut butter, liver	Glucose production, fat synthesis	Alcoholism	Dermatitis, tongue pain, anemia, depression	N/A
B_6 pyridoxine	Animal protein, spinach, broccoli, bananas, salmon	Protein metabolism, neurotransmitter synthesis, hemoglobin	Adolescents, alcoholism	Headache, anemia, seizures, flaky skin, sore tongue	Nerve destruction
Folate	Green leafy vegetables, orange juice, grains, organ meats	DNA synthesis	Alcoholism, pregnancy	Megaloblastic anemia, sore tongue, diarrhea, mental disorders	N/A
B_{12} cobalamin	Animal foods	Folate metabolism, nerve function	Elderly, vegans	Megaloblastic anemia, poor nerve function	N/A
Vitamin C	Citrus fruits, strawberries, broccoli, greens	Collagen synthesis, hormone function, neurotransmitter synthesis	Alcoholism, elderly men	Scurvy (poor wound healing, petechiae, bleeding gums)	Diarrhea

Adapted from Wardlaw GM. *Perspectives in Nutrition*. 4th ed. New York: McGraw-Hill; 1999.

XII. METABOLIC DISORDERS

A. Lactose intolerance

1. Lactose is digested by lactase, which is produced in the small intestine.

2. The persistence of lactase production past the age of 12 is common only in northern European populations. For most of the world's population, lactase does not persist, and lactose-containing products are not well digested.

3. Symptoms of lactose intolerance include nausea, bloating, flatulence, diarrhea, cramping, and, occasionally, vomiting.

4. Lactose intolerance is easily managed by avoiding milk and dairy products or use of lactase enzyme tablets or drops.

B. Phenylketonuria

1. Phenylketonuria is a rare autosomal recessive inability to metabolize the protein phenylalanine.

2. Phenylalanine and its metabolites accumulate in the central nervous system, causing mental retardation and movement disorders.

3. Screening at birth is simple and allows early detection and management; delay in diagnosis (after age 3 years) will lead to irreversible brain damage.

4. Management is by a low-phenylalanine diet and tyrosine supplementation. Breast milk is low in phenylalanine, and special formulas are available. Strict control of protein intake is required for life.

Nephrology and Urology

Eric H. Vangsnes

6

I. RENAL FAILURE

A. Acute renal failure (ARF) (acute kidney injury [AKI])

1. General characteristics

   a. ARF refers to a syndrome of rapidly deteriorating glomerular filtration rate (GFR) with the accumulation of nitrogenous wastes (urea, creatinine) referred to as azotemia. Serum creatinine acutely increases by more than 0.5 mg/dL or more than 50% over baseline levels.

   b. It is important to distinguish between an acute insult and worsening of a chronic state. Of the many conditions that can result in ARF, two diseases account for the majority of cases: reduced renal perfusion and acute tubular necrosis.

   c. Causes are classified into three categories: prerenal, intrinsic renal, and postrenal (Table 6-1).

   d. ARF occurs in 5% of hospitalized patients and in up to 30% of critical care patients. The overall mortality rate for ARF is 10% to 50% depending on patient comorbidities and clinical setting.

2. Clinical features

   a. A thorough medical history can identify possible causes of ARF, such as procedures and medications as well as exposure to nephrotoxins, family history of renal disease, urologic disease, or contributing factors, such as hypertension, hypotension, volume loss, congestive heart failure (CHF), or diabetes.

   b. General symptoms include nausea, vomiting, diarrhea, pruritus, drowsiness, dizziness, hiccups, shortness of breath, anorexia, and hematochezia.

   c. Signs can reflect the underlying cause.

      (1) Tachycardia and hypotension may indicate prerenal causes.

      (2) A distended bladder, costovertebral angle tenderness, or enlarged prostate suggests postrenal causes.

      (3) Other signs include anuria or oliguria, change in volume status (weight), change in mental status, edema, weakness, dehydration, rashes, jugular venous distention, uriniferous odor, and ecchymosis.

3. Laboratory studies

   a. GFR is the key parameter to measure renal function. Serum creatinine or blood urea nitrogen (BUN) is less reliable, although more easily measured; creatinine and BUN are helpful for monitoring renal insufficiency and provide clues to cause.

   b. BUN provides an estimate of renal function, but is much more sensitive to dehydration, catabolism, diet, renal perfusion, and liver disease.

   c. Urinalysis is essentially normal in prerenal and postrenal causes of ARF with only a few hyaline casts. Granular casts, white blood cells (WBCs) and casts, red blood cells (RBCs) and casts, proteinuria, and tubular epithelial cells indicate intrinsic renal causes of ARF.

   d. Other blood and urine studies

      (1) Prerenal causes

         (a) Urine sodium less than 20 mEq/L

         (b) Fractional excretion of sodium (FE_{Na}) less than 1%

         (c) Urine osmolality 500 mOsm

         (d) Elevated BUN to plasma Cr ratio (20:1)

   e. If the presentation is unknown with respect to an acute episode versus a chronic problem, renal ultrasonography may be utilized to measure renal size. A kidney smaller than 10 cm indicates a chronic problem.

      (2) Intrinsic renal causes

         (a) Increased urine sodium greater than 40 mEq/L

         (b) FE_{Na} greater than 1–2%

         (c) Urine osmolality of 250 to 300 mOsm

         (d) Decreased BUN to plasma Cr ratio (<15:1)

TABLE 6-1 **Causes of Acute Renal Failure**
Prerenal causes (60–70%)
Hypovolemia
Hypotension
Ineffective circulating volume (CHF, cirrhosis, nephrotic syndrome, early sepsis)
Aortic aneurysm
Renal artery stenosis or embolic disease
Intrinsic renal causes (25–40%)
Acute tubular necrosis
Nephrotoxins (NSAIDs, aminoglycosides, radiologic contrast)
Interstitial diseases (acute interstitial nephritis, SLE, infection)
Glomerulonephritis
Vascular diseases (polyarteritis nodosa, vasculitis)
Postrenal causes (5–10%)
Tubular obstruction
Obstructive uropathy (urolithiasis, BPH, bladder outlet obstruction)
CHF, congestive heart failure; NSAIDs, nonsteroidal anti-inflammatory drugs; SLE, systemic lupus erythematosus; BPH, benign prostatic hyperplasia.

(3) Postrenal causes: Urine sodium, FE_{Na}, osmolality, and BUN to Cr ratio can vary, depending on how long the obstruction has been present.

f. Many other abnormal laboratory findings are associated with loss of renal function, including azotemia, decreased creatinine clearance, metabolic acidosis, and hyperkalemia. Other blood chemistries and hematologic tests are abnormal, depending on the severity of disease.

4. Treatment

a. Treatment involves correction of the underlying problem. Examples include the following:

(1) Achievement of normal hemodynamics in prerenal states (intravenous [IV] fluids, improving cardiac output)

(2) Adjustment and avoidance of medications and nephrotoxic agents in intrarenal states

(3) Relief of urinary tract obstruction (ureteral stents, urethral catheter) in postrenal states

(4) Consideration of early intervention under the supervision of a nephrologist or intensivist for management of potential renal replacement therapy

b. Short-term dialysis should be implemented when serum creatinine exceeds 5 to 10 mg/dL. Other indications for dialysis include unresponsive acidosis, electrolyte disorders, fluid overload, or uremic complications.

B. Chronic kidney disease (CKD)

1. General characteristics

a. Definitions

(1) CKD is progression of ongoing loss of kidney function (GFR). CKD is classified into five stages based upon the estimated GFR. These stages have been developed by the National Kidney Foundation (NKF) to help provide an intervention plan for evaluation and management of each stage.

(a) Stage 1: Kidney damage with normal GFR greater than 90 mL/min/1.73 m^2 body surface area (BSA) and persistent albumiuria

(b) Stage 2: Kidney damage with mild decrease in GFR 60 to 89 mL/min/1.73 m^2 body surface area

(c) Stage 3: Moderate decrease in GFR 30 to 59 mL/min/1.73 m^2 BSA

(d) Stage 4: Severe decrease in GFR 15 to 29 mL/min/1.73 m^2 BSA

(e) Stage 5: Kidney failure with GFR less than 15 mL/min/1.73 m^2 BSA

(2) In stages 1 and 2, the patient is generally asymptomatic without an increase in BUN or serum creatinine; acid–base maintenance is adaptive through an increase in remaining nephron function.

(3) When the patient is in stage 3, he or she may still remain asymptomatic; however, serum creatinine and BUN increase. In addition, other hormones (parathyroid hormone [PTH], erythropoietin, calcitriol) become abnormal.

TABLE 6-2	Causes of Chronic Renal Failure

Diabetes mellitus

Hypertension

Glomerulonephritis

Polycystic kidney disease

Other causes

Primary glomerular diseases (membranous nephropathy, minimal change disease, IgA nephropathy)

Secondary glomerular diseases (sickle cell anemia, SLE)

Tubulointerstitial renal diseases (nephrotoxins, infection, multiple myeloma, HIV)

Chronic pyelonephritis (tuberculosis)

Vascular diseases (renal artery stenosis or obstruction)

Obstructive nephropathies (nephrolithiasis, prostate disease, neurogenic bladder)

SLE, systemic lupus erythematosus.

---

(4) In stage 4, the patient may become symptomatic with anemia, acidosis, hyperkalemia, hypocalcemia, and hyperphosphatemia. In stage 5, the patient is a candidate for renal replacement therapy.

b. Diabetes mellitus, hypertension, glomerulonephritis (GN), and polycystic kidney disease (PKD) are the most common causes (Table 6-2).

c. Patients with CKD generally progress to chronic renal failure.

(1) The rate of progression depends on the underlying cause, the effectiveness of treatments, and the individual patient.

(2) The 5-year survival rate for chronic renal failure is 35%.

2. Clinical features

a. Uremic symptoms may develop (stages 3 to 5) insidiously and include fatigue, malaise, anorexia, nausea, vomiting, metallic taste, hiccups, dyspnea, orthopnea, impaired mentation, insomnia, irritability, muscle cramps, restless legs, weakness, pruritus, easy bruising, and altered consciousness.

b. Signs include cachexia, weight loss, muscle wasting, pallor, hypertension, ecchymosis, sensory deficits, asterixis, and Kussmaul respirations.

3. Laboratory findings

a. Measurement of GFR is the gold standard. The Cockcroft–Gault formula (requires the patient age, body weight, and serum creatinine) or the Modification of Diet in Renal Disease (MDRD) equation (requires serum albumin, BUN as well as patient age, body weight, and serum creatinine) will give a fairly accurate prediction of GFR. The MDRD is probably more accurate. The MDRD also takes into account gender and ethnicity.

b. Proteinuria is a marker for kidney damage. Microalbuminuria appears early in the disease.

c. BUN and creatinine are elevated.

d. Hemoglobin and hematocrit, serum electrolytes, and urinalysis are abnormal.

4. Treatment is aimed at slowing the progression of CKD and treating reversible causes of acute deterioration.

a. Angiotensin-converting enzyme (ACE) inhibitors and angiotensin-receptor blockers (ARBs) slow the progression of renal dysfunction, particularly in proteinuric patients.

b. Managing comorbid conditions improves the outcome, including tight hypertensive control (BP >130/80), tight glycemic control in diabetic patients (HbA1C <7.5%), cholesterol-lowering therapy (goal low-density lipoprotein [LDL] <100 mg/dL), tobacco cessation, and weight control.

c. Erythropoietin, iron supplements, and antiplatelet therapy should be considered to maintain hemoglobin (11 to 12 g/dL) and bleeding time as needed.

d. Medical therapy requires careful drug dosing to adjust for decreased renal function.

e. Dietary management includes restriction of protein intake, adequate caloric intake, calcium and vitamin D supplements, and limitation of water, sodium, potassium, and phosphorus.

f. Need for hemodialysis, peritoneal dialysis, or kidney transplantation should be coordinated with nephrology service.

II. GLOMERULAR DISORDERS

A. Glomerulonephritis

1. General characteristics

   a. GN generally refers to damage of the renal glomeruli by deposition of inflammatory proteins in the glomerular membranes as the result of an immunologic response. The severity of disease is dictated by the degree of glomerular injury.

   b. About 60% of cases are in children 2 to 12 years of age.

   c. Prognosis is excellent in children and worse in adults, especially in those with preexisting renal disease.

2. Causes

   a. The major causes of GN are listed in Table 6-3.

   b. Causes are divided into focal GN, which is characterized by involvement of less than half the glomeruli, and diffuse GN, which affects most glomeruli.

3. Clinical features

   a. Hematuria is present; urine often is tea or cola colored.

   b. Oliguria or anuria is present.

   c. Edema of the face and eyes is present in the morning, and edema of the feet and ankles occurs in the afternoon and evening.

   d. Hypertension also is a common, but not an essential, clinical finding.

4. Laboratory findings

   a. Antistreptolysin O titer is increased in 60% to 80% of cases and should be considered if there is a possibility of a recent streptococcal infection. A common cause of GN is poststreptococcal infection (PSGN).

   b. Urinalysis reveals hematuria (>3 RBCs/HPF; also RBCs will often be misshapened [acanthocytes] due to their passage through the glomerulus as opposed to a normal-shaped RBC that could represent bleeding from the bladder or urethra), RBC casts, and proteinuria (1–2 g/24 hr).

   c. Serum complement (C3) levels are often decreased.

   d. Renal biopsy may be done to determine exact diagnosis or severity of disease.

5. Treatment

   a. Steroids and immunosuppressive drugs may be used to control the inflammatory response which is responsible for the damage. These are usually not needed in PSGN.

   b. Dietary management: Salt and fluid intake should be decreased.

   c. Dialysis should be performed if symptomatic azotemia is present.

   d. Medical therapy

      (1) ACE inhibitors are renoprotective (reduce urinary protein loss) in chronic GN.

      (2) Use medications as appropriate for hyperkalemia, pulmonary edema, peripheral edema, acidosis, and hypertension.

TABLE 6-3	Causes of Glomerulonephritis	
Type	**Children**	**Adults**
Focal	Benign hematuria	IgA nephropathy
	Henoch–Schönlein purpura	Hereditary nephritis
	Mild postinfectious GN	SLE
	IgA nephropathy	
	Hereditary nephritis	
Diffuse	Postinfectious GN	SLE
	Membranoproliferative GN	Membranoproliferative GN
		Rapidly progressive GN
		Postinfectious GN
		Vasculitis

GN, glomerulonephritis; SLE, systemic lupus erythematosus.

TABLE 6-4	Causes of Nephrotic Syndrome	
Primary Renal Disease		**Secondary Renal Disease**
Focal GN		Poststreptococcal GN
Focal glomerulosclerosis		SLE
IgA nephropathy		Malignancy
Membranoproliferative GN		Toxemia of pregnancy
Membranous glomerulopathy		Drugs and nephrotoxins
Mesangial proliferative GN		Lymphomas and leukemias
Minimal change disease		Diabetic glomerulosclerosis
Rapidly progressive GN		Amyloidosis
Congenital nephrotic syndrome		

GN, glomerulonephritis; SLE, systemic lupus erythematosus.

B. Nephrotic syndrome

  1. General characteristics

    a. Nephrotic syndrome is defined as excretion of more than 3.5 g of protein per $1.73\ m^2$ in 24 hours. It manifests with hypoalbuminemia, lipiduria, hypercholesterolemia, and edema. It can predispose to thrombosis secondary to loss of proteins S and C and antithrombin III.

    b. It can affect adults and children, depending on the underlying cause (Table 6-4).

    c. Prognosis depends on the specific cause and degree of renal damage. Complete remission is possible if the underlying disease is treatable.

  2. Clinical features

    a. Symptoms include malaise, abdominal distention, anorexia, facial edema/puffy eyelids, oliguria, scrotal swelling, shortness of breath, and weight gain.

    b. Signs include ascites, edema, hypertension, orthostatic hypotension, retinal sheen, and skin striae.

  3. Laboratory findings

    a. Urinalysis reveals proteinuria, lipiduria, glycosuria, hematuria, and foamy urine.

    b. Microscopic examination of the urine shows RBC casts, granular casts, hyaline casts, and fatty casts. Key finding in microscopic urinalysis is the oval fat body which is a renal tubular cell that has reabsorbed some of the excess lipids in the urine.

    c. Blood chemistry shows hypoalbuminemia, azotemia, and hyperlipidemia. Hyperlipidemia is secondary to the liver producing increased lipoproteins due to hypovolemia from the loss of intravascular volume (edema).

    d. C3 levels can be low or normal, depending on the cause.

  4. Treatment

    a. Medical therapy

      (1) ACE inhibitors should be used early in the course of the disease.

      (2) Judicious use of diuretics is recommended to reduce fluid accumulations.

    b. Dietary management

      (1) Sodium and fluid intake should be restricted.

      (2) Dietary protein and potassium intake can be normal but not excessive.

    c. Infections should be treated aggressively.

    d. Anticoagulants should be used if thromboses are present.

    e. Nephrotoxic drugs (e.g., nonsteroidal anti-inflammatory drugs (NSAIDs) aminoglycoside antibiotics) should be avoided.

    f. Some patients respond to steroid therapy.

    g. Frequent relapsers or steroid nonresponders may try cyclophosphamide or cyclosporine.

III. POLYCYSTIC KIDNEY DISEASE (PKD)

A. General characteristics

1. PKD is characterized by growth of numerous cysts in the kidneys. The cysts are made of epithelial cells from the renal tubules and collecting system. The cysts replace the mass of the kidneys, reducing function and leading to kidney failure.

2. Autosomal dominant PKD (ADPKD) is the most common form and almost always is bilateral. Symptoms typically develop during the fourth decade of life.

3. The less common autosomal recessive PKD (ARPKD) begins in utero and can lead to fetal and neonatal death. Surviving infants have significantly reduced life expectancy usually due to renal and hepatic failure.

4. An acquired form of cystic kidney disease (ACKD) occurs in individuals with long-term or end-stage renal disease (ESRD). It is more common in African American men than in other ethnicities.

B. Clinical features

1. The most common symptoms of ADPKD are back and flank pain (secondary to the massive enlargement of the kidneys and/or liver) and headaches (greater risk of intracranial aneurysms).

2. Hematuria, hypertension, recurrent urinary tract infection, weight loss, renal colic, as well as nausea and vomiting also may be present.

3. One or both kidneys may be palpable and feel nodular or tender. Cysts also may be present on the liver, pancreas, and other locations.

C. Laboratory findings

1. Anemia may be noted on complete blood count (CBC).

2. Urinalysis shows proteinuria, hematuria, and, commonly, pyuria and bacteriuria.

3. Imaging studies

   a. The diagnostic method of choice is ultrasonography which shows fluid-filled cysts.

   b. Plain-film radiography of the abdomen shows enlarged kidneys.

   c. Excretory infusion urography reveals multiple lucencies.

   d. Angiography shows bending of small vessels around cysts.

   e. Computed tomography (CT) shows large renal size and multiple thin-walled cysts.

D. Treatment

1. There is no cure for ADPKD; treatment is supportive to ease symptoms and prolong life.

2. General measures should include management of pain (secondary to cyst hemorrhage), control of hypertension (goal of <130/80 mm Hg through use of an ACE inhibitor or ARB), high intake of fluids, and a low-protein diet.

3. Infections should be treated vigorously with antibiotics (trimethoprim–sulfamethoxazole, fluoroquinolones, chloramphenicol, or vancomycin) that can penetrate the cyst wall.

4. Dialysis or transplantation should be considered when renal insufficiency becomes life threatening. Transplantation has been successful, and non-PKD kidneys do not develop cysts.

IV. NEPHROLITHIASIS

A. General characteristics

1. Nephrolithiasis (renal calculi) occur throughout the urinary tract and are common causes of pain, infection, and obstruction.

2. Stones

   a. They are caused by increased saturation (supersaturation) of urine with stone-forming salts (calcium, oxalate, and other solutes) or a possible lack of inhibitors (citrate) in the urine to prevent crystal formation. If either situation happens, then precipitation occurs and crystalluria develops.

   b. They typically are formed in the proximal tract and pass distally.

   c. They lodge at the ureteropelvic junction (UPJ; kidney stones), the ureterovesicular junction (UVJ; bladder stones), or the ureter at the level of the iliac vessels.

3. Nephrolithiasis commonly occurs during the third to fourth decade of life. The disease is two- to threefold more common in males than in females.

4. Four major types of stones exist.

   a. Calcium: 75% to 85% of stones are formations of calcium crystals; these stones are radiopaque.

b. Uric acid: 5% to 8% of stones are formed by precipitation of uric acid; these stones are radiolucent. These stones form in individuals with persistently acid urine with or without hyperuricemia.

c. Cystine: Less than 1% of stones are caused by an impairment of cystine transport; these stones are radiolucent. They occur only in autosomal recessive cystinuria.

d. Struvite: 10% to 15% of stones are formed by the combination of calcium, ammonium, and magnesium and are radiopaque. Formation is increased by urinary tract infections with urease-producing bacterium; therefore, this type is common in patients with abnormal urinary tract anatomy and urinary diversions and in those who require frequent catheterization.

5. Patients usually have complete return to health, but recurrences can occur. Frequency of recurrence has been up to 30% to 50% in 5 years.

B. Clinical features

1. Nephrolithiasis generally is asymptomatic until inflammation or complete or partial ureteral obstruction develops.

2. Clinical features of nephrolithiasis include unilateral back pain and renal colic that waxes and wanes.

3. Symptoms include hematuria, dysuria, urinary frequency, fever, chills, nausea, and vomiting.

4. Location can determine direction of pain and its radiation.

a. A stone in the upper ureter: The pain tends to radiate to the anterior abdomen.

b. A stone in the lower part of the ureter: The pain tends to radiate to the ipsilateral groin, testicle in men, or labia in women.

c. A stone lodged in the UVJ: Urinary frequency and urgency are noted as well as lower pelvic pain.

d. As the stone passes through the ureter it may mimic other acute conditions, for example, acute cholecystitis, acute appendicitis, acute cystitis, and diverticulitis.

5. Signs include diaphoresis, tachycardia, tachypnea, restlessness, costovertebral angle tenderness, and abdominal distention because of ileus.

C. Laboratory findings

1. Serum chemistries are usually normal; however, there may be a leukocytosis from infection or stress.

a. Urinalysis usually reveals microscopic or gross hematuria and may show leukocytes and/or crystals.

b. Urine culture should be performed to rule out infection.

2. Imaging modality of choice is the helical (spiral) CT. This does not require the use of radiocontrast and can detect stones as small as 1 mm.

3. Plain-film radiography of the abdomen can identify radiopaque stones; unfortunately, it may miss a small stone even if radiopaque.

4. Renal ultrasonography can only identify stones in the kidney, proximal ureter, or the UVJ.

5. An intravenous pyelogram (IVP) is rarely indicated in the treatment and evaluation of a patient with nephrolithiasis. If an IVP is considered, remember to make sure that the patient has normal renal function.

D. Treatment: All stones should undergo chemical analysis, as the type of stone may dictate additional treatment.

1. Stones measuring less than 5 mm

a. Many are likely to pass spontaneously and, in an otherwise healthy individual, may be managed on an outpatient basis.

b. The patient should drink plenty of fluids.

c. Strain urine to catch the stone and save it for analysis.

d. Use an adequate supply of analgesics.

e. An alpha blocker or calcium channel blocker may facilitate passage.

f. Follow up weekly or biweekly to monitor progress. Most stones that pass do so within 2 to 4 weeks of onset of symptoms.

2. Stones measuring 5 to 10 mm

a. These are less likely to pass spontaneously; patients should be considered for early elective intervention if no other complicating factors (e.g., infection, high-grade obstruction, solitary kidney, anatomic abnormality preventing passage, and intractable pain) are present.

b. Increased fluids and analgesics are needed.

c. Elective lithotripsy or ureteroscopy with stone basket extraction may be used.

3. Stones measuring greater than 10 mm

a. These are not likely to pass spontaneously; these patients are more likely to have complications.

b. The patient should be treated on an inpatient basis if he or she is unable to maintain adequate oral intake.

    c. Vigorous hydration should be maintained.

    d. Ureteral stent or percutaneous nephrostomy (gold standard) should be used if renal function is jeopardized.

    e. Urgent treatment with extracorporeal shock wave lithotripsy can be used for renal stones of less than 2 cm or for ureteral stones of less than 1 cm; ureteroscopic fragmentation also may be used. Percutaneous nephrolithotomy can be used for stones of greater than 2 cm.

  4. Analgesics should be administered, including morphine, meperidine, or ketorolac. Depending on stone makeup: antibiotics if signs of infection are present; hydrochlorothiazide to decrease urine calcium excretion; allopurinol to decrease urine uric acid excretion; and alkali to increase urine citrate excretion.

V. DISORDERS OF SALT AND WATER

  A. Hyper- and hyponatremia reflect disturbances in water homeostasis. Serum sodium accurately reflects changes in serum osmolality and, therefore, changes in free water balance.

  B. Disorders of water deficiency: hypernatremia

    1. General characteristics

      a. In hypernatremia, the water content of body fluid is deficient in relation to sodium content (serum sodium >145 mEq/L). There is either too much salt or not enough water.

      b. Hypernatremia generally results from either inadequate fluid intake or excess water loss. Causes include deficit of thirst, hypotonic fluid loss, urinary loss, gastrointestinal (GI) loss, insensible loss, burns, diuretic therapy, osmotic diuresis (hyperglycemia, mannitol administration), sodium excess, and diabetes insipidus (DI).

      c. It occurs commonly in the elderly and may occur in infants with diarrhea.

    2. Clinical features

      a. Neurologic manifestations result from alterations in the brain water content and include thirst, restlessness, irritability, disorientation, lethargy, delirium, convulsions, and coma. Brain cell shrinkage may be substantial and can cause damage to the supporting vasculature.

      b. Other findings include dry mouth and dry mucous membranes, lack of tears and decreased salivation, flushed skin, tachycardia, hypotension, fever, oliguria and anuria, hyperventilation, lethargy, and hyperreflexia.

    3. Laboratory findings

      a. By definition, plasma sodium will be greater than 145 mEq/L. Urine sodium is decreased if due to extrarenal losses and is elevated if due to renal losses or sodium excess. Urine is concentrated with extrarenal losses and diluted with DI.

      b. DI

        (1) Low urine sodium and polyuria usually indicate DI.

        (2) Antidiuretic stimulation does not increase urine osmolality in nephrogenic DI (see V.D, Diabetes insipidus).

      c. Hyperosmolar coma may be indicated by elevated serum glucose, decreased urine output, and increased urine osmolality.

    4. Treatment

      a. Hypernatremia should be treated on an inpatient basis.

      b. Identify the underlying cause and treat accordingly.

      c. Free water may be administered orally, which is the preferred route, or IV, as a 5% dextrose solution.

      d. Hypovolemia should be treated first (with isotonic saline) and the hypernatremia second.

      e. Dialysis should be implemented if sodium is greater than 200 mEq/L.

      f. Use caution during treatment because rapid correction of hypernatremia can cause pulmonary or cerebral edema, especially in patients with diabetes mellitus.

  C. Disorders of water excess: hyponatremia

    1. General characteristics

      a. Hyponatremia is defined as a plasma sodium concentration of less than 135 mEq/L. Signs and symptoms may not occur until the concentration falls below 125 mEq/L.

      b. Hyponatremia is the most common electrolyte disorder seen in the general hospital population secondary to the use of hypotonic fluid administration.

      c. Type is determined by the serum osmolality and volume status.

        (1) Hyponatremia with hypervolemia occurs in the setting of congestive heart failure, nephrotic syndrome, renal failure, and hepatic cirrhosis.

(2) Hyponatremia with euvolemia occurs with hypothyroidism, glucocorticoid excess, and syndrome of inappropriate antidiuretic hormone (SIADH) release.

(3) SIADH is defined as hypotonic hyponatremia; urine osmolality of greater than 100 mOsm/kg; normal cardiac, hepatic, thyroid, adrenal, and renal function; and absence of extracellular fluid volume deficit. Urine sodium is usually greater than 40 mEq/L.

(4) Hyponatremia with hypovolemia occurs with renal or nonrenal sodium loss.

(5) Table 6-5 provides an approach to the causes of hyponatremia.

2. Clinical features

a. Symptoms correlate to the sodium concentration and may include lethargy, disorientation, muscle cramps, anorexia, hiccups, nausea, vomiting, and seizures.

b. Signs include weakness, agitation, hyporeflexia, orthostatic hypotension, Cheyne–Stokes respirations, delirium, coma, or stupor.

3. Laboratory findings

a. Serum sodium of less than 135 mEq/L.

b. Plasma osmolality usually is decreased, except in cases of fluid redistribution due to hyperglycemia or proteinemia.

c. Urine sodium is increased or decreased, depending on the cause (Table 6-5).

d. If SIADH is suspected, CT may be done to rule out a central nervous system (CNS) disorder, and chest radiography may be done to rule out lung pathology.

4. Treatment

a. Treat hypovolemia on an inpatient basis, especially if symptomatic or if serum sodium is less than 125 mEq/L. Also consider consultation with nephrology and/or endocrinology.

b. Treat the underlying cause, which usually requires fluid restriction except in hypovolemic hyponatremia where isotonic saline is the treatment.

c. Monitor volume status.

TABLE 6-5	Differential Diagnosis of Hyponatremia

1. Is the plasma osmolality between 280 and 295 mOsm/kg?

   If yes, think isotonic hyponatremia (paraproteinemia, hypertriglyceridemia).

2. Is the plasma osmolality >295 mOsm/kg?

   If yes, think hypertonic hyponatremia (hyperglycemia).

3. Is the plasma osmolality <280 mOsm/kg?

   If yes, think hypotonic hyponatremia and measure the urine osmolality.

4. Is the urine osmolality <100 mOsm/kg?

   If yes, think excessive water intake (primary polydipsia).

5. Is the urine osmolality >100 mOsm/kg?

   If yes, think impaired renal diluting ability and assess the ECFV.

6. Does the ECFV appear normal?

   If yes, think endocrinopathies (hypothyroidism, glucocorticoid insufficiency), SIADH (drugs, tumors, CNS disorders, nausea, pain, stress), a reset osmostat, potassium depletion, or thiazide diuretics.

7. Is the ECFV decreased and the urine sodium increased (>20 mEq/L)?

   If yes, think renal solute loss (diuretics, osmotic diuresis, Addison's disease).

8. Is the ECFV decreased and the urine sodium decreased (<10 mEq/L)?

   If yes, think extrarenal sodium loss.

9. Is the ECFV increased and the urine sodium increased?

   If yes, think renal failure.

10. Is the ECFV increased and the urine sodium decreased?

    If yes, think edematous disorders (CHF, cirrhosis, nephrotic syndrome).

ECFV, extracellular fluid volume; SIADH, syndrome of inappropriate antidiuretic hormone; CNS, central nervous system; CHF, congestive heart failure.

    d. In severe symptomatic hyponatremia with sodium of less than 120 mEq/L, hypertonic saline may be used very cautiously.

      (1) Overly rapid correction can cause central pontine myelinolysis, resulting in neurologic damage.

      (2) Serum sodium levels should be checked hourly and neurologic status closely monitored.

    e. In chronic hyponatremia unresponsive to fluid restriction, demeclocycline may be used to induce nephrogenic DI but may cause nephrotoxicity in patients with cirrhosis. Vasopressin antagonists (conivaptan) may be considered in euvolemic or hypervolemic hyponatremia.

D. Diabetes insipidus

  1. General characteristics

    a. DI is a disorder of water.

    b. Neurogenic (or central) DI is caused by deficient secretion of arginine vasopressin (antidiuretic hormone, ADH) from the posterior pituitary.

    c. Nephrogenic DI is caused by kidneys that are unresponsive to normal vasopressin levels.

    d. Nephrogenic DI may be an inherited X-linked trait or acquired as a result of lithium therapy, hypokalemia, hypercalcemia, or renal disease.

  2. Clinical features

    a. Physical findings are associated with the primary cause.

    b. Polyuria (up to 12 L/day), nocturia, and polydipsia are the main symptoms.

  3. Laboratory findings

    a. Neurogenic (central) and nephrogenic DI can be distinguished by water deprivation and desmopressin (deamino-8-D-arginine vasopressin) testing. If the test results in reduced urine output, central DI is diagnosed.

    b. Urine osmolality of less than 250 mOsm/kg, despite hypernatremia, indicates DI.

  4. Treatment

    a. Neurogenic or central DI is best treated with parenteral or intranasal desmopressin.

    b. Diuretics, chlorpropamide, or carbamazepine can be used in patients with mild disease.

    c. Nephrogenic diabetes can be treated with hydrochlorothiazide or amiloride diuretics or indomethacin.

    d. Dietary measures, such as limiting salt and protein intake, can be helpful.

E. Volume depletion

  1. General characteristics

    a. Volume depletion occurs when body fluids are lost from the extracellular compartment at a rate that exceeds intake.

    b. Fluid can be lost from the GI tract, kidneys, or skin or from "third spacing" in the abdomen (i.e., ascites) or injured tissues (i.e., burns).

  2. Clinical features

    a. Volume-depleted patients become thirsty, and urinary output decreases.

    b. Mild volume depletion can cause increased heart rate, fatigue, and muscle cramps.

    c. Moderate fluid loss causes dizziness and hypotension when standing.

    d. Severe hypovolemia results in general hypotension, signs of ischemia and shock, as well as lethargy and confusion.

    e. Decreased skin turgor and dry mucous membranes are unreliable signs of hypovolemia in older adults.

  3. Laboratory testing

    a. Hematocrit and serum albumin may be increased.

    b. Urinary sodium decreases.

    c. Urea increases (secondary to urine stasis in the nephron), but there is little change in serum creatinine.

  4. Treatment

    a. Mild hypovolemia can be treated by increasing salt and water intake.

    b. Severe volume depletion can be treated with oral fluids containing electrolytes, glucose, and amino acids.

    c. IV fluids should be used when patients cannot tolerate oral solutions. Isotonic fluids should be given until tissue perfusion has improved.

VI. ELECTROLYTE DISORDERS

A. Disorders of potassium

1. Hyperkalemia

   a. General characteristics

      (1) Hyperkalemia refers to an elevated serum potassium level.

      (2) It may result from cellular redistribution from intracellular to extracellular compartment, potassium retention, impaired potassium excretion, or elevations caused by increased tissue breakdown. Hemolysis or thrombocytosis may cause spurious hyperkalemia.

      (3) It most commonly is associated with renal failure, ACE inhibitors, hyporeninemic hypoaldosteronism, cell death, and metabolic acidosis.

   b. Clinical features

      (1) Severe hyperkalemia can result in dysrhythmias and cardiac arrest.

      (2) Neurologic symptoms include numbness, tingling, weakness, and flaccid paralysis.

   c. Laboratory findings

      (1) Serum potassium level is greater than 5.0 mEq/L; serum creatinine and BUN should be measured to assess renal function. Urine potassium, creatinine, and osmolality can reveal decreased fractional excretion of potassium.

      (2) Electrocardiography (ECG) changes evolve as potassium rises to greater than 6 mEq/L.

         (a) Earliest ECG manifestation is peaking of the T waves (>6.5 mEq/L).

         (b) Flattening of the P wave, prolongation of the PR interval, and widening of the QRS complex are seen with more severe hyperkalemia (>7.0 mEq/L).

         (c) A final event is a sine-wave pattern with cardiac arrest (8.0 to 10.0 mEq/L).

   d. Treatment

      (1) Potentially life-threatening hyperkalemia should be treated first, and then the underlying cause discovered. Review the clinical situation, determine the acid–base status, and consider drug-induced conditions.

      (2) Potassium-sparing drugs and dietary potassium supplements should be discontinued. A low potassium diet is recommended.

      (3) In severe hyperkalemia with ECG changes, calcium gluconate should be given IV to antagonize the effects of hyperkalemia on the heart. Strict monitoring is required.

      (4) Sodium bicarbonate, glucose (D_{50}), and insulin may be administered to drive potassium back into the intracellular compartment. The onset of action is rapid but the duration short; therefore, serial potassium levels should be followed until correction is complete.

      (5) Sodium polystyrene sulfonate (Kayexalate), a cation-exchange resin, is used to remove potassium from the body when levels are extremely high. Hemodialysis may be required if above therapies fail.

2. Hypokalemia

   a. General considerations

      (1) Hypokalemia is defined as a decreased serum potassium level (<3.5 mEq/L).

      (2) It can result from a shift of potassium into the intracellular compartment or from potassium losses of extrarenal or renal origin.

      (3) It most commonly occurs with use of diuretics, renal tubular acidosis, or GI losses.

   b. Clinical features

      (1) Cardiovascular manifestations are the most important, resulting in ventricular arrhythmias, hypotension, and cardiac arrest.

      (2) Neuromuscular manifestations also occur, including malaise, skeletal muscle weakness, cramps, and smooth muscle involvement, leading to ileus and constipation.

      (3) Other manifestations include polyuria, nocturia, hyperglycemia and rhabdomyolysis.

   c. Laboratory findings

      (1) Serum potassium is less than 3.5 mEq/L.

      (2) ECG may reveal flattened or inverted T waves, increased prominence of U waves, depression of the ST segment, and ventricular ectopy.

      (3) The most helpful tests for causal workup include blood acid–base parameters, and urinary potassium and chloride levels.

d. Treatment

(1) Hypokalemia usually is not an emergency unless cardiac manifestations are present. In nonemergent conditions, oral potassium therapy is preferred, usually with potassium chloride.

(2) For emergent situations (serum potassium < 2.5 mEq/L or arrhythmias), IV replacement is indicated.

(3) Hypokalemia potentiates the effects of cardiac glycosides on myocardial conduction and may lead to digitalis intoxication. More aggressive potassium replacement may be required in this situation.

B. Disorders of calcium and phosphorus

1. General considerations

a. Mechanisms for calcium and phosphorus homeostasis are complex and carefully maintained by several interrelated and interdependent mechanisms. These involve vitamin D, the small intestine, renal tubules, PTH, and bone.

b. Increased PTH levels result in increased serum calcium and decreased phosphorus. Conversely, decreased levels of PTH result in decreased serum calcium and increased phosphorus.

c. Parathyroid disorders, chronic renal failure, and malignancy are the most common causes of disorders of calcium and phosphorus.

2. Hypercalcemia

a. General characteristics

(1) Hypercalcemia is a significant elevation in serum calcium after adjustment for albumin level (see below).

(2) This is one of the most common disorders of calcium and phosphorus, especially in hospitalized patients with malignancy (e.g., lung cancer; squamous cell carcinoma of the head, neck, esophagus; female genital tract carcinoma; multiple myeloma; lymphoma; renal cell carcinoma [RCC]).

(3) Other causes include vitamin D intoxication, hyperparathyroidism, and sarcoidosis.

b. Clinical features: Severity of symptoms depends on calcium level. Most patients are asymptomatic until serum calcium is greater than 12 mg/dl. Symptoms will also differ by the rapidity of onset of hypercalcemia, state of hydration, and underlying malignancy, if any.

(1) Symptoms include anorexia, nausea, constipation, polyuria, polydipsia, dehydration, and change in level of consciousness (lethargy, stupor, and coma).

(2) Signs of intravascular volume depletion (e.g., orthostatic hypotension and tachycardia) are frequent.

c. Laboratory studies

(1) Serum calcium is high.

(a) The calcium level must be corrected for albumin levels.

(b) Corrected calcium = measured total calcium + [0.8 × (4 − albumin)].

(2) Chest radiography may reveal an underlying pulmonary mass.

(3) Perform urinalysis for hematuria, an early sign of RCC.

(4) Erythrocyte sedimentation rate may be elevated in monoclonal gammopathy. Protein electrophoresis of serum or urine may be needed to confirm the diagnosis.

(5) A 24-hour urine collection must be done for calcium determination.

(a) An elevated urine calcium suggests malignant neoplastic or paraneoplastic process or hyperparathyroidism.

(b) A decreased urine calcium suggests primary hyperparathyroidism.

(6) Serum vitamin D levels. Elevations are consistent with vitamin D toxicity.

d. Treatment

(1) Isotonic saline should be used for volume repletion. Loop diuretics should be used if the patient is hypervolemic after volume repletion.

(2) Manage the underlying cause.

3. Hypocalcemia

a. General characteristics

(1) Hypocalcemia is more common than hypercalcemia, and it can be found in a significant number of critically ill patients.

(2) It commonly results from chronic disease (most common cause is CKD) or hypoparathyroidism. Although it typically presents in a mild, asymptomatic form, severe hypocalcemia can result in complete cardiovascular collapse.

  b. Clinical features

   (1) Symptoms include dry skin, brittle nails, pruritis, muscle cramping, shortness of breath, and numbness and tingling in the extremities. Severe cardiovascular manifestations include syncope and angina.

   (2) Signs include psoriasis, dry skin, and perioral numbness. Cardiovascular signs include wheezing, bradycardia, crackles, and a third heart sound.

   (3) Classic neurologic findings include the Trousseau's sign (carpal tunnel spasm after BP cuff applied for 3 minutes) and the Chvostek's sign (spasm of facial muscle after tapping facial nerve in front of ear). Other neurologic manifestations include irritability, confusion, dementia, and seizures.

  c. Laboratory studies

   (1) Hypocalcemia is defined as a corrected serum calcium level of less than 8.5 mEq/L.

   (2) Ionized calcium also should be measured. Magnesium, phosphate, albumin, liver function tests, and other electrolytes should be obtained.

   (3) BUN and creatinine should be measured to assess renal function.

  d. Treatment

   (1) Treat any emergent cardiovascular states.

   (2) Severe hypocalcemia should be replaced (intravenous calcium gluconate or calcium chloride).

   (3) Mild hypocalcemia can be treated on an outpatient basis with oral calcium and vitamin D supplements.

 4. Hyperphosphatemia and hypophosphatemia

  a. General characteristics

   (1) Hyperphosphatemia is most commonly secondary to CKD, while hypophosphatemia is secondary to diminished supply or absorption, or increased urinary losses or redistribution.

   (2) Hypophosphatemia can be classified by the serum level. Moderate is a serum level of 1.0 to 2.5 mg/dL and is usually asymptomatic. Severe is a serum level of 1 mg/dL or less.

   (3) Severe hypophosphatemia may lead to rhabdomyolyis, paresthesia, and encephalopathy.

  b. Treatment

   (1) Hyperphosphatemia secondary to CKD should be treated with dietary phosphorus restriction and oral phosphate binders. Calcium carbonate tablets may also help to reduce phosphate absorption 0.5 to 1.5 g three times daily with meals (500 mg tablets).

   (2) Hypophophatemia of chronic origin can be treated with oral phosphate repletion.

C. Disorders of magnesium

 1. Hypermagnesemia

  a. General characteristics

   (1) Hypermagnesemia is defined as plasma magnesium levels of greater than 2.5 mEq/L.

   (2) Most magnesium is stored in bone and muscle.

  b. Clinical features

   (1) Symptomatic hypermagnesemia rarely occurs, except in patients with CKD who are given magnesium-containing products, such as laxatives or antacids.

   (2) Hypermagnesemia can be iatrogenically induced as part of treatment in eclampsia or preterm labor.

   (3) Signs and symptoms reflect impaired neuromuscular transmission.

    (a) Initially, deep tendon reflexes are reduced.

    (b) Muscle weakness, hypotension, respiratory depression, and then cardiac arrest can follow with increasing magnesium levels.

    (c) Nausea, vomiting, and flushing also can occur.

  c. Laboratory tests

   (1) ECG shows widened QRS complex, prolonged PR interval, and prolonged Q-T interval.

   (2) Bleeding and clotting times are increased.

  d. Treatment

   (1) Administer 10 to 20 mL of 10% calcium gluconate IV over 10 minutes.

   (2) Saline diuresis and IV furosemide may increase excretion of magnesium.

   (3) Dialysis is effective in severe hypermagnesemia.

2. Hypomagnesemia

a. General characteristics

(1) Hypomagnesemia is defined as plasma magnesium levels of less than 1.5 mEq/L. Plasma levels do not reflect total body stores.

(2) Hypomagnesemia usually presents when total body stores are severely depleted. Depletion usually results from diminished intake and impaired absorption.

(3) It is most commonly associated with chronic alcoholism, chronic diarrhea, hypoparathyroidism, hyperaldosteronism, diuretic therapy, osmotic diuresis, and nutritional deficiencies (e.g., prolonged parenteral feeding, malnutrition).

b. Clinical features: Signs and symptoms include lethargy, anorexia, nausea and vomiting, weakness, tetany, and seizures.

c. Laboratory tests

(1) Hypokalemia, hypocalcemia and hypocalciuria commonly are associated with causes of magnesium depletion.

(2) ECG may show prolonged PR and QT intervals or widening of the QRS.

d. Treatment

(1) Administer oral magnesium oxide for chronic hypomagnesemia. Administer twice the estimated deficit over several days.

(2) In severe symptomatic hypomagnesemia, a magnesium sulfate solution (1 to 2 g) can be administered IV followed by an infusion of 6 g of magnesium sulfate over 1 L of fluids in 24 hours to replete magnesium stores. This may be repeated for up to 7 days.

(3) Magnesium sulfate may also be given intramuscularly (IM) in four divided doses (200 to 800 mg/day).

(4) Serum levels should be monitored for the development of hypermagnesemia.

VII. ACID–BASE DISORDERS

A. General characteristics

1. Disturbances in the acid–base equilibrium are common, especially in patients who are critically ill.

2. They may be respiratory (characterized by alterations in carbon dioxide [CO_2]) or metabolic (characterized by alterations in serum bicarbonate [HCO_3]). Table 6-6 summarizes the relationships.

3. pH

a. The pH usually is considered to be "normal" between 7.38 and 7.42; however, for mixed acid–base problems, a pH of 7.40 should be considered as the absolute normal. When dealing with mixed acid–base disorders, variations from a pH of 7.40 in either direction will indicate whether there is an underlying acidosis or alkalosis present.

b. A pH of less than 7.35 represents acidemia.

c. A pH of greater than 7.45 represents alkalemia.

d. A pH of 7.2 or lower represents severe acidemia.

e. A pH of 7.6 or greater represents severe alkalemia.

4. Compensation for changes in the hydrogen ion concentration (pH) will always occur in the buffering system, the lungs or kidneys. The degree of compensation depends on the duration of the disturbance and the functioning of the organ.

TABLE 6-6	Acid–Base Disorders		
Disorder	**pH**	**Carbon Dioxide (Pco₂)**	**Bicarbonate (HCO₃)**
Respiratory acidosis	Decreased (↓)	Increased (↑)[a]	Increased (↑)
Respiratory alkalosis	Increased (↑)	Decreased (↓)[a]	Decreased (↓)
Metabolic acidosis	Decreased (↓)	Decreased (↓)	Decreased (↓)[a]
Metabolic alkalosis	Increased (↑)	Increased (↑)	Increased (↑)

B. Respiratory acidosis

1. General characteristics

  a. Respiratory acidosis is defined as a primary increase in the partial pressure of CO_2 (PCO_2) in the blood (hypercapnia) and decreased blood pH. The normal compensatory response is a gradual slow increase in plasma bicarbonate by the kidneys.

  b. Respiratory acidosis results from the failure of the lung to excrete CO_2 that is generated through normal metabolism. It can be a result of alveolar hypoventilation leading to pulmonary CO_2 retention or of overproduction of CO_2 or a combination of both.

  c. The primary cause of respiratory acidosis includes all disorders that reduce pulmonary function and CO_2 clearance, such as primary pulmonary disease, neuromuscular disease (myasthenia gravis), primary CNS dysfunction (severe brain stem injury), and drug-induced hypoventilation. Other causes of respiratory acidosis include higher-than-normal carbohydrate loads and parenteral nutrition in critically ill patients.

2. Clinical features

  a. Metabolic encephalopathy, also known as hypercapnic encephalopathy, with headache and drowsiness is the most characteristic change. It should be remembered that with an ensuing hypercapnia a resultant hypoxemia also ensues. It is difficult to determine if the symptoms are a result of the hypercapnia or the hypoxemia.

  b. If not corrected, initial CNS symptoms may progress to stupor and coma.

3. Laboratory findings (the pH is decreased and the PCO_2 is increased)

  a. Acute CO_2 retention leads to an increase in blood PCO_2 with a minimal change in plasma bicarbonate content. Serum electrolyte levels are close to normal.

  b. After 2 to 5 days, renal compensation occurs, leading to increased hydrogen ion secretion and bicarbonate production in the distal nephron, after which the plasma bicarbonate level steadily increases.

4. Treatment

  a. The underlying disorder must be identified and corrected.

  b. A blood PCO_2 of greater than 60 mm Hg may indicate the need for assisted ventilation if CNS or pulmonary muscular depression is severe.

C. Respiratory alkalosis

1. General characteristics

  a. Respiratory alkalosis is defined primarily by decreased blood PCO_2 (hypocapnia) and increased blood pH.

  b. Respiratory alkalosis is the result of excessive elimination of CO_2 from increased ventilatory drive. The response of the kidneys is to gradually eliminate plasma bicarbonate.

  c. The causes of respiratory alkalosis include any disorders associated with inappropriately increased ventilatory rate and CO_2 clearance.

  d. Anxiety (hysterical hyperventilation) is the most common cause of respiratory alkalosis. Other causes include salicylate intoxication, hypoxia, intrathoracic disorders, primary CNS dysfunction, Gram-negative septicemia, liver insufficiency, and pregnancy. Respiratory alkalosis may also result from inappropriate ventilatory settings on a mechanical ventilator.

2. Clinical features

  a. Obvious hyperventilation usually is present, particularly when alkalosis is caused by cerebral or metabolic disorders.

  b. The breathing pattern in the anxiety-induced syndrome varies from frequent, deep, sighing respirations to sustained and obvious rapid, deep breathing.

  c. Acute alkalemia may produce a tetany-like syndrome, which may be indistinguishable from acute hypocalcemia. Paresthesia of the extremities, chest discomfort, light-headedness, and confusion may be present.

  d. Circumoral paresthesias, acroparesthesias (painful burning of hands and feet), giddiness, or light-headedness may occur.

3. Laboratory findings (pH is increased and the PCO_2 is decreased)

  a. In acute alkalosis, increased respiratory rate leads to a loss of CO_2 via the lungs, which in turn increases the blood pH.

  b. Within hours after an acute decrease in arterial PCO_2, hydrogen ion secretion in the distal nephron decreases, leading to a decrease in plasma bicarbonate. Serum chloride level becomes elevated to maintain electroneutrality.

4. Treatment

    a. The primary goal of therapy is to correct the underlying disorder. Rebreathing techniques such as breathing into a paper bag will quickly increase CO_2.

    b. Use of CO_2-enriched breathing mixtures or controlled ventilation may be required in cases of severe respiratory alkalosis (pH 7.6).

D. Metabolic acidosis

  1. General characteristics

    a. Metabolic acidosis is an elevation in the normal serum concentration of hydrogen ions (nonvolatile acids) that is initiated either by the loss of bicarbonate from or by the addition of hydrogen ions to the serum. Respiratory response is immediate with a compensatory increase in respiration.

    b. Several conditions may result in increased hydrogen ions in the serum.

      (1) These include lactic acidosis, diabetic ketoacidosis, starvation ketosis, and ethylene glycol, methanol, and salicylate intoxication; these conditions result in an increased anion gap (AG).

      (2) Hydrogen ions also may be retained in renal tubular acidosis, renal insufficiency, and adrenal insufficiency.

    c. Conditions that may result in the loss of bicarbonate include diarrhea, pancreatic or biliary drainage, and ureteral diversion; these conditions typically have a normal AG.

  2. Clinical features

    a. Hyperventilation is the earliest and most recognized sign, resulting from stimulation of the respiratory drive to blow off CO_2 (pulmonary compensation). Using Winter's formula ($P_{CO_2} = [1.5 \times \{HCO_3^-\}] + 8 \pm 2$) allows for calculation of the expected P_{CO_2} compensation in metabolic acidosis.

    b. Ventricular arrhythmias may occur.

    c. Neurologic symptoms range from lethargy to frank coma.

  3. Laboratory studies (bicarbonate follows the pH in metabolic acid–base disorders; in acidosis the pH and bicarbonate both go down)

    a. Complete evaluation of a suspected acid–base disorder should include electrolytes, arterial blood gases, and serum albumin.

    b. Arterial blood gas measurements reveal a pH less than 7.38, decreased plasma bicarbonate, and decreased P_{CO_2} (compensation).

    c. The AG should be calculated ($Na^+ - (HCO_3^- + Cl^-)$) to separate metabolic acidosis with an elevated AG from metabolic acidosis with a normal AG. The normal AG is 8 ± 4 mEq/L.

      (1) A normal AG acidosis can also be called hyperchloremic metabolic acidosis (chloride increases as bicarbonate decreases to maintain electroneutrality). Normal AG renal tubular acidosis can be divided into cases of the kidney failing to reabsorb bicarbonate or secrete acid.

      (2) When calculating the AG it must be remembered that the negative charge of albumin can have an impact on the overall AG. If hypoalbuminemia is present, for each 1.0 g/dL decrease in serum albumin the AG should be increased by 2.5 mEq/L.

      (3) Elevated AG acidosis can be broken down into four categories: lactic acidosis, ketoacidosis, toxins/drugs, and kidney failure.

  4. Treatment

    a. Identify and, if possible, remove the primary cause of the metabolic acidosis.

    b. Insulin therapy and volume repletion are the mainstays of therapy for diabetic ketoacidosis.

    c. Bicarbonate therapy can be considered if the pH is less than 7.20. Blood pH should be carefully monitored, because ongoing acid production may increase bicarbonate requirements.

E. Metabolic alkalosis

  1. General characteristics

    a. Metabolic alkalosis is defined as an increase in serum bicarbonate with no change in P_{CO_2}, causing an increase in extracellular pH to greater than 7.42. Generally, the kidney fails to excrete the excess HCO_3^-, thereby maintaining the alkalosis. The following formula allows calculation of expected CO_2 compensation:

      Expected $P_{CO_2} = (0.7 \times HCO_3) + 20 \pm 2$.

    b. Metabolic alkalosis and increased serum bicarbonate can be caused by loss of hydrogen (vomiting), addition of bicarbonate (hyperalimentation therapy), or disproportionate loss of chloride (diarrhea).

    c. Common causes include vomiting, nasogastric tube suctioning, villous adenoma, chloride diarrhea, diuretics, hypercalcemia, milk–alkali syndrome, mineralocorticoid excess, Bartter's and Gitelman's syndromes, and chloride and potassium depletion because of excessive steroids.

2. Clinical features

   a. Neurologic abnormalities are common. Symptoms reflecting low ionized calcium may be seen, which include paresthesias, carpopedal spasm, and light-headedness. Symptoms occasionally may progress to confusion, stupor, and coma.

   b. Symptoms arising from volume depletion frequently are present; weakness, muscle cramps, and postural dizziness may develop.

   c. Abnormalities secondary to potassium depletion may lead to polyuria, polydipsia, and muscle weakness.

3. Laboratory studies (the pH is up and the bicarbonate is also elevated)

   a. Arterial blood gas measurements reveal pH greater than 7.42, increased serum bicarbonate, and increased P_{CO_2} (pulmonary compensation).

   b. Urine chloride concentrations can distinguish between hypovolemic hypochloremic patients with a decreased urine chloride concentration (<20 mEq/L) and volume-expanded patients with mineralocorticoid excess who have urine chloride concentrations of greater than 30 mEq/L.

4. Treatment

   a. Interventions to increase renal excretion of bicarbonate are the most effective therapy for metabolic alkalosis. Additional consideration should be given to the volume status of the patient as well.

   b. Chloride-responsive conditions (e.g., gastric fluid loss, diuretic therapy) are treated with solutions containing sodium chloride to repair the sodium and chloride deficits.

   c. Chloride-resistant conditions (e.g., mineralocorticoid excess) can be successfully treated by removing an adrenal adenoma, if present, or by using spironolactone, an aldosterone antagonist.

VIII. URINARY TRACT INFECTION

A. Cystitis

1. General characteristics

   a. Cystitis is an infection of the normal bladder most commonly caused by coliform bacteria (especially *Escherichia coli*, which accounts for 80% to 85% of cases) and occasionally Gram-positive bacteria (enterococci).

   b. The route of infection typically is ascending from the urethra. It is more common in women.

2. Clinical features

   a. Irritative voiding symptoms (frequency, urgency, dysuria) are common, as is suprapubic discomfort.

   b. Gross hematuria may occur. Symptoms in women often may appear following sexual intercourse.

   c. Physical examination may elicit suprapubic tenderness, but examination often is unremarkable.

3. Laboratory studies

   a. Urinalysis shows pyuria, bacteriuria, and varying degrees of hematuria.

   b. Urine culture is positive (>10^3 cfu/mL) for the offending organism.

   c. Imaging is warranted only if pyelonephritis, recurrent infections, or anatomic abnormalities are suspected.

4. Treatment

   a. Uncomplicated cystitis in women can be treated with short-term antimicrobial therapy.

      (1) The suggested regimen is a fluoroquinolone for 3 to 5 days.

      (2) Resistant *Escherichia coli* are common, but trimethoprim/sulfamethoxazole can be used as an alternative to a quinolone in susceptible strains.

   b. Uncomplicated cystitis is rare in men.

   c. Fluids should be encouraged. Preventive measures include proper hygiene, urine acidification and voiding after intercourse.

   d. Hot sitz baths or urinary analgesics (phenazopyridine) may provide symptomatic relief. Patients should be warned that phenazopyridine will discolor the urine (dark orange or reddish).

B. Pyelonephritis

1. General characteristics

   a. Acute pyelonephritis is an infectious inflammatory process involving the kidney parenchyma and renal pelvis. Bacteremia may occur in up to 10% of cases; however, this is more common in diabetics and elderly women.

   b. Gram-negative bacteria are the most common causative agents, including *Escherichia coli* (85%), *Proteus* sp., *Klebsiella* sp., *Enterobacter* sp., and *Pseudomonas* sp. The infection usually ascends from the lower urinary tract.

   c. Chronic pyelonephritis is the result of progressive inflammation of the renal interstitium caused by bacterial infection, and occurs in patients with anatomic urinary tract abnormalities such as vesicoureteral reflux.

2. Clinical features
   a. Symptoms include fever, flank pain, shaking chills, and irritative voiding symptoms. Nausea, vomiting, and diarrhea are not uncommon.
   b. Young children may have fever and abdominal discomfort.
   c. Signs include fever and tachycardia. Costovertebral angle tenderness usually is pronounced.

3. Laboratory studies
   a. CBC shows leukocytosis and left shift.
   b. Urinalysis shows pyuria, bacteriuria, and varying degrees of hematuria. WBC casts may be seen.
   c. Urine culture (which should be obtained before beginning antibiotics) will demonstrate heavy growth of the offending agent.
   d. In complicated pyelonephritis, renal ultrasonography may show hydronephrosis secondary to obstruction.

4. Treatment
   a. In the outpatient setting, treatment with quinolones or trimethoprim/sulfamethoxazole for 1 to 2 weeks has shown to be effective in immunocompetent patients. Immunocompromised patients should be treated for a longer duration.
   b. Hospital admission is required for patients with severe infections or complicating factors, such as older age, comorbid conditions, signs of obstruction, or inability to tolerate oral antibiotics.
   c. IV fluoroquinolones or ampicillin and gentamicin should be initiated while waiting for sensitivity results. IV antibiotics should be continued for 24 to 48 hours after the patient becomes afebrile; oral antibiotics are then given to complete a minimum of 2 weeks of therapy.
   d. Failure to respond warrants ultrasound imaging to exclude complicating factors such as stones or possible abscess formation that may require prompt intervention.
   e. Follow-up urine cultures are mandatory 1 to 2 weeks following treatment.

C. Prostatitis
1. General characteristics
   a. Acute bacterial prostatitis is caused by ascending infection of Gram-negative rods into the prostatic ducts.
   b. Chronic bacterial prostatitis may be associated with evolution or recurrence of an acute bacterial infection. Its route of infection is the same as for acute prostatitis. The same Gram-negative organisms are most commonly responsible. *Enterococcus* may be identified less often.
   c. Chronic nonbacterial prostatitis is the most common of the prostatitis syndromes, and its cause is unknown. It may represent a noninfectious inflammatory disorder, perhaps with an autoimmune origin, and is a diagnosis of exclusion. It often is associated with the term *chronic pelvic pain syndrome*.
   d. Prostatic abscess is an uncommon complication of acute bacterial prostatitis.

2. Clinical features
   a. Acute infection is characterized by sudden onset of high fever, chills, and low back and perineal pain.
   b. Chronic infection has more variable symptoms, ranging from asymptomatic to acute symptomatology.
   c. All forms of prostatitis present with irritative bladder symptoms (frequency, urgency, dysuria) and some obstruction.
   d. The prostate is swollen and tender.

3. Laboratory studies
   a. Urinalysis reveals pyuria.
   b. Prostatic fluid culture typically is positive for *Escherichia coli* in acute infections. Chronic infection is characterized by recurrence of the same organism or enterococcus. In nonbacterial prostatitis, cultures are negative.
   c. The four-glass localization test is the classic means of distinguishing a chronic prostate infection from another urinary tract infection. Urine samples are taken at initial void, midstream, and after prostatic massage; prostatic secretions account for the fourth sample. Assessment of the samples helps to localize the nidus of infection. This test should be avoided in a patient suspected to have acute prostatitis.

4. Treatment
   a. Antibiotics are the most effective treatment for bacterial infections. Hospitalization may be indicated in acute prostatitis. Treatment with parenteral antibiotics (gentamycin and ampicillin) may be needed until culture results are available and the patient is afebrile for 24 to 48 hours.
      (1) For men younger than 35 years, ofloxacin for 10 days or ceftriaxone, 250 mg IM, followed by 10 days of doxycycline is recommended.

(2) In men older than 35 years, a fluoroquinolone or trimethoprim/sulfamethoxazole may be used for 10 to 14 days.

(3) Some experts suggest that 3 to 4 weeks of treatment is necessary to effectively eradicate the acute infection.

(4) In chronic prostatitis, ciprofloxacin for 4 weeks, ofloxacin for 6 weeks, or trimethoprim/sulfamethoxazole for 1 to 3 months can be used.

(5) Antibiotics are not effective in nonbacterial prostatitis.

   b. NSAIDs are effective analgesics.

   c. Chronic, recurrent, or resistant prostatitis with or without prostatic calculi may require transurethral resection of the prostate for ultimate resolution.

D. Orchitis

1. General characteristics

   a. Orchitis commonly is caused by ascending bacterial infection from the urinary tract.

   b. It occurs in 25% of postpubertal males who have mumps infection.

2. Clinical features

   a. Testicular swelling and tenderness, usually unilateral, occur.

   b. Fever and tachycardia are common.

3. Laboratory studies

   a. Urinalysis reveals pyuria and bacteriuria with bacterial infection.

   b. Cultures are positive for suspected organisms.

   c. Ultrasonography is useful if abscess or tumor is suspected.

4. Treatment

   a. If mumps is the cause, symptomatic relief with ice and analgesia should be provided.

   b. If bacteria are the cause, the orchitis should be treated like epididymitis.

   c. Carefully evaluate any scrotal masses.

E. Epididymitis

1. General characteristics

   a. Epididymitis is infection of the epididymis acquired by retrograde spread of organisms through the vas deferens.

   b. In men younger than 35 years, chlamydia and gonococci are the most common organisms.

   c. In men older than 35 years, *Escherichia coli* is the most common organism.

2. Clinical features

   a. Epididymitis presents with heaviness and dull, aching discomfort in the affected hemiscrotum, which can radiate up the ipsilateral flank. History of the patient may reveal heavy lifting, trauma, or sexual activity.

   b. The epididymis is markedly swollen and exquisitely tender to touch, eventually becoming a warm, erythematous, enlarged scrotal mass. As the disease progresses, it may become difficult to distinguish the testes from the epididymis.

   c. The patient may have fever and chills.

   d. The Prehn's sign (relief of pain with scrotal elevation) is a classic sign, but it is not very reliable.

3. Laboratory studies

   a. Urinalysis reveals pyuria and bacteriuria.

   b. Cultures show positive results for suspected organisms.

4. Treatment

   a. In men younger than 35 years, ceftriaxone, 250 mg IM, plus doxycycline, 100 mg twice per day orally for 10 days, may be administered for gonococci or chlamydia.

   b. In men older than 35 years, ciprofloxacin 500 mg twice per day orally for 10 to 14 days may be used.

   c. Supportive care may include bed rest, scrotal elevation, and analgesics.

IX. BENIGN PROSTATIC HYPERPLASIA

A. General characteristics

1. Proliferation of the fibrostromal tissue of the prostate can lead to compression of the prostatic urethra, creating an obstruction of the urinary outlet.

TABLE 6-7	**American Urological Association BPH Scoring Index**					
	Score					
Over About the Past Month	**Never**	**<1 in 5 Times**	**<50% of the Time**	**About 50% of the Time**	**>50% of the Time**	**Almost Always**
How often have you had a sensation of not emptying your bladder completely after you finish urinating?	0	1	2	3	4	5
How often have you had to urinate again <2 hr after you finished urinating?	0	1	2	3	4	5
How often have you stopped and started again several times when urinating?	0	1	2	3	4	5
How often have you found it difficult to postpone urination?	0	1	2	3	4	5
How often has your urinary stream been weak?	0	1	2	3	4	5
How often have you had to push or strain to begin urination?	0	1	2	3	4	5
How many times did you most typically get up to urinate between going to bed at night and waking in the morning?	None = 0	Once = 1	Twice = 2	3 times = 3	4 times = 4	≥5 times = 5
American Urological Association symptom score = Total _____						

0–7 points: Symptoms are considered mild.
8–19 points: Symptoms are considered moderate.
20–35 points: Symptoms are considered severe.
Reprinted with permission from Barry MJ, Fowler FJ Jr, O'Leary MP, et al. The American Urological Association symptom index for benign prostatic hyperplasia. *J Urol.* 1992;148(5):1549–1557. Copyright © Elsevier.

    2. Benign prostatic hyperplasia (BPH) is a disease of older men; the mean age of onset is 60 to 65 years.

B. Clinical features

    1. The symptom complex is referred to as prostatism, which includes symptoms of obstruction and irritation. The American Urological Association (AUA) symptom index is beneficial to assess symptom severity prior to and throughout any treatment regimen (Table 6-7).

    2. Obstructive symptoms include decreased force of urinary stream, hesitancy and straining, postvoid dribbling, and sensation of incomplete emptying.

    3. Irritative symptoms include frequency, nocturia, and urgency.

    4. Recurrent urinary tract infections and urinary retention also can occur.

    5. Digital rectal examination typically reveals an enlarged prostate.

C. Laboratory studies

    1. Prostate-specific antigen (PSA) typically is slightly elevated.

    2. Other tests are done to evaluate for renal damage, infection, and prostate or bladder cancer, as suspected.

D. Treatment

    1. Men with mild to moderate symptoms may choose watchful waiting and frequent monitoring.

    2. Options for medical therapy include α-adrenergic agonists and 5α-reductase inhibitors.

    3. Procedures that may be used to relieve obstruction include use of balloon dilation, microwave irradiation, and stent placements.

    4. Surgical treatment is transurethral resection of prostate or transurethral incision of prostate.

X. INCONTINENCE

A. General characteristics

    1. Urinary incontinence is defined as the unintentional leakage of urine at inappropriate times.

2. Women experience incontinence twice as often as men. Older women experience it more often than younger women.

3. Incontinence can be classified based on the underlying pathophysiologic mechanism.

   a. Urge incontinence results from bladder contractions that cannot be controlled by the brain.

   b. Stress incontinence is caused by dysfunction of the urethral sphincter, allowing urine to leak with increased intra-abdominal pressure.

   c. Overflow incontinence occurs when urinary retention leads to bladder distention and overflow of urine through the urethra.

   d. Functional incontinence is untimely urination caused by physical or cognitive disability, preventing a person from reaching a toilet.

   e. Mixed incontinence is a combination of elements of both stress and urge incontinence.

B. Clinical features

   1. Reversible causes of incontinence, such as medication side effects, recent prostatectomy, excess fluid intake, atrophic vaginitis, fecal impaction, urinary tract infection, impaired mobility, and glycosuria, should be identified.

   2. The principal symptom of urge incontinence is a strong desire to void, followed by loss of urine.

   3. Overactive bladder disorder is a related symptom complex characterized by frequency of urination, urgency to urinate, and nocturia. Patients may present with or without urge incontinence.

   4. The principal symptom of stress incontinence is leakage of urine with increased intra-abdominal pressure, such as with sneezing, coughing, or laughing.

   5. Untreated overflow incontinence can lead to hydronephrosis and obstructive nephropathy.

   6. Incontinence is common with neurologic diseases (stroke, Parkinson's disease, or dementia), metabolic disorders (hypoxemia, diabetic neuropathy), and pelvic disorders (uterine prolapse).

C. Laboratory findings

   1. Urinalysis can identify diabetes-related glycosuria or acute urinary tract infection.

   2. Postvoid residual urine volume should be measured to identify urinary retention.

   3. Simple urodynamic studies such as cystometry (instillation of water into the bladder) can identify bladder contractions and should be considered.

   4. Stress test, ultrasonography, cystoscopy, and cystographic studies may also be used to determine anatomic abnormalities.

D. Treatment

   1. Pelvic floor muscle training (or Kegel exercises), electrical muscle stimulation, biofeedback, and bladder training can be used to improve the strength and control of the pelvic muscles. Pessaries or implants can help decrease stress incontinence.

   2. Anticholinergic medications, such as oxybutynin or tolterodine, are effective for urge incontinence. Estrogen can be used for stress incontinence. Oral or vaginal estrogen may be used; if used for long term, progestin should be added to prevent endometrial hyperplasia.

   3. Tolterodine and oxybutynin can be used for overactive bladder.

   4. Catheterization, either intermittent or indwelling, can be used for overflow incontinence.

   5. Although surgical treatments often are the last resort, they are very effective for stress incontinence.

XI. NEOPLASMS OF THE URINARY TRACT

A. Prostate cancer

   1. General characteristics

      a. Prostate cancer is a common, generally slow-growing, malignant neoplasm of the adenomatous cells of the prostate gland that can lead to urinary obstruction and metastatic disease. The majority of prostate cancers originate in the peripheral zone (outer portion of the prostate palpable on rectal examination), followed by the transitional zone (portion of prostate surrounding the majority of the urethra [BPH symptomatology]), and lastly the central zone (portion of prostatic urethra with ejaculatory ducts).

      b. A disease of aging, it rarely is seen in men younger than 40 years.

      c. The cause is unknown. Risk factors may include genetic predisposition, hormonal influences, dietary and environmental factors, and infectious agents.

   2. Clinical features

      a. Many cases are not clinically apparent.

   b. Symptoms of urinary obstruction or irritative voiding symptomatology may occur if the tumor has invaded into the urethra, bladder neck, or trigone of the bladder.

   c. In advanced disease, patients may present with bone pain from metastases, possible spinal cord impingement if the vertebral bodies are involved.

   d. The prostate may be enlarged, nodular, and asymmetric.

3. Laboratory studies

   a. PSA usually is elevated in patients with prostate cancer.

   b. Pathologic examination of tissue removed for treatment of obstructive prostatic hyperplasia reveals that 10% have malignancy.

   c. Transrectal ultrasonography reveals hypoechoic lesions in the prostate (peripheral zone).

   d. Biopsy confirms the diagnosis of adenocarcinoma and allows histologic grading (Gleason grading system, based on architectural pattern), which can provide prognostic information. The Gleason grading system adds together the primary and secondary grades of the tumor, resulting in a final score of 2 to 10. The total score can be used for prognostic purposes, with a higher score indicating a worse prognosis than a lower score.

4. Treatment

   a. Appropriate treatment depends on the staging, which is done by abdominal and pelvic CT or magnetic resonance imaging (MRI), pelvic lymphadenectomy, and bone scan.

   b. Low-grade tumors that are well differentiated may not require any treatment, whereas higher-grade tumors more typically are aggressive and, therefore, should be managed more aggressively.

   c. Stage A and B disease (tumor confined to the prostate) may be treated with radical retropubic prostatectomy, brachytherapy, or external beam radiation therapy.

   d. Stage C disease (tumor with local invasion) is treated similar to stage A and B disease, but with reduced effectiveness.

   e. Stage D disease (distant metastases) is treated with hormonal manipulation using orchiectomy, antiandrogens, luteinizing hormone–releasing hormone agonists, or estrogens. Chemotherapy has limited usefulness, and palliative treatment is given for advanced disease.

B. Bladder cancer

1. General characteristics

   a. Causal factors for bladder cancer include exposure to tobacco; occupational carcinogens from rubber, dye, printing, and chemical industries; schistosomiasis; exposure to cyclophosphamide; and chronic infections.

   b. Uroepithelial tumors (most [98%] are transitional cell carcinomas [TCC]) account for 3% of cancer deaths in the United States. Bladder carcinoma is three times more common in men than in women, and it usually occurs in patients 40 to 70 years of age.

2. Clinical features

   a. Painless hematuria is the most common presenting symptom.

   b. Bladder irritability and infection are other presenting symptoms.

3. Laboratory findings

   a. CBC and blood chemistry should be done to evaluate for infection and renal function.

   b. Cystoscopy, which has an accuracy rate of nearly 100%, is the definitive diagnostic procedure. Biopsy confirms the pathologic diagnosis.

   c. Radiologic procedures include IV urogram, pelvic and abdominal CT, chest radiography, bone scan, and retrograde pyelography for renal pelvic or ureteral tumors and staging.

4. Treatment

   a. Treatment depends on the stage.

   b. Superficial lesions are treated with endoscopic resection and fulguration, followed by cystoscopy every 3 months. Recurrent or multiple lesions can be treated with intravesical instillation of thiotepa, mitomycin-C, or bacillus Calmette–Guérin (BCG).

   c. Radical cystectomy is used for recurrent cancer, diffuse TCC in situ, and for tumors that have invaded the muscle.

   d. Combination chemotherapy has been used in bladder-sparing trials with or without radiation therapy. External beam irradiation therapy is typically reserved for those individuals who are not surgical candidates due to significant comorbid medical conditions.

C. Renal cell carcinoma

1. General characteristics

   a. RCC is the most common type of renal malignancy. It accounts for 3% of all adult cancers.

   b. RCC is more common in men, usually affecting those older than 55 years. Incidence is higher in black men than in men of all other races.

   c. The cause is unknown, but cigarette smoking is consistently linked to RCC.

   d. There are forms of hereditary RCC including von Hippel–Lindau disease and hereditary papillary renal carcinoma.

   e. Patients on hemodialysis and peritoneal dialysis have a higher risk of developing RCC in association with cystic changes of the kidney.

2. Clinical features

   a. RCC is associated with a wide range of presenting signs and symptoms and often is called the "internists' tumor."

   b. The most common symptom is gross or microscopic hematuria, followed by pain or an abdominal mass. The classic triad of gross hematuria, flank pain, and a palpable mass, however, occurs only in a small percentage of patients.

   c. RCC is associated with paraneoplastic syndromes, including erythrocytosis, hypercalcemia, hypertension, and hepatic dysfunction in the absence of hepatic metastases.

3. Laboratory findings

   a. Normochromic anemia occurs in nearly one-third of patients with RCC. An elevated erythrocyte sedimentation rate has been reported in up to 75% of patients.

   b. Patients presenting with hematuria should undergo ultrasonography to rule out a stone.

   c. CT scanning is the primary technique for diagnosing RCC. Other confirming studies can include MRI and arteriography.

4. Treatment

   a. Treatment depends on the Furman grade (I, II, III) and stage (TNM) of the tumor; therefore, a thorough evaluation is required.

   b. Radical nephrectomy is the primary treatment for localized disease (stage T1–T3a lesions). Neoadjuvant or adjuvant radiation therapy has not been shown to prolong survival for early stage lesions.

   c. Radiation therapy is an important method of palliation in patients with disseminated disease to the brain, bone, and lungs. Radical nephrectomy has little role in advanced disease.

   d. Hormonal therapy and chemotherapy have shown little effect.

   e. Medications, such as α-interferon and interleukin, have been successful in reducing the growth of some RCCs, including some with metastasis.

D. Wilms' tumor

1. General characteristics

   a. Wilms' tumor, also known as nephroblastoma, is the most common solid renal tumor of childhood.

   b. Most occur in healthy children, but about 10% occur in children with recognized malformations.

   c. Most cases of Wilms' tumor are curable, but on histologic study, about 5% of patients have anaplasia, which is associated with a poorer prognosis. The incidence of anaplasia increases with age.

2. Clinical features

   a. The most common sign is an asymptomatic abdominal mass found by a family member or during physical examination.

   b. Symptoms at presentation might include anorexia, nausea and vomiting, fever, abdominal pain, or hematuria.

   c. Hypertension caused by elevated renin levels can occur.

3. Laboratory findings

   a. Urinalysis may show hematuria, and anemia may be present.

   b. Ultrasonography is the initial study of choice to evaluate abdominal masses.

   c. Abdominal CT is performed in patients with suspected Wilms' tumors to assess tumor extension and regional lymph nodes. MRI also can provide information regarding tumor extension.

   d. Chest radiography is used to evaluate the presence of metastases in the lungs.

4. Treatment
   a. The goal of therapy is to provide the highest possible cure rate with the lowest treatment-related morbidity.
   b. The most effective therapy is a multimodal approach that incorporates surgery, chemotherapy, and in some patients, radiation therapy.
   c. Radical nephrectomy with lymph node sampling is the treatment of choice in surgically resectable tumors. Unresectable tumors should undergo preoperative biopsy followed by chemotherapy.
   d. Wilms' tumor is chemosensitive and responsive to dactinomycin, vincristine, and doxorubicin.
   e. Radiation therapy is added for higher-stage tumors (stages III and IV) and for tumors with focal anaplasia.

E. Testicular cancer
   1. General characteristics
      a. Testicular cancer is the most common malignancy in young men.
      b. Risk factors include history of cryptorchidism or a previous history of testicular cancer.
   2. Clinical features
      a. More than 90% of patients present with a painless, solid, testicular swelling. Patients may also complain of heaviness in the testicle. Occasionally, patients with painful testicular masses are erroneously diagnosed as having epididymitis or orchitis.
      b. Para-aortic lymph node involvement can present as ureteral obstruction.
      c. Patients also may present with abdominal complaints from an abdominal mass or with pulmonary symptoms from multiple nodules.
   3. Laboratory studies
      a. Scrotal ultrasonography may reveal a suspicious intratesticular echogenic focus.
      b. Radiologic studies for staging include radiography of the chest and CT of the chest, abdomen, and pelvis. CT scan of the chest remains controversial, as pulmonary metastasis is often detected by chest X-ray (CXR).
      c. Tumors are classified pathologically as seminomatous (35%) or nonseminomatous (65%). Subtypes of nonseminomatous include embryonal carcinoma (20%), teratoma (5%), mixed cell type (40%), and choriocarcinoma (<1%).
      d. Elevated blood levels of α-fetoprotein or α-human chorionic gonadotropin are diagnostic for nonseminomatous germ cell tumors; the majority of patients with seminoma have normal levels.
   4. Treatment
      a. Treatment depends on pathology and stage. Staging is based on the degree of lymph node spread.
         (1) Orchiectomy is performed for diagnostic and therapeutic reasons.
         (2) Seminomatous tumors are radiosensitive; nonseminomatous tumors are radioresistant.
      b. Nonseminomatous tumors
         (1) Stage I disease limited to the testis can be treated with nerve-sparing retroperitoneal lymph node dissection or rigorous surveillance without surgery or chemotherapy.
         (2) Stage II tumors can be treated with surgery or chemotherapy.
         (3) Stage III disease should be treated with surgery and chemotherapy.
      c. Seminomatous tumors
         (1) The mainstay of therapy for stage I disease isolated to the testis is radiation therapy to the para-aortic and ipsilateral iliac nodal areas.
         (2) Therapy for stages IIa and IIb adds increased radiation to the affected nodes.
         (3) Therapy for stages IIc and III is chemotherapy.

XII. MALE REPRODUCTIVE DISORDERS

A. Phimosis
   1. General characteristics
      a. It is characterized by the inability to retract the foreskin over the glans penis.
      b. Phimosis may be congenital or acquired.
         (1) Congenital phimosis is identified in children and adolescents and usually is physiologic.
         (2) Acquired phimosis is more typical in adults and is usually caused by poor hygiene and chronic balanitis. Consider evaluation for possible diabetes in men with chronic infections.

2. Clinical features

    a. Erythema with tenderness and possible purulent drainage.

    b. Inability to retract the foreskin over the glans penis.

    c. Obstructed urinary stream, hematuria, or pain of the prepuce can indicate more severe constriction.

3. Laboratory findings: None usually required.

4. Treatment

    a. As long as it is asymptomatic, a congenital phimosis should be left alone, as the preputial opening will gradually widen as the child gets older.

    b. If symptomatic, referral for circumcision usually is necessary.

    c. Antibiotics with broad-spectrum drugs is indicated if infection is present. Steroidal creams or nonsteroidal ointments may be of benefit.

B. Paraphimosis

  1. General characteristics

    a. Paraphimosis is defined as entrapment of the foreskin behind the glans penis.

    b. Frequent catheterizations without reducing the foreskin can lead to paraphimosis.

    c. Forcibly retracting a constricted foreskin (phimosis) for cleaning or catheterization can lead to paraphimosis.

    d. Vigorous sexual activity can predispose men to paraphimosis.

  2. Clinical features

    a. Pain, edema, tenderness, and erythema of the glans and foreskin are present.

    b. Identification of any encircling foreign bodies, such as hair, clothing, rubber bands, or metallic objects, is important.

  3. Laboratory findings: None required.

  4. Treatment

    a. Paraphimosis should be reduced emergently.

      (1) Manual reduction should be tried initially. Firmly squeeze the glans for 5 minutes to reduce the tissue edema and decrease the size of the glans and then try to bring the foreskin back over the glans.

      (2) Surgical techniques to incise the restricted foreskin can be used if manual reduction fails.

    b. Inability to reduce a paraphimosis requires emergent urologic referral.

    c. After reduction, referral for circumcision is necessary, because the condition is likely to recur.

C. Erectile dysfunction

  1. General characteristics

    a. Erectile dysfunction is defined as the consistent inability to maintain an erect penis with sufficient rigidity to allow sexual intercourse. It is part of a broader classification of sexual dysfunctions.

    b. Normal erections require intact parasympathetic and somatic nerve supply, unobstructed arterial inflow, adequate venous constriction, hormonal stimulation, and psychological desire. Disorders of any of these systems may result in impotence.

    c. Most cases of male erectile disorders have a primary organic rather than a psychogenic cause. Nearly all cases have a secondary psychogenic component.

    d. This condition affects millions of American men, and its incidence is age related.

    e. Major predictors of erectile dysfunction include hypertension, diabetes mellitus, hyperlipidemia, and cardiovascular disease.

  2. Clinical features

    a. The medical history must be adequately evaluated. Medications such as some antihypertensives (e.g. beta-blockers) may be the cause of erectile dysfunction; switching to another antihypertensive agent may resolve the problem.

    b. A sexual history should be taken, including detailed information on timing and frequency of sexual relations, partners, presence of morning erections, ejaculation, and the ability to masturbate. The International Index of Erectile Function (IIEF) is a validated questionnaire useful to determine baseline erectile function.

    c. Past medical history should document presence of hypertension, diabetes, endocrine disease, medications, pelvic surgery, or trauma.

    d. Physical examination should look for penile deformities (e.g., Peyronie's disease [fibrous plaque causing penile curvative]), testicular atrophy, hypertension, peripheral neuropathy, and other signs of endocrine, vascular, or neurologic abnormalities.

3. Laboratory findings
   a. CBC, urinalysis, lipid profile, thyroid function tests, serum testosterone, glucose, and prolactin screening should be done, depending on the suspected cause.
   b. Measurement of follicle-stimulating hormone and luteinizing hormone may be required for patients with abnormalities of testosterone or prolactin.
   c. Nocturnal penile tumescence testing can be done to differentiate between organic and psychogenic impotence. Patients with psychogenic impotence have normal nocturnal erections of adequate frequency and rigidity.
   d. Direct injection of vasoactive substances into the penis induces erections in men with intact vascular systems.
   e. Patients who do not achieve erections with injections may undergo studies to evaluate the arterial and venous vasculature, such as ultrasonography of the cavernous arteries, pelvic arteriography, and cavernosonography.

4. Treatment
   a. True psychogenic causes can be treated with behaviorally oriented sex therapy. Patients with organic causes of impotence may also benefit from counseling.
   b. Phosphodiesterase-5 (PDE-5) inhibitor therapy is considered the mainstay of treatment for erectile dysfunction. Sildenafil, vardenafil, and tadalafil are the drugs currently indicated for erectile dysfunction.
   c. Side effects of PDE-5 therapy can include headache, flushing, dyspepsia, rhinitis, and visual disturbances and possible priapism. PDE-5 should be avoided in patients taking nitrates as the combination may cause a significant drop in blood pressure.
   d. For men in whom PDE-5 therapy is ineffective or inappropriate, there are other treatments, including use of vacuum constriction devices, injected or inserted vasoactive substances, and penile prostheses. Patients with disorders of the arterial system are candidates for arterial reconstruction.

D. Scrotal masses
   1. Hydrocele
      a. General characteristics: A hydrocele is a mass of the fluid-filled congenital remnants of the tunica vaginalis, usually resulting from a patent processus vaginalis.
      b. Clinical features
         (1) A soft, nontender fullness of the hemiscrotum that transilluminates.
         (2) The mass may wax and wane in size; an indirect hernia may be concurrently present.
      c. Laboratory studies: Few laboratory studies are warranted for hydrocele.
         (1) Urinalysis with microscopic analysis is negative.
         (2) Ultrasonography rarely is indicated but can distinguish between hydrocele, spermatocele, and testicular tumors.
      d. Treatment: Elective repair as clinically indicated.
   2. Spermatocele
      a. General characteristics
         (1) A spermatocele typically is a painless cystic mass containing sperm.
         (2) Most spermatoceles are less than 1 cm in size.
         (3) They lie superior and posterior and are distinct from the testes.
         (4) Some may simulate a solid tumor.
      b. Clinical features: Palpable, round, firm cystic mass with distinct borders, free floating above the testicle, which transilluminates. The mass may be tender.
      c. Laboratory studies
         (1) Needle aspiration should not be performed.
         (2) Scrotal ultrasonography provides a very accurate diagnosis.
      d. Treatment
         (1) No medical treatment required.
         (2) Large spermatoceles can be surgically removed or sclerosed.

E. Testicular torsion
   1. General characteristics
      a. The testis is abnormally twisted on its spermatic cord, thus compromising arterial supply and venous drainage of the testis, leading to testicular ischemia.

b. This condition is most common in prepubertal and postpubertal young males (12 to 18 years), especially with a history of cryptorchidism (late descent of the testes).

2. Clinical features

a. Sudden onset of severe unilateral pain and scrotal swelling are present.

b. Testis is painful to palpation; testicle and scrotum are edematous. There is no relief with elevation of the testicle (negative Prehn's sign).

3. Laboratory findings

a. Testicular torsion is a clinical diagnosis.

b. If the diagnosis is equivocal, do not wait for laboratory studies.

c. Doppler ultrasonography demonstrates decreased blood flow to the affected spermatic cord and testis.

d. Radioisotope scan demonstrates decreased uptake in the affected testes.

4. Treatment

a. Mild analgesics may be administered once the diagnosis is made.

b. This is a surgical emergency. Manual detorsion (twisting the testes outward and laterally) may be attempted by experienced clinicians, but whether this is successful or not, surgery will be required. If the affected testicle is corrected within a 6-hour time frame, there is a greater chance of salvaging the testicle. Surgical detorsion and orchiopexy are the definitive therapies.

c. Emergent surgical intervention on the affected testis must be followed by elective surgery (orchiopexy) on the contralateral testis, which also is at risk of torsion.

F. Varicocele

1. General characteristics

a. Varicocele is the formation of a venous varicosity within the spermatic vein (pampiniform plexus).

b. The left spermatic vein has an increased incidence of varicosity because the vein is longer than the right and joins the left renal vein at right angles.

2. Clinical features

a. A chronic, nontender mass that does not transilluminate is seen, usually on the left side.

b. The lesion has the consistency of a "bag of worms," increases in size with Valsalva, and decreases in size with elevation of the scrotum or supine position.

3. Laboratory studies

a. No laboratory studies are required.

b. If the diagnosis is inconclusive, Doppler sonography is the diagnostic method of choice.

4. Treatment: Surgical repair (left spermatic vein ligation) can be performed if the varicocele is painful or if it appears to be a cause of infertility.

I. MENSTRUAL DISORDERS

A. Amenorrhea

1. General characteristics

   a. Primary amenorrhea is the absence of spontaneous menstruation by age 16.

   b. Secondary amenorrhea

   (1) In a woman who has previously menstruated, secondary amenorrhea is defined as the absence of menses for 6 months or longer.

   (2) In a woman with oligomenorrhea, secondary amenorrhea is defined as the absence of menses for 12 months.

   c. The most common cause of secondary amenorrhea is pregnancy; amenorrhea not caused by pregnancy occurs in fewer than 5% of women during their lifetime.

   d. Women who fail to menstruate in the presence of estrogen stimulation of the endometrium are at increased risk for endometrial cancer.

2. Clinical features

   a. Primary amenorrhea is divided into four categories based on clinical features.

   (1) Amenorrhea in a woman with no secondary sexual characteristics suggests gonadal agenesis or dysgenesis, ovarian resistance syndrome, galactosemia, gonadotropin-releasing hormone (GnRH) deficiency, constitutional pubertal delay, a central nervous system mass lesion, stress, or hyperprolactinemia.

   (2) Amenorrhea in a woman with breast development but no pubic or axillary hair suggests androgen insensitivity.

   (3) Amenorrhea in a woman with normal secondary sexual characteristics suggests imperforate hymen, transverse vaginal septum, or cervical or mullerian agenesis.

   (4) Amenorrhea in a woman with incompletely developed sexual characteristics suggests a tumor of the hypothalamus or pituitary, hypothyroidism, premature ovarian failure, or hyperprolactinemia.

   b. Secondary amenorrhea

   (1) Pregnancy is the most common cause of secondary amenorrhea.

   (2) Signs and symptoms associated with drug use, stress, significant weight change, or excessive exercise may be present and alert the clinician to the cause.

   (3) In women with normal estrogen, the cause is likely to be Asherman's syndrome (intrauterine synechiae) or polycystic ovary syndrome (PCOS).

   (4) In hypoestrogenic women, causes include central nervous system tumor, stress, hyperprolactinemia, hypophysitis, Sheehan's syndrome, and premature ovarian syndrome.

   (5) Galactorrhea may be present, indicating prolactinemia.

3. Laboratory studies

   a. A pregnancy test is advisable.

   b. Serum follicle-stimulating hormone (FSH), estrogen, prolactin, and testosterone levels are often necessary to make the correct diagnosis.

   c. A progesterone challenge test will determine the presence or absence of sufficient estrogen.

   d. Other tests may be indicated, including thyroid studies, magnetic resonance imaging (MRI) or computed tomography (CT) of the hypothalamus and pituitary or pelvis, genetic testing, and pelvic and transvaginal ultrasonography.

4. Treatment: Depends on the underlying cause.

B. Dysmenorrhea

1. General characteristics

   a. Primary dysmenorrhea is painful menstruation caused by excess prostaglandin E_2 secretion in the menstrual fluid, leading to painful uterine contractions; prostaglandin E_2 causes smooth muscle contraction, leading to nausea, vomiting, and diarrhea. Onset is usually within 3 to 6 months of menarche.

    b. Secondary dysmenorrhea is painful menstruation caused by an identifiable clinical condition, usually a disease of the uterus or pelvis (e.g., endometriosis, adenomyosis, uterine fibroids, pelvic inflammatory disease, use of an intrauterine device [IUD]). It usually affects women older than 25 years and may involve prostaglandins.

    c. Dysmenorrhea affects more than half of women of reproductive age at some point during their reproductive years and is a cause of recurrent disability in 10% to 15% of women during their early reproductive years.

    d. The incidence of primary dysmenorrhea peaks during the late teens and early 20s; the incidence of secondary dysmenorrhea increases with age.

2. Clinical features

    a. Women with primary dysmenorrhea have cramping in the central lower abdomen or pelvis radiating to the back or thighs, beginning before or at the onset of menses, and lasting for 1 to 3 days. Physical examination is normal.

    b. Symptoms of secondary dysmenorrhea are similar but also may include bloating, menorrhagia, and dyspareunia. It is less related to the first day of flow.

    c. Adenomyosis (implantation of endometrial tissue in the myometrium) results in a tender, symmetrically enlarged, "boggy" uterus.

3. Laboratory studies

    a. The diagnosis of primary dysmenorrhea is established on the basis of history and physical examination.

    b. Specific tests for secondary dysmenorrhea target possible pelvic pathology.

4. Treatment

    a. Primary dysmenorrhea

        (1) Start nonsteroidal anti-inflammatory drugs (NSAIDs) just before the expected menses and continue for 2 to 3 days.

        (2) Oral contraceptives, application of heat, and regular exercise also reduce pain.

        (3) Resistant cases may respond to tocolytic agents, calcium channel blockers, or progestogens.

    b. Secondary dysmenorrhea

        (1) Obvious underlying conditions should be treated and IUDs removed.

        (2) Symptomatic treatment may be sufficient.

        (3) Hysteroscopy, dilation and curettage (D&C), and laparoscopy allow both diagnosis and treatment.

C. Premenstrual syndrome (PMS)

1. General characteristics

    a. PMS lacks agreed-on diagnostic criteria, pathophysiologic mechanisms, and optimal treatment.

    b. Hypothesized causes include abnormal levels of estrogen, progesterone, cortisone, prolactin, antidiuretic hormone, endogenous opiates, melatonin, serotonin, and/or prostaglandins; vitamin and mineral deficiencies; reactive hypoglycemia; menstrual toxins; and psychological, social, evolutionary, and genetic factors.

    c. The reported incidence is 10% to 90%, and it is debilitating in 10%. The prevalence is greatest during the fourth and fifth decades. Seventy percent of women have some premenstrual symptoms.

    d. Fewer than 4% of women meet criteria for premenstrual dysphoric disorder. This diagnosis indicates premenstrual symptoms severe enough to cause dysfunction in daily living.

    e. An association exists among postpartum depression, perimenopausal depression, other affective disorders, and PMS.

2. Clinical features

    a. Symptoms are associated with the menstrual cycle and begin 1 to 2 weeks before menses (i.e., during the luteal phase) and end 1 to 2 days after the onset of menses.

    b. A monthly symptom-free period during the follicular phase (i.e., from day 1 of menses to ovulation) must exist (Fig. 7-1).

    c. The most common complaints are mood alteration and psychological effects (e.g., irritability, anxiety, depression, sleep and appetite changes, poor concentration, fatigue, insomnia).

    d. Symptoms related to fluid retention include edema, weight gain, and breast pain.

    e. Bloating, constipation, and backache also may occur.

    f. Symptoms are consistent month to month within the same patient, although they vary widely woman to woman.

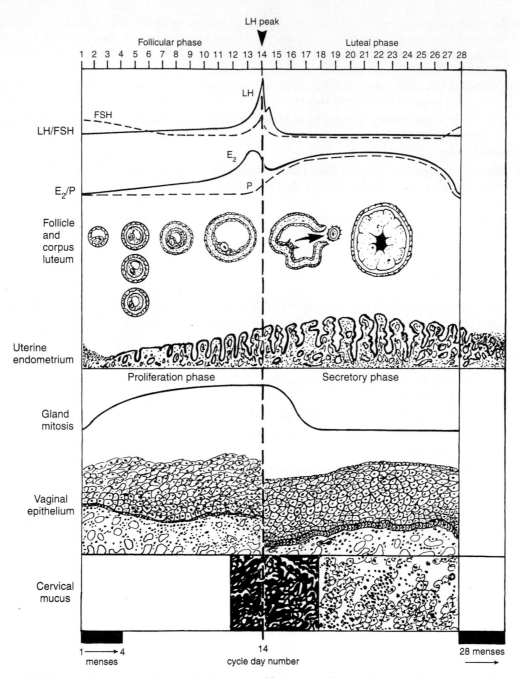

FIGURE 7-1 Composite changes in tissues and hormones during the reproductive cycle. E_2, prostaglandin E_2; FSH, follicle-stimulating hormone; LH, luteinizing hormone; P, progesterone. (From Beckmann CB, Ling FW, Smith RP, et al., eds. *Obstetrics and Gynecology*. 5th ed. Baltimore: Lippincott Williams & Wilkins; 2006:348.)

3. Laboratory studies
   a. Tests include daily charting of symptoms; the specific constellation of symptoms is less important than their cyclical pattern of occurrence.
   b. Thyroid studies and complete blood count (CBC) are used to rule out thyroid disease and anemia.
4. Treatment
   a. Women should be treated on the basis of individual risk factors and symptoms. Education for the patient and her family is essential.
   b. Lifestyle modification includes caffeine reduction, salt restriction, low-fat and high–complex carbohydrate intake, emphasis on fresh foods, increased exercise, relaxation tapes, and stress reduction.

    c. Drug treatment

       (1) Pyridoxine (vitamin B_6) and evening primrose oil show no benefit over placebo in clinical trials but relieve breast tenderness and depression in some women; some preliminary studies show the benefits of calcium carbonate, magnesium, vitamin B_6, and vitamin E supplementation.

       (2) Oral contraceptives may improve, worsen, or not change symptomatology; clinical studies have not shown progesterone to be useful.

       (3) Diuretics (e.g., spironolactone) may be used for fluid retention symptoms; bromocriptine may help relieve mastalgia.

       (4) NSAIDs are useful for pain but also seem to relieve other symptoms.

       (5) Selective serotonin reuptake inhibitors (SSRIs) have proven to be beneficial in some patients; anxiolytics, including buspirone and cyclic alprazolam, may relieve anxiety.

D. Menopause

  1. General characteristics

    a. By definition, menopause is the last menses; perimenopause (usually lasting 3 to 5 years) is the time surrounding it; the climacteric is that portion of the aging process where a woman moves from her reproductive years to her nonreproductive years.

    b. Mean age at natural menopause is 51.5 years; 95% of women stop menstruating between 44 and 55 years. Smoking is associated with early menopause.

    c. The subjective experience of menopause varies by individual and is influenced by cultural expectations and life circumstances.

    d. Premature menopause (spontaneous premature ovarian failure) is cessation of menses before age 40.

    e. The ovaries continue to produce testosterone and androstenedione; estrone is the predominant postmenopausal circulating estrogen.

  2. Clinical features

    a. Vasomotor symptoms vary in intensity; when they occur frequently at night, they may cause insomnia, tiredness, and irritability. They resolve in 2 to 3 years (3 to 6 weeks with estrogen replacement therapy).

    b. Urogenital atrophy may cause poor vaginal lubrication, dyspareunia, dysuria, urge incontinence, pelvic relaxation, atrophic cystitis, caruncles (small elevation of the mucous membrane around the vaginal opening), pruritus, leucorrhea, petechiae, and easy bleeding.

    c. Accelerated bone loss may result in osteoporosis.

    d. Estrogen-related cardiovascular protection declines.

    e. One of the most disabling effects is changes in the sleep cycle.

    f. The skin thins and becomes less elastic, and facial hair may increase. Hair loss increases and nails become brittle.

    g. Confusion, loss of memory, lethargy, inability to cope, depression, and loss of interest in sex have been associated with menopause. Causes are not clear, but symptoms may be relieved with hormone administration.

  3. Laboratory studies: FSH of greater than 30 mIU/mL is diagnostic of menopause.

  4. Treatment

    a. Women should be treated on the basis of individual risk factors and symptoms.

    b. Lifestyle modifications may ameliorate symptoms and decrease risks.

    c. Combined hormone replacement therapy is effective in reducing symptoms but appears to increase the risks for cardiovascular disease, breast cancer, and cognitive changes. Other possible risks include migraine and gallbladder disease.

    d. Contraindications include undiagnosed vaginal bleeding, acute vascular thrombosis, and history of estrogen-dependent tumors.

    e. Calcium and vitamin D supplementation, bisphosphonates, selective estrogen receptor modulators (SERMs), or calcitonin may be used in women at risk for osteoporosis; lifestyle modifications may also decrease risk.

    f. Topical estrogens may improve urogenital symptoms, but any unopposed estrogen administration places a woman at increased risk for endometrial cancer.

II.   UTERINE DISORDERS

  A. Dysfunctional uterine bleeding (DUB)

    1. General characteristics

      a. DUB is abnormal uterine bleeding in the absence of an anatomic lesion, usually caused by a problem with the hypothalamic–pituitary–ovarian hormonal axis.

    b. DUB most commonly occurs shortly after menarche and during perimenopause because of increased anovulatory cycles.

    c. Other causes include PCOS, exogenous obesity, and adrenal hyperplasia.

  2. Clinical features: Abnormal bleeding with an unremarkable physical examination in a very young or perimenopausal woman.

  3. Laboratory studies

    a. CBC, possibly iron studies, prothrombin time (PT) and partial thromboplastin time (PTT), urinary human chorionic gonadotropin (hCG) level, documentation of ovulation, thyroid function tests, serum progesterone level, liver function tests, and prolactin and serum FSH levels are needed.

    b. Pap smear, endometrial biopsy, pelvic ultrasonography, hysterosalpingography, hysteroscopy, and/or D&C may be indicated based on history and physical examination.

  4. Treatment

    a. Treatment depends on severity of bleeding and may include observation, iron therapy, and volume replacement. Acute hemorrhage may necessitate intravenous (IV) or oral (po) high-dose estrogens.

    b. Cyclic estrogens with progestins added to the last 10 to 15 days of the reproductive cycle for 3 to 6 months may establish a normal pattern.

    c. Oral contraceptives

      (1) Oral contraceptives should not be used in women who smoke or who have hypertension, diabetes, history of vascular disease, breast cancer, liver disease, or focal headaches.

      (2) Older women without risk factors can be prescribed oral contraceptives.

    d. Cyclic progestins alone may be used in younger patients.

    e. D&C may be both diagnostic and curative.

    f. Refractory cases may require endometrial ablation or vaginal hysterectomy.

B. Leiomyomata (uterine fibroids)

  1. General characteristics

    a. Fibroids are more common in black women and those with a positive family history.

    b. Fibroids depend on estrogen and appear with increased frequency in women who have endometrial hyperplasia, anovulatory states, and estrogen-producing ovarian tumors.

    c. Women with fibroids have a fourfold increase in the risk of endometrial cancer.

    d. Fibroids may mask other lethal tumors; they undergo malignant transformation in 0.1% to 0.5%.

  2. Clinical features

    a. Most women have no symptoms but do have a firm, enlarged, irregular uterine mass. Some will have symptoms of pressure or fullness in the pelvis.

    b. Menorrhagia, metrorrhagia, intermenstrual bleeding, and dysmenorrhea are common. Bleeding is the most common presenting symptom.

    c. The risk of spontaneous abortion is increased.

  3. Diagnostic procedures may include ultrasonography, D&C, saline hysteroscopy, MRI, intravenous urography, hysterosalpingography, and laparoscopy.

  4. Treatment

    a. Observation is recommended in most cases of leiomyomata.

    b. Symptomatic patients may undergo myomectomy, hysterectomy, or D&C.

    c. GnRH agonists and mifepristone may reduce tumor size; in women with small leiomyomata, GnRH agonists may restore fertility.

    d. Use of arterial embolization as a treatment for fibroids is increasing.

C. Endometrial cancer

  1. General characteristics

    a. Postmenopausal women make up 75% of patients; median age at presentation is 58 years.

    b. There are two types of endometrial cancer: estrogen dependent, which generally is found in younger, perimenopausal women, and estrogen independent, which is found in older, postmenopausal woman; adenocarcinoma is the most common type.

    c. Prognosis is influenced by histologic appearance, age (older women have poorer outcomes), and extent of spread.

    d. Endometrial cancer is the most common gynecologic malignancy and the fourth most common malignancy in women in the United States.

    e. Risk factors include obesity, nulliparity, infertility, late menopause, diabetes mellitus, unopposed estrogen stimulation, hypertension, gallbladder disease, and chronic tamoxifen use; it is not related to sexual history.

    f. White women are more likely to develop endometrial carcinoma than black women.

    g. Oral contraceptives seem to have a protective effect.

    h. Hyperplasia may be simple or complex and may occur with or without atypia.

  2. Clinical features

    a. The cardinal symptom is inappropriate uterine bleeding (90% of patients).

    b. Obesity, hypertension, and diabetes mellitus may be present.

  3. Laboratory and diagnostic testing

    a. Women with postmenopausal bleeding should have a Pap smear, endocervical curettage, and endometrial biopsy. Endometrial biopsy has an accuracy rate of 90% to 95%.

    b. Other tests include fractional D&C and transvaginal ultrasonography.

  4. Treatment

    a. Total hysterectomy combined with bilateral salpingo-oophorectomy is the basis of treatment and staging.

    b. Radiotherapy may be indicated.

    c. Recurrence is treated with high-dose progestins or antiestrogens.

D. Endometriosis

  1. General characteristics

    a. Endometriosis is a condition in which endometrial glands and stroma are found outside the endometrial cavity. Most sites are found in the pelvis or on the ovary (60%), but they also may be distant (e.g., lung).

    b. It most commonly occurs in nulliparous women in their late 20s or early 30s. First-degree relatives have a 7% chance of developing endometriosis.

    c. Infertility is common. Endometriosis is found in 25% to 34% of infertile women.

  2. Clinical features

    a. Endometriosis presents with dysmenorrhea, deep-thrust dyspareunia, dyschezia (difficulty passing bowel movement), intermittent spotting, and pelvic pain.

    b. Signs include tender nodularity of the cul-de-sac and uterine ligaments and a fixed uterus.

    c. The degree of endometriosis does not correlate with symptomatology.

  3. Laboratory and diagnostic testing: Diagnostic testing for endometriosis includes ultrasonography and laparoscopy or laparotomy.

  4. Treatment

    a. Endometriosis treatment is based on severity of symptoms, location and severity of disease, and desire for childbearing.

    b. In women with few symptoms, expectant management may suffice.

    c. NSAIDs and prostaglandin synthetase inhibitors may relieve discomfort.

    d. Surgery may be conservative or definitive; large endometriomas must be resected.

    e. Treatment with danazol or a GnRH agonist around surgery improves fertility.

    f. Combined oral contraceptives or progestins may relieve symptoms.

E. Adenomyosis

  1. General characteristics

    a. Adenomyosis is the extension of endometrial glands into the uterine musculature.

    b. It is not thought to be related to endometriosis.

  2. Clinical features

    a. Adenomyosis may present with severe secondary dysmenorrhea, but many patients are asymptomatic.

    b. The classic patient is middle aged and parous with severe secondary dysmenorrhea and menorrhagia and a symmetrically enlarged uterus.

     3. Laboratory testing

       a. Pelvic ultrasonography may detect adenomyosis.

       b. Pregnancy should be ruled out.

       c. Endometrial biopsy, fractional D&C, or hysteroscopy in a patient with suspected adenomyosis will rule out endometrial cancer.

     4. Treatment

       a. Adenomyosis may be treated with D&C, a GnRH agonist, or mifepristone; hysterectomy is the definitive therapy.

       b. Hormonal treatment has not been successful.

  F. Prolapse

     1. General characteristics

       a. Prolapse of the uterus typically occurs after pregnancy, labor, and vaginal delivery but also may occur in nulliparas.

       b. Prolapse is less common in Asian and African American women than in white women.

       c. Any condition that increases intra-abdominal pressure may predispose a woman to prolapse, including obesity, chronic cough, and repetitive heavy lifting.

       d. Systemic problems such as obesity, asthma, and chronic obstructive pulmonary disease (COPD) and local factors such as pelvic tumors and ascites predispose to prolapse.

       e. Iatrogenic causes include failure to correct pelvic support defects during surgery.

     2. Clinical features

       a. Symptoms vary but usually are worse after prolonged standing or late in the day and are relieved by lying down. These include vaginal fullness, lower abdominal aching, or low back pain.

       b. Uterine prolapse is graded as 0 (no descent) to 4 (through the hymen).

       c. With moderate prolapse, patients describe a falling-out sensation or a feeling of sitting on a ball.

       d. Most prolapses are accompanied by cystocele, rectocele, or enterocele.

     3. Laboratory testing is not indicated.

     4. Treatment

       a. Nonsurgical approaches include weight reduction, smoking cessation, pelvic muscle exercises, and use of a vaginal pessary.

       b. Surgical treatment relieves symptoms, restores normal anatomic relationships and visceral function, and allows coitus.

III. OVARIAN DISORDERS

  A. Ovarian cysts

     1. General characteristics

       a. Cysts are the most common ovarian growths.

       b. Most cysts are functional; these include follicular, corpus luteum, and, much less commonly, theca lutein cysts.

     2. Clinical features: Cysts may present as asymptomatic masses, with pain and menstrual delay or with hemorrhage because of rupture.

     3. Diagnostic studies: Cysts usually are confirmed by pelvic ultrasonography.

     4. Treatment

       a. Follow for one or two cycles in premenopausal women with cysts smaller than 8 cm. Persistent cysts warrant further investigation.

       b. Large or persistent cysts require laparoscopic evaluation.

       c. Cysts in postmenopausal women are presumed to be malignant until proven otherwise.

       d. Oral contraceptives have not been validated in treating functional cysts.

  B. Polycystic ovary syndrome (PCOS)

     1. General characteristics

       a. Formerly known as Stein–Leventhal syndrome, PCOS is the most common cause of androgen excess and hirsutism.

       b. Patients with PCOS have bilaterally enlarged polycystic ovaries, amenorrhea or oligomenorrhea, and infertility.

      c. Patients usually have a normal puberty and adolescence, followed by progressively longer episodes of amenorrhea.

    d. The underlying abnormality is thought to be hypothalamic pituitary dysfunction and insulin resistance, although the pathophysiology is not entirely clear. A genetic predisposition exists.

    e. Patients are at increased risk for endometrial hyperplasia and carcinoma because of unopposed estrogen stimulation.

  2. Clinical features

    a. Half of patients with PCOS are hirsute, and many show truncal obesity.

    b. Patients usually present for treatment of hirsutism or infertility. Others present with intractable acne or menstrual irregularities (oligomenorrhea or amenorrhea).

    c. Acanthosis nigricans sometimes is found.

    d. Impaired glucose tolerance is present in 30% of patients; frank diabetes mellitus (type 2) is present in 8%.

  3. Laboratory studies

    a. Ultrasonography may demonstrate a characteristic "string of pearls" appearance within the ovaries.

    b. Laboratory testing reveals mildly elevated serum androgen levels, increased LH/FSH ratio, lipid abnormalities, and insulin resistance.

  4. Treatment

    a. Weight reduction improves hirsutism, lipid and glucose parameters, and fertility.

    b. Hirsutism is treated with androgen-lowering agents, including oral contraceptives.

    c. Infertility usually is treated with clomiphene citrate; in refractory cases, wedge resection of the ovary is used.

    d. Lipid abnormalities and insulin resistance should be managed medically.

C. Ovarian cancer

  1. General characteristics

    a. High-risk women are older, nulliparous, white, and have a positive family history of ovarian or endometrial cancer.

    b. Long-term oral contraceptive use may be protective because of the suppression of ovulation.

    c. A leading cause of death, ovarian cancer is the fifth most common cancer in U.S. women and the third most common gynecologic malignancy, with the highest mortality rate; 60% of patients die within 5 years.

    d. Ten percent of patients have a genetic predisposition; 90% of cases are sporadic.

    e. Hereditary ovarian cancer has two forms: breast and ovarian cancer syndrome (BOC) or hereditary nonpolyposis colorectal cancer syndrome (HNPCC).

  2. Clinical features

    a. Diagnosis often is delayed because of lack of specific symptoms. Women may present with ascites, abdominal distention, vague gastrointestinal (GI) symptoms, or a fixed mass.

    b. Most patients are diagnosed between 40 and 60 years of age.

  3. Laboratory studies

    a. The *BRCA1* gene is associated in 5% of cases; cancer antigen 125(CA-125) may be used to follow treatment, particularly in postmenopausal women.

    b. An association exists with mutations in the *P53* tumor suppressor gene.

    c. Transvaginal or abdominal ultrasonography is useful in distinguishing benign from potentially malignant masses.

  4. Treatment: This involves surgery plus chemotherapy and radiotherapy.

IV. CERVICAL DYSPLASIA AND NEOPLASIA

A. General characteristics

  1. Human papillomavirus (HPV) infection (especially types 16, 18, 31, 33, and 45) is strongly linked to cervical neoplasia; types 6 and 11 are linked to condylomata acuminate; 80% of cervical intraepithelial neoplasia (CIN) lesions and 90% of invasive cervical carcinomas show the presence of HPV.

  2. HPV infection alone is probably not sufficient for development of CIN; cofactors play a strong role. Other risk factors include early age at first intercourse, early childbearing, multiple sexual partners or a high-risk sex partner, history of sexually transmitted disease, low socioeconomic status, African American heritage, and cigarette smoking.

  3. Atypical changes at the transformation zone of the cervix initiate CIN, the preinvasive phase of cervical cancer. The transformation zone is involved in 95% of cases.

    a. Mild dysplasia (CIN-1) may progress to moderate dysplasia (CIN-2), severe dysplasia (CIN-3), and carcinoma in situ (CIS); may stay the same; or may regress.

      b. About one-third of patients with CIN-3 develop microinvasive and frankly invasive carcinoma.

      c. CIN most commonly occurs in women in their 20s, CIS in those aged 25 to 35 years, and cervical cancer after age 40.

B. Clinical features

  1. Most women with abnormal Pap smears or other screening tests have no symptoms.

  2. Advanced or invasive cervical cancer may cause abnormal vaginal bleeding and vaginal discharge, and tumor may be seen on clinical examination.

  3. The mean age at diagnosis is 47 years overall but 39 years in lower socioeconomic status groups.

C. Laboratory studies

  1. Pap smear, liquid-based specimen, and other cytologic screening techniques are highly effective and should begin within three years of becoming sexually active or reaches age 21, whichever comes first. Annual Pap smear reduces the incidence of invasive cervical carcinoma by 95%.

  2. Abnormal cytologic screenings (Table 7-1) indicate a need for further diagnostic testing; repeat smear may be sufficient to evaluate mild changes.

      a. Biopsy of suspicious lesions is mandatory.

      b. Colposcopy with biopsies is the most appropriate technique for histologic evaluation.

      c. Conization is used when the results of colposcopy are unsatisfactory or endocervical curettage scrapings indicate severe disease.

  3. HPV DNA testing is now standard.

D. Treatment is based on the classification of disease.

  1. Mild lesions may resolve spontaneously.

  2. Preinvasive neoplasia may be treated with electrocautery or cryocautery, laser therapy, conization, large-loop excision of transitional zone, or loop electrodiathermy excision procedure (LEEP).

  3. Hysterectomy and pelvic lymphadenectomy or radiation therapy is indicated for more severe abnormalities.

  4. Gardasil is a vaccine against HPV associated with cervical cancer. The Centers for Disease Control and Prevention has recommended that all girls aged 11 to 12 years receive the series of three injections over 6 months; it is available to all women aged 9 to 26 years. It prevents four types of HPV in those not previously exposed, targeting HPV that causes 70% of all cervical cancers and 90% of genital warts. Boosters may be needed every 5 years, but final word is not known.

V. VAGINAL AND VULVAR DISORDERS

A. Pelvic organ prolapse

  1. General characteristics

      a. Pelvic organ prolapse refers to protrusion of the pelvic organs into or out of the vagina.

      b. Organ prolapses may occur in isolation but usually are combined.

      c. Prolapse may result from excessive stretching of pelvic fascia, ligaments, and muscles during pregnancy, labor, and delivery; from increased intra-abdominal pressure; or from iatrogenic factors.

      d. Anterior vaginal prolapse includes cystocele or cystourethrocele.

      e. Apical includes uterovaginal or vaginal vault prolapse.

      f. Posterior includes enterocele and rectocele.

  2. Clinical features

      a. The amount of discomfort and other symptoms varies among patients. Most symptoms are worse after standing and late in the day and may be relieved by lying down.

      b. Grading of prolapse: 0 = no descent, 1 = descent between normal position and ischial spines, 2 = descent between ischial spines and hymen, 3 = descent within hymen, and 4 = descent through hymen.

  3. Laboratory studies are not indicated.

  4. Treatment includes pelvic floor exercises, vaginal pessaries, and surgical treatment.

B. Neoplasm of the vulva and vagina

  1. General characteristics

      a. Neoplasia in this area is the rarest of the gynecologic neoplasms.

      b. Most vulvar malignancies are squamous cell carcinomas and occur in postmenopausal women (mean age at diagnosis, 65 years).

TABLE 7-1 The 2001 Bethesda System for Reporting Cervical and Vaginal Cytologic Diagnoses

Specimen type
  Conventional smear (Pap smear), liquid based, or other type
Adequacy of the specimen
  Satisfactory for evaluation
  Unsatisfactory for evaluation (specify reason)
General categorization (optional)
  Negative for intraepithelial lesion or malignancy
  Epithelial cell abnormality (see *Interpretation/result*)
  Other (see *Interpretation/result*)
Automated review
Ancillary testing
Interpretation/result
  Negative for intraepithelial lesion or malignancy
    Organisms
      Trichomonas vaginalis
      Fungal organisms morphologically consistent with *Candida* spp.
      Shift in flora suggestive of bacterial vaginosis
      Bacteria morphologically consistent with *Actinomyces* spp.
      Cellular changes associated with herpes simplex virus
  Other nonneoplastic findings
    Reactive cellular changes associated with inflammation (includes typical repair)
    Radiation
    Intrauterine device
    Glandular cells status posthysterectomy
    Atrophy
  Other
    Endometrial cells (in a woman >40 years of age)
Epithelial cell abnormalities
  Squamous cell
    ASC-US; cannot exclude HSIL (ASC-H)
    LSIL, encompassing HPV, mild dysplasia, CIN
    HSIL, encompassing moderate and severe dysplasia, CIN-2 and -3, CIS
    Squamous cell carcinoma
  Glandular cells
    Atypical (AGC)
      Endocervical cells
      Endometrial cells
      Glandular cells NOS
    Atypical, favor neoplastic
      Endocervical cells
      Glandular cells NOS
  Endocervical AIS
  Adenocarcinoma
    Endocervical
    Endometrial
    Extrauterine
    NOS
Other malignant neoplasms (specify)
Educational notes and suggestions (optional)

ASC-US, atypical squamous cells of undetermined significance; HSIL, high-grade squamous intraepithelial lesion; ASC-H, atypical squamous cells, cannot rule out a high-grade lesion; LSIL, low-grade squamous intraepithelial lesion; HPV, human papilloma virus; CIN, cervical intraepithelial neoplasia; CIS, carcinoma in situ; AGC, atypical glandular cells; NOS, not otherwise specified; AIS, adenocarcinoma in situ.

    c. Primary vaginal neoplasms are rare and far less common than cervical or vulvar neoplasms.

    d. Women with in utero exposure to diethylstilbestrol (DES) are at increased risk for clear cell adenocarcinoma of the vagina.

    e. Metastatic vaginal cancers arise from the urethra, Bartholin's gland, rectum, bladder, endometrial cavity, endocervix, kidney, or other distant site.

    f. Vaginal melanoma also occurs.

2. Clinical features

    a. Vulvar cancer more often is found in women who are obese and who have hypertension, diabetes mellitus, and arteriosclerosis. A history of chronic vulvar itching is common.

    b. Vulvar cancer in younger women is associated with HPV infection and smoking; 25% of patients have coexisting cervical carcinoma.

    c. Most vaginal intraepithelial neoplasms occur in the upper one-third of the vagina and are asymptomatic; the most common presenting problems are postmenopausal bleeding or bloody discharge.

    d. DES-exposed women may have vaginal adenosis and structural changes of the cervix, vagina, and upper genital tract, leading to increased risk of miscarriage, premature delivery, and ectopic pregnancy.

3. Laboratory studies

    a. Application of acetic acid or staining with toluidine blue may help to direct biopsies of suspicious vulvar lesions.

    b. Vaginal biopsy for suspected vaginal invasive neoplasm should be directed by colposcopy or Lugol staining.

    c. Clear cell adenocarcinoma is diagnosed by careful inspection and palpation of the vagina and cervix, followed by biopsies.

4. Treatment

    a. Local excision, topical 5-fluorouracil, and laser therapy are used for early vulvar lesions.

    b. Surgical excision is required for most vaginal neoplasms; primary vaginal cancer is treated with radiotherapy.

    c. For clear cell lesions, radical hysterectomy and vaginectomy or radiation therapy is effective.

VI. BREAST DISORDERS

A. Benign breast disorders

1. General characteristics

    a. Mastodynia (mastalgia), or breast tenderness, is common, often cyclical, and increases in women taking contraceptive pills or hormone replacement therapy.

    b. Mastitis, or breast infection, and breast abscesses most often are caused by *Staphylococcus aureus* and occur primarily, but rarely, in primigravid lactating women.

    c. Abscesses also may result from secondary infection of a galactocele.

    d. Fibrocystic changes (the most frequent benign condition of the breast) include cysts, papillomatosis, fibrosis, adenosis, and ductal epithelial hyperplasia.

    e. Fibroadenomas are the second most common benign breast disorder and occur in young women; they are more common in black women.

2. Clinical features

    a. Persistent, noncyclic breast pain suggests underlying cancer; cyclic pain suggests luteal phase tenderness.

    b. Mastitis and abscesses present with tenderness, heat, significant fever, chills, and other flu-like symptoms. Usually one quadrant or a lobule of one breast is affected.

    c. Fibroadenomas typically are round, firm, smooth, discrete, mobile, and nontender.

    d. Fibrocystic changes are most common in women 30 to 50 years of age and may present as asymptomatic masses or as painful and tender masses. Pain, size fluctuation, and multiple lesions distinguish fibrocystic changes from carcinoma.

3. Laboratory studies

    a. Mammography, ultrasonography, and biopsy may be indicated for breast complaints; however, young women's breasts usually are radiodense. Ultrasonography differentiates between solid and cystic masses.

    b. Because *Staphylococcus aureus* is present in approximately 50% of patients with mastitis, culture of purulent material or milk usually is not done.

    c. In suspected cysts, fine-needle aspiration is both diagnostic and therapeutic; cysts usually contain straw-colored fluid.

    d. In a woman younger than 25 years, a fibroadenomatous mass should be biopsied.

4. Treatment

   a. Treat mastodynia with reassurance, vitamin B_6, bromocriptine, tamoxifen, or danazol.

   b. Treat mastitis with a penicillinase-resistant antibiotic (cloxacillin, dicloxacillin, nafcillin) or a cephalosporin and hot compresses. Breast-feeding may continue, because the source is likely to be the infant's oropharynx.

   c. Surgical treatment may be required for abscesses or duct ectasia.

   d. Many types of fibrocystic breast problems need no treatment other than a supportive bra. Aspirate cysts and excise fibroadenomas.

   e. The role of caffeine restriction in the treatment of fibrocystic changes is controversial; some patients respond to low-salt diet, vitamin E supplementation, or hydrochlorothiazide premenstrually.

   f. Fibroadenomas may be excised or managed expectantly.

B. Breast neoplasms

   1. General characteristics

      a. Breast cancer is the most common female malignancy and the second leading cause of death from cancer in women.

      b. Most women with breast cancer have no identifiable risk factors other than female sex and increasing age (mean age at diagnosis, 60 to 61 years); *BRCA1* and *BRCA2* genes are associated with 5% to 10% of cases of breast cancer but appear in only 1% of the population.

      c. Associated factors include nulliparity, early menarche, late menopause, long-term estrogen or radiation exposure, and delayed childbearing.

      d. Women with first-degree relatives with breast cancer are at increased risk, especially if the cancer was premenopausal or bilateral or found in two of these relatives.

      e. Breast cancer increases the risk of endometrial cancer and vice versa.

      f. Ductal carcinomas account for 80% to 85% of breast cancers; the remainder are lobular carcinomas. Lobular CIS and atypical ductal hyperplasia predispose to cancer.

      g. Paget's disease is a ductal carcinoma presenting as an eczematous lesion of the nipple.

      h. All invasive lobular carcinomas and two-thirds of ductal carcinomas are estrogen-receptor positive.

   2. Clinical features

      a. Breast cancer most often presents as a single, nontender, firm, immobile mass; 45% occur in the upper outer quadrant and 25% under the nipple and areola.

      b. Early carcinoma may also appear with mammographic changes and no palpable masses.

      c. Rarer presentations include nipple discharge or retraction, dimpling, breast enlargement or shrinkage, skin thickening or peau d'orange skin, eczematous changes, breast pain, fixed mass, axillary node enlargement, ulcerations, arm edema, and palpable supraclavicular nodes.

   3. Diagnostic studies

      a. A combination of physical examination, mammography (the best screening tool), and fine-needle or sterotactic core-needle biopsy is highly accurate in establishing the diagnosis. Open biopsy may be required.

      b. Ultrasonography and excisional biopsy may be indicated. Biopsy specimen should undergo estrogen and progesterone receptor analysis as well as histologic analysis.

   4. Treatment

      a. Staging should occur before treatment begins.

      b. Breast conservation therapy (lumpectomy), modified radical mastectomy, and partial mastectomy have equivalent survival rates when surgery is followed by radiation therapy.

      c. Adjuvant chemotherapy and/or hormonal manipulation benefit some women.

      d. Tamoxifen is used to treat women with estrogen receptor–positive disease and postmenopausal women.

VII. CONTRACEPTIVE METHODS

A. Traditional methods

   1. Coitus interruptus, postcoital douching, and use of household wraps are ineffective and unreliable.

   2. Lactational amenorrhea may be effective in delaying conception for 6 months after birth if the woman breast-feeds exclusively and amenorrhea is maintained.

3. Periodic abstinence methods rely on abstinence from just before the time of ovulation until 2 to 3 days thereafter; pregnancy rates for these methods average 5 to 25 per 100 woman-years.

   a. Calendar methods predict the day of ovulation based on average menstrual patterns, are based on the relative constancy (14-day) of the luteal phase, and have a 35% failure rate.

   b. The basal body temperature method requires recording daily vaginal or rectal temperature before any activity is undertaken. A slight drop in temperature occurs 24 to 36 hours after ovulation, then rises by 0.3°C to 0.48°C, remaining at a plateau for the rest of the cycle.

   c. Combining the calendar and basal body temperature methods for contraception results in only 5 pregnancies per 100 couples per year.

   d. The cervical mucous method requires daily evaluation of the mucus; fertile mucus resembles egg white.

   e. The symptothermal method combines the cervical mucous and basal body temperature methods; it is probably the most reliable periodic abstinence method.

B. Oral hormonal contraceptives are the most effective reversible means of pregnancy prevention.

   1. All oral contraceptives contain synthetic steroids (similar to natural estrogens and progestins) used in doses and combinations that inhibit ovulation.

      a. The estrogen component is usually ethinyl estradiol or mestranol.

      b. The progestin component is one of the 19-nortestosterones, including norethindrone acetate, norethindrone, levonorgestrel, ethynodiol diacetate, desogestrel, norgestimate, DL-norgestrel, gestodene, and drospirenone.

   2. Use of combined estrogen–progestin pills begins with the onset of menses or the following Sunday; active pills are taken for 21 days, followed by 7 days of no pills or placebos. A newer method allows for 84 days of active pills; this results in limiting menses to four times per year. Theoretical failure rate for combination pills is less than 1%; actual rates are 4% to 6%

   3. Withdrawal bleeding begins within 3 to 5 days of the last active pill.

   4. Minipills (progestin only) are half as effective as combination pills and may cause amenorrhea. They are most useful in lactating woman and in those older than 40 years.

   5. Noncontraceptive advantages

      a. Less benign breast disease, iron deficiency anemia, and pelvic inflammatory disease as well as fewer ovarian cysts.

      b. Protection against ectopic pregnancy; reduced risk of ovarian and endometrial cancer; reduced dysmenorrhea and menorrhagia; and improvements in hirsutism, acne, and symptoms of endometriosis. Oral contraceptives also may protect against rheumatoid arthritis.

   6. Disadvantages

      a. Increased risk of thromboembolic disease, particularly in smokers, and abnormal lipids.

      b. Possible increased risk of breast cancer and, rarely, hypertension, cholelithiasis, and benign liver tumors.

   7. Adverse effects

      a. Missed periods, intermenstrual bleeding, bloating, acne, nausea, headaches, and weight gain.

      b. Most of these problems resolve within the first few months of use and are rare with current low-dose formulations.

C. Injected, implanted, and transdermal hormonal contraceptives

   1. Intramuscular (IM) injection of a depot formulation of synthetic sex hormones may be pure progestin or a combination of progestin and estrogen; both inhibit anterior pituitary function.

      a. The most common is medroxyprogesterone acetate, 150 mg every 90 days.

      b. The failure rate is 0.3% in the first year.

      c. Fertility rates return to normal within 18 months of discontinuation.

   2. The Norplant system relies on the implantation of six rods that release levonorgestrel. Efficacy is very good, but side effects are common, including menstrual irregularity, headache, and weight gain.

   3. The transdermal patch is applied once a month. It is not effective in women who weigh more than 200 lbs.

   4. A hormone-impregnated vaginal ring is inserted for 3 weeks and then removed for 1 week; withdrawal bleeding should occur.

D. IUDs

   1. The mechanism of action is unknown, but leukocyte aggregation may produce an environment that is hostile to a fertilized ovum.

2. Two devices currently are available in the United States.
   a. Progestasert (usable for 1 year)
   b. Copper T (usable for 10 years)
3. Failure rates are less than 1% per year for copper T and 1% to 1.5% for Progestasert.
4. IUDs usually are inserted during menses.
5. Disadvantages and adverse effects include uterine perforation; higher incidence of spontaneous abortion if pregnancy occurs; increased risk of ectopic pregnancy, cramping, or bleeding with menses; and risk of pelvic infection.
6. Absolute contraindications include current pregnancy, undiagnosed vaginal bleeding, acute infection, past salpingitis, and suspected gynecologic malignancy.
7. Relative contraindications include nulliparity, previous ectopic pregnancy or sexually transmitted disease, multiple sexual partners, severe dysmenorrhea, uterine abnormalities, anemia, valvular heart disease, and young age.

E. Barrier methods include the male and female condoms, cervical caps, and diaphragms, which provide some additional protection against sexually transmitted infections. The common spermicides are nonoxynol-9 and octoxynol-3.

F. Emergency (postcoital) contraception is provided by high-dose estrogen–progestin or progestin-only tablets given within 72 hours of unprotected intercourse. It may be effective up to 5 days after unprotected intercourse. Nausea and vomiting is a frequent adverse effect of the former. Another method is postcoital insertion of an IUD.

G. Other methods of controlling fertility include induced abortion and sterilization.

VIII. INFERTILITY

A. General characteristics
   1. Infertility generally is defined as a failure to conceive after 1 year of unprotected intercourse. Surveys estimate that up to 15% of reproductive-age couples in the United States are infertile. Prevalence ranges from 7% to 28%, increasing as a woman ages.
   2. Female factors include ovulatory (central, peripheral, metabolic), pelvic (infection, structural, endometriosis), and cervical (congenital, acquired) causes.
   3. Male factors include endocrine and anatomic disorders, abnormal spermatogenesis or motility, and sexual dysfunction.

B. Clinical examination typically is normal.

C. Laboratory studies
   1. Semen analysis should precede any other testing as a normal analysis excludes most male factors.
   2. Basal body temperature, ovulation prediction tests, and progesterone levels confirm ovulation.
   3. Luteal phase endometrial biopsy, FSH levels, prolactin, and thyroid-stimulating hormone tests may be helpful.
   4. Postcoital testing measures sperm survival.
   5. Hysterosalpingography determines tubal patency and uterine abnormalities.
   6. Other tests that may be useful include laparoscopy, sperm penetration assay, sperm antibody testing, ultrasonography, and hysteroscopy.

D. Treatments currently have an overall success rate of about 85%.
   1. Clomiphene citrate, 50 to 100 mg for 5 days beginning on day 3, 4, or 5 of the cycle, should be given to anovulatory women to promote ovulation.
   2. Artificial insemination is an alternative for couples with abnormal postcoital tests.
   3. Other treatments depend on the cause of the infertility, the couple's resources, and the age of the woman.
   4. Assisted reproductive technologies include in vitro fertilization, gamete intrafallopian transfer, zygote intrafallopian transfer, and surrogate options.

IX. PELVIC INFLAMMATORY DISEASE

A. General characteristics
   1. Pelvic inflammatory disease includes acute salpingitis (gonococcal or nongonococcal), IUD-related pelvic cellulitis, tubo-ovarian abscess, and pelvic abscess.
   2. It usually is polymicrobial (mixed aerobic and anaerobic). Most are bacterial, but viral, fungal, or parasitic causes are known.
   3. Complications include infertility and ectopic pregnancy.

B. Clinical features

1. Lower abdominal and pelvic pain typically is bilateral. Nausea (with or without vomiting), headache, and lassitude are common. Fever may or may not be present.

2. Examination reveals lower abdominal and pelvic pain and cervical motion tenderness (chandelier sign). Purulent discharge and inflammation of Bartholin's or Skene's glands may be present.

3. An adnexal mass may indicate a tubo-ovarian abscess.

C. Laboratory studies

1. DNA probes for gonorrhea and chlamydia have largely replaced Gram staining and culture of any discharge.

2. Transvaginal ultrasonography is helpful in differentiating acute and chronic inflammation or the presence of adnexal masses.

3. Diagnostic culdocentesis or laparoscopy may be required.

D. Treatment

1. Women with mild disease can be treated as outpatients with antibiotics, antipyretics, analgesics, and bed rest; if present, an IUD should be removed.

2. Women with severe disease should be hospitalized for IV antibiotic therapy and possible surgery.

3. Sex partners should be evaluated and treated.

Obstetrics

Lori Parlin Palfreyman

8

I. ROUTINE PRENATAL CARE AND PRENATAL DIAGNOSTIC TESTING

A. Routine prenatal care

1. General characteristics

a. An initial obstetric history includes subjective symptoms and signs (Table 8-1) of pregnancy as well as the patient's general medical, obstetric, and family history (Table 8-2).

b. The due date or expected date of confinement (EDC) can be calculated using the Nägele's or McDonald's rule: Start at the first day of last menstrual period (LMP), go back 3 months and add 7 days. For example, if the LMP is January 15, go back 3 months to October 15, and add 7 days, making the EDC October 22. This is based on a 28-day menstrual cycle and must be adjusted for shorter or longer cycles.

c. The patient's obstetric history can be expressed as gravida (G; number of total pregnancies) and parity (P; number of deliveries). The parity is denoted as a sequence of four digits (P_ _ _ _) signifying the number of term infants (37 to 42 weeks of gestation), premature deliveries (20 to 36 weeks of gestation), abortions (therapeutic and/or spontaneous, occurring before 20 weeks of gestation), and living children.

d. The initial visit should take place 6 to 8 weeks after the LMP. Generally, a woman is examined every 4 weeks until the 28th week of gestation, every 2 to 3 weeks up to 36 weeks of gestation, and then weekly thereafter.

e. After the initial visit, each subsequent prenatal visit includes a focused history and examination, including assessment of general health, diet, activity, compliance with vitamins, maternal weight gain, edema, fetal movement, and blood pressure; check of fundal height starting at 20 weeks' gestation and fetal heart tones starting at 10 weeks' gestation; and a urinalysis for glucosuria and proteinuria. Vaginal examination to assess cervical dilation is added after 37 weeks or as indicated.

2. Clinical features

a. Uterine growth throughout pregnancy (Fig. 8-1)

(1) At 20 weeks, the fundus is at the umbilicus.

(2) From 21 weeks on, the height of the uterine fundus should correlate roughly to the number of weeks of gestation.

b. Fetal heart tones can be appreciated beginning at 10 to 12 weeks using a handheld Doppler; normal fetal heart rate is 120 to 160 bpm.

c. Quickening, or the first awareness of fetal movement, usually occurs at 18 to 20 weeks in a primigravida and as early as 14 to 18 weeks in a multigravida.

d. Common complaints, such as backache, increasing varicosities, heartburn, hemorrhoids, and fatigue, can be associated with an otherwise healthy pregnancy.

B. Laboratory and prenatal screening and diagnostic testing

1. Table 8-3 lists the most common laboratory and prenatal testing by gestational age. All women should be offered screening tests regardless of maternal age.

2. First-trimester screening and diagnostic testing

a. Maternal blood levels of pregnancy-associated plasma protein A (PAPP-A) and free β-human chorionic gonadotropin (free β-hCG): Abnormally low PAPP-A and abnormally high free β-hCG indicate increased risk of trisomy 21 and other genetic disorders.

b. Ultrasound for establishing or confirming EDC and detecting multiple gestations: Ultrasound can detect fetal heart activity as early as 5 to 6 weeks after the LMP.

c. Nuchal translucency screening test (also known as a nuchal fold scan)

(1) Ultrasound measurement of the nuchal space is performed at 10 to 13 weeks. It screens for trisomies 13, 18, and 21 as well as for Turner's syndrome.

(2) Indications for nuchal translucency screening are listed in Table 8-4.

(3) If an abnormally wide measurement for gestational age is detected, chorionic villus sampling (CVS) or amniocentesis is offered.

(4) The combination of nuchal translucency measurement and PAPP-A and β-hCG screening can detect 82% to 87% of trisomy 21 disorders.

TABLE 8-1	**Manifestations of Pregnancy**

Symptoms
  Amenorrhea
  Nausea/vomiting
  Breast tenderness
  Quickening (fetal movement)
    Nullipara: 18–20 weeks
    Multipara: 14–16 weeks
  Easy fatigability
  Urinary frequency, nocturia, infection

Signs
  Chadwick's sign (bluish discoloration of vagina and cervix)
  Increased basal body temperature
  Skin changes
    Melasma/chloasma (dark patches on face)
    Linea nigra
  Positive pregnancy test
  Hagar's sign (softening between fundus and cervix)
  Uterine growth
    12 weeks: at symphysis pubis
    16 weeks: midway between pubis and umbilicus
    20 weeks: at umbilicus
    After 20 weeks: 1 cm for every week of gestation
  Fetal heart tones
  Palpation of fetus
  Ultrasonography of fetus

TABLE 8-2	**Patient History on Initial Prenatal Office Visit**

Menstrual history
  Last menstrual period

Present pregnancy
  See Table 8-1

Previous pregnancies
  Vaginal vs. cesarean section
  Complications
  Size of baby, Apgar scores

Medical history
  Cardiovascular
  Asthma
  Systemic lupus erythematosus
  Bleeding disorders
  Seizure disorders

Surgical history
  Abdominal surgery
  Pelvic surgery

Family history
  Chromosomal abnormalities
  Mental retardation
  Diabetes

Social history
  Alcohol
  Drugs
  Diet

Adapted from DeCherney AH, Nathan L. *Current Diagnosis and Treatment Obstetrics and Gynecology.* 10th ed. New York: McGraw-Hill Companies; 2007.

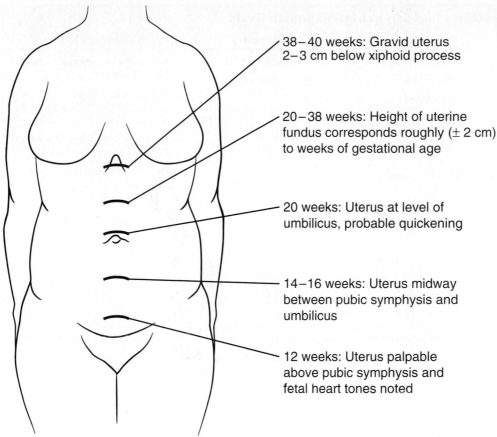

FIGURE 8-1 Uterine size and position throughout gestation.

38–40 weeks: Gravid uterus 2–3 cm below xiphoid process

20–38 weeks: Height of uterine fundus corresponds roughly (± 2 cm) to weeks of gestational age

20 weeks: Uterus at level of umbilicus, probable quickening

14–16 weeks: Uterus midway between pubic symphysis and umbilicus

12 weeks: Uterus palpable above pubic symphysis and fetal heart tones noted

  d. Chorionic villus sampling
  (1) CVS is performed between 10 and 13 weeks; a catheter or needle is used to biopsy placental cells.
  (2) Indications for CVS are listed in Table 8-4.
  (3) The advantage of CVS is its ability to be performed during the first trimester, allowing the option of a first-trimester termination if a major malformation is detected. Also, preliminary results are available within 48 hours after the procedure. CVS is considered a diagnostic not screening test.
  (4) The disadvantage of CVS is that, unlike amniocentesis, CVS specimens cannot be used in α-fetoprotein (AFP) testing for neural tube defects. Also, the risk of spontaneous abortion after CVS is slightly higher than that after amniocentesis (0.5% to 1% vs. 0.25% to 0.5%).
3. Second-trimester screening and diagnostic testing
  a. Maternal serum levels of unconjugated estriol, AFP (a major circulating protein of the early fetus), and inhibin A: Abnormally low unconjugated estriol and AFP and abnormally high inhibin A indicate increased risk of trisomy 21 and other genetic disorders.
  (1) Abnormally high levels of AFP indicate increased risk for neural tube defects. AFP can detect up to 75% to 85% of open neural tube defects, such as spina bifida and anencephaly.
  (2) Combining the first-trimester maternal serum blood tests with second-trimester maternal serum blood tests can detect 94% to 96% of trisomy 21 disorders.
  b. Ultrasound is an accurate modality checking for fetal viability, correlating appropriate growth in relation to gestational age, checking for placental status and location, and checking amniotic fluid level.
  (1) It also can be used to help detect lethal malformations and as a follow-up to abnormal prenatal blood work screening tests.

TABLE 8-3	Prenatal Laboratories and Screening/Diagnostic Tests			
1st Prenatal Visit	**First Trimester**	**Second Trimester**	**Third Trimester**
CBC	PAPP-A	Unconjugated estriol	Screen for gestational diabetes (24–28 weeks)
Blood type and Rh	Free β-hCG	Maternal serum AFP	
Rubella titer	Ultrasound	Inhibin A	In unsensitized Rh patients, repeat antibody titers (followed by Rh immunoglobulin) (28 weeks)
Hepatitis B serum antigen	Nuchal translucency (10–13 weeks)	Ultrasound	
Cultures for chlamydia and gonorrhea, as needed		Amniocentesis (15–18 weeks)	Vaginal–rectal culture for group B streptococci (35 weeks)
Offer all women HIV testing	CVS (10–13 weeks)		Hemoglobin and hematocrit (35 weeks)
Offer all couples screening for cystic fibrosis, sickle cell, other conditions per maternal and paternal history			NST
Urinalysis			Ultrasound
Coombs' test (irregular antibody screen)			Biophysical profile
Serologic testing for syphilis			
Pap smear			

CBC, complete blood count; PAPP-A, pregnancy-associated plasma protein A; β-hCG, β-human chorionic gondatropin; AFP, α-fetoprotein; CVS, chorionic villi sampling; NST, nonstress test.
Suggestions from the American College of Obstetricians and Gynecologists. ACOG Practice Bulletin. Clinical management guidelines for obstetrician gynecologists. *Obstet Gynecol.* 2007;109(1):217–226.

   c. Amniocentesis involves the withdrawal of amniotic fluid via needle under ultrasound guidance for prenatal diagnosis.

     (1) It is usually performed between 15 and 18 weeks of gestation.

     (2) Indications for amniocentesis are listed in Table 8-4.

     (3) There is a lower risk of spontaneous abortion following second-trimester amniocentesis than following first-trimester CVS (0.25% to 0.5% vs. 0.5% to 1%). Also, amniocentesis can offer a wider array of genetic testing.

     (4) The disadvantage of amniocentesis is that it is performed during the second trimester; therefore, if termination of the pregnancy is chosen, a more complicated procedure is involved. Also, results from the test are not available for a minimum of 7 days.

  4. Third-trimester screening for fetal well-being

    a. External Doppler monitor, along with an external stress gauge for uterine contractions (together called the nonstress test [NST]), is used near term to monitor fetal well-being. It also is used to assess risks for those with preexisting maternal conditions and pregnancies with complications.

     (1) Baseline fetal heart rate is 120 to 160 bpm.

TABLE 8-4	Indications for Nuchal Translucency Screening, Chorionic Villus Sampling, or Amniocentesis
Maternal age of 35 years or older
Previous child with chromosomal abnormality
Patient or father of baby with chromosomal anomaly
Family history of chromosomal anomaly
Neural tube defect risk (amniocentesis only)
Abnormal first-trimester or second-trimester maternal serum screening tests

(2) A normal (reactive) NST requires two accelerations of fetal heart rate in 20 minutes of up to 15 bpm from the baseline heart rate for a duration of 15 seconds and the absence of decelerations.

(3) Contractions usually decrease the flow of blood to the placenta. This is poorly tolerated by the stressed fetus and leads to hypoxia and concomitant relative bradycardia.

(4) Decelerations are defined as a decline in fetal heart rate of 15 bpm or lasting more than 15 seconds or a slow return to baseline. Persistent late decelerations, which begin *after* the peak of the contraction, are nonreassuring and warrant intervention.

b. Ultrasonography is used late in pregnancy to monitor fetal well-being in the form of a scored examination (biophysical profile [BPP]).

(1) The BPP examines five parameters including NST, amniotic fluid level, gross fetal movements, fetal tone, and fetal breathing.

(2) Each parameter has a maximum of 2 points; a total of 10 points is possible.

II. COMPLICATIONS OF PREGNANCY

A. Ectopic pregnancy

1. General characteristics

   a. Ectopic pregnancy is the implantation of a pregnancy anywhere but the endometrium.

   b. More than 95% of ectopic pregnancies occur in the fallopian tube, and 55% of tubal pregnancies occur in the ampulla of the tube.

   c. The most common cause of ectopic pregnancy is occlusion of the tube secondary to adhesions.

   d. The most common risk factors for ectopic pregnancy include a history of a previous ectopic pregnancy, previous salpingitis (caused by pelvic inflammatory disease), previous abdominal or tubal surgery, use of an intrauterine device, and assisted reproduction.

2. Clinical features

   a. The presentation of ectopic pregnancy is widely variable and may depend on the site of implantation.

   b. The classic presentation includes unilateral adnexal pain, amenorrhea or spotting, and tenderness or mass on pelvic examination (Table 8-5). Other symptoms may include dizziness or syncope as well as gastrointestinal (GI) distress.

   c. Signs and symptoms associated with a ruptured ectopic pregnancy are severe abdominal or shoulder pain associated with peritonitis, tachycardia, syncope, and orthostatic hypotension.

3. Laboratory studies

   a. Serum levels of hCG normally double every 48 hours. If serial increases of hCG are less than expected, ectopic gestation should be suspected until the diagnosis has been definitively excluded.

   b. Transvaginal ultrasonography is diagnostic in 90% of cases of ectopic gestation.

   c. Women with an hCG titer of greater than 1,500 mU/mL should show evidence of a developing intrauterine gestation on transvaginal ultrasound. If no such evidence is found, ectopic pregnancy is the clinical diagnosis.

TABLE 8-5	Signs and Symptoms Associated with Ectopic Pregnancy
Signs/Symptoms	**% of Cases**
Pain	80
Abnormal menstruation	75
Tachycardia, hypotension	75
Pelvic mass	30–50
Dizziness or syncope	30–50
Shock	10
Gastrointestinal symptoms	Often

Adapted from McPhee SJ, Papadakis MA. *Current Medical Diagnosis and Treatment*. 48th ed. New York: McGraw-Hill Companies; 2009; and DeCherney AH, Nathan L. *Current Diagnosis and Treatment Obstetrics and Gynecology*. 10th ed. New York: McGraw-Hill Companies; 2007.

4. Treatment

   a. Medical treatment with methotrexate, a folic acid analog, can be used to treat up to 80% of ectopic gestations when diagnosed early. Criteria for methotrexate treatment include a serum hCG titer of less than 5,000 mU, ectopic mass less than 3.5 cm on ultrasound, a patient who is hemodynamically stable, and a patient who is deemed to be compliant for follow-up.

   b. Surgical treatment involves removal of the ectopic gestation using laparoscopy or laparotomy.

      (1) Laparoscopy is the preferred method.

      (2) Laparotomy usually is reserved for patients with known significant abdominal adhesions or those who are clinically unstable.

   c. Follow-up testing using serum hCG levels or pelvic examination is crucial to exclude any remaining evidence of pregnancy.

B. Spontaneous abortion

   1. General characteristics

      a. Abortion is the termination of pregnancy, by any means, before 20 weeks of gestation.

      b. Spontaneous abortion is the spontaneous, premature expulsion of the products of conception; it occurs in up to 15% to 20% of clinically recognized pregnancies.

      c. Eighty percent of spontaneous abortions occur during the first trimester of pregnancy; of these, up to 50% are associated with chromosomal abnormalities.

      d. Possible maternal factors that increase the risk of spontaneous abortion include smoking, infection, maternal systemic disease, immunologic parameters, and drug use.

   2. Clinical features

      a. Table 8-6 indicates the various classifications of spontaneous abortion.

      b. Bleeding is variable on examination.

      c. Uterine size often does not correlate appropriately to the LMP, and the fundus of the uterus may be boggy or tender.

   3. Laboratory studies

      a. Serial hCG titers, serum progesterone, or serial ultrasonography may be required to confirm a viable pregnancy.

      b. Ultrasound findings in a nonviable pregnancy may include inappropriate development or interval growth, poorly formed or unformed fetal pole, and fetal demise.

      c. Blood type and Rh status are necessary tests to preclude Rh sensitization in the mother.

   4. Treatment

      a. If the pregnancy has been definitively determined to be no longer viable, the uterus must be emptied.

      b. If the pregnancy is early and the patient is managed expectantly (allow the products of conception to pass naturally), careful follow-up with pelvic examinations, serial hCG titers, and transvaginal ultrasonography can be used to determine whether the abortion is complete.

      c. Dilation and curettage also may be necessary to ensure complete emptying of the uterus or as one form of induced abortion. Morbidity is caused by uterine perforation or cervical laceration.

TABLE 8-6	Classification of Spontaneous Abortions[a]		
Type	Vaginal Bleeding	Cervix Open	Products of Conception Passed
Threatened	Yes	No	No
Inevitable	Yes	Yes	Not yet, but no way to maintain pregnancy
Incomplete	Yes	Yes	Partial
Complete	Yes	Yes	Yes
Missed	No	No	No (fetal demise has occurred without symptoms)

[a]Three or more consecutive abortions is classified as recurrent, and any abortion with associated sepsis is classified as septic.

d. Immunoglobulin should be administered to Rh-negative women in the event of either an elective or spontaneous abortion.

e. Septic or infected abortion requires complete evacuation of the uterine contents, medical support, and antibiotics.

C. Gestational trophoblastic disease (GTD)

1. General characteristics

a. GTD is a spectrum of diseases arising from the placenta and includes complete and partial hydatidiform moles, placental site invasive moles, trophoblastic tumors, and choriocarcinomas.

b. GTD is divided into benign and malignant forms. A hydatidiform mole (also called a molar pregnancy) is the benign form of GTD.

2. Hydatidiform moles are divided into complete and incomplete molar pregnancies. Complete molar pregnancies are the most common form of GTD.

a. Complete hydatidiform moles are characterized by an empty egg and the appearance of "grapelike vesicles" or a "snowstorm pattern" on ultrasound. Approximately 20% progress to malignancy.

b. Partial hydatidiform moles have a fetus present, but the fetus is nonviable. Less than 5% progress to malignancy.

3. Clinical features: A complete or partial molar pregnancy most commonly presents with abnormal vaginal bleeding, uterine size greater than dates, hyperemesis gravidarum, or preeclampsia-like symptoms before 20 weeks of gestation.

4. Laboratory studies

a. With complete molar pregnancy, the hCG level often is greater than 100,000 mU/mL. Persistently elevated levels of hCG may indicate gestational trophoblastic tumor.

b. Ultrasonography of a complete hydatidiform mole shows a characteristic "grape-like vesicles" or "snowstorm" appearance consistent with the swelling of the chorionic villi. Ultrasonography may aid in establishing the diagnosis of a partial molar pregnancy.

5. Treatment

a. Treatment depends on tumor classification. Benign tumors and low-risk metastatic tumors can be treated with chemotherapy. Metastatic high-risk tumors require a combination of chemotherapy with or without adjuvant radiation and surgery.

b. Surgical treatment includes suction curettage (for those desiring to preserve fertility) and hysterectomy. These treatments all carry high cure rates of 80% to 100%.

c. After evacuation, patients must be monitored with serial hCG to assure return to baseline and to diagnose and manage sequelae properly. Contraception is recommended for 6 to 12 months after remission.

D. Multiple gestation

1. General characteristics

a. The overall incidence of multiple births in the United States is 3% and has been increasing during the past 30 years, in part as a result of the use of assisted reproductive techniques and ovulation induction. Twins occur in 1 out of every 80 births.

b. With multiple gestations, all the same symptoms of pregnancy generally occur, but they often are more severe. Prenatal visits should occur more frequently than with single gestations.

c. Types

(1) Two-thirds of twins are dizygotic, or fraternal (i.e., formed by the fertilization of two ova). The incidence of dizygotic twins is increased in those with a family history of twins, those taking fertility drugs, mothers with above-average weight and height, and African American women.

(2) Monozygotic twins (i.e., those formed from the fertilization of one ovum) occur randomly and are associated with fetal transfusion syndrome and discordant fetal growth.

d. Maternal complications

(1) The most common complications of multiple gestation are spontaneous abortion and preterm birth.

(2) Other problems that occur with greater frequency are preeclampsia and anemia.

e. Fetal complications include intrauterine growth restriction, cord accidents, death of one twin, congenital anomalies, abnormal or breech presentation, and placental abruption or previa.

E. Gestational diabetes

1. General characteristics

 a. Gestational diabetes mellitus is carbohydrate intolerance of variable severity that is only present during pregnancy.

 b. The lifetime risk of developing diabetes after pregnancy in women who have had gestational diabetes is increased to greater than 50% (vs. 5% in the general population). If insulin is required during the pregnancy, there is a 50% risk of developing diabetes within 5 years from the pregnancy.

 c. Recurrence of gestational diabetes is common, occurring in 60% to 90% of subsequent pregnancies.

 d. Maternal complications associated with gestational diabetes mellitus include preeclampsia, hyperacceleration of general diabetic complications, and traumatic birth, including shoulder dystocia.

 e. Fetal complications associated with gestational diabetes mellitus include macrosomia, prematurity, fetal demise, and delayed fetal lung maturity.

2. Clinical features

 a. Patients with gestational diabetes usually are asymptomatic.

 b. Risk factors for the development of gestational diabetes include a history of a previous large-for-gestational-age infant, obesity, age older than 25 years, glucosuria, a family history of diabetes, or being a member of the following ethnic groups: African American, Asian, Hispanic, or American Indian.

3. Laboratory studies

 a. Screening recommendations

 (1) Screen high-risk women during the first prenatal visit to check for preexisting diabetes, then conduct a repeat screening at 24 to 28 weeks.

 (2) All other women should be screened at 24 to 28 weeks.

 (3) Screening consists of administering a nonfasting 50-g glucose challenge test, followed by a serum glucose level 1 hour later. If the 1-hour serum glucose value is greater than 130 mg/dL, a 3-hour glucose tolerance test is performed. Glycosylated hemoglobin (HgbA1c) is not recommended as a screening method in gestational diabetes.

 (4) The 3-hour glucose tolerance test consists of a 100-g glucose load in the morning after an overnight fast. Serum glucose levels are taken at fasting and then at 1, 2, and 3 hours after the glucose load. If two or more of the values are abnormal, the patient is diagnosed with gestational diabetes (Table 8-7).

 b. Antepartum testing using BPPs and NSTs often is used in gestational diabetes beginning at 34 weeks of gestation.

 c. Women who have had gestational diabetes should be screened at 6 weeks postpartum for diabetes and at yearly intervals thereafter.

4. Treatment

 a. Careful management of gestational diabetes with diet and exercise is essential.

 b. Patients with gestational diabetes must check their blood glucose levels after fasting overnight and after each meal. At each office visit, the patient's home glucose levels should be reviewed, and if necessary, a fasting or a 2-hour postprandial blood glucose measurement should be done during the office visit.

 c. Patients who have fasting blood glucose measurements of greater than 105 mg/dL or 2-hour postprandial blood sugar measurements of greater than 120 mg/dL may require insulin. Oral hypoglycemic agents are not used.

TABLE 8-7	Diagnosis of Gestational Diabetes Mellitus with a 100-g Oral Glucose Load[a]	
Test	**Results (mg/dL)**	
Fasting	95	
1 hr	180	
2 hr	155	
3 hr	140	

Adapted from McPhee S, Papadakis MA. *Current Medical Diagnosis and Treatment.* 48th ed. New York: McGraw-Hill Companies; 2009.

[a]Two or more of the venous plasma concentrations must be met or exceeded for a positive diagnosis. The test should be done in the morning after an overnight fast of between 8 and 14 hr and after at least 3 days of unrestricted diet and unlimited physical activity.

    d. To help avoid the development of diabetes later in life, the patient should be advised to obtain and maintain ideal body weight. Annual evaluations of fasting glucose concentrations are recommended.

F. Preterm labor and delivery

  1. General characteristics

    a. Preterm delivery is the delivery of a viable infant before 37 weeks gestation and occurs in 8% to 10% of births.

    b. Preterm delivery is the most common cause of neonatal deaths not resulting from congenital malformations.

    c. Low-birth-weight infants born prematurely often have significant developmental delays, cerebral palsy, and lung disease.

    d. The cause of preterm labor is poorly understood. Risk factors include smoking, cocaine use, uterine malformations, cervical incompetence, infection (vaginal group B streptococci or urinary tract infection), and low prepregnancy weight.

    e. Complications of maternal or fetal health, such as hypertension, diabetes mellitus, infection, premature rupture of membranes, or abruptio placentae, are associated with preterm delivery.

  2. Clinical features

    a. Preterm labor is defined as regular uterine contractions (>4 to 6/hr) between 20 and 36 weeks of gestation and the presence of one or more of the following signs:

      (1) Cervical dilatation of 2 cm or greater at presentation

      (2) Cervical dilatation of 1 cm or greater on serial examinations

      (3) Cervical effacement of greater than 80%

    b. Late symptoms of preterm labor include painful or painless contractions, pressure, menstrual-like cramps, watery or bloody discharge, and low back pain.

  3. Laboratory studies

    a. Ultrasonography is sometimes used to examine the length of the cervix.

    b. Examination of the cervicovaginal secretions for fetal fibronectin, a glycoprotein, has been used as a marker for preterm labor. Its absence has a negative predictive value of 93% to 97% for delivery within 7 to 14 days.

    c. Vaginal cultures and urinalysis with culture and sensitivity also should be obtained.

  4. Treatment

    a. Management techniques include bed rest, oral or intravenous (IV) hydration, antibiotics to treat subclinical infection, steroids administered to the mother to enhance fetal lung maturity, and tocolytics, if indicated.

    b. Tocolytics are used in an attempt to stop contractions.

      (1) Magnesium sulfate ($MgSO_4$) inhibits myometrial contractility mediated by calcium. Side effects include nausea, fatigue, and generalized muscle weakness.

        (a) $MgSO_4$ can lead to decreased reflexes, respiratory depression, and cardiac collapse.

        (b) In the case of $MgSO_4$ toxicity, calcium gluconate can be given.

      (2) β-Mimetic adrenergic agents, including ridodrine and terbutaline, stimulate β-receptors to relax smooth muscle to decrease uterine contractions. Side effects include maternal and fetal tachycardia, emesis, headaches, and pulmonary edema.

      (3) Calcium channel blockers inhibit smooth muscle contractility by decreasing intracellular Ca^{2+} ions, which therefore relax uterine muscle. Side effects include maternal hypotension and tachycardia.

    c. The goal in treatment of these patients is to identify those at risk and to diagnose the condition before labor is irreversibly established. Cervical cerclage (i.e., closure of cervix by mechanical means) is an option for women with known cervical incompetence or a history of preterm birth.

  5. Prevention: For women with a history of preterm delivery, weekly injections of 17α-hydroxyprogesterone caproate from 16 to 36 weeks gestation can substantially reduce the rate of recurrent preterm birth.

G. Premature rupture of membranes (PROM) and preterm premature rupture of membranes (PPROM)

  1. General characteristics

    a. PROM is rupture of the amniotic membranes before the onset of labor at or beyond 37 weeks of gestation, and it occurs in approximately 8% of all pregnancies. Most women (90%) will go into spontaneous labor within 24 hours after PROM.

    b. PPROM occurs before 37 weeks of gestation and precedes 30% to 40% of all preterm deliveries.

    c. The major risk associated with both PROM and PPROM is infection (chorioamnionitis and endometritis). This risk increases with time and hastens delivery.

    d. Cord prolapse also can occur with ruptured membranes if the head is not well engaged.

2. Clinical features

    a. Symptoms of ruptured membranes are a gush or persistent leakage of fluid from the vagina, vaginal discharge, and, occasionally, simply pelvic pressure.

    b. Ruptured membranes can be confirmed with direct visualization of pooling using a sterile speculum, use of nitrazine paper, and the fern test. Ultrasonography can be used to check the amniotic fluid index.

    c. Digital examination should be avoided unless delivery is imminent.

    d. Cord prolapse is identified as a ropelike, soft, elongated mass on speculum or bimanual examination.

3. Treatment

    a. PROM (after 37 weeks)

      (1) If expectant management is feasible, the patient should be hospitalized and the fetus carefully monitored.

      (2) Active management of PROM involves induction with prostaglandin cervical gel or oxytocin. The goal of this treatment is to expedite delivery to decrease rates of infection.

    b. PPROM (20 to 36 weeks)

      (1) If there is no sign of maternal or fetal infection or distress, expectant management is preferred. The patient should be admitted to the hospital and put on strict bed rest.

      (2) If under 34 weeks of gestation, steroids (betamethasone) should be administered to enhance fetal lung maturity.

      (3) Antibiotics often are administered to prevent infection and help prolong the pregnancy, because they have been shown to decrease infant mortality.

      (4) NST and BPP should be performed daily to assess fetal well-being.

      (5) Amniocentesis can be performed to check for lung maturity.

      (6) If there is any indication of maternal or fetal infection or distress, delivery of the fetus is warranted.

H. Hypertension in pregnancy

1. Chronic hypertension is hypertension that presents before 20 weeks gestation.

2. Pregnancy-induced hypertension (PIH) is hypertension that presents after 20 weeks gestation but has no other associated symptoms.

    a. Chronic hypertension and PIH are treated in the same manner: monthly ultrasonography to check for intrauterine growth retardation, serial blood pressure and urine protein, and weekly NST during the third trimester.

    b. The basic underlying pathophysiology of PIH is thought to be vasospasm or arteriolar constriction.

    c. Medication for chronic hypertension and PIH is only given in severe cases. Methyldopa is the treatment of choice, with labetalol as an alternative.

3. Preeclampsia/eclampsia

    a. General characteristics

      (1) To be diagnosed as preeclampsia/eclampsia, the symptoms must occur after 20 weeks gestation. It most often occurs near term but can occur up to 6 weeks postpartum.

      (2) Preeclampsia is the classic triad of hypertension, edema, and proteinuria, but edema is no longer necessary for the diagnosis. Preeclampsia is categorized into mild or severe preeclampsia (Table 8-8).

      (3) HELLP syndrome is the presence of severe preeclampsia with the addition of **H**emolysis, **E**levated **L**iver enzymes, and **L**ow **P**latelets.

      (4) Eclampsia is severe preeclampsia with the addition of seizures.

      (5) The most common risk factor for preeclampsia is nulliparity. Other risk factors include extremes of age (<20 or >35 years), multiple gestation, diabetes, and chronic hypertension.

      (6) Maternal complications of preeclampsia include progression to eclampsia or HELLP syndrome, abruptio placentae, renal failure, cerebral hemorrhage, pulmonary edema, and disseminated intravascular coagulation.

      (7) Fetal complications include hypoxia, low birth weight, preterm delivery, and perinatal death.

TABLE 8-8	Classification of Mild vs. Severe Preeclampsia	
	Mild Preeclampsia	**Severe Preeclampsia**
Blood pressure	>140/90 mm Hg but <160/110 mm Hg, *or* increase of 30 mm Hg systolic and 15 mm Hg diastolic from prepregnancy blood pressure on at least two occasions at least 6 hr apart while the patient is on bed rest	>160–180 mm Hg systolic or >110 mm Hg diastolic on two occasions at least 6 hr apart while the patient is on bed rest
Proteinuria	>300 mg/24 hr but <5 g/24hr	5 g/24 hr or catheterized urine with 4+ on dipstick
Uric acid	>4.5 mg/dL	Much greater than 4.5 mg/dL
Creatinine	Normal	Elevated
Liver enzymes	Normal	Elevated AST, ALT, LDH
Symptoms/signs	Hyperreflexia	Headaches Blurred vision Scotomas Clonus Right upper quadrant pain

AST, aspartate aminotransferase; ALT, alanine aminotransferase; LDH, lactate dehydrogenase.
Adapted from McPhee S, Papadakis MA. *Current Medical Diagnosis and Treatment.* 48th ed. New York: McGraw-Hill Companies; 2009; and DeCherney AH, Nathan L. *Current Diagnosis and Treatment Obstetrics and Gynecology.* 10th ed. New York: McGraw-Hill Companies; 2007.

    b. Clinical features
        (1) Symptoms include edema of the face and hands, sudden weight gain, headache, visual disturbances, nausea, vomiting, right upper quadrant pain, and decreased urine output.
        (2) Signs include hypertension, proteinuria, and hyperreflexia.
    c. Laboratory studies
        (1) Sterile urine protein, 24-hour urine protein level, complete blood count (CBC), fibrinogen, and prothrombin time (PT)/partial thromboplastin time (PTT) are followed.
        (2) Chemistry panel, including liver enzymes, creatinine, and uric acid levels, aids in identifying risk for complications.
    d. Treatment
        (1) Delivery of the infant is the ultimate treatment for hypertensive disorders of pregnancy.
        (2) Mild preeclampsia
            (a) If the patient is reliable, she may be followed up as an outpatient. Alternatively, the patient may be hospitalized with expectant management. Whether or not the patient is followed as an in- or outpatient, delivery through induction is indicated after 37 weeks of gestation.
            (b) MgSO$_4$, administered by IV drip, is the first-line medication for inpatient management to decrease chance of seizures. MgSO$_4$ should be continued for 24 hours after delivery.
            (c) Hydralazine or labetalol sometimes is given for acute management of high blood pressure.
            (d) Betamethasone is given before 34 weeks of gestation to enhance fetal lung maturity.
        (3) Severe preeclampsia or eclampsia is an indication for prompt delivery regardless of gestational age.
I. Rh incompatibility
  1. General characteristics
    a. If the infant's blood type is not identical to the mother's blood type, the mother may develop antibodies against the infant's blood (i.e., Rh sensitization). For example, if mother is Rh negative and fetus Rh positive, the mother may develop antibodies against the infant's blood, and hemolysis can occur.
    b. The most common problem of mismatched blood involves the rhesus D factor (Rh factor). Approximately 15% of the population is Rh negative. Although 98% of isoimmunizations are secondary to the Rh factor, 43 other antigens exist.
    c. Rh immunoglobulin (Rho-Gam) is administered routinely at 28 to 29 weeks of gestation to all Rh-negative mothers for prophylactic protection. After delivery, if the baby is found to be Rh positive, the mother receives

Rho-Gam again to protect subsequent pregnancies. When Rho-Gam is given, it helps to prevent development of these antibodies to the infant's blood in 99% of cases.

    d. The most common time of maternal–fetal blood mixing is at delivery. However, Rho-Gam should be administered after any event that may allow fetal cells to enter maternal circulation such as ectopic pregnancy, spontaneous or therapeutic abortion, CVS, amniocentesis, or trauma. The Apt or Kleihauer-Betke (KB) test measures occurrence and degree of fetomaternal hemorrhage.

    e. If antibodies develop, they will attack subsequent Rh-incompatible infants and can lead to severe fetal anemia and death (fetal hydrops).

  2. Laboratory studies

    a. Routine prenatal blood work should include blood type, Rh factor, and Coombs' test for antibodies.

    b. Antibody titers of less than 1:16 probably will not adversely affect the pregnancy.

    c. In a sensitized pregnancy, a combination of Coombs' test, amniocentesis, and ultrasonography is used to follow the developing fetus for evidence of distress or fetal hydrops.

  3. Treatment

    a. Routinely give Rh immunoglobulin (Rho-Gam), 300 mg, to Rh-negative, nonimmunized women at 28 weeks of gestation and within 72 hours of delivering an Rh-positive infant.

    b. Rh immunoglobulin also is to be administered at amniocentesis and other instances of potential uterine bleeding, as noted previously.

    c. Massive fetal–maternal hemorrhage may require larger doses of immunoglobulin.

J. Abruptio placentae

  1. General characteristics

    a. Abruptio placentae is the premature separation of a normally implanted placenta after the 20th week of gestation but before birth.

    b. Abruptio placentae is the most common cause of third-trimester bleeding.

    c. Several risk factors are known for the development of abruptio placentae: trauma, smoking, hypertension, decreased folic acid, cocaine use, alcohol (>14 drinks/wk), uterine anomalies, high parity, previous abruption (recurrence rate is 10% to 17%), and advanced maternal age.

    d. Types of abruption include external abruption (more common, less severe), where blood escapes from the uterus, and concealed abruption (less common, more severe), where blood is retained between the detached placenta and the uterus. Figure 8-2 depicts common types.

    e. Abruption can lead to liberation of tissue thromboplastin or consumption of fibrinogen, thereby activating the extrinsic clotting mechanism. This could eventually lead to disseminated intravascular coagulation.

  2. Clinical features

    a. Painful vaginal bleeding occurs in the majority of cases (85%).

    b. Uterine, abdominal, or back pain is a frequent symptom of abruptio placentae and, if bleeding is concealed, may be the only symptom.

    c. The uterus becomes hypertonic, irritable, or tender when the placenta has abrupted.

    d. Evidence of fetal distress may or may not be present, depending on the degree of separation.

    e. Complications of abruptio placentae, in addition to the obvious compromise of placental blood flow to the fetus and hemorrhage, are renal failure, coagulation failure, and death.

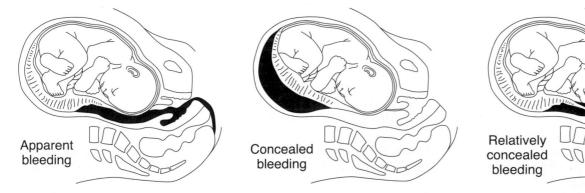

Apparent bleeding   Concealed bleeding   Relatively concealed bleeding

FIGURE 8-2 Types of abruptio placentae: external (apparent) and concealed.

3. Laboratory studies

   a. Diagnosis is almost always clinical.

   b. Ultrasonography is not reliable in establishing the diagnosis of this problem.

4. Treatment

   a. Delivery of the fetus and placenta is the definitive treatment of abruptio placentae. However, ultimate management depends on the degree of separation and the age and viability of the fetus.

   b. Blood type, cross-match, and coagulation studies are indicated in an unstable patient, as is placement of a large-bore IV line.

   c. Cesarean section most often is the preferred route for delivering the infant in cases of abruptio placentae.

K. Placenta previa

1. General characteristics

   a. Placenta previa occurs when the placenta partially or completely covers the cervical os.

   b. Performing a digital examination in a patient with placenta previa is contraindicated because it can incite severe bleeding.

   c. Placenta previa occurs in 0.3% to 0.5% of pregnancies and is associated with advanced age, smoking, high parity, and any process that could cause scarring of the lower uterine segment (e.g., cesarean delivery).

2. Clinical features

   a. Painless vaginal bleeding is the hallmark of placenta previa.

   b. Bleeding may continue from the placenta's implantation site after delivery, because the lower uterus contracts poorly.

3. Laboratory studies

   a. Ultrasonography is the test of choice for establishing the diagnosis of placenta previa.

   b. When the patient is hemodynamically unstable, studies for blood type, cross-match, and coagulation should be ordered; a large-bore IV line should be placed.

4. Treatment

   a. Before term, watchful waiting is warranted if the patient is stable.

   (1) Blood transfusion may be necessary while waiting for fetal maturity.

   (2) Placenta previa often is diagnosed before 20 weeks of gestation (on routine ultrasound). Up to 50% of affected placentas "migrate" up the uterine wall, however, because of growth during the pregnancy, so they are not ultimately misplaced at term.

   (3) Patients with previa should abstain from vaginal penetration.

   b. Cesarean section is the preferred method of delivering the infant in cases of placenta previa.

III. LABOR AND DELIVERY

A. Routine vaginal labor and delivery

1. General characteristics

   a. Approximately 20% of perinatal morbidity and mortality occurs during the intrapartum period in otherwise healthy pregnancies.

   b. Most infants present with a vertex (head-down) presentation. However, other possibilities include breech, face, transverse, and compound (arm or leg).

2. Clinical features

   a. Cervical examination to assess labor

   (1) Dilatation: opening of the cervical os, expressed in centimeters (fully dilated is 10 cm)

   (2) Effacement: cervical softening and thinning out, expressed as a percentage (up to 100%)

   (3) Station

      (a) Location of the presenting part (usually the head) in relation to the maternal ischial spines

      (b) The level at the spines is denoted as "0" station. Stations above the spines are expressed in negative numbers (e.g., −1 cm, −2 cm), and stations below the spine in positive numbers (e.g., +1 cm, +2 cm).

   b. Stages of labor

   (1) The first stage of labor begins at the onset of true, regular contractions and ends at full dilatation. The length of the first stage of labor generally is 6 to 20 hours for nulliparous women and 2 to 14 hours for multiparous women (or 1 to 1.5 cm/hr).

(2) The second stage of labor begins at full dilatation and ends with the delivery of the infant. The length of the second stage of labor generally is 30 minutes to 3 hours (average, 50 minutes) for primiparous women and 5 to 60 minutes (average, 20 minutes) for multiparous women.

(3) The third stage of labor begins after the delivery and entails separation and expulsion of the placenta. The length of the third stage of labor is 0 to 30 minutes but usually is about 5 minutes.

(4) The hour after delivery sometimes is called the fourth stage and is critical in assessing and treating tears, lacerations, and hemorrhage.

   c. Bloody show, which is the passage of a small amount of blood-tinged mucus that has been plugging the cervical os, often precedes true labor.

   d. Amniotic fluid rupture can occur before or during the first stage of labor.

3. Laboratory studies

   a. On admission, urinalysis for protein, glucose, and hematocrit should be obtained.

   b. Fetal monitoring is used in labor to assess the fetus' response to labor.

   (1) An external fetal monitor is attached to the maternal abdomen and assesses an estimated fetal heart rate via transmitted sound waves.

   (2) An internal fetal monitor is an electrode attached to the infant's head and gives the most accurate fetal heart rate pattern because it transmits the true R wave (as with an electrocardiogram) of electroactivity. The cervix must be dilated at least 2 cm and membranes ruptured to attach an internal fetal monitor.

   (a) Accelerations of an increase of 15 bpm for 15 seconds above the normal baseline heart rate (120 to 160 bpm) are reassuring and denote fetal well-being.

   (b) Early decelerations mirror the images of the contractions and denote fetal head compression. They often are present as a woman approaches the second stage of labor and are considered to be benign.

   (c) Variable decelerations are rapid drops in fetal heart rate with a return to baseline with variable shape and no identifiable pattern. They often occur with cord compression and, if mild or infrequent, are benign.

   (d) Late decelerations are fetal heart rate drops during the second half of the contractions. They denote uteroplacental insufficiency and always are worrisome.

   (e) When a nonreassuring fetal heart rate is present, the following management is appropriate: stop oxytocin (if applicable), change maternal position, administer oxygen via face mask, and measure fetal scalp pH.

4. Treatment

   a. Regular cervical examinations for dilation, station, and effacement are necessary to check the progress of labor.

   b. Continued blood pressure, temperature, and pulse readings are critical to exclude late preeclampsia and infection.

   c. Analgesia is offered to provide comfort and prevent fatigue.

   d. After crowning of the presenting part, pressure applied from the coccygeal region upward will extend the head at the proper time and help to protect the perineal musculature.

   e. When the head has been delivered, the baby can be suctioned with a rubber suction bulb.

   f. When the rest of the body passes, the cord is clamped and cut.

   g. Episiotomy (surgical incision to prevent traumatic tearing) is sometimes used to protect the perineum as the head crowns for such indications as a large baby or a short perineum.

   h. Signs of placental separation include umbilical cord lengthening, a fresh show of blood flow, fundus rising, and the uterus becoming firm and globular.

   i. The infant is suctioned, kept warm, and assessed for Apgar score at 1 and 5 minutes after delivery (Table 8-9).

   j. The placenta and umbilical cord should be examined to ensure that the entire placenta and membranes are passed and that the cord contains three vessels (two arteries and one vein).

   k. Oxytocin is sometimes used in the third stage of labor to reduce blood loss by stimulating the contractions.

B. Abnormal labor and delivery

1. General characteristics

   a. Dystocia, or abnormal labor, occurs when the cervix fails to dilate progressively over time and the fetus fails to descend.

		Points		
TABLE 8-9 **Apgar Scoring**[a]				
Letter	**Sign**	**0**	**1**	**2**
A	Activity (muscle tone)	Absent	Arms and legs flexed	Active movement
P	Pulse	Absent	<100 bpm	>100 bpm
G	Grimace (reflex irritability)	No response	Grimace	Sneezes, coughs, pulls away
A	Appearance (skin color)	Blue-gray, pale all over	Pink, except extremities	Pink all over
R	Respiration	Absent	Slow, irregular	Good, crying

[a]A score is determined for each sign at 1 and 5 min after birth; if there are problems with the neonate, a score is determined at 10 min as well. Scores are classified as follows: 7–10 = normal; 4–7 = may require some resuscitative measures; ≤3 = immediate resuscitation required.

Adapted with permission from Childbirth.org. Apgar scoring for newborns. Copyright © 1994–2007 by Childbirth.org. Available at: www.childbirth.org/articles/apgar.html. Accessed June 9, 2003.

    b. Common causes include abnormalities with the pelvis, powers, or passenger.

        (1) Pelvis refers to the passage through the pelvic structures. Sometimes, the pelvis is not large enough to allow the infant to pass through, which denotes cephalopelvic disproportion.

        (2) Powers refer to the contractions, which are needed to dilate the cervix and expel the infant. If the contractions are inadequate, oxytocin (Pitocin) can be given IV to enhance labor.

        (3) Passenger refers to the baby. The head usually is the biggest part. The bigger the baby is in relation to the pelvis, the larger the likelihood of cephalopelvic disproportion.

2. Clinical features

    a. Inability to deliver vaginally after full cervical dilation is a good marker of true dystocia.

    b. Macrosomia, nonvertex presentation, and the adequacy of the pelvis can be evaluated by clinical examination before the onset of labor.

3. Treatment

    a. Inadequate uterine contractions can be augmented with oxytocin after the maternal pelvis and fetus are assessed.

    b. If maternal pushing is inadequate, rest or assisted delivery with vacuum extraction or forceps may be used. Forceps or vacuum extractors are used to shorten the second stage of labor and may be indicated for fetal distress or maternal indications only if the head is engaged and the cervix is fully dilated.

    c. Dystocia is a leading indication for cesarean section.

    d. If the baby is in a nonvertex presentation, external version with ultrasound guidance can be attempted after 37 weeks of gestation.

C. Cesarean delivery and vaginal birth after cesarean delivery (VBAC)

1. General characteristics

    a. Cesarean section is defined as the birth of the fetus through an incision in the abdominal and uterine walls and constitutes 21% to 25% of deliveries in the United States.

    b. The most frequent indications for cesarean section are repeat cesarean (one-third of cesareans), dystocia or failure to progress, breech presentation, and fetal distress.

    c. The success rate of VBAC depends on the indications for and the number of the previous cesarean sections.

        (1) When dystocia was the indicator for a previous cesarean delivery, the rate of successful VBAC is the lowest. Conversely, women who have a cesarean delivery for malpresentation (e.g., breech) have a higher rate of success with VBAC.

        (2) Although the incidence of uterine rupture in a VBAC after use of a low transverse incision is relatively low (0.2% to 1.5%), it can lead to death of the fetus and significantly increased morbidity and mortality of the mother.

    d. Risks of cesarean section include a greater likelihood of thromboembolic events, increased bleeding, and development of infection.

    e. With each subsequent cesarean section, the risk of complications is higher.

2. Treatment

    a. Prophylactic antibiotics often are used after a cesarean section to prevent infection.

     b. A low transverse uterine incision usually is made because of the decreased blood loss associated with its use, the ease of repair, and the lower likelihood of rupture compared with that of a classical incision (incidence with a classical incision is 4% to 9%). A classical incision is vertical through the entire length of the uterus.

D. Induction of labor

  1. General characteristics

     a. Induction of labor can be done by medical or surgical means.

     b. Induction of labor is considered when prolongation of pregnancy might expose the mother or fetus to complications and when vaginal delivery is not contraindicated (Table 8-10).

  2. Methods

     a. Early induction of labor (when minimal dilation or effacement has occurred) is initiated with prostaglandin gel put directly on the cervix; it may be repeated once in 12 hours. This helps to soften or "ripen" the cervix.

     b. Later induction (when the cervix is dilated <1 cm and some effacement has occurred) is initiated with oxytocin (Pitocin) given IV, with systematic increases in the oxytocin level until strong contractions are occurring approximately every 3 minutes.

     c. Amniotomy, or artificially rupturing the membranes with a small hook, also can induce labor.

E. Postpartum hemorrhage

  1. General characteristics

     a. Postpartum hemorrhage is defined as blood loss requiring transfusion or a 10% decrease in hematocrit between admission and the postpartum period. It is the third leading cause of maternal mortality in advanced gestation.

     b. Early postpartum hemorrhage occurs less than 24 hours after delivery and is associated with abnormal involution of the placental site, cervical or vaginal lacerations, and retained portions of placenta.

     c. Late postpartum hemorrhage occurs more than 24 hours after delivery to 6 weeks postpartum and most commonly is caused by subinvolution of the uterus, retained products of conception, or endometritis.

  2. Clinical features

     a. Complaints of increased bleeding after delivery signal a need to evaluate for hemorrhage.

     b. A subinvoluted uterus will feel enlarged and soft on examination, and the patient may present with complaints of increased bleeding, pain, fever, and foul-smelling lochia.

  3. Laboratory studies

     a. Hemoglobin and hematocrit tests are necessary to quantify complaints of bleeding.

     b. Ultrasonography sometimes can detect obvious retained placental fragments.

  4. Treatment

     a. Initially, uterine massage and compression can be used.

TABLE 8-10 **Induction of Labor**		
Indications	**Relative Contraindications**	**Absolute Contraindications**
Prolonged pregnancy	Breech presentation	Cephalopelvic disproportion
Diabetes mellitus	Oligohydramnios	Placenta previa
Rh isoimmunization	Multiple gestation	Uterine scar from previous classical cesarean section
Preeclampsia	Prematurity	
Premature rupture of membranes	Grand multiparity	Transverse lie
	Previous cesarean section with transverse scar	Myomectomy
Chronic hypertension		
Placental insufficiency	Fetal macrosomia	
Suspected intrauterine growth retardation		

Adapted from DeCherney AH, Nathan L. *Current Diagnosis and Treatment Obstetrics and Gynecology.* 10th ed. New York: McGraw-Hill Companies; 2007.

  b. Establish IV access and prepare blood components.

  c. Use of IV oxytocin, ergonovine, methylergonovine, or prostaglandins often is first-line treatment for early postpartum hemorrhage.

  d. Subinvolution of the uterus often responds to oral agents that increase uterine contraction (e.g., methylergonovine maleate, ergonovine maleate). Antibiotic treatment also may be necessary.

  e. Postpartum hemorrhage may require surgical intervention, depending on the cause and severity.

F. Endometritis

 1. General characteristics

  a. Endometritis most commonly occurs after cesarean section or when membranes are ruptured more than 24 hours before delivery.

  b. Findings most commonly present 2 to 3 days postpartum. Fever higher than 38.3°C (101°F) and uterine tenderness are highly suspicious for endometritis.

  c. Adnexal tenderness, peritoneal irritation, and decreased bowel sounds may occur.

 2. Laboratory studies

  a. White blood cell (WBC) count commonly is more than 20,000/mcL.

  b. Causative bacteria vary widely from hospital to hospital, but anaerobic streptococci are most common.

  c. Urinalysis also should be performed.

 3. Treatment

  a. Antibiotics are administered until afebrile for 24 hours.

   (1) Clindamycin plus gentamicin is the first-line treatment.

   (2) Ampicillin is added if there is no response in 24 to 48 hours.

   (3) Metronidazole is added if sepsis is present.

  b. A single dose of antibiotic at the time of cord clamping reduces the incidence of endometritis.

IV. PUERPERIUM

A. Definition: The 6-week period after delivery is known as the puerperium or the postpartum period.

B. Normal puerperium

 1. General characteristics

  a. Immediately after delivery, the uterus is at the level of the umbilicus.

   (1) After 2 days, the uterus shrinks or involutes.

   (2) After 2 weeks, it descends into the pelvic cavity.

   (3) By 6 weeks, it is back to its antenatal size.

  b. Lochia, or bleeding that occurs after delivery, represents the sloughing off of decidual tissue. It can last for 4 to 5 weeks postpartum.

  c. In a nonbreastfeeding mother, menses resume 6 to 8 weeks postpartum. In contrast, breastfeeding mothers typically are anovulatory and may remain amenorrheic for the duration of lactation.

 2. Clinical features

  a. The first postpartum visit should be approximately 6 weeks after delivery. This should include a thorough history with attention to bleeding, breast- or bottle-feeding, pelvic pain, sexual and contraceptive history, bowel and bladder function, and emotional well-being.

  b. On pelvic examination at 6 weeks, the perineum should be well healed and the uterus back to its pregravid size.

  c. Occasionally, a lactating mother will have atrophic vaginitis.

 3. Laboratory studies

  a. During the first postpartum visit, hemoglobin and hematocrit are sometimes performed as dictated by history.

  b. If the patient had developed gestational diabetes, a fasting blood glucose should be ordered.

 4. Treatment

  a. It is important to emphasize contraceptive counseling at the postpartum examination.

  b. Vitamin supplementation should be continued for the nursing mother.

  c. Atrophic vaginitis can be treated with vaginal estrogen as needed.

9 Rheumatology and Orthopaedics (Musculoskeletal System)

Jennifer Joseph

I. ARTHRITIS/RHEUMATOLOGIC CONDITIONS

A. Osteoarthritis (OA)

1. General characteristics

   a. OA is the most common arthropathy among adults, particularly the elderly.

   b. OA is characterized as progressive loss of articular cartilage with reactive changes in the bone, resulting in pain and destruction of the joint.

   c. Among persons aged 40 years or older, 90% display radiographic signs of the disease.

2. Clinical features

   a. Decreased range of motion (ROM), joint crepitus, and pain gradually worsening throughout the day are features of OA.

   b. Common sites of involvement are the distal interphalangeal (DIP) joint (Heberden's nodes), proximal interphalangeal (PIP) joint (Bouchard's nodules), wrist, hip, knee, and spine. The metacarpophalangeal (MCP) joints (except the thumb), ankle, and elbow are usually spared.

   c. Joints can become unstable during the late stages of OA.

3. Laboratory studies and imaging

   a. Laboratory tests are nonspecific.

   b. Radiographs show asymmetric narrowing, subchondral sclerosis, cysts, and marginal osteophytes.

4. Treatment

   a. Weight reduction, moderate physical activity, acetaminophen, nonsteroidal anti-inflammatory drugs (NSAIDs), intra-articular steroids and viscosupplement injections, bracing, canes, and quadriceps strengthening may be useful in managing OA.

   b. Total joint replacement may be indicated in advanced cases. Osteotomy and surgical arthrodesis generally do not have long-term benefit.

B. Rheumatoid arthritis (RA)

1. General characteristics

   a. RA is a chronic disease with synovitis affecting multiple joints and other systemic extra-articular manifestations.

   b. Females are affected more often than males (3:1 ratio), with onset typically occurring between 40 and 60 years of age. The juvenile form occurs in patients younger than 16.

   c. A cascade of events leads to joint destruction. Hyperplastic synovial tissue (pannus) may erode cartilage, subchondral bone, articular capsule, tendons, and ligaments.

2. Clinical features

   a. See Table 9-1 for diagnostic criteria of RA. To make the diagnosis, four of the criteria must be present.

   b. The DIP joints are usually spared.

   c. Extra-articular manifestations of RA include changes in the skin, lungs, kidneys, eyes, liver, blood system, and heart. Osteoporosis is frequently diagnosed.

3. Laboratory studies and imaging

   a. Aspiration and joint fluid analysis are useful laboratory tests to quantify inflammation and exclude the presence of gout or septic arthritis (Table 9-2).

   b. Erythrocyte sedimentation rate (ESR) and C-reactive protein (CRP) are elevated.

   c. Rheumatoid factor (RF) and anti-CCP antibodies are positive in 70% to 80% of patients; levels may be low in early disease.

   d. Soft-tissue swelling and juxta-articular demineralization are seen on radiography.

TABLE 9-1	**Rheumatoid Arthritis Diagnostic Criteria**

Morning stiffness lasting >1 hr for at least 6 weeks

Arthritis and soft-tissue swelling of >3 joints, present for at least 6 weeks

Arthritis of the hand joints, present for at least 6 weeks

Symmetric arthritis, present for at least 6 weeks

Subcutaneous nodules in specific places (over bony prominences, extensor surfaces, or juxta-articular regions)

Rheumatoid factor at a level above the 95th percentile

Radiologic changes suggestive of joint erosion or bony decalcification

Adapted from Arnett FC, Edworthy SM, Bloch DA, et al. The American Rheumatism Association 1987 revised criteria for the classification of rheumatoid arthritis. *Arthritis Rheum.* 1988;31(3):315–324.

4. Treatment
   a. Consultation with a rheumatologist is recommended for initiation of treatment and development of a long-term plan.
   b. Physical and occupational therapy should be implemented.
   c. Pharmacologic management should be early and aggressive to reduce pain, preserve function, and prevent deformity.
      (1) NSAIDs may be used in conjunction with disease-modifying antirheumatic drugs (DMARDs).
      (2) DMARDs are begun as soon as the diagnosis is made.
         (a) Methotrexate is frequently the initial DMARD.
         (b) Other DMARDs include corticosteroids, sulfasalazine, antimalarials, and leflunomide.
         (c) Newer biologic treatments include etanercept, abatacept, rituximab, infliximab, and adalimumab.
         (d) Combination therapy may be required.
   d. Reconstructive surgery is indicated for severe cases.
C. Childhood-onset idiopathic arthritis
   1. General characteristics
      a. Childhood-onset idiopathic arthritis is characterized by chronic synovitis and a number of extra-articular manifestations (fever, rash, weight loss, other organ involvement).
      b. Females are affected more often than males (2:1 ratio) and have an earlier age of onset (females, 1 to 3 years of age; males, 8 to 12 years of age).
      c. Forms of arthritis include systemic (15%), pauciarticular (50%), and polyarticular (35%).
   2. Clinical features
      a. Systemic (Still's disease; juvenile rheumatoid arthritis [JRA])
         (1) This type is characterized by spiking fevers (39 to 40°C; 102.2–104°F), myalgias, polyarthralgias, and a typical salmon-pink maculopapular rash appearing in the evening and with the fever.
         (2) The rash may be elicited by scratching the skin in susceptible areas (Koebner's phenomenon).
         (3) There are minimal articular findings, but hepatosplenomegaly, lymphadenopathy, leukocytosis, pericarditis, or myocarditis may occur.

TABLE 9-2	**Differentiation of Joint Fluid Analysis**			
	Color	**WBCs (/μL)**	**PMNs (%)**	**Culture**
Osteoarthritis	Yellow	200–300	25	Negative
Rheumatoid arthritis (or other inflammatory conditions)	Yellow to opalescent	3,000–50,000	25–50	Negative
Septic	Yellow to green	>50,000	75	Positive

WBCs, white blood cells; PMNs, polymorphonucleocytes.

    b. Pauciarticular: This type is characterized by involvement of four or fewer medium to large joints. Patients are also at risk for development of asymptomatic uveitis that may lead to blindness if they have a positive antinuclear antibody (ANA) test.

    c. Polyarticular

        (1) This type resembles adult RA with its symmetric involvement and involves five or more of the small and large joints.

        (2) Systemic symptoms include low-grade fever, fatigue, rheumatoid nodules, and anemia.

3. Laboratory studies and imaging

    a. There are no specific diagnostic tests for JRA, but 10% to 15% of patients have a positive RF; anti-CCP antibody test may be positive as well.

        (1) ESR and CRP are increased or normal with the systemic type.

        (2) The ANA test may be increased in the pauciarticular type and indicates a tendency for uveitis.

    b. Imaging studies may be similar to those for adults with soft-tissue swelling and periarticular osteoporosis findings. Joint destruction is less frequent.

4. Treatment

    a. Some NSAIDs and physical and occupational therapy are most beneficial. Methotrexate or leflunomide may be used as second-line agents, early on, if there is no improvement with NSAIDs.

    b. Monitor children with JRA for any growth abnormalities, nutritional deficiencies, and school/social impairment.

    c. Seventy-five percent to 80% remit without serious disability. Patients who are RF positive are at greatest risk of progressing to disabling arthritis into adulthood.

D. Other types of arthritis

  1. Infectious (septic) arthritis

    a. General characteristics and clinical features

        (1) The hematogenous spread of bacteremia, periarticular osteomyelitis, infection caused by diagnostic or therapeutic procedure (e.g., intra-articular injection), or infection elsewhere (e.g., cellulitis, bursitis) may lead to infectious arthritis. Bacterial septic arthritis usually involves a single joint (most commonly the knee, followed by hip, shoulder, ankle, and wrist) in 90% of cases.

        (2) *Staphylococcus aureus* is the most common pathogen in joint infections.

        (3) Sexually active young adults are at risk for septic arthritis caused by infection with *Neisseria gonorrhoeae*.

        (4) Patients usually present with acute swelling, fever, joint warmth and effusion, tenderness to palpation, and increased pain with minimal ROM in the involved joint.

    b. Laboratory studies and imaging

        (1) Synovial fluid should be collected. See Table 9-2 for typical characteristics of septic arthritis. Forty percent of patients will have a positive blood culture.

        (2) Radiographs usually only show soft-tissue swelling.

    c. Treatment

        (1) Aggressive treatment with intravenous (IV) antibiotics is required.

        (2) Arthrotomy (surgical opening into a joint to drain and debride the infection) and arthrocentesis (puncture of joint space with a needle for synovial fluid analysis and culture) often are required. Arthrotomy is definitely required for infection involving the hip joint; it usually is not required when *Neisseria gonorrhoeae* is the infecting organism.

        (3) Oral antibiotics should follow the IV antibiotics for an additional 7 to 10 days.

  2. Psoriatic arthritis

    a. General characteristics: This is an inflammatory arthritis with skin involvement usually preceding joint disease by months to years.

    b. Clinical features

        (1) The course usually is mild and intermittent, affecting a few joints.

        (2) Symmetric arthritis resembles RA and may involve the hands and feet. Pitting of the nails and onycholysis are seen.

        (3) Sausage-finger appearance (caused by arthritis and tenosynovitis of the flexor tendon) is a common feature.

    c. Laboratory studies and imaging

      (1) ESR is elevated; normocytic normochromic anemia is seen.

      (2) Hyperuricemia may occur when skin involvement is severe.

      (3) RF is normal.

      (4) "Pencil in cup" deformities of the proximal phalanx are demonstrated on radiography.

    d. Treatment

      (1) NSAIDs are sufficient for mild cases.

      (2) Methotrexate is beneficial for both the skin inflammation and the arthritis. Corticosteroids and antimalarials should be avoided.

      (3) Reconstructive surgery (arthrodesis or joint replacement) is indicated for painful end-stage arthropathy.

  3. Reactive arthritis (Reiter syndrome)

    a. General characteristics

      (1) Reactive arthritis is a seronegative arthritis that presents with a tetrad of urethritis, conjunctivitis, oligoarthritis, and mucosal ulcers.

      (2) It is often seen as a sequelae to sexually transmitted infections (chlamydial urethritis or ureaplasma) or gastroenteritis (*Shigella*, *Salmonella*, *Yersinia*, or *Campylobacter*).

    b. Clinical features

      (1) Patients may have asymmetric arthritis that involves large joints usually below the waist (i.e., knee and ankle); mucocutaneous lesions (balanitis, stomatitis), urethritis, and conjunctivitis are common.

      (2) The gender ratio is 1:1 after enteric infections and 9:1 after sexually transmitted infections, with a male predominance. It is the leading cause of nontraumatic monoarthritis.

    c. Laboratory studies and imaging

      (1) Fifty percent to 80% of patients are HLA-B27 positive.

      (2) Synovial fluid is usually culture negative.

      (3) Evidence of permanent and progressive joint disease may be present on radiography.

    d. Treatment

      (1) Physical therapy and NSAIDs are the mainstay of treatment.

      (2) Antibiotics given at the time of infection will reduce the chance of developing the disorder but do not alleviate the symptoms of the reactive arthritis.

E. Gout

  1. General characteristics

    a. Gout is a systemic disease of altered purine metabolism and subsequent sodium urate crystal precipitation into synovial fluid.

    b. It is more common in men than in women (9:1) until menopause, after which the ratio approaches parity.

  2. Clinical features

    a. The most common feature is initial attack of the metatarsal phalangeal joint of the great toe (podagra); it is the presenting manifestation in 70% of cases.

    b. Other joints of the feet, ankles, and knees are commonly affected.

    c. Pain, swelling, redness, and exquisite tenderness develop suddenly at and surrounding the joint. In chronic gout, tophi (chalky deposits of urate crystals) may form adjacent to the joint and are considered diagnostic.

  3. Laboratory studies

    a. Joint fluid analysis is diagnostic if rod-shaped, negatively birefringent urate crystals are seen. The diagnosis of gout also may be inferred by clinical examination.

    b. Serum uric acid level of greater than 8 mg/dL is suspicious but not diagnostic.

  4. Imaging: Characteristic erosions make the diagnosis of gout highly suspect.

  5. Treatment

    a. Elevation and rest may alleviate symptoms. Dietary modifications stressing decreased ingestion of purines and alcohol can reduce elevated urate levels.

b. Pharmacotherapy

(1) NSAIDs generally are the initial drug of choice (i.e., indomethacin, 25 to 50 mg three times daily, until symptoms resolve).

(2) Corticosteroid injections are recommended for accessible joints; oral prednisone (or adrenocorticotropic hormone [ACTH]) may be used if other medicines are not tolerated and septic arthritis has been ruled out.

(3) Management between acute attacks can be achieved with colchicine, probenicid, sulfapyrazone, allopurinol, or febuxostat.

F. Calcium pyrophosphate dehydrate (CPPD) disease (pseudogout)

1. General characteristics

a. Pseudogout affects peripheral joints, usually in the lower extremity, and results from intra-articular deposition of calcium pyrophosphate.

b. Acute presentations may mimic gout; recurrent and abrupt onset of attacks is characteristic.

2. Clinical features

a. Painful inflammation results when crystals are shed into the joint.

b. The joints most commonly involved are the knee, wrist, and elbow.

3. Laboratory studies and imaging

a. Rhomboid-shaped calcium pyrophosphate crystals that are negatively birefringent are found in joint aspiration.

b. Radiographs show fine, linear calcifications in cartilage (chondrocalcinosis).

4. Treatment: NSAIDs, colchicine, and intra-articular steroid injections may be beneficial.

G. Systemic lupus erythematosus (SLE)

1. General characteristics

a. SLE is an autoimmune disorder characterized by inflammation and positive ANAs and involvement of multiple organs.

b. SLE commonly affects women of childbearing age. Prevalence also is found among certain familial and ethnic groups (most common in African American women).

2. Clinical features

a. The diagnosis of SLE is based on the presence of certain criteria (Table 9-3).

b. Diagnosis requires at least four criteria to be met, including a significantly high-titer ANA.

c. Drug-induced lupus must be ruled out. Some drugs may cause a lupus-like syndrome, including procainamide, hydralazine, isoniazid, methyldopa, quinidine, and chlorpromazine. If the offending agent is stopped, the symptoms typically resolve. These patients have positive antihistone antibodies.

TABLE 9-3	**Diagnostic Criteria for Systemic Lupus Erythematosus**
Malar rash	
Discoid rash	
Photosensitivity	
Oral ulcers	
Arthritis	
Serositis (heart, lungs, or peritoneal)	
Renal disease (proteinuria, cellular casts)	
ANA	
Hematologic disorders (hemolytic anemia, leucopenia, leukocytosis, thrombocytopenia)	
Immunologic disorders (LE cell, anti-DNA, anti-Sm, false-positive serologic test for syphilis)	
Neurologic disorders (seizures or psychosis in absence of any other cause)	

ANA, antinuclear antibody; LE, lupus erythematosus.

Adapted from Tan EM, Cohen AS, Fries JF, et al. The 1982 revised criteria for the classification of systemic lupus erythematosus. *Arthritis Rheum.* 1982;25:1271–1277.

3. Laboratory studies
   a. Routine laboratory studies should include complete blood count (CBC), blood urea nitrogen (BUN), creatinine, urinalysis, ESR, and serum complement (C3 or C4).
   b. Antibodies to Smith antigen, double-stranded DNA, or depressed levels of serum complement may be used as markers for progression of the disease.
   c. ANA is present (99%), but low titers have a low predictive value.
4. Treatment
   a. Regular exercise and sun protection are important for all patients.
   b. NSAIDs are often used for musculoskeletal complaints.
   c. Antimalarials (hydroxychloroquine or quinacrine) may be used for musculoskeletal complaints and cutaneous manifestations.
   d. Corticosteroids
      (1) Topical or intralesional preparations are often used for cutaneous manifestations.
      (2) Low- or high-dose oral corticosteroids are used for disease flares and tapered as symptoms resolve.
   e. Methotrexate is used at low doses for arthritis, rashes, serositis, and constitutional symptoms.

H. Polymyositis
1. General characteristics
   a. Polymyositis is an inflammatory disease of striated muscle affecting the proximal limbs, neck, and pharynx. The skin also can be affected (dermatomyositis).
   b. Other organ systems affected include joints, lungs, heart, and gastrointestinal (GI) tract.
   c. Cause is unknown, but there is a strong association with an occult malignancy.
   d. Women are more commonly affected than men (3:1).
2. Clinical features may include: insidious, painless, proximal muscle weakness; dysphagia; skin rash (malar or heliotrope); polyarthralgias; and muscle atrophy.
3. Laboratory studies
   a. The muscle enzymes creatine phosphokinase (CPK) and aldolase will be elevated.
   b. Muscle biopsy should be performed and will show myopathic inflammatory changes.
4. Treatment: Polymyositis is treated with high-dose steroids, methotrexate, or azathioprine until symptoms resolve.

I. Polymyalgia rheumatica
1. General characteristics
   a. Polymyalgia rheumatica is characterized by pain and stiffness in the neck, shoulder, and pelvic girdles and is accompanied by constitutional symptoms (e.g., fever, fatigue, weight loss, depression).
   b. It affects women twice as often as men and usually presents in patients older than 50 years.
   c. Cause is unknown. It is associated with temporal arteritis in up to 30% of cases.
2. Clinical features
   a. Stiffness usually is the predominant feature, being severe after rest and in the morning.
   b. Musculoskeletal symptoms usually are bilateral, proximal, and symmetrical.
   c. Giant cell (temporal) arteritis must be ruled out. It characteristically presents with scalp tenderness, jaw claudication, headache, and temporal artery tenderness and may lead to vision loss.
3. Laboratory studies: ESR is markedly elevated (>50 mm/hr).
4. Treatment: Patients respond quickly to low-dose corticosteroid therapy, which may be required for up to 2 years and slowly tapered. Higher doses are required if giant cell arteritis is present.

J. Polyarteritis nodosa
1. General characteristics
   a. Small and medium artery inflammation involving the skin, kidney, peripheral nerves, muscle, and gut occurs.
   b. The male to female ratio is 3:1.
   c. Onset generally is between 40 and 60 years, although it may occur in every age group.
   d. Cause is unknown, but association with hepatitis B is seen in up to 30% of patients.

2. Clinical features

    a. Fever, anorexia, weight loss, abdominal pain, peripheral neuropathy, arthralgias, and arthritis are commonly seen.

    b. Skin lesions, including palpable purpura and livedo reticularis, occur in some patients.

    c. Hypertension, edema, oliguria, and uremia may be present in patients with renal involvement.

3. Laboratory studies

    a. The diagnosis usually is established by vessel biopsy or angiography.

    b. Elevated ESR and CRP and proteinuria may be present as well as a positive hepatitis B surface antigen (HBsAg).

    c. Presence of antineutrophil cytoplasmic antibody (ANCA) is suggestive but not diagnostic of polyarteritis nodosa.

4. Treatment

    a. Initial management is with high doses of corticosteroids.

    b. Cytotoxic drugs and immunotherapy also may be used. Concomitant treatment of hepatitis B may be required.

    c. Hypertension should be treated if present.

K. Systemic sclerosis (scleroderma)

  1. General characteristics

    a. Scleroderma is of unknown cause and is characterized by deposition of collagen in the skin and, less commonly, in the kidney, heart, lungs, and stomach.

    b. The female to male ratio is 4:1.

    c. The peak age of onset is between 30 and 50 years.

  2. Clinical features

    a. There are two types of scleroderma: *diffuse,* which affects the skin as well as the heart, lungs, GI tract, and kidneys, and *limited,* which mostly affects the skin of the face, neck, and distal elbows and knees and late in the disease causes isolated pulmonary hypertension.

    b. Skin involvement occurs in 95% of patients. Changes most often begin with swelling in the fingers and hands and may spread to involve the trunk and the face.

    c. Raynaud's phenomenon, vasospasm of the digital arteries, is seen in 75% of patients.

    d. Calcinosis, Raynaud's phenomenon, esophageal dysfunction, sclerodactyly, and telangiectasias (CREST) syndrome is associated with limited scleroderma.

    e. Patients usually present with skin changes, polyarthralgias, and esophageal dysfunction.

  3. Laboratory studies

    a. ANA is present in 90% of patients with diffuse scleroderma.

    b. Anticentromere antibody is associated with limited scleroderma.

    c. Patients should be monitored for development of hypertension, heralding kidney involvement.

  4. Treatment

    a. There is no cure for scleroderma.

    b. Treatment is aimed at organ-specific disease processes (i.e., proton pump inhibitors for reflux disease, angiotensin-converting enzyme [ACE] inhibitors for renal disease, avoidance of triggers and treatment with calcium channel blockers for Raynaud's, and immunosuppressive drugs for pulmonary hypertension).

L. Sjögren's syndrome

  1. General characteristics

    a. Sjögren's syndrome is an autoimmune disorder that destroys the salivary and lacrimal glands (exocrine glands).

    b. It also may be a secondary complication to a preexisting connective tissue disorder such as RA, SLE, polymyositis, or scleroderma.

    c. It is most often diagnosed in middle-aged females.

  2. Clinical features

    a. Mucous membranes are most affected. Dry mouth (xerostomia) and dry eyes (xerophthalmia or keratoconjunctivitis sicca) are characteristic features of primary Sjögren's syndrome.

    b. The parotid glands also may be enlarged.

3. Laboratory studies

   a. RF is present in 70% of cases, ANA in 60%, anti-Ro antibodies in 60%, and anti-La antibodies in 40% of cases.

   b. A Schirmer's tear test evaluates tear secretions by the lacrimal glands. Wetting of less than 5 mm of filter paper placed in the lower eyelid for 5 minutes is positive for decreased secretions.

   c. Biopsy of the lower lip mucosa confirms lymphocytic infiltrate and gland fibrosis.

4. Treatment: Management is mainly symptomatic, with the goal of keeping mucosal surfaces moist. This can be achieved by using artificial tears and saliva, increased oral fluid intake, and ocular and vaginal lubricants. Pilocarpine may increase saliva flow.

M. Fibromyalgia syndrome

1. General characteristics

   a. The fibromyalgia syndrome is a central pain disorder whose cause and pathogenesis are poorly understood.

   b. Fibromyalgia can occur with RA, SLE, and Sjögren's syndrome.

2. Clinical features

   a. Patients have nonarticular musculoskeletal aches, pains, fatigue, sleep disturbance, and multiple tender points on examination.

   b. Anxiety, depression, headaches, irritable bowel syndrome, dysmenorrhea, and paresthesias are associated with this condition.

3. Laboratory studies

   a. Fibromyalgia is recognized by the typical pattern of pain and other symptoms as well as by exclusion of contributory or underlying diseases such as hypothyroidism, hepatitis C, and vitamin D deficiency.

   b. There are no routine laboratory markers; it often is a diagnosis of exclusion.

   c. Abnormality of the T-cell subsets has been described.

4. Treatment

   a. Selective serotonin reuptake inhibitors (SSRIs), selective serotonin and norepinephrine reuptake inhibitors (SSNRIs), and tricyclic antidepressants (TCAs) have all been shown to be helpful in subsets of patients with fibromyalgia.

   b. Pregabalin (Lyrica) is the only drug that is FDA-approved specifically for the treatment of fibromyalgia. Studies report reduced pain and improved sleep. Side effects, however, include fatigue, trouble concentrating, sleepiness, and edema.

   c. Aerobic exercise improves conditioning and has been shown to improve functioning as long as overtraining is avoided.

   d. Patient education, stress reduction, sleep assistance, and treatment of psychological problems may alleviate some symptoms.

II.   BONE AND JOINT DISORDERS

A. Tendinitis and tenosynovitis

1. General characteristics

   a. Tendinitis refers to inflammation of the tendon.

   b. Tenosynovitis is inflammation of the enclosed tendon sheath.

   c. Common causes include overuse injuries and systemic disease (e.g., arthritides).

2. Clinical features

   a. Tendinitis and tenosynovitis commonly appear in the following sites: rotator cuff, supraspinatus, biceps, flexor carpi ulnaris, flexor carpi radialis, flexor digitorum, patella, hip adductor, and Achilles.

   b. Tendinitis and tenosynovitis generally occur together, causing pain with movement, swelling, and impaired function.

   c. The conditions may resolve over several weeks, but recurrence is common.

3. Treatment

   a. Ice, rest, and stretching help to relieve inflammation.

   b. NSAIDs may alleviate pain but do not penetrate the tendon circulation adequately. An injection with corticosteroids combined with anesthesia and administered alongside the tendon may be beneficial. Intratendon injection should be avoided because of the risk of rupture.

   c. Excision of scar tissue and necrotic debris may be performed if conservative measures are unsuccessful. The scar tissue is caused by repetitive microtrauma to the tissue.

B. Bursitis

  1. General characteristics

    a. Bursitis is an inflammatory disorder of the bursa (a thin-walled sac lined with synovial tissue).

    b. The inflammation is caused by trauma or overuse.

  2. Clinical features

    a. The common sites of presentation are subacromial, subdeltoid, trochanteric, ischial, iliopsoas, olecranon, and prepatellar and suprapatellar (housemaid's knee).

    b. Pain, swelling, and tenderness may persist for weeks.

  3. Treatment of bursitis includes prevention of the precipitating factors, rest, NSAIDs, and steroid injections.

C. Osteomyelitis

  1. General characteristics

    a. Osteomyelitis is an inflammation of the bone caused by a pyogenic organism (most commonly *Staphylococcus aureus*) and is described by duration (acute, chronic), cause (hematogenous, exogenous, surgical, true contiguous spread), site (spine, hip, other), extent (size of defect), and type of patient (infant, child, adult, immunocompromised host).

    b. Types

      (1) Acute hematogenous osteomyelitis most commonly affects the long bones of children.

      (2) Patients with sickle cell anemia are at risk for salmonella osteomyelitis.

      (3) Osteomyelitis is termed *chronic hematogenous osteomyelitis* when, after the original acute infection has completed appropriate treatment (antibiotics, surgery), viable colonies of bacteria harbored in necrotic and ischemic tissue cause a recurrence of infection.

      (4) Exogenous osteomyelitis results from open fracture or surgery.

  2. Clinical features

    a. Acute hematogenous osteomyelitis

      (1) Pain, loss of motion, and soft-tissue swelling occur.

      (2) Drainage is rare.

    b. Chronic hematogenous osteomyelitis

      (1) Recurrent acute flare-ups of tender, warm, sometimes swollen areas occur, and patients often complain of malaise, anorexia, fever, weight loss, and night sweats as well as pain and drainage from a sinus tract (an abnormal channel permitting escape of exudate to the surface).

      (2) Bone necrosis, soft-tissue damage, and bone instability can occur.

  3. Laboratory studies and imaging

    a. White blood cell (WBC), CRP, and ESR may be mildly elevated in acute and chronic osteomyelitis, although normal results are possible.

    b. Identification of the infectious organism by blood culture or bone biopsy is best.

    c. Radiographic evidence of osteomyelitis lags behind symptoms and pathologic changes by 7 to 10 days. Ultrasonography can be useful for early detection of acute osteomyelitis.

    d. Late sequestra (i.e., dead bone surrounding granulation tissue) and involucrum (i.e., periosteal new bone) take several weeks to months to appear.

    e. Magnetic resonance imaging (MRI) shows the changes before plain-film radiography or bone scan.

  4. Treatment

    a. Acute osteomyelitis is treated with a 3-week course of antibiotics (typically 1 week IV and 2 weeks oral).

    b. Chronic osteomyelitis is treated with a minimum of 4 weeks to 24 months of IV and PO antibiotics depending on the organism involved and the comorbidities of the patient.

    c. Immobilization and surgical drainage may be indicated. Attention to open wounds must be a part of the treatment as well as removal of any hardware present.

    d. Surgical treatment may be required to remove sequestra, sinus tract, infected bone, and scar tissue.

D. Neoplasms

  1. General characteristics

    a. Carcinomas of the prostate, breast, lung, kidney, and thyroid are the primary carcinomas that most commonly metastasize to the bone. The spine is the most common site of bony metastases.

  b. Incidence

  (1) Benign tumors of the bone and soft tissue are more common than primary malignant tumors.

  (2) Enchondroma (cartilaginous tumor) is the most common primary benign bone neoplasm of the hand and is asymptomatic unless complicated by pathologic fracture.

  (3) Lipomas (soft, nontender, movable mass) and ganglions (soft, nontender, transilluminant mass, usually on the dorsum of the hand or wrist) are common benign soft-tissue masses.

  (4) Mucous cysts are ganglia originating from the DIP joint and often are associated with Heberden's nodules.

  (5) Soft-tissue sarcomas occur three times more often than primary bone malignancies.

  (6) The most common types of primary sarcomas of bone are chondrosarcoma, Ewing's sarcoma, and osteosarcoma.

  (7) Multiple myeloma is the most common primary malignant bone tumor.

  c. Age groups

  (1) Ewing's sarcoma is found in patients between 5 and 25 years of age, usually in the diaphyses of long bones, ribs, and flat bones. Osteosarcomas are most common in individuals 10 to 20 years of age, arising in the metaphyseal area of the long bones.

  (2) In adults 60 years of age or older, metastatic carcinoma is the most common source of bone lesion. Chondosarcomas also increase in incidence in adults older than 60 years and can present within the central metaphyseal area.

2. Clinical features

  a. Night pain often is associated with malignancy.

  b. A painful mass attached to bone is likely to be malignant; however, some malignant tumors are nonpainful.

  c. Severe pain preceded by dull, aching pain may indicate pathologic fracture.

  d. Systemic symptoms, such as fever, weight loss, anorexia, or fatigue, should be noted.

  e. Rule out areas of metastases, such as the lungs, breasts, prostate, thyroid, and kidneys.

3. Laboratory studies

  a. Routine laboratory studies are noncontributory, but with suspected malignancy, routine labs can provide a baseline for patients who will need chemotherapy.

  b. Alkaline phosphatase and lactate dehydrogenase are elevated when the bone is broken down and remodeled.

  c. Serum and urine protein electrophoresis studies can detect the specific abnormal globulin of multiple myeloma.

  d. Biopsy is essential to diagnose whether benign or malignant, the cell type, and the grade of lesion.

  (1) Open incisional biopsy is best and should be done by a specialist.

  (2) The capsule is then closed tightly to prevent bleeding and local spread.

4. Imaging studies

  a. Radiology

  (1) Radiographic signs may help to distinguish benign from malignant tumors, because certain tumors have a characteristic appearance.

  (2) Radiography also may help to determine a tumor's location and may narrow the diagnostic possibilities.

  b. Computed tomography (CT) is used to determine if pulmonary metastasis is present.

  c. MRI is used to determine the local extent of a tumor.

  d. Bone scans can evaluate distant osseous metastasis and noncontiguous tumor or skip lesions. They are not diagnostic in multiple myeloma.

5. Treatment

  a. The goals of treatment are to relieve pain and maintain function.

  b. For benign tumors, simple excision is the treatment.

  c. Malignant neoplasms

  (1) Wide surgical resection is used when feasible.

  (2) The success of chemotherapy, either alone or in conjunction with radiation therapy, depends on the type of tumor, its location, and whether metastasis has been found.

  (3) Limb salvage (using cadaver allograft or endoprosthetic devices) is part of definitive treatment.

  (4) Radiation therapy followed by local resection is the common treatment for soft-tissue sarcomas.

E. Osteoporosis

1. General characteristics

a. Osteoporosis is a disease of abnormal bone remodeling.

(1) It is characterized by a decrease in total bone volume; although the bone that is present is normal, it is less dense.

(2) This decrease in mass leads to an increased susceptibility to fractures.

b. Osteoporosis is divided into two categories, primary and secondary:

(1) Primary osteoporosis is further divided.

(a) Type I (postmenopausal) occurs primarily in women, but can occur in men. It is the most prevalent form of primary osteoporosis.

(b) Type II (senile) occurs in both men and women.

(2) Secondary osteoporosis is recognized by conditions in which bone is lost because of the presence of other diseases (malignancies, corticosteroid use, GI disorders, or hormonal imbalances).

c. Risk factors include those that are modifiable (alcoholism, smoking, low body weight, sedentary lifestyle, low calcium and vitamin D intake, corticosteroid use, recurrent falls) and nonmodifiable (advanced age, Caucasian or Asian race, female gender).

2. Clinical features

a. Type I commonly is associated with loss of estrogen in postmenopausal women and with testosterone deficiency in men.

(1) The trabecular bone primarily is affected.

(2) The vertebrae, hip, and distal radius are the most common fracture sites.

b. Patients older than 75 years with poor calcium absorption are at high risk for type II.

(1) Both trabecular and cortical bone are affected.

(2) The hip and pelvis are the most common fracture sites.

3. Laboratory studies and imaging

a. Calcium, phosphate, alkaline phosphatase, and serum protein electrophoresis should be done and serum markers should be considered as well to rule out other secondary causes of osteoporosis (i.e., hyperthyroidism, hyperparathyroidism, Cushing's syndrome, hematologic disorders, malignancy, and vitamin D deficiency).

b. Dual-energy x-ray absorptiometry is the most helpful way to measure bone density with the least amount of radiation. Screening bone density is recommended in the following groups:

(1) Postmenopausal women younger than 65 years who have one or more additional risk factors

(2) All postmenopausal women older than 65 years

(3) Postmenopausal women who present with fractures

(4) All women considering therapy for other conditions in which the bone mineral density will affect that decision

(5) Women who have been on hormone replacement therapy (HRT) for prolonged periods

(6) Men who experience fractures after minimal trauma

(7) Patients with evidence of osteopenia on radiography or a disease known to increase risk for osteoporosis

(8) Patients with RA

c. Radiographs show features of decreased bone density when 30% bone loss is present.

4. Treatment

a. Preventative measures include weight-bearing exercise, adequate calcium, vitamin D and phosphorus intake, smoking cessation, and limited alcohol intake.

b. At present, the bisphosphonate class of drugs are considered to be first-line treatment for osteoporosis. These drugs must be taken on an empty stomach, and the patient must be able to sit upright for half an hour.

c. HRT, which is estrogen alone or in combination with progesterone, may be used to treat osteoporosis. HRT carries a risk for myocardial infarction (MI), stroke, breast cancer, and thromboembolic events, so the risks must be weighed against the benefits when considering this treatment.

d. Selective estrogen receptor modulators (SERMs) may also be used in the treatment of osteoporosis; however, the risk for deep venous thrombosis is increased.

     e. Nasal or subcutaneous calcitonin may be used but is not considered first-line treatment for osteoporosis.

     f. Teriparatide has shown great promise in the treatment of osteoporosis, but it is not recommended to be used longer than 2 years.

III.   FRACTURES, DISLOCATIONS, SPRAINS, AND STRAINS

  A. Classification of fractures

    1. Examples of location are proximal, middle, and distal third.

    2. Examples of direction are transverse (at a right angle to the axis of the bone), spiral (bone has a twisted appearance; also called torsion), oblique (fracture line between horizontal and vertical direction), comminuted (splintered or crushed), and segmental (double).

    3. Examples of alignment are angulation (deviation from straight line) and displacement (abnormal position of fracture fragments), such as dorsal displacement of the bone fragment in a Colles' fracture of the wrist and volar displacement of the bone fragment in a Smith's fracture of the wrist; both may be complicated by injury to the median nerve or radial artery.

    4. Examples of associated factors are open fracture (disruption of the skin), closed fracture (skin is intact), and dislocation (displacement of bone from a joint).

  B. Imaging studies

    1. Plain-film radiographs are sufficient to visualize most fractures.

     a. Both anteroposterior (AP) and lateral films should be taken to ensure visualization of the bony structures 90 degrees away from each other.

     b. Concurrent fractures also may be seen at the joints proximal and distal to the fracture (e.g., distal tibia, proximal fibula, dome of the talus, lateral malleolus).

    2. Radionucleotide bone scanning shows increased uptake at the site of an occult fracture or stress fracture (common in athletes and associated with disuse osteopenia when weight bearing starts after long periods of immobilization).

    3. CT is now a better diagnostic method than plain-film radiography or bone scans. It allows visualization of the bone's articular surface otherwise obscured by overlying structures (e.g., carpal bones, elbow, tibial plateau).

    4. CT is helpful in establishing the diagnosis of pelvic, facial, or intra-articular fractures.

    5. MRI is the study of choice to diagnose an occult hip fracture.

  C. Treatment

    1. The following types of fractures are initially treated with analgesics, immobilization, and emergent referral to an orthopaedist after adequate stabilization of the patient.

    2. Open fractures

     a. Any bleeding fracture should be considered an open fracture until proven otherwise.

     b. Ideally, open fractures must be debrided and irrigated (in the operating room) within 4 to 8 hours of injury.

     c. IV antibiotics (first- and second-generation cephalosporins and aminoglycosides) should be administered for 48 hours after fracture and for 48 hours after surgical procedures. Always inquire about tetanus status.

     d. Immobilization and fixation should be performed to preserve function.

    3. Intra-articular fractures (the fracture line enters a joint cavity)

     a. Open treatment may be indicated to restore and maintain articular congruity.

     b. When stable, consider active ROM.

    4. Femur fractures

     a. Treat femoral neck fractures with percutaneous screws or hemiarthroplasty, femoral shaft fractures with intramedullary rods or plates, and intertrochanteric fractures with sliding hip screw fixation or a long gamma nail.

     b. There is significant potential for hemorrhage with fractures of the femur.

    5. Fractures of the tibia and fibula in adults

     a. Fractures of the tibia and fibula are associated with ligamental, meniscal, and vascular injuries.

     b. For simple fractures, closed reduction with cast placement is appropriate; for more complicated or unstable fractures, open reduction combined with internal fixation (ORIF) is required.

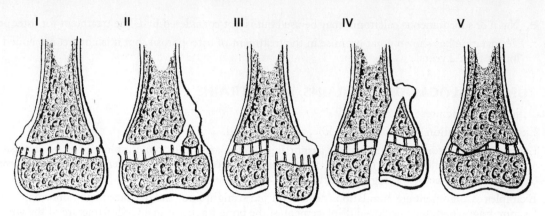

FIGURE 9-1 The Salter–Harris classification of fractures involving the physis. **I:** Fracture through epiphyseal plate. **II:** Epiphyseal fracture with associated metaphyseal fragment. **III:** Fracture through the epiphysis into the articular surface. **IV:** Fracture through the distal metaphysis, epiphyseal plate, and epiphysis. **V:** Impaction of the epiphyseal plate. (From Jarrell BE, Carabasi RA III. *NMS Surgery.* 3rd ed. Baltimore: Williams & Wilkins, 1996; redrawn with permission from Salter RB, Harris WR. Injuries involving the epiphyseal plate. *J Bone Joint Surg Am.* 1963;45:587.)

D. Fractures in children

  1. The physis, or growth plate, is more susceptible to fracture than to injury to attached ligaments.

    a. Swelling and tenderness over the physis are the common findings when fractured.

    b. Growth plate fractures are classified with the Salter–Harris classification system (Fig. 9-1).

    c. Comparison films may be helpful and should be obtained as part of any pediatric fracture workup.

  2. Incomplete fractures occur when the line of fracture does not continue through to the other side of the bone.

    a. Torus fractures (buckle fractures) occur when one side of the cortex buckles as a result of a compression injury (e.g., falling on an outstretched hand). It differs from a greenstick fracture by the mechanism of injury and sometimes buckles on both sides of the bone. Treatment is 4 to 6 weeks in a cast.

    b. Greenstick fractures

      (1) These fractures occur in long bones when bowing causes a break in one side of the cortex.

      (2) When the angulation of the fracture is less than 15 degrees, a long arm or leg cast can be applied for 4 to 6 weeks.

      (3) Fractures with angulation of greater than 15 degrees need referral to an orthopaedic surgeon.

  3. When radiographs of a young child show multiple fractures at various stages of healing, abuse should be suspected and the child referred to a protective agency.

E. Dislocations and subluxations

  1. General characteristics

    a. Dislocation is total loss of congruity that occurs between the articular surfaces of the joint.

    b. Subluxation is any less serious loss of congruity, or a less than complete dislocation.

  2. Sites of dislocation

    a. Common sites of dislocation are the anterior shoulder, posterior hip (a common complication of a posterior dislocation is osteonecrosis of the femoral head), and dislocations of the posterior elbow.

    b. Less common sites of dislocation are the navicular and subtalar joints, as part of a combination of Lisfranc fracture (a dislocation of the tarsometatarsal joint complex), and the second metatarsal joint (often one metatarsal is fractured at the base and the others are dislocated).

  3. Treatment

    a. After assessment of the neurovascular status, most dislocations are treated with closed reduction.

    b. Dislocations that reduce spontaneously require immobilization for 2 to 4 weeks, followed by ROM activity and return to normal activity.

c. If associated fractures or interposed soft tissues are present, the patient needs to undergo open reduction and internal fixation.

d. It is imperative to assess the neurovascular status pre- and postreduction as well as get postreduction radiographs to assure adequate reduction.

F. Strains and sprains

1. A strain is an injury to the bone–tendon unit at the myotendinous junction or the muscle itself.

2. A sprain involves collagenous tissue, such as ligaments or tendons.

3. A strain or sprain injury often follows a sudden stretch.

a. It can lead to avulsion of tendon (e.g., mallet finger avulsion or stretch of the terminal extensor tendon, which is treated with extensor splinting for 6 weeks).

b. It also can lead to ligamentous sprain (e.g., stretch of the anterior talofibular ligament (ATL), which causes the common ankle sprain).

4. Treatment: Both strains and sprains require supportive therapy: rest, ice, compression, elevation, and support/bracing (RICES).

IV. DISORDERS OF THE HEAD AND NECK

A. Temporomandibular joint (TMJ) disorder

1. General characteristics

a. TMJ disorder, which is the most common cause of facial pain, involves pain that affects the TMJ and muscles of mastication.

b. Causes

(1) Neuropsychologic components, such as psychologic stress, may play a role.

(2) Joint capsulitis from bruxism, such as grinding of teeth, clenching of teeth, and posturing of the jaw, may cause TMJ disorder.

(3) Hypermobility syndrome and malocclusion may lead to pain in the jaw area.

2. Clinical features

a. Pain is aggravated by movement of the jaw.

b. There may be restricted ROM; a click or pop may be felt or heard.

3. Imaging studies

a. Initial radiographic studies are normal.

b. Arthritis is a late finding.

c. Other systemic causes need to be ruled out, such as OA, RA, growth abnormalities, and tumor.

4. Treatment

a. Most cases resolve without identification of the cause.

b. Suggestion of conservative lifestyle changes and behavior modification can be helpful.

c. Referral to a specialist, such as an odontologist or oral and maxillofacial surgeon, is required if the symptoms warrant.

B. Neck pain

1. General characteristics

a. Spondylosis is the most common condition affecting the cervical spine.

(1) Degenerative changes occur in the disk, most frequently in C5-6, with the formation of osteophytes and disk narrowing.

(2) Later, facet joints and the joints of Luschka are affected.

(3) Paresthesias and numbness occur in the fingers. Pain increases with extension and decreases with flexion of the neck.

b. Compression by central disk protrusion or osteophytes may cause long-tract signs (e.g., clonus, Babinski's sign) and gait disturbance.

2. Treatment

a. Conservative treatment involves the use of a cervical collar, traction, physical therapy, and analgesics.

b. In advanced disease, cervical fusion or diskectomy may be necessary.

C. Other conditions of the neck
   1. Whiplash and extension injury are common causes of pain and can last 18 months or longer.
      a. Injury occurs as a result of a rear impact, with rapid extension followed by flexion of the cervical spine.
      b. Treatment includes a soft cervical collar (2 to 3 days), application of ice or heat, analgesics, and gentle active ROM very soon after injury.
   2. Rheumatoid spondylitis of the neck is found in most of the patients with adult RA.
      a. Ligamentous stretching causes progressive atlantoaxial and midcervical subluxation.
      b. Surgical stabilization is often necessary.

V. DISORDERS OF THE SHOULDER AND UPPER EXTREMITY

A. Shoulder pain
   1. Shoulder pain can be referred pain caused by cervical spondylosis.
   2. Pain, if localized to a particular area of the shoulder, may be the site of pathology; referred pain is diffuse and cannot be well localized.

B. Rotator cuff syndrome
   1. General characteristics
      a. This syndrome occurs with eccentric overload (e.g., a throwing athlete), underlying glenohumeral instability, poor muscle strength, and training errors.
      b. A common cause in adults is impingement of the supraspinatus tendon as it passes beneath the subacromial arch.
   2. Clinical features
      a. Dull aching in the shoulder is the main clinical feature.
      b. The pain is caused by inflammation, fibrosis, and tears.
      c. The pain may interfere with sleep and is exacerbated by abduction of the arm.
   3. Laboratory studies and imaging
      a. Radiographs are helpful in ruling out calcific tendinitis, glenohumeral or acromioclavicular arthrosis, and bone tumors.
      b. Arthrography or MRI can be used to diagnose tears.
   4. Treatment
      a. Aggravating factors, such as repetitive throwing, other overhead activities, and improper mechanics, must be avoided.
      b. NSAIDs may help to alleviate inflammation and pain.
      c. Local steroid injections may be considered.
      d. Physical therapy may provide relief. Begin nonoperative management of cuff tears with a ROM and strengthening program.
      e. Arthroscopic subacromial decompression should be considered for adults with persistent impingement.
      f. If the patient is still symptomatic after conservative treatment, surgical repair should be considered.

C. Shoulder dislocations
   1. General characteristics
      a. Fall on outstretched arm in abduction and extension is the most common cause of shoulder dislocation.
      b. Anterior shoulder dislocations are more common than posterior shoulder dislocations.
   2. Clinical features
      a. Patient usually presents supporting the affected extremity with the other arm.
      b. Loss of shoulder contour is observed, with the elbow pointing outward (anterior dislocation).
      c. Careful neurovascular assessment must be performed to rule out axillary, musculocutaneous nerve, brachial plexus, or axillary artery injury before reduction attempts.
   3. Diagnostic imaging should include an AP view of the shoulder as well as a transthoracic "Y" view. Humeral head deformities (Hill–Sachs lesions) may be noted in recurrent dislocations. Bankart's lesion, a tear of the glenoid labrum, may be picked up on MRI.

    4. Treatment includes reduction and immobilization.

        a. As with all orthopaedic reductions, postreduction films should be obtained and neurovascular status should be assessed.

        b. Immobilization by sling and swath (Velpaeu's sling) is recommended for all. For patients younger than 40 years, therapy should begin after 3 weeks, and for those older than 40 years, therapy should begin after 1 week.

D. Other conditions of the shoulder

    1. Adhesive capsulitis (frozen shoulder) is an inflammatory process that may follow injury to the shoulder or arise on its own (common in diabetes).

        a. It is characterized by pain and restricted glenohumeral movement.

        b. Arthrography may show decreased volume of the joint capsule and capsular contraction.

        c. Treatment includes NSAIDs, passive ROM, and, occasionally, manipulation under anesthesia.

    2. OA of the humeral head can be secondary to osteonecrosis, trauma, septic arthritis, and endocrine disorders or neuropathic disorders.

        a. Pain, stiffness, and limited ROM are features of the condition.

        b. Radiographs show osteophytes and joint space narrowing.

        c. Treatment includes NSAIDs, cortisone injections, activity modification, and debridement or total joint replacement in severe cases.

    3. Rupture of the long head of the biceps tendons

        a. This rupture can occur as a result of spontaneous or forced overload.

        b. In the elderly, this rupture may be caused by degeneration or attritional changes.

        c. Treatment: Rupture is managed by surgical repair.

E. Fractured clavicle

    1. General characteristics

        a. This is the most common fracture in children and adolescents.

        b. It is usually caused by a fall on an outstretched arm.

        c. It can be found in up to 3% of live births as a result of trauma.

    2. Clinical features

        a. Visible deformity usually is present.

        b. The arm is supported by the contralateral extremity.

        c. Look for brachial plexus injuries (pain, weakness, reflex and sensory abnormalities).

        d. The proximal portion may be displaced superiorly because of the attachment of the sternocleidomastoid muscle.

    3. Imaging studies: An AP view generally will visualize the fracture.

    4. Treatment

        a. In children, the figure-of-eight sling is used for 4 to 6 weeks.

        b. In adults, a sling for 6 weeks is generally enough to treat the fracture.

F. Acromioclavicular separations

    1. General characteristics

        a. Acromioclavicular separation is also referred to as a "separated shoulder."

        b. It involves a "tearing" of the acromioclavicular and/or coracoclavicular ligaments.

        c. It is usually caused by a fall on or impact to the tip of the shoulder.

    2. Clinical features: Patients may have a clinically apparent step off at the acromioclavicular joint.

    3. Imaging studies

        a. An AP view of both shoulders usually is necessary.

        b. Mild separations may require stress films that are obtained while the patient holds a weighted object to reveal the separation.

    4. Treatment

        a. Conservative management is possible for mild to moderate injuries, because they can be managed with a sling and analgesia.

        b. More severe injuries usually will require operative repair.

G. Humeral head fractures

1. General characteristics

  a. Most fractures of the proximal humerus occur in older patients with osteoporosis.

  b. The female to male ratio is 2:1.

2. Clinical features

  a. Pain, swelling, and tenderness, especially in the region of the greater tuberosity, are the most common findings.

  b. Ecchymosis typically does not appear until after 24 to 48 hours.

  c. The patient will hold the affected extremity against the chest wall.

  d. Look for injuries to the brachial plexus and/or axillary artery.

3. Imaging studies

  a. AP, lateral, and "Y" view typically are diagnostic.

  b. Humeral fractures are assessed most commonly by the Neer classification. Displaced fractures are two-part, three-part, or four-part based on whether or not the fracture parts (e.g., head, greater tuberosity, lesser tuberosity, shaft) are involved.

4. Treatment

  a. Closed reduction with the application of a sling and swath (Velpaeu's sling) can treat most nondisplaced fractures. Early mobilization with pendulum exercises is indicated to prevent frozen shoulder.

  b. ORIF is reserved for the management of displaced fractures.

H. Humeral shaft fractures

1. General characteristics

  a. The mechanism of injury includes motor vehicle accidents, fall on an outstretched hand, and penetrating injuries, such as gunshot wounds.

  b. The degree of comminution and amount of soft-tissue injury relate directly to the amount of energy causing the fracture.

2. Clinical features

  a. Pain, arm swelling, deformity, and shortening are all possible initial complaints.

  b. Radial nerve injury should be looked for carefully.

3. Imaging studies: AP and lateral views that include the elbow and shoulder should be performed.

4. Treatment

  a. Initial treatment usually is the application of a coaptation splint.

  b. The coaptation splint can be followed by a hanging cast, Sarmiento's brace, or operative repair.

5. Complications: Fractures of the humeral shaft may be associated with radial nerve injury at the time of fracture or during reduction.

I. Supracondylar humerus fractures

1. General characteristics: The usual mechanism of fracture is a fall on the outstretched hand with hyperextension of the elbow.

2. Clinical features

  a. Initially, patients may have pain with minimal swelling. Extension of swelling around the elbow is a delayed finding.

  b. Full neurovascular examination must be performed. Special attention to brachial artery injuries should be given. The brachial artery is the most spastic artery in the body and can lead to Volkmann's ischemic contractures.

3. Imaging studies

  a. AP and lateral views generally are sufficient to make the diagnosis.

  b. In children, always obtain comparative views.

4. Treatment

  a. Treatment involves closed reduction in the operating room with posterior splint application for displaced fractures in children.

  b. Adults should have ORIF.

5. Complications
   a. Besides Volkmann's ischemic contractures, injuries to all three nerves have been described.
   b. Varus (gunstock) or valgus deformities of the elbow also may result from arrest of the medial or the lateral growth plate, respectively.

J. Hand and wrist pain
   1. OA and RA are the most common painful conditions of the hand and wrist.
      a. OA commonly affects the carpometacarpal joint of the thumb and DIP joints.
      b. OA of the wrist can be posttraumatic or follow osteonecrosis of the lunate (Kienböck's disease).
   2. Clinical features
      a. OA presents with Heberden's nodes and mucous cysts in DIP joints and Bouchard's nodes in PIP joints.
      b. RA causes soft-tissue swelling that is symmetrical and primarily affects the MCP and PIP joints, usually sparing the DIP joints.
      c. Dupuytren's disease affects the palmar aponeurosis, ring, little, and middle fingers, causing painful nodules, pitting, and contractures.
   3. Treatment
      a. Nonsurgical treatment includes heat, stretching, ultrasound therapy, and steroid injections.
      b. Surgical release is indicated for contractures of the metacarpal phalangeal joint that are greater than 30 degrees and for proximal phalangeal contractures of any degree, pain (rare), or nerve compression (digital).

K. Carpal tunnel syndrome
   1. General characteristics
      a. Carpal tunnel syndrome, the most common mononeuropathy, involves compression of the median nerve under the transverse carpal ligament.
      b. It can be precipitated by premenstrual fluid retention, early RA with thickening of the synovial tendon sheath, acromegaly, pregnancy, repetitive flexion or extension of the wrist (e.g., production line work, keyboard work), and alcohol abuse.
   2. Clinical features
      a. Classic findings of night pain, numbness, paresthesias (sparing the little finger), clumsiness, and weakness are seen.
      b. Thenar atrophy may occur late in the disease.
      c. Tinel's sign (tingling with percussion over the volar aspect of the wrist) may be noted.
      d. Phalen's test (symptoms with full flexion of the wrist for >1 minute) may be positive.
   3. Laboratory studies: Electromyography (EMG) and nerve conduction velocity (NCV) studies may help confirm the diagnosis when considered with the clinical presentation.
   4. Treatment
      a. Activity modification, volar wrist splint, and NSAIDs (except in pregnancy) make up the initial recommended treatment.
      b. Steroid injections may be used.
      c. Surgical intervention may be needed to decompress the nerve.

L. Fractures and dislocations of the hand
   1. A boxer's fracture is a fracture of the metacarpal neck of the fourth or fifth finger.
      a. Examination reveals loss of prominence of the knuckle with tenderness and pain.
      b. Inspect for a puncture wound over the metacarpal phalangeal joint. If the fracture was caused by a punch to another's mouth, it also may be necessary to treat with antibiotics (*Eikenella corrodens* is an organism specific to the human mouth).
      c. Fractures with 25 to 30 degrees of angulation should be reduced with the application of an ulnar splint with follow-up in 1 to 2 weeks.
   2. A Colles' fracture is a distal radius fracture with dorsal angulation.
      a. It is the most common injury of the wrist, and results from a fall onto the dorsiflexed hand, described as a silver fork deformity.
      b. Cast immobilization is adequate after reduction in most cases.

    3. Gamekeeper's thumb is a sprain or tear of the ulnar collateral ligament of the thumb.

      a. There usually is a history of a sprained thumb or a fall on the hand.

      b. Examination reveals ligamentous laxity of the ulnar collateral ligament, with instability and weakness of pinch.

      c. Surgical repair is indicated for a complete rupture; a partial rupture may be treated by immobilization with a thumb spica cast.

M. Lateral epicondylitis ("tennis elbow")

  1. General characteristics

    a. Most common overuse injury of the elbow

    b. Most common during the fourth decade of life

    c. It involves the tendinous insertion of the extensor carpi radialis brevis

  2. Clinical features

    a. Pain on lifting objects, primarily when the arm is pronated

    b. Duplicate pain by having patients extend their elbow, hold the forearm in the pronated position, and then extend the fingers and wrist against resistance

  3. Imaging studies

    a. AP and lateral views of the elbow may demonstrate osteophytes overlying the lateral epicondyle.

    b. MRI is useful in demonstrating tendon disruption.

  4. Treatment

    a. Cessation of the provocative activity for at least 6 weeks is probably the most important component in the treatment.

    b. Counterbalance braces (tennis elbow braces) are beneficial.

    c. Instruct the patient to pick up objects with the extremity in supination.

    d. Physical and occupational therapy are important adjuncts to care.

    e. Steroid injections may give short-term relief but do not offer long-term treatment.

    f. NSAIDs frequently are used. Because anti-inflammatory agents are being used more for their analgesic effect, their role as an anti-inflammatory is controversial.

    g. Surgery is reserved for those patients who fail at least 6 months of conservative management.

N. Medial epicondylitis ("golfer's elbow" or "baseball elbow")

  1. General characteristics: This affects the flexor–pronator muscles at their origin, anterior to the medial epicondyle.

  2. Clinical features

    a. A history of repetitive stress is obtained in most patients.

    b. Pain is reproduced by resisted pronation or flexion of the wrist.

    c. Patients may complain of paresthesias in the distribution of the ulnar nerve.

  3. Imaging studies: MRI typically is not indicated but is useful for assessing the ulnar nerve.

  4. Treatment

    a. Conservative management, including cessation of precipitating activity, NSAIDs, and physical and occupational therapy, most commonly is used.

    b. A medial counterforce brace frequently is applied.

    c. Surgical intervention to debride the epicondyle usually is not necessary but is an option.

O. Olecranon bursitis

  1. General characteristics

    a. It is caused either by an acute injury or by repetitive trauma to the olecranon bursa.

    b. Less frequently, it can result from breaks in the skin, leading to a septic cause. The most common organism is *Staphylococcus aureus.*

  2. Clinical features

    a. Swelling overlying the olecranon process is the most common finding. This swelling may be mildly painful, but in chronic cases, it usually is painless.

    b. ROM usually is preserved.

3. Imaging studies generally are not indicated unless there is a significant history of trauma or a fracture is suspected.

4. Treatment

   a. Avoid continued trauma to elbow and use ace wrap for compression. Aspiration of the bursa is not recommended unless infection is suspected.

   b. NSAIDs and warm compresses are used for their analgesic properties.

   c. Surgical removal of the bursa is reserved for septic bursal sacs that are nonresponsive to conservative management.

P. Radial head injuries

1. General characteristics

   a. Fractures of the radial head result from a fall on the outstretched hand.

   b. Subluxation of the radial head in children, or nursemaid's elbow, is caused by excessive longitudinal traction. It is most common before the age of 4. The radial head slips anteriorly room the elbow out of the annular ligament.

2. Clinical features

   a. Fractures of the radial head present with pain over the lateral aspect of the elbow that worsens with forearm rotation. They are the most common fracture of the elbow in adults.

   b. Children who have sustained a subluxation of the radial head usually present with the extremity fully pronated, partially flexed, and held tightly to the side.

3. Imaging studies

   a. AP and lateral films of the elbow usually are sufficient to establish the diagnosis. Displacement of the anterior fat pad and presence of a posterior fat pad imply the presence of a hemarthrosis. CT is useful in determining the degree of comminution.

   b. AP and lateral films usually are performed to rule out fracture in children who are suspected of having a subluxed radial head.

4. Treatment

   a. Treatment of radial head fractures depends on the type of fracture.

   b. Radial head subluxations can be reduced by holding the affected arm just above the wrist and just below the elbow. The practitioner then places the thumb of the proximal hand over the radial head while fully supinating and flexing the forearm and applying posteriorly directed pressure. The objective is to effect a "screwing" action and place the radial head back within the annular ligament.

Q. Scaphoid (navicular) fracture

1. General characteristics

   a. The scaphoid bone is the most commonly fractured carpal bone.

   b. Blood supply is from the radial artery by way of lateral and distal branches. The proximal pole of the scaphoid has a poor blood supply that is further compromised with fractures through the waist of the bone; this can lead to avascular necrosis or nonunion of the scaphoid.

2. Clinical features

   a. Cardinal finding is pain over the anatomic snuffbox.

   b. Swelling over the region in association with ecchymosis implies a fracture–dislocation.

   c. It is often confused with a "sprain" of the wrist, so clinical suspicion is key.

3. Imaging studies

   a. AP, lateral, and scaphoid views should be ordered. If negative initially, films may be repeated after 2 to 3 weeks, at which time the fracture may become apparent.

   b. Bone scan or MRI can be used to make diagnosis at the time of injury.

4. Treatment

   a. A delay in diagnosis should be avoided. Suspicion of scaphoid fracture without radiologic evidence should be treated as a fracture in a long-arm thumb spica cast until bone scan or MRI can be performed.

   b. The initial treatment for a displaced scaphoid fracture is long-arm thumb spica cast and then referral to an orthopaedic surgeon. A short-arm thumb spica cast is used for nondisplaced fractures with referral to an orthopaedic specialist.

   c. Displacement of 1 mm or greater requires ORIF.

5. Complications include nonunion of the fracture or development of avascular necrosis. In avascular necrosis, radiography may reveal a ground-glass appearance of the proximal pole or an increased bone density.

R. de Quervain's disease

    1. Clinical characteristics

        a. de Quervain's disease is a stenosing tenosynovitis involving the abductor pollicis longus and extensor pollicis brevis.

        b. It is more common in females older than 30 years and in diabetics.

    2. Clinical features

        a. Pain and tenderness occur at the wrist and base of the thumb. Radiation of pain up the forearm is common.

        b. Swelling and thickening of the tendon sheath may be appreciated during examination.

        c. The patient places the thumb within his or her fist, and the wrist is then ulnarly deviated, reproducing the pain (Finkelstein's test).

    3. Imaging studies: Not usually required

    4. Treatment

        a. Conservative treatment for at least a month using a thumb spica splint, NSAIDs, and physical/occupational therapy is required.

        b. Injection of steroid into the tendon sheath can be employed if conservative measures fail. No more than three injections should be given before referral to an orthopaedist.

        c. Surgical decompression of the first dorsal compartment may be required in cases that are resistant to all conservative measures.

VI. DISORDERS OF THE BACK

A. Low back pain and sciatica

    1. General characteristics

        a. The most common causes of low back pain are prolapsed intervertebral disk and low back strain.

        b. When back pain is unrelated to the mechanical use of the back, it can be referred from the intra-abdominal, pelvic, or retroperitoneal areas.

    2. Clinical features

        a. Pain originating in the back and radiating down the leg suggests nerve root irritation.

        b. Pain from musculoskeletal causes may be localized to an area of point tenderness.

        c. Sciatica (pain in the distribution of the sciatic nerve) is pain felt in the buttock, posterior thigh, and postero-lateral aspect of the leg around the lateral malleolus to the lateral dorsum of the foot and the entire sole.

        d. Unilateral low back and buttock pain that gets worse with standing in one position may have sacroiliac joint involvement.

        e. Pain in the elderly that is increased by walking and is relieved by leaning forward suggests spinal stenosis.

    3. Laboratory studies and imaging

        a. Radiography of the spine in nontraumatic low back pain often is not required when pertinent directed history and physical examination reveal no sign of a serious condition. Red flags that indicate a need for urgent radiography include fever, weight loss, morning stiffness, history of IV drug or steroid use, trauma, history of cancer, saddle anesthesia, loss of anal sphincter tone, or major motor weakness.

        b. CT is helpful in demonstrating bony stenosis and identifying lateral nerve root entrapment.

        c. MRI can be useful in identifying cord pathology, neural tumors, stenosis, herniated disks, and infections.

    4. Treatment

        a. Short-term relative rest (maximum of 2 days) with support under the knees and neck and administration of NSAIDs or analgesics are the first components of treatment.

        b. Progressive ambulation to normal activities may follow if pain has subsided.

        c. A fitness program, including postural exercises (e.g., McKenzie exercises for disk derangement), should be implemented for back rehabilitation.

        d. If no improvement occurs in 6 weeks, perform further evaluation with bone scan, CT, MRI, or EMG and a medical workup to rule out spinal tumor or infection.

        e. If studies are normal, continue back rehabilitation.

        f. When conservative treatment fails, consider surgical intervention (~5% of those who present with low back pain).

B. Scoliosis and kyphosis

1. Scoliosis

   a. General characteristics

      (1) Scoliosis is defined as lateral curvature of the spine.

      (2) Some curves are secondary to underlying causes (i.e., upper or lower motor neuron disease, myopathies).

      (3) Idiopathic adolescent scoliosis is the most common spinal deformity evaluated by a clinician.

      (4) Girls between onset of the puberty growth spurt and cessation of spinal growth are at the greatest risk for idiopathic scoliosis.

      (5) The vertebrae at the apex of the curve are used for its description. Right thoracic curves (T7 or T8) are the most common, followed by the double major (right thoracic, left lumbar), left lumbar, and right lumbar.

      (6) A thoracic curve to the left is rare; other spinal cord pathology needs to be ruled out before making a diagnosis of scoliosis.

   b. Clinical features

      (1) Physical examination reveals asymmetry in the shoulder and iliac height; asymmetric scapular prominence; and a flank crease with forward bending, showing right thoracic and left lumbar prominence.

      (2) Gait and neurologic examination are normal.

      (3) Curves of less than 20 degrees, diagnosed less than 2 years postmenarche, and Risser stage 2 to 4 are less likely to progress than are other curves.

   c. Imaging

      (1) Single, standing AP radiographs should be obtained when a patient has scoliometer (a device used for measuring curves) readings of greater than 5 degrees.

      (2) Vertebral levels are identified on radiography.

         (a) The greatest anterior tilt is measured by the Cobb's method (measurement is perpendicular to the end plate of the most tilted [end] vertebra).

         (b) Curves of greater than 15% are significant.

      (3) Accurate measurement is best performed by an orthopaedic specialist.

   d. Treatment

      (1) Curves of 10 to 15 degrees are treated by 6- to 12-month follow-up with clinical evaluation and possibly x-rays.

      (2) Curves of 15 to 20 degrees need serial AP radiographic follow-up every 3 to 4 months for larger curves and every 6 to 8 months for smaller curves or for patients near the end of growth.

      (3) Curves of 20 degrees or greater need referral to an orthopaedist for continuous monitoring and management (bracing, electrical stimulation, or surgery).

2. Kyphosis

   a. General characteristics

      (1) Kyphosis is defined as increased convex curvature of the thoracic spine.

      (2) Scoliosis also is present in one-third of patients with kyphosis.

      (3) Juvenile kyphosis (Scheuermann's disease) is idiopathic osteochondrosis of the thoracic spine.

      (4) Tuberculosis of the spine (the most common extrapulmonary location of tuberculosis after the lymph nodes) causes progressive kyphosis (Pott's disease).

   b. Clinical features

      (1) When several vertebrae are involved, there is a round back appearance; when only one vertebra is involved, there is an angular curve.

      (2) If the curve is a result of faulty posture, it will disappear with spinal flexion.

      (3) Excessive lumbar lordosis is common.

   c. Imaging: Standing lateral films

   d. Treatment

      (1) Curves of 45 to 60 degrees should be observed every 3 to 4 months and exercises prescribed for lumbar lordosis and the thoracic spine.

      (2) Curves of greater than 60 degrees or with persistent pain can be treated using a Milwaukee brace.

      (3) Surgery is indicated when curvature is unresponsive to conservative treatment.

C. Spinal stenosis
   1. General characteristics
      a. Spinal stenosis is nerve compression caused by narrowing of the spinal canal or neural foramina.
      b. Types
         (1) Central stenosis (compression of the thecal sac) can be idiopathic or developmental.
         (2) Lateral stenosis (impingement of the nerve root lateral to the thecal sac) often accompanies central stenosis or is an isolated entity in young adults and the middle-aged.
      c. Spinal stenosis usually is symptomatic in late middle age and is more common in men than in women.
   2. Clinical features
      a. Neural claudication and exacerbation of pain with walking is typical. The pain is relieved by leaning forward.
      b. Variable back and leg pain may occur.
   3. Imaging
      a. Radiographs show soft-tissue and thecal narrowing.
      b. Plain CT, postmyelographic CT, and MRI are standard imaging modalities.
   4. Treatment
      a. Conservative management includes rest, isometric abdominal exercises, pelvic tilt, flexion exercises, NSAIDs, and weight reduction.
      b. Lumbar epidural corticosteroid injections provide symptomatic relief; 25% of patients will gain sustained relief of symptoms following steroid injection.
      c. Decompression and fusion are indicated when studies are positive for neural compressive pathology and quality of life is unacceptable to the patient.

D. Ankylosing spondylitis (AS)
   1. General characteristics
      a. AS is a seronegative spondyloarthropathy that progresses to fusion of the vertebrae.
      b. This condition involves onset of back pain, stiffness, and hip pain during the third and fourth decades of life and is seen more often in men than in women.
      c. This disorder affects the sacroiliac joint symmetrically and the spine in a progressively ascending manner.
   2. Clinical features
      a. Lumbar motion is restricted.
      b. Limited motion in the shoulders and hips, synovitis of the knees, plantar fasciitis, and Achilles tendinitis are seen.
      c. Patients also have hip contractures and fixed cervical, thoracic, and lumbar hyperkyphosis.
      d. Fracture of the fused osteopenic spine may occur (commonly cervical), as may sciatica.
      e. Extra-articular manifestations may occur, including uveitis, cardiac abnormalities, and interstitial lung disease.
      f. Noninvasive tests for spine and thoracic mobility include the Schober's test, thoracolumbar rotation and flexion, finger-to-floor distance, cervical rotation, occiput–wall distance, and chest expansion.
   3. Laboratory studies and imaging
      a. Elevated levels of ESR and CRP are seen. Ninety percent of white and 50% of black patients with AS are HLA-B27 positive.
      b. Sacroiliitis is an early radiographic finding. The "bamboo appearance" on radiography occurs because of radiographic obliteration and marginal syndesmophyte ossification of the paraspinal ligaments.
      c. Generalized osteopenia of the spine may be seen.
   4. Treatment
      a. The mainstay of treatment is physical therapy with emphasis on posture, extension exercises, and breathing exercises. Swimming is considered the best overall exercise.
      b. NSAIDs can be used for stiffness and pain.
      c. Spine fractures need intervention and stabilization.

E. Cauda equina syndrome
   1. General characteristics: This is a rare condition involving a large midline disk herniation that compresses several nerve roots, usually at L4 to L5 level.

2. Clinical features

    a. Bowel and bladder function is severely impaired.

    b. Leg pain, numbness, saddle anesthesia, and/or paralysis are noted.

3. Treatment: This is a surgical emergency requiring immediate referral.

VII. DISORDERS OF THE HIP AND LOWER EXTREMITY

  A. Aseptic necrosis of the hip

    1. General characteristics

      a. Aseptic necrosis (also known as osteonecrosis or avascular necrosis) of the hip results from loss of blood supply to the trabecular bone which causes a collapse of the femoral head.

      b. It can occur at any age but is seen with greater frequency during the third to fifth decades of life and often is bilateral.

      c. In children, it is known as Legg–Calvé–Perthes (LCP) disease; it typically develops in children aged 2 to 11 years, with a peak incidence between 4 and 8 years of age.

      d. The cause generally is unknown, but it often is seen in patients with a history of trauma, steroid use, alcohol abuse, RA, radiation therapy, and SLE.

    2. Clinical features

      a. Dull ache or throbbing pain localized to the groin, lateral hip, or buttocks.

      b. Pain with weight bearing and activity that is relieved with rest.

      c. Loss of rotation (internal and external) or abduction and an antalgic limp.

      d. Children with LCP usually present with persistent pain, a limp, and loss of motion, particulary internal rotation and abduction.

      e. Adverse outcomes include secondary OA, femoral head collapse, and disability.

    3. Imaging

      a. MRI is the study of choice for early detection.

      b. Radiography may be normal early in the course of adult disease; later, progression of necrosis may reveal a crescent sign in lateral films.

      c. Bone scans are useful but are less sensitive than MRI.

      d. Radiography should be done early in children and may show soft-tissue swelling, joint distension, increased bone density, fragmentation, or a deformed femoral head, all various stages of the disease.

    4. Treatment

      a. Protected weight bearing for early stage disease is considered to be a temporary treatment. Alendronate has been used to prevent early collapse.

      b. Surgical options range from core decompression to total hip replacement.

      c. In children the treatment is protected weight bearing. Little benefit has been shown from bracing.

  B. Slipped capital femoral epiphysis (SCFE)

    1. General characteristics

      a. SCFE is a weakening of the epiphyseal plate of the femur, resulting in a displacement of the femoral head. It may be bilateral.

      b. It typically presents in children between 10 and 16 years of age.

      c. Boys are affected more often than girls, and there is a higher incidence in African Americans, the athletically inclined, and obese children.

      d. Most cases of SCFE are idiopathic, but in the younger child, consider a metabolic cause (hypothyroidism or hypopituitarism).

    2. Clinical features include a history of insidious hip, thigh, or knee pain associated with a painful limp.

    3. Imaging: Lateral radiographs show posterior and medial displacement of the epiphysis. SCFE is best assessed with the patient in the frog-leg lateral pelvis or lateral hip view.

    4. Treatment

      a. Definitive treatment for chronic SCFE is pinning in situ.

      b. The child should be placed on crutches and should avoid weight bearing before and after surgery.

C. Meniscal injuries
1. General characteristics
   a. Meniscal injury occurs with excessive rotational force of the femur on the tibia.
   b. The medial meniscus is injured most often.
   c. Injuries may be isolated or may occur with other ligamentous ruptures.
2. Clinical features
   a. Patients report joint line pain on the side of the injury, which may be palpable during examination.
   b. Inability to fully extend the knee is described as locking.
   c. The patient may describe a feeling of the knee giving way.
   d. Swelling occurs gradually, over several hours.
   e. Walking up and down stairs or squatting is difficult and may be painful.
   f. The McMurray's and Apley's tests may be helpful in detecting a meniscal tear.
3. Imaging
   a. Radiography usually is negative.
   b. MRI often makes the diagnosis of a meniscal tear, but occasionally arthroscopy is required for diagnosis.
4. Treatment
   a. Initial treatment is conservative: activity modification, NSAIDs, quadriceps strengthening exercises, and time.
   b. Indications for arthroscopy include persistent symptoms unresponsive to conservative treatment or irreducible locking.
D. Osgood–Schlatter disease
1. General characteristics
   a. Osgood–Schlatter disease is apophysitis of the tibial tubercle caused by trauma or overuse.
   b. The age of onset is between 8 and 15 years. Males are affected two to three times more often than females.
   c. A self-limited disease, it usually heals when the epiphysis closes.
2. Clinical features
   a. Patients complain of anterior knee pain, with localized pain and swelling over the tibial tubercle.
   b. Pain typically is related to activity and is relieved with rest.
3. Imaging: Lateral radiography usually is normal but may show fragmentation at the tibial tubercle.
4. Treatment
   a. The patient should abstain from physical activity for as long as several months.
   b. Stretching, ice, and NSAIDs after exercise are indicated.
E. Cruciate ligament injuries
1. General characteristics
   a. The anterior cruciate ligament (ACL) is more commonly injured than the posterior cruciate ligament (PCL).
   b. ACL injury is commonly associated with a pivoting motion during running, jumping, or cutting activities.
   c. Women are affected more often than men.
2. Clinical features
   a. Patients usually report hearing a pop and complain of knee instability.
   b. Hemarthrosis develops quickly within 3 to 4 hours.
   c. Lachman's test is the most sensitive for diagnosing an ACL tear.
3. Imaging
   a. Radiographs are done to rule out associated fracture.
   b. MRI is useful as an adjunct to physical exam to diagnose an ACL tear.
4. Treatment
   a. Nonoperative treatment with physical therapy and bracing is appropriate in patients who do not participate in competitive activities or who do not report instability with desired activities.
   b. Surgical reconstruction with autograft or allograft is appropriate in patients who are younger than 40 years of age, those who participate in competitive activities, or those who report instability with desired activities.
   c. Complications from surgery may include limited or loss of full ROM or anterior knee pain.

F. Ankle sprain/strain

1. General characteristics

 a. Ankle sprains are one of the most common sports-related injuries; 85% result from an inversion injury.

 b. Ankle sprains most often involve the lateral ligaments, particularly the anterior talofibular ligament (ATL).

2. Clinical features

 a. Patients will often report hearing a pop and will present with ecchymosis and tenderness of the lateral ankle.

 b. Stability of the ankle can be assessed using the anterior drawer test.

3. Imaging: Radiography should be done to rule out a fracture, especially if the patient is unable to bear weight or has tenderness to palpation over a bone.

4. Treatment

 a. Treatment should be tailored to the severity of the sprain, but always should include "RICE" (rest, ice, compression, elevation).

 b. Patients should use crutches for the first 48 to 72 hours, and a brace should be used for support.

 c. Referral to physical therapy may speed up recovery. Length of recovery could be 3 to 4 months.

G. Achilles tendonitis

1. General characteristics

 a. Pain is attributed to inflammation and degeneration of the Achilles tendon and its attachment to the calcaneus.

 b. It is common in runners and in patients who suddenly increase their activity level.

 c. It is considered an overuse injury and is usually the result of improper stretching and training.

 d. If untreated, it may result in rupture of the Achilles tendon.

2. Clinical features

 a. Patients usually report a gradual onset of pain during activity or after activity is completed.

 b. The pain is located on the posterior calf, 2 to 6 cm above the insertion of the Achilles tendon.

 c. Patients will be tender over the posterior calf above the calcaneus and will report pain on passive dorsiflexion and resisted plantar flexion.

 d. Ankle ROM and strength should be normal.

 e. Thompson's test should be done to rule out Achilles tendon rupture.

3. Imaging

 a. Radiographs may show a soft-tissue shadow and calcifications along the tendon and its insertion.

 b. MRI may show hypertrophy of the Achilles tendon or help rule out a rupture.

4. Treatment: The patient should be started on a regimen of NSAIDs and physical therapy for stretching and strengthening exercises.

H. Bunions (hallux valgus)

1. General characteristics

 a. The most common deformity of the metatarsophalangeal (MTP) joint is hallux valgus; it is the result of a lateral deviation of the proximal phalanx.

 b. Bunions are more common in women than in men (10:1). They are often caused by wearing tight, pointed shoes.

 c. Other causes include congenital deformity and systemic diseases such as RA.

2. Clinical features

 a. Patients will often complain of medial eminence pain, metatarsal head pain, deformities of the toes, and the inability to find shoes that fit.

 b. Exam may show a hallux valgus deformity, MTP enlargement, and pain and crepitation on movement of the MTP joint.

 c. Patients may also have limited ROM and pain on extreme ROM of the MTP joint.

3. Imaging

 a. Weight-bearing radiography of the foot will show the valgus deformity of the proximal phalanx; an angle of greater than 15 degrees is considered abnormal.

4. Treatment
   a. Encourage patients to buy shoes with a wide toe box and to use pads on the medial eminence of the bunion deformity or between the first and second toes if they are rubbing together.
   b. Surgical treatment is for severe deformity or pain that is not relieved with conservative measures.

I. Morton's neuroma
   1. General characteristics
      a. Morton's neuroma is a result of traction of the interdigital nerve against the transverse metatarsal ligament causing degeneration of the nerve and chronic inflammation.
      b. It usually affects the third web space and is more common in women than in men (10:1).
   2. Clinical features
      a. Patients complain of pain and localized numbness when walking and standing, which is relieved with rest.
      b. Pain is usually localized to the web space and, often, a mass is palpable.
      c. Squeezing the forefoot will often reproduce the symptoms.
   3. Imaging
      a. Plain radiography is normal.
      b. MRI is sensitive but not usually needed, as the diagnosis is made clinically.
   4. Treatment
      a. Conservative treatment using a soft metatarsal pad and shoes with a wide toe box are helpful.
      b. Steroid injections into the web space can be helpful.
      c. Surgical removal of the neuroma is possible in cases that are not resolved with conservative treatment, but the patient should be aware that both toes will be chronically numb.

J. Plantar fasciitis
   1. General characteristics
      a. Plantar fasciitis is very common in runners and overweight patients.
      b. It is caused by microscopic tears in the plantar fascia at the calcaneal origin.
   2. Clinical features
      a. Patients will complain of pain with the first few steps in the morning and heel pain at night.
      b. Exam will show pain at the calcaneal origin and an inflexible Achilles tendon.
   3. Imaging
      a. Plain radiography is typically normal, but may reveal a calcaneal fracture or bone spur.
      b. MRI may reveal calcifications of the plantar fascia.
   4. Treatment
      a. Conservative treatment is recommended for 6 to 12 months, including physical therapy for stretching of the plantar fascia and the Achilles tendon, heel pads, arch supports, and massage of the area with a tennis ball.
      b. Steroid injections should be used with caution due to the risk of rupture of the plantar fascia.
      c. Surgery is reserved for extreme cases.

Endocrinology

Rebecca Lovell Scott

I. THYROID DISORDERS

A. Hyperthyroidism (thyrotoxicosis)

1. General characteristics

a. Hyperthyroidism involves elevated thyroid hormone concentrations and may be caused by excess production, leakage, or exogenous hormone administration.

b. The most common cause (90% of cases) is Graves' disease.

(1) Graves' disease is an autoimmune disorder in which autoantibodies attach to thyroid-stimulating hormone (TSH) receptors and stimulate thyroid hyperfunctioning. It most often occurs in women (8:1) who are 20 to 40 years of age.

(2) A familial tendency exists, as does an association with HLA-B8 and HLA-DR3.

(3) Graves' disease also may be found in individuals with other autoimmune disorders (e.g., pernicious anemia, myasthenia gravis, diabetes mellitus [DM]).

(4) Persons with Graves' disease are at increased risk of Addison's disease, alopecia areata, celiac disease, cardiomyopathy, and hypokalemic periodic paralysis.

c. Other causes include toxic adenomas; subacute (de Quervain's) and postpartum thyroiditis; pregnancy; exogenous thyroid hormone ingestion; trophoblastic tumors and, rarely, pituitary tumors; and administration of amiodarone, which causes either active elaboration of excessive thyroid hormone (type I) or destructive thyroiditis (type II).

d. Thyroid storm is the abrupt onset of more florid symptoms of thyrotoxicosis.

2. Clinical features

a. Symptoms include heat intolerance, sweating, weight loss (or gain), increased appetite, nervousness, loose stools, frequent urination, muscle cramps, irritability, fatigue, weakness, dyspnea on exertion, and menstrual abnormalities (typically excess bleeding).

b. Patients also may have sinus tachycardia or atrial fibrillation, premature atrial contractions, palpitations, precordial chest pain, cardiomyopathy, warm moist skin, fine hair, stare, onycholysis, fine resting finger tremor, lid lag, hyperreflexia, and muscle weakness.

c. Hyperthyroidism caused by Graves' disease

(1) Patients may have a goiter, frequently with a bruit.

(2) Between 20% and 40% of patients will have mild ophthalmopathy (chemosis, conjunctivitis, proptosis), and between 5% and 10% will have severe ophthalmopathy (exophthalmos, possibly diplopia, corneal drying). Risk is higher in smokers. Changes may be asymmetric.

(3) Pretibial myxedema occurs in 3% of patients.

d. Ophthalmopathy also occurs in persons with type I amiodarone-induced thyrotoxicosis.

e. Findings may be limited to one organ system and may include isolated atrial fibrillation, psychosis, or myopathies.

f. Complications include atrial fibrillation, hypercalcemia, osteoporosis, impotence, nephrocalcinosis, decreased libido, gynecomastia, and decreased sperm count.

g. Chronic thyrotoxicosis may cause osteoporosis, clubbing, and finger swelling.

h. About 15% of Asian or Native American men with thyrotoxicosis may develop hypokalemic periodic paralysis lasting 7 to 72 hours, often after intravenous (IV) dextrose, oral carbohydrate, or vigorous exercise.

i. Thyroid storm

(1) Thyroid storm follows stressful illness, thyroid surgery, or radioactive iodine administration.

(2) It presents with high fever, tachycardia, vomiting, diarrhea, dehydration, marked weakness, and muscle wasting; extreme restlessness, confusion, delirium, and emotional lability may also occur.

(3) Although rare, its mortality rate is high.

3. Laboratory studies
   a. Laboratory studies are based on levels of thyroid hormones. TSH is secreted by the pituitary gland and stimulates thyroid hormone production. Thyroid hormone levels are affected by severe illness, cirrhosis, nephrotic syndrome, a variety of drugs, high-estrogen states, and acute psychiatric illness.
   b. In primary hyperthyroidism, TSH (the most sensitive indicator of thyroid disease) is low.
   c. Serum thyroxine (T_4), triiodothyronine (T_3), free T_4, free T_4 index, and thyroid resin uptake usually will be elevated.
   d. TSH receptor antibody and antithyroglobulin or antithyroperoxidase antibody levels usually are high in Graves' disease; serum antinuclear antibody and anti–double-stranded DNA antibodies usually are elevated without signs/symptoms of related conditions.
   e. In subacute thyroiditis, erythrocyte sedimentation rate may be elevated.
   f. Thyroid radioactive iodine uptake and scan reveal high uptake in Graves' disease and toxic multinodular goiter.
   g. Magnetic resonance imaging (MRI) of the orbits is preferred for evaluation of ophthalmopathy.
4. Treatment
   a. β-Blockers (primarily propranolol) control symptoms (tachycardia, tremor, diaphoresis, anxiety, palpitations) in any hyperthyroid episode and are the initial treatment of choice for thyroid storm and periodic paralysis.
   b. Thiourea drugs (methimazole or propylthiouracil)
      (1) These drugs control hyperthyroidism within several weeks and are taken for 12 to 24 months.
      (2) They are useful in preparing patients for surgery or radioactive iodine treatment.
      (3) Propylthiouracil is the drug of choice for pregnant and breast-feeding women.
      (4) Thiourea drugs are associated with lower risk of posttreatment hypothyroidism compared to other medical or surgical treatments.
      (5) Agranulocytosis is a rare complication.
   c. Radioactive iodine (^{131}I) ablation is preferred to surgery for permanent control, particularly in the elderly; it is contraindicated in pregnancy. Surgery is preferred for pregnant women, patients with large goiters, and when malignancy is likely.
   d. Iodinated contrast agents provide temporary treatment and may be helpful in highly symptomatic patients. T_3 levels may drop by more than 50% in 24 hours.
   e. Ophthalmopathy responds best to intravenous methylprednisolone, but may respond to high-dose, tapered prednisone treatment, particularly in nonsmokers. Retrobulbar radiation treatment or optic nerve decompression surgery may be indicated.
   f. Atrial fibrillation is not likely to convert electrically while the patient is hyperthyroid.
      (1) Digoxin may be used in large doses, and β-blockers with caution.
      (2) Anticoagulation with warfarin is used to prevent thromboembolism.
      (3) Congestive heart failure must be treated as usual, along with aggressive treatment for hyperthyroidism.
   g. Thyroid storm is a life-threatening emergency requiring prompt and specific treatment. The treatment for thyroid storm includes administration of β-blockers and hydrocortisone, supportive therapy, and attempts to control hyperthyroidism with a thiourea drug, followed by iodide.
B. Hypothyroidism and myxedema
   1. General characteristics
      a. Hypothyroidism almost always results from autoimmune thyroiditis, previous thyroid surgery, or radiation therapy.
      b. Hashimoto's thyroiditis (autoimmune thyroiditis, chronic lymphocytic thyroiditis) frequently leads to hypothyroidism.
   2. Clinical features
      a. Thyroiditis is often subclinical; if clinical, signs and symptoms tend to be vague and nonspecific.
      b. Common complaints include fatigue, lethargy, anorexia, constipation, depression, menstrual abnormalities, muscle stiffness, memory impairment, cold intolerance, and dry skin.
      c. Signs include peripheral edema, weight gain, thinning hair, weakness, hypotension, bradycardia, hyporeflexia, dementia, and psychosis.

3. Laboratory studies
   a. TSH will be elevated in primary disease.
   b. Low total T_4 and free T_4 are likely; T_3 may be normal.
   c. Presence of antithyroid peroxidase and antithyroglobulin antibodies in the serum confirms autoimmune disease.
4. Treatment with synthetic T_4 is best monitored by serial TSH levels.

C. Thyroiditis
   1. General characteristics
      a. Hashimoto's (chronic lymphocytic) thyroiditis is the most common thyroid disorder in the United States and may be associated with other autoimmune or polyglandular syndromes. It often is associated with other autoimmune disorders.
         (1) It affects 1% of the population and 5% of those over age 65 years. It tends to be familial and is more common in women (6:1) and patients with hepatitis C.
         (2) Frequency is increased with excess dietary iodine supplementation and exposure to head and neck radiation during childhood.
         (3) Certain drugs, such as amiodarone, interleukins, and interferon, are also associated with thyroiditis.
      b. Subacute (granulomatous, de Quervain's, giant cell) thyroiditis may present either with acute symptoms or silently and accounts for about 5% of clinical disease.
         (1) It is most common in young or middle-aged women.
         (2) A viral cause is suspected; the incidence peaks in summer.
      c. Postpartum thyroiditis occurs soon after parturition and usually resolves completely.
      d. Suppurative (infectious) and Riedel's (invasive fibrous, woody, ligneous) thyroiditis are rare.
   2. Clinical features
      a. In Hashimoto's thyroiditis, the thyroid is diffusely enlarged, firm, and finely nodular; changes may be asymmetric.
         (1) Signs and symptoms usually are of hypothyroidism (more likely in smokers), but transient thyrotoxicosis may occur.
            (a) It usually is not painful, although neck tightness occurs.
            (b) Depression and chronic fatigue are common and may persist after treatment.
            (c) Autoimmune xerostomia and keratoconjunctivitis may occur, as may mild myasthenia gravis. It is also associated with inflammatory bowel and celiac disease.
         (2) In elderly women (10% of cases), the gland is atrophic and fibrotic.
      b. Subacute thyroiditis presents as an acute, painful glandular enlargement with dysphagia, low-grade fever, fatigue, and malaise. Radiation of pain to the ears is common. It is most common in young and middle-aged women.
         (1) Patients may have thyrotoxicosis followed by hypothyroidism.
         (2) Manifestations last from weeks to months and usually resolve within 12 months.
      c. Postpartum thyroiditis manifests with hyperthyroidism 1 to 6 months after delivery and lasts for 1 to 2 months.
      d. Fever, pain, redness, and a fluctuant neck mass are common in suppurative thyroiditis associated with bacterial, fungal, or parasitic causes.
   3. Laboratory studies
      a. Testing for Hashimoto's disease involves screening for serum antithyroid peroxidase and antithyroglobulin antibodies, which will confirm autoimmune disease. The increase in T_4 is greater than that of T_3; TSH levels are suppressed.
      b. Ultrasonography helps distinguish thyroiditis from goiter or nodules and helps guide fine-needle biopsies of suspicious nodules; color-flow Doppler ultrasonography is used to distinguish thyroiditis from Graves' disease. Radioactive iodine uptake may also be helpful.
   4. Treatment is based on specific manifestations.
      a. Hashimoto's thyroiditis requires lifelong replacement with thyroid hormone for hypothyroidism or large goiter, with watchful waiting in others.
      b. Subacute thyroiditis is treated with aspirin; other treatment is directed at symptoms.
      c. Postpartum thyroiditis may not require therapy; propranolol is used for cardiac symptoms.
      d. Suppurative thyroiditis requires antibiotic therapy and surgical drainage.

D. Thyroid cancer

   1. General characteristics

      a. The most common form (80% of cases) is papillary carcinoma; other forms are follicular (14%), medullary (3%), anaplastic (2%), and lymphoma/metastatic disease (3%).

      b. Women are affected three times more often than men; the incidence increases with age.

      c. Cancer usually presents as a single nodule; however, only 5% of all palpable thyroid nodules are malignant.

      d. Cancer risk is associated with childhood neck or head irradiation or exposure to radioactive isotopes of iodine, with peak occurrence 20 to 25 years later.

      e. Papillary, follicular, medullary, and anaplastic cancers are all associated with genetic mutations and translocations.

      f. One-third of medullary carcinomas are sporadic, one-third familial, and one-third associated with multiple endocrine neoplasia (MEN) type 2. Families of patients with medullary disease should have genetic testing.

      g. Papillary carcinoma is usually the least aggressive and anaplastic the most aggressive.

   2. Clinical features

      a. Patients most often present with painless neck swelling and have a single, palpable, nontender, firm nodule. Hoarseness, neck discomfort, and dysphagia also may occur.

      b. The nodule may enlarge over a short period.

      c. Patients may have evidence of metastatic disease, including thyrotoxicosis.

      d. The gland often is stony and hard.

      e. Medullary carcinoma causes flushing, diarrhea, fatigue, and Cushing's syndrome; anaplastic carcinoma has signs of pressure or invasion, such as recurrent laryngeal nerve palsy (hoarseness).

   3. Laboratory studies

      a. Thyroid function tests often are normal; TSH should be measured to exclude primary thyroid disease.

      b. Serum thyroglobulin is often elevated in metastatic papillary and follicular cancers.

      c. Fine-needle biopsy is essential.

      d. Medullary tumors have high serum calcitonin and carcinoembryonic antigen.

      e. Hot nodules on radionuclide scanning usually are benign.

      f. Ultrasonography of the neck is useful in determining size, location, and local metastasis; other possible tests include radioisotope scanning, chest radiography, MRI, computed tomography (CT), and positron-emission tomography (PET).

   4. Treatment

      a. Surgical resection and near-total thyroidectomy are indicated, followed by radiation for anaplastic disease. Monitor for postoperative hypocalcemia.

      b. T_4 therapy prevents hypothyroidism and reduces the risk of recurrence.

      c. Radioactive iodine ablation is used for residual disease.

      d. Metastatic bone disease is treated with external radiation and brain metastasis with gamma knife radiation therapy.

II. PARATHYROID DISORDERS

A. Hypoparathyroidism and pseudohypoparathyroidism

   1. General characteristics

      a. Hypoparathyroidism most commonly is found after thyroidectomy, but it also may be caused by heavy metal toxicity, granulomas, Riedel's thyroiditis, tumors, infection, autoimmune problems, or, rarely, neck irradiation.

      b. Functional disease may occur in the presence of magnesium deficiency.

      c. Pseudohypoparathyroidism results from a group of diseases characterized by hypocalcemia caused by renal resistance to parathyroid hormone.

      d. DiGeorge's syndrome includes hypoparathyroidism plus congenital facial and cardiac anomalies.

      e. Hypoparathyroidism is a possible manifestation of polyglandular autoimmunity type 1.

   2. Clinical features

      a. Acute disease causes tetany, carpopedal spasm, cramping, convulsions, circumoral and distal extremity tingling, and irritability.

    b. Positive Chvostek's sign (facial muscle contraction after tapping the facial nerve) and Trousseau's phenomenon (carpal spasm with blood pressure cuff inflation) as well as cataracts and teeth and nail defects indicate associated hypocalcemia.

    c. Findings in patients with chronic disease include lethargy, anxiety, parkinsonism, mental retardation, personality changes, and blurred vision caused by cataracts.

    d. Dry skin, loss of eyebrow hair, brittle nails, and hyperreflexia may be present.

3. Laboratory and diagnostic studies

    a. Corrected serum calcium, urinary calcium, and parathyroid hormone levels are low.

    b. Serum magnesium may be low.

    c. Serum phosphate will be high; alkaline phosphatase will be normal.

    d. CT or radiography of the skull may show dense bones and basal ganglia calcifications.

    e. Electrocardiographic (ECG) findings include prolonged QT intervals and T-wave abnormalities.

    f. Slit-lamp examination may show early posterior lenticular changes.

    g. Radiography may demonstrate chronic increased bone mineral density, especially in the lumbar spine.

4. Treatment

    a. Emergency treatment for tetany includes airway maintenance and slow administration of IV calcium gluconate.

    b. Maintenance therapy includes oral calcium (1 to 2 g/day) and vitamin D preparations to keep serum calcium at 8 to 8.6 mg/dL. Calcitriol is also used.

    c. Magnesium supplementation may be required.

    d. Transplantation of cryopreserved parathyroid tissue may restore normocalcemia.

    e. Monitoring of treatment includes measurement of serum and urine calcium levels.

    f. Phenothiazines and furosemide should be avoided.

B. Hyperparathyroidism

1. General characteristics

    a. This condition is more common in women (3:1) compared to men and in those older than 50 years.

    b. Causes include parathyroid adenoma (80%) and, less commonly, hyperplasia or carcinoma. Multiglandular disease and carcinoma are more common in persons younger than 30 years.

    c. Many malignancies also cause hypercalcemia and have clinical findings similar to those of hyperparathyroidism.

2. Clinical features

    a. Hypercalcemia of hyperparathyroidism most commonly is identified on routine chemistry panels in asymptomatic patients; abnormal screening studies should be repeated.

    b. Patients may have polydipsia and polyuria caused by hypercalcemia-induced nephrogenic diabetes insipidus (DI).

    c. Excessive calcium and phosphate excretion may lead to renal stones, and nephrocalcinosis and renal failure may occur.

    d. Bone pain and arthralgias are common; cortical bone or diffuse bone demineralization, trabecular bone increase, pathologic fractures, and cystic bone lesions may occur (jaw is most common). Pathologic fractures are more common than in the general population.

    e. Mild hypercalcemia is likely to be asymptomatic; if the hypercalcemia is more severe, it causes thirst, anorexia, nausea, vomiting, abdominal pain, constipation, fatigue, anemia, weight loss, peptic ulcer disease, pancreatitis, hypertension, and depressed deep tendon reflexes.

    f. Depression, increased need for sleep, muscle weakness, fatigability, paresthesias, pruritus, disorientation, cognitive impairment, psychosis, and coma occur in severe disease.

    g. Signs and symptoms can be summarized as "bones, stones, abdominal groans, psychic moans, with fatigue overtones."

    h. Secondary hypercalcemia is caused by many malignant tumors (e.g., breast, lung, pancreas, uterus) and, in older persons, by multiple myeloma.

    i. Other secondary causes of hypercalcemia include granulomatous disorders, calcium or vitamin D ingestion, familial hypocalciuric hypercalcemia, adrenal insufficiency, hyperthyroidism, certain medications, prolonged bed rest, and acute renal failure.

3. Laboratory studies

   a. Hypercalcemia (Ca^{2+} >10.5 mg/dL) is the hallmark; serum phosphate often is less than 2.5 mg/dL.

   b. Urine calcium excretion generally is low for the degree of hypercalcemia. Excess loss of phosphate in the urine occurs, and serum phosphate is low to normal.

   c. Elevated parathyroid hormone levels confirm the diagnosis.

   d. Vitamin D levels should be determined with a serum 25-OH vitamin D level.

   e. All patients should be screened for familial benign hypocalciuric hypercalcemia with a 24-hour urine for calcium and creatinine before treating for hyperparathyroidism.

   f. ECG findings may include prolonged PR interval, shortened QT interval, bradyarrhythmias, heart block, and asystole.

4. Treatment

   a. Surgical treatment is recommended for symptomatic and certain asymptomatic patients. Hypocalcemia is a common complication, as is transient hyperthyroidism.

   b. Medical treatment includes intensive hydration, inhibitors of bone resorption (i.e., bisphosphonates), calcium-receptor agonists, and avoidance of immobility; postmenopausal estrogen supplementation and propranolol may be helpful. Cautious administration of vitamin D may be indicated.

   c. Patients should avoid thiazide diuretics, large doses of vitamins A and D, and calcium-containing antacids and supplements.

III. DIABETES MELLITUS

A. General characteristics

   1. DM describes a group of disorders characterized by disordered metabolism and inappropriate hyperglycemia. This may be due to deficiencies in insulin secretion, inadequate response to insulin, or both.

   2. Most patients with diabetes have type 1 (1,000,000 patients in the United States) or type 2 (17.2 million patients in the United States).

   3. Rare types of diabetes include maturity-onset diabetes of the young (MODY), diabetes caused by mutant insulins or insulin receptors, diseases of the exocrine pancreas, endocrinopathies, drug and chemical induced diabetes, and other genetic syndromes.

   4. Insulin resistance syndrome (metabolic syndrome, syndrome X) is a constellation of hyperglycemia, hyperinsulinemia, dyslipidemia (including elevated triglycerides and decreased high-density lipoprotein [HDL]), and hypertension; it predisposes patients to coronary artery disease (CAD) and stroke. Patients also may have hyperuricemia and abdominal obesity, as well as prothrombotic and proinflammatory states.

   5. Diabetic retinopathy is the leading cause of blindness among people in the United States who are older than 60 years. Other ocular problems include premature cataracts and glaucoma.

   6. Diabetic nephropathy causes approximately one-third of end-stage renal disease in the United States. Patients with type 1 DM have a 30% to 40% chance, whereas those with type 2 DM have a 15% to 20% chance of serious renal disease.

   7. Patients with diabetes have accelerated large vessel atherosclerosis, putting them at increased risk for stroke and CAD. Large vessel atherosclerosis in diabetic patients also is the cause of at least half of the nontraumatic lower extremity amputations in the United States.

   8. Neuropathy is the most common complication of DM.

      a. It commonly causes a characteristic peripheral symmetric polyneuropathy but may cause a peripheral mononeuropathy or mononeuropathy multiplex.

      b. Painful foot neuropathy may be physically and emotionally disabling.

      c. Nerve damage also causes autonomic dysfunction, leading to erectile dysfunction, atonic bladder, and delayed gastric emptying.

   9. Skin changes associated with DM include candidal infections, slow wound healing, necrobiosis lipoidica diabeticorum, and acanthosis nigricans.

B. Type 1 DM

   1. General characteristics

      a. Type 1 occurs most often in young people (before school age or near puberty) of normal or low weight, particularly among individuals of Scandinavian ancestry; nonautoimmune type 1 disease occurs primarily in those of Asian or African origin.

    b. There is little or no endogenous insulin secretion.

        (1) Plasma glucagon is elevated.

        (2) Pancreatic B cells fail to respond to stimuli and undergo autoimmune destruction. If untreated, this is a catabolic state with ketosis.

    c. Most type 1 DM is an autoimmune disease (90%), with 95% of patients having HLA-DR3 or HLA-DR4 antigens. HLA-DQ genes are even more specific, and 85% of patients have islet cell antibodies. Sixteen other genetic regions related to risk also have been identified. It is estimated that genetic factors account for one-third of the susceptibility to DM and environmental factors for two-thirds.

    d. Extrinsic factors hypothesized to affect pancreatic B-cell function include mumps and Coxsackie B4 virus infection, toxic chemicals, and destructive cytokines and antibodies.

2. Clinical features

    a. The most common findings include polydipsia, polyuria, nocturia, and rapid weight loss despite normal or increased appetite, associated with a random plasma glucose of 200 mg/dL or greater.

    b. Blurred vision is common; pruritus, weakness, postural hypotension, paresthesias, and vulvovaginitis may occur.

    c. Untreated type 1 DM results in diabetic ketoacidosis, leading to anorexia, nausea, vomiting, dehydration, stupor, and, ultimately, coma. Fruity breath suggests ketoacidosis.

3. Laboratory studies

    a. A random plasma glucose of more than 200 mg/dL with classic symptoms or fasting levels of 126 mg/dL or greater on more than one occasion is diagnostic.

    b. Most patients with new-onset type 1 DM will have a severely elevated glucose, warranting no further diagnostic study; suspected cases may be confirmed by glucose tolerance testing.

    c. Patients are likely to have glucosuria; they also may have ketonemia and/or ketonuria.

    d. Hemoglobin A1 (glycosylated hemoglobin, HbA1) reflects glycemic control over the preceding 8 to 12 weeks; this test should not be used for diagnosing diabetes.

        (1) Levels of HbA1c (the major form) are highly specific and are used to follow treatment.

        (2) Serum fructosamine reflects control over the preceding 1 to 2 weeks, resulting in more rapid change than HbA1c. This test should be complementary to glycosylated hemoglobin and not substitutive.

    e. Patients should use a portable glucometer to monitor control; continuous monitoring systems are available but expensive.

    f. Well-controlled type 1 DM results in normal lipid values.

    g. Patients with DM should also be closely monitored for risk of cardiovascular disease.

4. Treatment

    a. Diet is central to management.

        (1) Diet must be individualized according to the patient's activity level, food preferences, and need to attain and maintain ideal weight.

        (2) Patients with type 1 DM should follow a well-balanced diet and may apply the principles of carbohydrate counting, often administering 1 U of short or rapidly acting insulin for each 10 to 15 g ingested in addition to basal insulin needs.

            (a) Carbohydrates should comprise 45% to 65% of the diet, protein 10% to 35% of total daily calories, and fat 25% to 35% with less than 7% saturated.

            (b) Cholesterol should be limited to fewer than 33 mg/day or less.

        (3) A diet high in soluble fiber improves glucose through slowed absorption and improves cholesterol levels; insoluble fiber improves colonic transit.

        (4) Patients should coordinate meals and snacks with exercise and insulin administration.

        (5) Artificial sweeteners appropriate for patients with diabetes include aspartame, saccharin, sucralose, and acesulfame potassium.

    b. Insulin may be delivered by subcutaneous injection, injector pens, or insulin pump.

        (1) Glycemic response depends on depth of injection, injection site, proximity of site to muscles being exercised, and ambient temperature.

        (2) Regular insulin is absorbed most rapidly from the abdomen, but any site with loose skin may be used. Analog insulins are less affected by site of injection.

    (3) Human insulin causes markedly less antibody response than animal insulin and is available in regular or neutral protamine hagedorn (NPH) formulations.

    (4) Analog insulins include rapid-acting (lispro, aspart, glulisine) and long-acting (glargine, detemir) forms.

    (5) Rapid-acting insulins (lispro, aspart, glulisine) reach peak serum values in 1 hour and have a 4-hour duration of action; they may be taken 20 minutes before a meal.

    (6) Regular insulin is short acting and is used an hour before meals; the effect appears in 30 minutes, peaks in 60 minutes, and lasts for 5 to 7 hours. IV administration is useful in diabetic ketoacidosis and in perioperative management of patients with diabetes.

    (7) NPH insulin is a longer-acting form with onset of action in 2 to 4 hours, peak effect in 8 to 10 hours, and duration of action of less than 24 hours (range 18 to 24 hours), often requiring two injections per day. NPH is often used in combination with regular or lispro insulin for improved control.

    (8) Glargine is given once a day for basal coverage, but cannot be mixed with other human insulins due to its acidity. It lasts for about 24 hours without peaks.

    (9) Detemir has a 17-hour duration of action and may be given daily or twice daily for basal coverage.

  c. Daily aspirin (81 to 325 mg) reduces the risk of diabetic atherothrombosis.

  d. Careful foot care, moderate exercise, meticulous personal hygiene, and prompt treatment of infection are imperative.

  e. Pancreas transplant is becoming more common but is not considered standard therapy at this time.

C. Type 2 DM

  1. General characteristics

    a. Type 2 DM, a heterogeneous group of diseases, occurs most often in middle-aged or older people; however, it is increasingly found in younger persons.

    b. Overweight and obesity are the strongest contributing factors. Distribution of fat to the upper body is associated with the highest risk, and exercise and weight loss decrease the risk.

    c. Type 2 DM has a strong genetic component, but a specific gene has not yet been identified.

    d. In the United States, type 2 DM accounts for more than 90% of diabetes cases and is found more often in African Americans, Hispanics, Pima Indians, and Pacific Islanders.

    e. In type 2 DM, insulin levels are high enough to prevent ketoacidosis, but tissues are resistant. Impaired pancreatic B-cell response to glucose also often is present. Resistance is increased with aging, sedentary lifestyle, and abdominovisceral obesity.

    f. Untreated type 2 DM can lead to hyperosmolar nonketotic states.

  2. Clinical features

    a. Many patients have polyuria and polydipsia; ketonuria and weight loss are rare.

    b. Patients also may present with fatigue, pruritus, recurrent candidal vaginitis, chronic skin infections, blurred vision, or poor wound healing.

    c. Many patients, particularly those who are obese, have few symptoms; DM is discovered during routine laboratory testing. Distribution of fat to the upper body is associated with increased risk; measuring waist-to-hip ratio is useful in monitoring treatment.

    d. Women who have delivered large-for-gestational age babies or had polyhydramnios, preeclampsia, or unexplained fetal loss are at increased risk.

  3. Laboratory studies

    a. The diagnostic criteria for type 2 DM are the same as those for type 1 DM: random glucose greater than 200 mg/dL or fasting glucose greater or equal to 126 mg/dL on more than one occasion.

    b. An oral glucose tolerance test may be needed in symptomatic patients, with fasting glucose levels between 100 and 125 mg/dL.

    c. HbA1c and fructosamine are used to monitor chronic control.

    d. Diabetic dyslipidemia includes high triglycerides, low HDL, and alteration of low-density lipoprotein (LDL) to smaller, denser particles. It is very common in type 2 DM.

    e. Impaired fasting glucose (glucose of 100 to 125 mg/dL in fasting state) and impaired glucose tolerance (glucose of 140 to 199 mg/dL 2 hours after 75 g oral glucose) are considered strong risk factors for the development of type 2 DM. These individuals benefit most from primary prevention efforts (diet, weight loss, and exercise).

4. Treatment
   a. Diet must be individualized, as for type 1 DM. In obese patients, the goal should be weight loss, which may restore insulin responsiveness.
   b. Cholesterol, protein, fat, fiber, and artificial sweetener recommendations are the same as in type 1 DM.
   c. Regular exercise also is correlated with better glucose control.
   d. Oral hypoglycemic agents potentiate insulin secretion.
      (1) The most commonly used oral hypoglycemic agents are the sulfonylureas; of these, glyburide, glipizide, and glimepiride are second-generation agents with few drug interactions. They are associated with weight gain and increased risk of hypoglycemia.
      (2) Other, newer insulin-stimulating drugs are repaglinide and nateglinide.
   e. Metformin, which reduces hepatic glucose production, may be used as a first- or second-line agent. It is considered first line in obese persons with mild disease. It decreases glucose levels without the risk of hypoglycemia, assists with weight loss, and decreases triglycerides, but is contraindicated in patients at risk for lactic acidosis, those with serum creatinine greater than 1.5 mg/dL (males) or greater than 1.4 mg/dL (females) or abnormal creatinine clearance. It is associated with gastrointestinal (GI) side effects.
   f. Thiazolidinediones (pioglitazone preferred due to questions about rosiglitazone's potential for causing cardiac disease) sensitize peripheral tissues to insulin and may be used either alone or in combination with a sulfonylurea, metformin, or insulin. They reduce glucose without increasing the risk for hypoglycemia but are contraindicated in patients with congestive heart failure (NY Heart Association stage 3 or 4 in particular) or liver disease.
   g. α-Glucosidase inhibitors (acarbose, miglitol) delay absorption of carbohydrate from the intestine, thereby decreasing glucose in the bloodstream. Their major side effects are GI symptoms.
   h. Exenatide lowers blood glucose via slowing of gastric emptying, stimulating the pancreatic insulin response to glucose, and prevents glucagon release after meals. It must be injected. Adverse effects include nausea and pancreatitis; it is contraindicated in patients with gastroparesis. Exenatide is associated with weight loss.
   i. Sitagliptin has a low risk of hypoglycemia and does not cause nausea and vomiting; serious allergic reactions (anaphylaxis, Stevens–Johnson syndrome) have occurred.
   j. Approximately one-third of patients with type 2 DM require insulin, either alone or in combination with other agents.
   k. Acceptable glucose levels are 70 to 130 mg/dL before meals and after an overnight fast and 180 mg/dL or less at 1 hour and less than 150 mg/dL at 2 hours postprandially. Patients should monitor glucose levels regularly.
   l. Careful foot care, moderate exercise, meticulous personal hygiene, and prompt treatment of infection are imperative.
   m. Daily aspirin (81 to 325 mg) reduces the risk of diabetic atherothrombosis. Careful monitoring and treatment of blood pressure to a goal of less than 130 systolic and less than 80 diastolic is essential to reduce the risk of cardiovascular disease. Hyperlipidemia should be treated with a goal of less than 100 mg/dL LDL and greater than 50 mg/dL HDL.
   n. Annual ophthalmologic exams are recommended to monitor for diabetic retinopathy.
   o. Annual urine albumin and serum creatinine is also recommended; early identification and treatment will reduce risk or slow progression of diabetic nephropathy.
   p. Aggressive insulin management of a patient with not-so-tightly controlled type 2 diabetes while the patient is hospitalized has been associated with increased morbidity. More research is needed in this area.
D. Hypoglycemia
   1. General characteristics
      a. Fasting hypoglycemia occurs secondary to some endocrine disorders, liver malfunction, and renal failure; primary hypoglycemia is caused by either hyperinsulinism (e.g., exogenous administration, insulinoma) or extrapancreatic tumors.
      b. Postprandial or reactive hypoglycemia is classified as early (2 to 3 hours after eating) or late (3 to 5 hours after eating).
      c. Other causes include GI surgery/dumping syndrome, functional, β-cell dysfunction, alcohol related, factitious, immunopathologic, and drug induced.
   2. Clinical features
      a. Symptoms begin at plasma glucose levels of 60 mg/dL; cognitive impairment begins at 50 mg/dL.
      b. Fasting hypoglycemia often is subacute or chronic and presents with neuroglycopenia.
      c. Postprandial hypoglycemia usually is acute and presents with sweating, palpitations, anxiety, and tremulousness.

    d. The Whipple's triad consists of a history of hypoglycemic symptoms, a fasting blood glucose of 40 mg/dL or less, and immediate recovery on administration of glucose.

  3. Laboratory studies depend on the suspected cause.

  4. Treatment is directed at the underlying cause.

IV. ADRENAL DISORDERS

A. Chronic adrenocortical insufficiency (Addison's disease)

  1. General characteristics

    a. The most common cause is autoimmune destruction of the adrenal cortex (80% of cases).

    b. It may occur alone or as part of polyglandular autoimmune (PGA) syndrome or genetic disorders such as adrenoleukodystrophy.

    c. Pituitary failure causes secondary adrenocortical insufficiency.

    d. Tuberculosis is a leading cause of Addison's disease in areas of prevalence.

    e. Adrenal crises may be precipitated by infection, trauma, surgery, stress, lymphoma, metastatic cancer, amyloidosis, scleroderma, hemochromatosis, or cessation of corticosteroid medication.

  2. Clinical features

    a. Addison's disease begins insidiously with nonspecific problems, such as fatigue and weakness. Anorexia and weight loss usually are present, as is irritability/anxiety.

    b. Most patients have myalgias and arthralgias; many have GI symptoms. Amenorrhea is common in females.

    c. Many patients develop sensory hypersensitivities.

    d. Some patients crave salt.

    e. Orthostatic hypotension is common. Systolic BP less than 110 mm Hg is found in 90% of patients.

    f. Delayed deep tendon reflexes are found.

    g. Hyperpigmentation is found only in primary disease (i.e., when adrenocorticotropic hormone [ACTH] is elevated). This is most marked in skin creases, pressure areas, and nipple areas.

    h. Other findings include small heart, hyperplasia of lymphoid tissues, scant axillary and pubic hair, and hypogonadism.

    i. Addisonian crisis is heralded by hypotension, acute pain (abdomen, low back), vomiting, diarrhea, dehydration, hypotension, and altered mental status. If untreated, it can be fatal.

  3. Laboratory studies

    a. Laboratory findings include hyperkalemia (only in primary disease), hyponatremia, hypoglycemia, hypercalcemia, and low blood urea nitrogen (BUN).

    b. Neutropenia, mild anemia, relative lymphocytosis, and eosinophilia may occur.

    c. Low (<3 μg/dL) 8:00 AM plasma cortisol accompanied by elevation of the plasma ACTH (>200 pg/mL) is diagnostic. Low levels of ACTH indicate secondary disease.

    d. The simplified cosyntropin stimulation test also is diagnostic. A serum cortisol rise of more than 20 μg/dL after administration of cosyntropin is normal; anything less is suspicious.

    e. Antiadrenal antibodies will be present in 50% of patients; antithyroid antibodies are found in 45% of patients.

    f. Serum dehydroepiandrosterone (DHEA) levels are less than 1,000 ng/mL; a level higher than this excludes Addison's disease.

    g. Chest radiography and abdominal CT scanning may be indicated for suspected secondary disease.

  4. Treatment

    a. Primary disease is treated with oral hydrocortisone or prednisone; many patients also require fludrocortisone acetate for its sodium-retaining effect.

    b. DHEA may be given to women who have adrenal insufficiency.

    c. Addisonian crisis requires aggressive IV saline, glucose, and glucocorticoids as well as treatment of underlying cause.

B. Cushing's disease and syndrome (hypercortisolism)

  1. General characteristics

    a. Cushing's syndrome may be exogenous or endogenous. The exogenous form is caused by chronic excess glucocorticoid, most commonly from corticosteroid drugs used to treat other diseases.

b. Cushing's disease is caused by excess secretion of ACTH by the pituitary, often resulting from a small, benign pituitary adenoma.

   (1) Cushing's disease is the major cause of endogenous Cushing's syndrome.

   (2) It is most common in premenopausal women.

c. Adrenocortical tumors and nonpituitary ACTH-producing tumors (most often small cell lung carcinoma) also may cause Cushing's syndrome.

2. Clinical features

a. Hypercortisolism may present as obesity, hypertension, and thirst and polyuria with or without glycosuria.

   (1) Obesity is centripetal, and extremities may appear wasted.

   (2) Fat deposition also causes the characteristic buffalo hump, moon facies, and supraclavicular pads.

b. The most specific signs are proximal muscle weakness and pigmented striae more than 1 cm wide; patients may present with backache and headache.

c. Oligomenorrhea or amenorrhea and erectile dysfunction are common.

d. Disorders of calcium metabolism may cause osteoporosis, vertebral fractures, hypercalciuria, and kidney stones. Avascular necrosis may occur.

e. Impaired wound healing, acne, easy bruisability, and superficial skin infections occur.

f. Psychiatric symptoms range from emotional lability to psychosis.

3. Laboratory studies

a. Excretion of free cortisol in the urine of greater than 125 mg/dL in 24 hours is diagnostic, as is greater than 95 mcg of cortisol per gram of creatinine.

b. Salivary cortisol assays are now available.

c. In Cushing's disease, the overnight dexamethasone suppression test will result in a plasma cortisol of greater than 10 μg/dL (<5 μg/dL is normal).

d. The cortisol excretion test and plasma cortisol test should be confirmed with a low-dose dexamethasone suppression test. False positives are caused by rifampin, phenytoin, primidone, phenobarbital, carbamazepine, fenofibrate, estrogens, and pregnancy.

e. Plasma ACTH of less than 20 pg/mL suggests adrenal tumor; higher levels suggest pituitary or ectopic production.

f. MRI is preferred to identify pituitary tumors. CT may show adrenocortical or other tumors. Somatostatin receptor scintigraphy is useful in detecting occult tumors.

g. Hyperglycemia, impaired glucose tolerance, and hypokalemia (without hypernatremia) are not unusual.

4. Treatment

a. Treatment of Cushing's disease is transsphenoidal resection of the pituitary adenoma and hydrocortisol replacement; an alternative is gamma knife radiosurgery.

b. Surgical removal of tumors is the treatment of choice for Cushing's syndrome.

c. Radiation and chemotherapy may be used for nonresectable tumors.

d. Adrenal inhibitors also can be used.

   (1) Metyrapone and/or ketoconazole may suppress hypercortisolism.

   (2) Parenteral octreotide suppresses ACTH in one-third of cases.

V. PITUITARY DISORDERS

A. Acromegaly or gigantism

   1. General characteristics

   a. Acromegaly almost always is caused by a pituitary adenoma and involves excessive growth hormone.

   b. It usually is sporadic but may be familial; it also may be part of multiple endocrine neoplasia (MEN) type 1.

   2. Clinical features

   a. Excessive growth of hands, feet, jaw, and internal organs occurs in acromegaly.

   b. Gigantism occurs if disease ensues before closure of the epiphyses.

   c. Other features include doughy, moist handshake; macroglossia; carpal tunnel syndrome; deep, coarse voice; obstructive sleep apnea; goiter; hypertension and cardiomegaly; weight gain and insulin resistance; arthralgias and arthritis; colon polyps; hyperhydrosis; cystic acne; acanthosis nigricans; headaches; spinal stenosis; temporal hemianopsia; decreased libido; erectile dysfunction; and menstrual abnormalities.

3. Laboratory studies

   a. Serum prolactin, insulinlike growth factor I, glucose, liver enzymes, BUN, TSH, free T$_4$, inorganic phosphorus, and calcium are measured after an overnight fast.

   b. Serum growth hormone is measured 1 hour after glucose syrup ingestion.

   c. Radiology

      (1) MRI is superior to CT for pituitary adenomas, which are present in 90% of patients with acromegaly.

      (2) Radiography may show enlarged sella turcica, thickened skull, tufting of the terminal phalanges, and thickening of the heel pad.

4. Treatment

   a. Treatment generally is endoscopic transnasal transsphenoidal pituitary microsurgery to remove the adenoma.

   b. Dopamine agonists are used in patients who fail surgery.

   c. Somatostatin analogs are beneficial for persistent disease.

   d. Pegvisomant, a growth hormone receptor antagonist, provides symptomatic relief and normalizes insulinlike growth factor I in about 90% of patients.

   e. Stereotactic radiosurgery is used for treatment failures.

B. Dwarfism

1. General characteristics: The prototype chondroplasia is achondroplasia, the most common nonlethal type.

2. Clinical features

   a. Achondroplastic dwarfs

      (1) These dwarfs have short limbs, long and narrow trunks, large heads with midface hypoplasia, and prominent brows.

      (2) They have delayed motor milestones and fall below normal height standards.

      (3) Intelligence is normal.

      (4) Neurologic complications, bowing of the legs, obesity, dental problems, and frequent otitis media are common.

   b. A substantial reduction in height may occur in children who have type I DM.

   c. Although not usually apparent at birth, pituitary dwarfism may present in male infants with hypoglycemia and micropenis.

   d. Children with constitutional growth delay are small but otherwise of normal appearance.

3. Laboratory studies: The achondroplasia group of disorders are all caused by mutations in the *FGFR3* gene.

4. Treatment

   a. Surgical correction of orthopaedic problems is indicated in achondroplasia.

   b. Use of human growth hormone is controversial.

C. Diabetes insipidus

1. General characteristics

   a. DI is uncommon and caused by deficiency of or resistance to vasopressin (antidiuretic hormone [ADH]).

   b. Primary DI may be familial (genetic) or sporadic.

   c. Secondary DI is due to hypothalamic or pituitary pathology caused by tumor, anoxic encephalopathy, surgery, accidental trauma, infection, sarcoidosis, multifocal Langerhans cell granulomatosis, or metastatic disease.

   d. Vasopressinase-induced DI may be seen during late pregnancy and the puerperium.

   e. Nephrogenic DI occurs in the presence of normal secretion of vasopressin with inappropriate response by the kidney.

2. Clinical features

   a. Intense thirst with fluid intake of 2 to 20 L/day, craving for ice water, and large-volume polyuria are most common; other possible presentations are hypernatremia and dehydration.

   b. Unremitting enuresis may be present in partial disease.

3. No single laboratory study can diagnose DI.

   a. Serum tests include glucose, BUN, calcium, uric acid, potassium, and sodium.

b. Urine collection for 24 hours is needed for volume, glucose, and creatinine; dipstick testing shows a low specific gravity, usually less than 1.006.

c. Central DI may be confirmed with a vasopressin challenge test.

4. Treatment

   a. Desmopressin acetate is the treatment of choice for central DI and DI associated with pregnancy and the puerperium.

   b. Mild cases may require no treatment except adequate hydration.

   c. Central and nephrogenic DI respond partially to hydrochlorothiazide with potassium.

   d. Nephrogenic DI may respond to indomethacin, either alone or in combination with hydrochlorothiazide, desmopressin, or ameloride.

VI. OTHER ENDOCRINE DISORDERS

A. Metabolic bone disease

   1. Osteoporosis (see Chapter 9)

   2. Osteomalacia and rickets

      a. General characteristics

         (1) Osteomalacia and rickets are diseases of defective mineralization.

         (2) Osteomalacia is found in adults and rickets is found in children.

         (3) Both most often are caused by a deficiency of vitamin D; they also may be caused by calcium or phosphate deficiency or aluminum toxicity. Other causes include disorders of bone matrix and inhibitors of mineralization.

         (4) Phenytoin, carbamazepine, valproate, and barbiturates may induce osteomalacia.

      b. Clinical features

         (1) Patients with osteomalacia present with diffuse muscle weakness (especially in the pelvic girdle), fractures following minor or no trauma, and bone pain.

         (2) Children develop permanent skeletal deformities.

      c. Laboratory studies

         (1) In osteomalacia, radiography shows generalized decrease in bone density; Milkman lines or Looser zones (pseudofractures) are diagnostic.

         (2) Both osteomalacia and rickets may be diagnosed by bone biopsy, although biopsy is not usually necessary.

         (3) Hypocalcemia, hypocalciuria, hypophosphatemia, secondary hyperparathyroidism, increased alkaline phosphatase, and decreased 25-OH vitamin D may be present.

      d. Treatment

         (1) Some patients require ergocalciferol (50,000 U by mouth twice per week for 6 to 12 months, followed by 1,000 to 2,000 U daily) to treat vitamin D deficiency.

         (2) Phosphate supplementation and vitamin D are required for renal phosphate wasting.

         (3) Oral calcium should be given with meals to treat nutritional calcium deficiency.

         (4) Aluminum-containing antacids should be discontinued.

         (5) Patients on phenytoin should be treated prophylactically.

   3. Paget's disease of bone (osteitis deformans)

      a. General characteristics

         (1) Paget's disease of bone involves localized dysplastic bone formation.

         (2) It affects 1% to 2% of adults and 5% to 11% of those in their 80s. Prevalence is highest among the elderly in the northeastern United States.

         (3) Patients may have a family history of Paget's disease.

         (4) In 1% to 3% of patients, long-standing lesions transform into osteosarcoma.

      b. Clinical features

         (1) Most patients (three-quarters) are asymptomatic.

         (2) Bone and joint pain often is the first symptom.

            (a) Common sites of involvement are spine, pelvis, femur, humerus, tibia, and skull.

        (b) Patients may present with pathologic fractures or other symptoms related to the site (e.g., headache, increased hat size, warmth).

    (3) Patients also may have bowed tibias and kyphosis.

    (4) Mixed sensorineural/conductive deafness is the most common neurologic finding.

    (5) Cardiac output may increase and progress to failure.

  c. Laboratory studies

    (1) Serum calcium and phosphate are normal; alkaline phosphatase is high.

    (2) Hypercalciuria is common, and urinary hydroxyproline is elevated in active disease.

    (3) Hypercalcemia occurs in patients on bed rest.

    (4) The extent of the disease should be determined by skeletal radiography (dense, expanded bone; fissures in long bone) and bone scans.

  d. Treatment

    (1) Prompt cyclic administration of bisphosphonates (alendronate, tiludronate, risedronate, zoledronic acid, or pamidronate) is the treatment of choice.

    (2) Nasal calcitonin–salmon (miacalcin) is an alternative treatment.

B. Dyslipidemia

  1. General characteristics

    a. Dyslipidemias are highly associated with atherosclerosis, especially CAD.

    b. Reducing total cholesterol in patients with known cardiovascular disease reduces total mortality in both men and women and middle-aged and older patients; in patients without cardiovascular disease, results are less conclusive.

    c. LDL cholesterol is associated with increased risk of atherosclerotic heart disease, and HDL cholesterol is associated with decreased risk.

    d. Hypertriglyceridemia is a risk factor for CAD, especially in women and diabetics. Severe elevations can cause pancreatitis.

    e. Genetic forms of dyslipidemia are rare, but patients with a history of familial hypercholesterolemia, familial combined hyperlipidemia, familial hyperchylomicronemia, or dysbetalipoproteinemia must be screened.

    f. Secondary hyperlipidemia has many possible causes including diabetes, alcohol use, hypothyroidism, hypercortisolism, acromegaly, obesity, sedentary lifestyle, renal and liver problems, estrogens, thiazide diuretics, and β-blockers.

  2. Clinical features

    a. Most patients have no symptoms or signs.

    b. Eruptive and tendinous xanthomas are common with hyperlipidemia and usually indicate a genetic cause.

    c. Nearly two-thirds of all people with xanthelasmas (the commonest form of xanthomas, affecting the eyelids) have normal lipid profiles.

    d. Patients with severe hypercholesterolemia may develop premature arcus senilis; lipemia retinalis is seen with triglyceride levels of greater than 2,000 mg/dL.

  3. Laboratory studies

    a. Patients with any evidence of cardiovascular disease or who have a coronary heart disease (CHD) risk equivalent should be screened with a fasting complete lipid profile; those without cardiac risk factors should be screened with at least a measurement of total cholesterol.

    b. Screening for patients with no evidence of cardiovascular disease and no other risk factors should begin at 35 years of age for men and 45 years of age for women.

    c. Risk factors for cardiovascular disease include family history, hypertension, cigarette smoking, DM, low HDL cholesterol, older age, and male gender.

    d. Screening may include total cholesterol alone, total and HDL cholesterol, or LDL and HDL cholesterol levels.

  4. Treatment

    a. Nonpharmacologic therapy

      (1) Initial dietary changes should include reducing total dietary fat to 25% to 30% and saturated fat to less than 7% of calories; some diets reduce fat even further. The Mediterranean diet reduces LDL cholesterol without reducing HDLs. Dietary cholesterol should not exceed 200 mg daily.

      (2) Soluble fiber, garlic, soy, pecans, plant sterols, and vitamin C also may help to reduce LDL cholesterol. Modest alcohol use may improve the lipid profile.

(3) The diet should be high in antioxidant-containing fruits and vegetables.

(4) Patients should be encouraged to increase aerobic exercise to increase levels of HDL.

b. Pharmacologic treatment

(1) Patients with high LDL cholesterol and a significant risk of CAD should take aspirin, 81 to 325 mg daily, unless contraindicated. This will reduce the risk of thromboembolism.

(2) Niacin is associated with reduced long-term mortality and has an optimal effect on lipids, but it is poorly tolerated at full doses because of flushing of the skin.

(3) Resins that bind bile acids in the intestine include cholestyramine, cholesevelam, and colestipol. These resins reduce the incidence of coronary events in middle-aged men, but they have no effect on total mortality.

(4) 3-Hydroxy-3-methylglutaryl–coenzyme A reductase inhibitors (HMG–CoA inhibitors [statins]) include lovastatin, pravastatin, simvastatin, fluvastatin, rosuvastatin, and atorvastatin.

    (a) These inhibit the rate-limiting enzyme in formation of cholesterol.

    (b) They also reduce CAD and total mortality in secondary prevention.

    (c) Myositis is a known side effect, especially in patients also taking niacin or a fibrate.

(5) Fibric acid derivatives include gemfibrozil and fenofibrate.

    (a) They reduce synthesis and increase breakdown of very low density lipoproteins.

    (b) Their side effects include cholelithiasis, hepatitis, and myositis.

(6) Ezetimibe blocks intestinal absorption of dietary and biliary cholesterol and may be used as monotherapy or in combination with a statin.

11 Neurology

William H. Marquardt

I. CEREBROVASCULAR DISEASE

A. Stroke

1. General characteristics

   a. Stroke is the third most common cause of death in the United States and the most disabling neurologic disorder.

   b. The overall incidence of stroke has decreased over the past three decades, likely secondary to increased awareness and a more aggressive focus on prevention.

   c. The incidence of stroke increases with age and is higher in men than in women and in blacks than in whites.

   d. The major risk factors for stroke include hypertension, hypercholesterolemia, diabetes, oral contraceptives, cigarette smoking, heavy alcohol use, AIDS, and elevated blood homocysteine levels.

   e. A previous stroke increases the susceptibility to additional strokes.

   f. Ischemic strokes account for 80% of all strokes. Two-thirds of ischemic strokes are thrombotic and one-third embolic. Emboli commonly arise from the heart, aortic arch, or large cerebral arteries.

   g. Hemorrhagic strokes, which usually are secondary to hypertension, account for 20% of strokes.

2. Clinical features

   a. Signs and symptoms of stroke begin abruptly and, by definition, last longer than 24 hours. They correlate with the area of the brain that is supplied by the affected vessel, especially with ischemic events.

   b. In most cases, hemiparesis or hemisensory deficit is revealed on history and physical examination. One can localize the lesion to one side, contralateral to these deficits.

   c. Strokes involving the anterior circulation (anterior choroidal, anterior cerebral, middle cerebral arteries), which supplies the cortex, subcortical white matter, basal ganglia, and the internal capsule, commonly are associated with hemispheric signs and symptoms (aphasia, apraxia, hemiparesis, hemisensory losses, visual field defects).

   d. Strokes involving the posterior circulation (vertebral and basilar arteries), which supplies the brain stem, cerebellum, thalamus, and portions of the temporal and occipital lobes, commonly are associated with evidence of brain stem dysfunction (coma, drop attacks, vertigo, nausea, vomiting, ataxia).

   e. Thrombotic strokes evolve in a stepwise fashion and often are preceded by transient ischemic attacks (TIAs). Embolic strokes occur abruptly and without warning. Hemorrhagic strokes are less predictable because of complications of blood dispersion, cerebral edema, and increased intracranial pressure.

3. Laboratory studies

   a. Routine blood tests include complete blood count (CBC), erythrocyte sedimentation rate, platelet count, prothrombin time (PT), partial thromboplastin time (PTT), cholesterol and lipids, and blood glucose level.

   b. Additional blood tests may include Venereal Disease Research Laboratory (VDRL) test for syphilis, antinuclear antibodies, and antiphospholipid antibodies depending on patient risk factors. Blood cultures should be considered if endocarditis is suspected.

   c. Computed tomography (CT) is recommended during the acute phase and is the best modality for differentiating ischemic versus hemorrhagic stroke.

   d. Additional imaging tests to evaluate stroke patients include magnetic resonance imaging (MRI), carotid ultrasonography, echocardiography, and angiography.

   e. Electrocardiography may reveal arrhythmia or a recent myocardial infarction as the possible source of embolus.

   f. Lumbar puncture and angiography should be reserved for patients with suspected hemorrhage or vascular malformations.

4. Treatment

   a. Acute treatment is aimed at reversing the ischemia and salvaging tissue in the core and surrounding penumbra.

   b. Thrombolytic therapy (recombinant tissue plasminogen activator) is given to reduce the extent of deficit; it is most effective within 3 hours of symptoms but can be attempted up to 12 hours.

      (1) The major complication is bleeding.

      (2) Contraindications include evidence or suspicion of intracranial bleed; recent intracranial surgery; serious head trauma or previous stroke; history of intracranial bleed or known bleeding diathesis; uncontrolled hypertension (>185/>110); seizure at stroke onset; active internal bleeding; intracranial neoplasm; AVM or aneurysm; heparin use within 48 hours; platelet count <1000,000/mm^3.

  c. Antiplatelet therapy is initiated for ischemic stroke and TIA, whereas anticoagulant therapy is indicated in the setting of cardiac embolus.

  d. Endarterectomy may be indicated if 70% to 99% stenosis of the common or internal carotid artery is present.

  e. Hemorrhagic stroke is treated with conservative and supportive measures, including management of hypertension and antiedema therapy (mannitol and corticosteroids). Endovascular repair and surgical clipping or coil embolization are options available for some patients with specific anatomic foci.

  f. Supportive therapy, follow-up physical therapy, and social supports are important.

B. Transient ischemic attack (TIA)

  1. General characteristics

    a. TIAs are noted most frequently in older patients and those at risk for vascular disease.

    b. Sudden onset of focal neurologic deficits is secondary to disturbance of cerebral circulation.

    c. TIAs typically relate directly to either the carotid or the vertebral vascular distribution.

    d. Most TIAs only last for a few minutes, but symptoms may persist for more than 1 hour. By definition, symptoms resolve completely within 24 hours.

    e. Although TIAs are brief and transient, one-third of these patients will have a stroke within 5 years, making assessment and treatment important in prevention.

  2. Clinical features

    a. If the TIA is related to a disturbance in carotid circulation, patients may demonstrate contralateral hand–arm weakness with sensory loss, ipsilateral visual symptoms or aphasia, or amaurosis fugax. Carotid bruit may be present, but with a high-grade stenosis (95%), it may be absent.

    b. Those experiencing vertebrovascular TIA may demonstrate diplopia, ataxia, vertigo, dysarthria, cranial nerve palsies, lower extremity weakness, dimness or blurring of vision, perioral numbness, or drop attacks.

    c. The differential diagnosis of TIA includes generalized seizure, migraine, syncope, hypoglycemia in patients using insulin or oral hypoglycemic agents, and mass lesions.

  3. Diagnostic studies

    a. Arteriography is the definitive study, but magnetic resonance angiography also is used and is less invasive.

    b. CT or MRI will exclude a possible small cerebral hemorrhage.

    c. Cardiac workup should be done to exclude arrhythmia and new murmurs. The heart is a very common source of emboli.

    d. A hematologic workup must be done to identify coagulopathies.

      (1) A normal erythrocyte sedimentation rate will effectively rule out temporal arteritis.

      (2) Other studies include CBC with differential, cholesterol, PT, PTT and antiphospholipids.

    e. Other studies to evaluate possible cardiogenic or carotid emboli are two-dimensional echocardiography, electrocardiography, and carotid Doppler imaging.

  4. Treatment

    a. Because a TIA may indicate an impending stroke, prophylactic antiplatelet therapy is initiated when the TIA is not cardiogenic. This therapy might include aspirin, ticlopidine, clopidogrel, sulfinpyrazone, or dipyridamole.

    b. Cardiogenic TIA requires anticoagulation, initially with intravenous (IV) heparin for those who are admitted to the hospital and with warfarin for long-term therapy.

    c. Carotid endarterectomy may be indicated in patients with anterior circulation TIAs and moderate- to high-grade carotid stenosis on the side appropriate to account for the symptoms.

    d. Vital adjunctive therapies include control of blood pressure, serum cholesterol, blood glucose, and atrial fibrillation. Patients also must be urged to discontinue cigarette smoking, avoid excessive use of alcohol, and lose weight if appropriate.

C. Cerebral aneurysm/subarachnoid hemorrhage

  1. General characteristics

    a. A ruptured cerebral arterial aneurysm or, less commonly, an arteriovenous malformation (AVM), causes bleeding into the subarachnoid space.

b. Ruptured saccular (berry) aneurysm accounts for approximately 75% of nontraumatic cases of subarachnoid hemorrhage (SAH) and has a mortality rate of 50%. It most often occurs during the fifth and sixth decades of life, with an approximately equal gender distribution.

c. Risk factors for developing aneurysms include smoking, hypertension, and hypercholesterolemia. They are also associated with polycystic kidney disease and coarctation of the aorta.

d. Intracranial AVM accounts for less than 10% of SAHs. Most AVMs are congenital. AVM occurs twice as often in men and typically is diagnosed during the second to fourth decades.

2. Clinical features

a. The classic SAH presents as sudden onset of an unusually severe, generalized headache, which patients may describe as "the worst headache I've had in my life." The headache may be followed by nausea and vomiting and an altered state of consciousness.

b. The headache may remain unchanged for several days and subside only slowly over 1 to 2 weeks.

c. Frequently, blood pressure rises precipitously as a result of the hemorrhage.

d. Patients with SAH may develop a temperature of up to 102°F (38.9°C) and frequently display confusion, stupor, coma, and nuchal rigidity or other signs of meningeal irritation.

e. A herald bleed, or aneurysmal leak, occurs in up to 40% of patients, producing a less severe but atypical headache and accompanied by focal neurologic signs resulting from pressure on the brain or cranial nerves.

3. Laboratory studies

a. CT is the initial investigational modality for suspected SAH; more than 90% of patients with aneurysmal rupture will be identified in this way.

b. Evaluation of cerebrospinal fluid (CSF) reveals markedly elevated opening pressures and grossly bloody fluid.

c. Cerebral angiography should be done to evaluate the entire vasculature when convenient, because as many as 20% of individuals will have multiple aneurysms.

d. Electroencephalography (EEG) may indicate the side or site of hemorrhage or may show only diffuse, nonspecific changes.

4. Treatment

a. Supportive medical treatment involves prevention of elevated arterial or intracranial pressures that might lead to rerupture of the affected vessel. It also may include strict bed rest, mild sedation, or administration of stool softeners to prevent straining.

b. Management of hypertension is important, but care must be taken to prevent hypotension and inadequate cerebral perfusion.

c. Surgical management includes the clipping or wrapping of aneurysms, depending on the clinical state of the patient, and removal or embolization of an AVM by intra-arterial catheter.

II. SEIZURE DISORDERS

A. General characteristics

1. Idiopathic seizures usually begin between 5 and 20 years of age and have no specific cause.

2. Secondary seizures may result from congenital abnormalities or perinatal injury, metabolic disorders, trauma, tumors, vascular disease, infectious diseases, or degenerative diseases, such as Alzheimer's disease.

3. Seizures are transient disturbances of cerebral function caused by abnormal paroxysmal neuronal discharges in the brain.

4. Seizures are characterized as either generalized or partial, depending on whether the disturbance affects the entire brain or only a portion.

5. Status epilepticus, either convulsive or nonconvulsive, is diagnosed when seizures fail to cease spontaneously or recur so frequently that full consciousness is not restored between successive episodes.

B. Clinical features

1. Generalized seizures are characterized by a sudden loss of consciousness and are either convulsive (grand mal or tonic–clonic) or nonconvulsive (absence).

a. Generalized convulsive seizures are associated with a postictal obtundation and confusion lasting for minutes to hours.

b. Generalized nonconvulsive seizures are associated with only minor motor activity, such as blinking.

c. Differential diagnosis includes syncope, cardiac dysrhythmias, brain stem ischemia, and pseudoseizure.

2. Partial seizures

    a. Simple partial seizures are not accompanied by an impairment of consciousness. There may be isolated tonic or clonic activity of a limb or transient altered sensory perception, which may spread to include the entire side of the body in a "jacksonian march."

    b. Complex partial (temporal lobe) seizures often are characterized by an aura (transient abnormalities in sensation, perception, emotion, or memory), followed by impaired consciousness lasting for seconds to minutes. Nausea or vomiting, focal sensory perceptions, and focal tonic or clonic activity may accompany a complex seizure.

    c. Differential diagnosis includes TIA, rage attack, or panic attack.

C. Laboratory studies

    1. In generalized absence seizures, EEG typically shows generalized spikes and associated slow waves.

    2. In simple partial seizures, EEG may show a focal rhythmic discharge at the onset of the seizure, but, occasionally, no ictal activity will be seen.

    3. EEG in complex partial seizures often reveals interictal spikes or spikes associated with slow waves in the temporal or frontotemporal areas.

    4. Other laboratory studies, such as CBC, blood glucose, liver and renal functions, and serologic test for syphilis, are indicated to evaluate potential metabolic or toxic causes.

D. Treatment

    1. Correction of hyponatremia, hypoglycemia, or drug intoxication may be all that is necessary to control seizures.

    2. Anticonvulsant therapy typically is not indicated in the setting of a single unprovoked seizure in a patient with a normal neurologic examination and normal brain imaging and EEG.

    3. The goal of medical therapy is to prevent seizures by using a single agent in progressive doses until seizures are controlled or toxicity occurs.

        a. Generalized convulsive, simple partial, and complex partial seizures typically are treated with carbamazepine, phenytoin, and valproic acid; phenobarbital and primidone are less effective. Newer anticonvulsants, such as gabapentin, topiramate, lamotrigine, oxcarbazepine, levetiracetam, and zonisamide, also are effective.

        b. Felbamate typically is reserved for patients who are unresponsive to other medications or combinations because of serious potential side effects, including aplastic anemia and hepatic failure.

        c. Valproic acid or ethosuximide is used for generalized nonconvulsive (absence) seizures.

    4. Because of the possibility of permanent brain damage secondary to hyperthermia, circulatory collapse, or excitotoxic neuronal damage, status epilepticus is a medical emergency.

        a. Immediate management must ensure a patent airway, including positioning the patient to prevent aspiration of stomach contents.

        b. Management of hyperthermia, related to increased motor activity and high levels of circulating catecholamines, may include a cooling blanket or induction of motor paralysis with a neuromuscular blocking agent.

        c. Diazepam or lorazepam is administered IV until the seizure stops; a loading dose of phenytoin or fosphenytoin also is given.

III. MULTIPLE SCLEROSIS (MS)

A. General characteristics

    1. MS is characterized by inflammation associated with multiple foci of demyelination in the central nervous system (CNS) white matter.

    2. Patients with MS typically follow either a relapsing–remitting pattern of episodes or a primary progressive course. A secondary progressive form also is seen, in which the relapsing–remitting pattern changes to one of progressive degeneration.

    3. MS is thought to be an immunologic disorder associated with CNS immunoglobulin production and alteration of T lymphocytes. A viral infection may act as a precipitant.

    4. Based on numerous studies of twins, familial cases, and the association with specific HLA antigens (HLA-DR2), a genetic relationship is considered to be likely.

    5. MS typically begins between 18 and 45 years of age; women are affected more often than men.

B. Clinical features

    1. Patients initially may present with any of an array of symptoms, including focal weakness, numbness or tingling, optic neuritis, diplopia, focal neuralgias, balance problems, or urinary symptoms.

    2. Symptoms last for days to weeks and affect different areas over different events.

3. Patients often develop cognitive and psychological deficits.

4. The diagnosis must be questioned if signs and symptoms are not related to multiple areas of the CNS over time.

C. Laboratory studies

1. The diagnosis cannot be based exclusively on laboratory findings.

2. MRI with gadolinium is very effective for visualizing white matter lesions in the CNS.

3. CSF can reveal a sterile inflammation with a mild lymphocytosis or slight protein elevation, elevated immunoglobulin G index, oligoclonal bands, and increased myelin basic protein.

4. Visual-, auditory-, and somatosensory-evoked potentials are helpful for assessing nerve transmission.

D. Treatment

1. Corticosteroids may hasten maximal recovery from acute exacerbations. High-dose IV corticosteroids often are used in the setting of optic neuritis.

2. Interferon-β decreases the frequency of relapses, especially moderate and severe attacks.

3. Daily subcutaneous injections of glatiramer acetate also decrease the frequency of relapses, especially in mild disease.

4. Several studies suggest that immunosuppressive agents such as cyclophosphamide or azathioprine may arrest the course of the secondary progressive form.

5. Otherwise, therapy is symptomatic.

   a. Amantadine and pemoline can improve fatigue.

   b. Baclofen and diazepam improve spasticity.

   c. Several agents may relieve urologic dysfunction.

IV. DEMENTIA

A. General characteristics

1. Dementia is characterized by a progressive impairment of intellectual functioning, with compromise in at least two of the following spheres of mental activity: language, memory, visuospatial skills, emotional behavior, personality, and cognition.

2. Alzheimer's disease is the most common form of dementia; other forms include vascular dementias, dementia due to other degenerative disorders (Parkinson's, Huntington's, other), frontotemporal dementia, and dementia due to infection (HIV, Creutzfeldt–Jakob), toxins, depression, or hydrocephalus.

B. Alzheimer's disease

1. General characteristics

   a. Alzheimer's disease is the most common cause of chronic dementia, constituting 60% to 80% of patients with dementia.

   b. Risk factors include older age, family history, lower education level, and female gender.

   c. The disease is characterized by steadily progressive memory loss and other cognitive deficits and typically begins during the sixth or seventh decade of life.

   d. Prevalence doubles every 5 years in the older population, reaching 30% to 50% at age 85.

   e. Genetic factors have been identified, and familial cases have been mapped to chromosomes 1, 14, 19, and 21.

   f. Alzheimer's disease has a characteristic pathology consisting of intracellular neurofibrillary tangles and extracellular neuritic plaques.

2. Clinical features

   a. The diagnosis can be established when an otherwise alert patient exhibits progressive memory loss and other cognitive deficits, such as disorientation, language difficulties, inability to perform complex motor activities, inattention, visual misperception, poor problem-solving abilities, inappropriate social behavior, or hallucinations.

   b. Intellectual decline should be present in two or more areas of cognition and documented by a mental status examination or similar scale.

   c. Formal neuropsychological testing can help to confirm the suspected diagnosis and document the progression of disease.

3. Laboratory studies

   a. Laboratory tests include CBC, heavy metal screens, serum electrolytes, calcium, glucose, thyroid-stimulating hormone, vitamin B_{12}, renal and liver function tests, and drug and alcohol levels. These labs are completed to rule out treatable causes as well as to establish a baseline.

   b. MRI or CT is helpful only in ruling out other treatable causes of dementia.

4. Treatment
   a. Standard medical therapy, initially in low doses, is useful in treating insomnia, agitation, and depression.
   b. A trial of acetylcholinesterase inhibitors, such as tacrine, donepezil, galantamine, or rivastigmine, may improve memory function. Memantine is a *N*-methyl-D-aspartic acid (NMDA) receptor antagonist that is thought to regulate glutamate and has been approved for use in severe Alzheimer's disease.
   c. The patient will require vigilant family supervision. Day care centers and respite care are adjuncts to family supervision.

C. Vascular dementia
   1. General characteristics
      a. Between 15% and 20% of patients with a chronic dementia have a vascular dementia, usually referred to as multi-infarct dementia, which includes lacunar and multiple cortical infarcts.
         (1) Multi-infarct dementia is more common in men than in women.
         (2) It is associated with hypertension, with or without a history of TIA or stroke.
      b. A similar percentage of patients (15% to 20%) have evidence of both vascular and Alzheimer-type dementia; the correct diagnosis for the large majority of these patients is Alzheimer's disease.
   2. Clinical features
      a. Vascular dementia usually manifests as forgetfulness in the absence of depression and inattentiveness. Symptoms typically occur in a stepwise fashion.
      b. Social graces may be well maintained, so mental status testing is important to establish the diagnosis.
      c. Progression of the disease leads to loss of computational ability, problems with word finding and concentration, difficulty with routine daily activities, and, ultimately, complete disorientation and social withdrawal.
   3. Laboratory studies: Laboratory testing and imaging are useful only in establishing other treatable causes of dementia.
   4. Treatment
      a. Control of hypertension and metabolic disorders may help to slow the progression of symptoms.
      b. As in Alzheimer's disease, standard medical regimens can be used to treat insomnia, agitation, or depression.
      c. Caregivers should identify and reduce home hazards and arrange, as necessary, community services or preparation of an advance directive.

D. Frontotemporal dementia
   1. General characteristics
      a. This clinical syndrome is secondary to degeneration of the frontal lobe of the brain and may include the temporal lobe.
      b. Etiologies include Pick's disease, dementia associated with amyotrophic lateral sclerosis, and others.
   2. Clinical features
      a. Frontal lobe symptoms include behavioral symptoms (euphoria, apathy, disinhibition) and compulsive disorders.
      b. Several primitive reflexes (frontal release signs) are often elicited, including the palmomental, palmar grasp, and rooting reflexes.
   3. Laboratory studies
      a. MRI often reveals frontal lobe and/or anterior temporal lobe atrophy but in early cases may appear normal.
      b. Positron-emission tomography (PET) scans classically show frontal and/or anterior temporal hypometabolism, which helps to differentiate from Alzheimer's associated with biparietal hypometabolism.
   4. Treatment
      a. Supportive care is essential as there is no curative treatment.
      b. Behavioral symptoms may require treatment, such as selective serotonin reuptake inhibitors (SSRIs) for depression.

E. Pseudodementia
   1. General characteristics
      a. *Pseudodementia* is a term that describes patients with psychiatric illness who appear to be demented.
      b. It is often seen as part of a major depression episode.
   2. Clinical characteristics
      a. Patients typically complain of memory problems, but attention span and concentration appear intact while appearing upset or distressed.
      b. In true dementia, the patient will often give wrong answers, have poor attention and concentration, and appear indifferent or unconcerned.

V. HEADACHE

A. Tension headache

1. General characteristics

   a. Tension headaches were once thought to be caused by muscle contraction. Current theory relates tension headaches to abnormal neuronal sensitivity.

   b. There may be an associated history of significant stress or minor trauma to the head or neck.

   c. Tension headache is the most frequent type of headache and can be very costly due to loss of productivity.

2. Clinical features

   a. Tension headaches are typified by a band-like pain around the head or generalized head pain. Discomfort usually is reported as steady or aching (nonpulsatile) and is not associated with focal neurologic symptoms. It typically is bilateral and without photophobia, phonophobia, nausea, or vomiting.

   b. Pain may be episodic or chronic. Stress, sleep deprivation, hunger, and eyestrain are typical precipitants.

   c. There may be tenderness of the posterior cervical and occipital muscles or the scalp, but the physical examination generally is normal.

3. Laboratory studies

   a. Routine laboratory tests are helpful only in ruling out concurrent illness or an underlying rheumatologic condition.

   b. Imaging studies, lumbar puncture, or EEG is done only if there is a high index of suspicion for a structural lesion.

4. Treatment

   a. Medical treatment generally is with simple analgesics, such as aspirin, acetaminophen, or nonsteroidal anti-inflammatory drugs (NSAIDs). If not effective, a trial of antimigrainous agents may be employed.

   b. When appropriate, local heat and muscle relaxants may be employed for muscle-tension discomfort. Physical therapy and stress reduction techniques also are helpful.

   c. In the setting of depression or significant stress or chronic recalcitrant tension headaches, antidepressants or psychotherapy may be indicated.

B. Migraine headache

1. General characteristics

   a. Migraine headaches more typically present unilaterally, with throbbing or pulsating discomfort. Patients often identify migraine triggers, including chocolate, red wine, hard cheeses, monosodium glutamate, hormonal changes, exertion, fatigue, and stress.

   b. Patients often relate a family history of migraine disease. Women are affected more commonly than men; migraines often follow the menstrual cycle pattern.

   c. The pathophysiology of migraines classically has been attributed to intracranial vasospasm followed by extracranial vasodilatation. More current theories relate to dysfunction of the trigeminovascular system, resulting in the perivascular release of substance P.

   d. Migraine often is associated with other diseases, such as seizure disorders, essential tremor, Tourette's syndrome, depression, anxiety, and stroke.

2. Clinical features

   a. Migraine with aura (formerly called classic migraine) presents with an aura commonly involving visual changes, field cuts, or flashing lights affecting one's visual hemifield.

      (1) The throbbing pain often is contralateral to the aura and associated with the other symptoms that are seen in migraine without aura.

      (2) Migraine with aura also can be associated with transient neurologic deficits and hemisensory loss.

   b. Migraine without aura (formerly called common migraine) frequently is accompanied by nausea, vomiting, photophobia, phonophobia, and anorexia.

   c. Patients also exhibit irritability and fatigue.

   d. Migraine patients often retreat to quiet, dark rooms and prefer to lie quietly.

3. Laboratory studies

   a. Routine laboratory tests are done only to help rule out other concurrent disorders.

   b. Imaging studies or lumbar puncture is done only in select clinical settings and then only to rule out causes of acute secondary headache.

4. Treatment

    a. Mild to moderate migraine headache

        (1) Abortive therapy may include aspirin, acetaminophen, NSAIDs, or isometheptene. A variety of products may be combined with caffeine, which has an adjunctive effect.

        (2) Subsequent measures for migraine might include serotonin-receptor agonists, such as the triptans (e.g., sumatriptan, zolmitriptan, rizatriptan, naratriptan, almotriptan, frovatriptan, eletriptan). Various forms of the ergotamines also are useful.

    b. In the setting of frequent migraine headache, prophylactic measures may be employed.

        (1) Medical prophylaxis for migraine might include β-blockers, tricyclic antidepressants, calcium channel blockers, NSAIDs, valproic acid, or topiramate.

        (2) Biofeedback therapy often is employed in migraine patients in the hope of reducing the number of headaches by helping patients deal more effectively with stress.

        (3) Botox injections may be helpful in patients with severe, intractable migraine.

    c. Patients with triggers should avoid exposure.

    d. Psychotherapy and stress reduction may be helpful.

C. Cluster headache

  1. General characteristics

    a. Cluster headaches (migrainous neuralgia) are severe, unilateral, periorbital headaches that last for 30 to 90 minutes and occur several times a day over a period of weeks to months.

    b. The typical patient with cluster headaches is a middle-aged man, often without a family history of headache or migraine.

    c. Cluster headache may have a vascular etiology, and evidence suggests a disturbance of serotonergic mechanisms.

  2. Clinical features

    a. The unilateral pain of cluster headache often is accompanied by ipsilateral lacrimation, conjunctival injection, nasal congestion, and myosis and ptosis.

    b. Patients with cluster headache often pace incessantly around the room, because the pain is severe and not relieved by rest.

  3. Laboratory studies

    a. As in other headache syndromes, laboratory studies only help to identify other concurrent conditions and to rule out other causes of acute head and facial pain.

    b. Imaging studies or lumbar puncture is indicated only in specific clinical settings and to rule out other causes of acute cephalgia.

  4. Treatment

    a. Abortive and symptomatic therapy for cluster headaches includes administration of 100% oxygen, injectable forms of ergotamines or sumatriptan, and analgesics (e.g., intranasal butorphanol).

    b. Prophylactic therapy for cluster headaches includes valproate, cyproheptadine, lithium, calcium channel blockers, and oral corticosteroids.

VI. MOVEMENT DISORDERS

A. Benign essential (familial) tremor

  1. General characteristics

    a. The cause of benign essential tremor is unknown. It often is inherited in an autosomal dominant manner and may thus be called familial tremor.

    b. Tremor may begin at any age.

    c. It is enhanced by emotional stress; small quantities of alcohol commonly provide dramatic, temporary relief from the tremor.

    d. Although the tremor may interfere with manual skills, it causes only minimal disability.

  2. Clinical features

    a. Patients with benign essential tremor display a rhythmic, 6- to 8-Hz, to-and-fro movement, usually of the upper extremities but sometimes of the head (titubation).

    b. Speech also may be affected if the laryngeal muscles are involved.

  3. Laboratory studies: No laboratory testing is needed or warranted.

4. Treatment

   a. Low doses of a β-blocker, usually propranolol, may be useful in controlling tremor but, unless tremor is associated only with certain circumstances and intermittent dosing is adequate, will have to be used indefinitely.

   b. Primidone may be useful in controlling tremor if propranolol fails.

B. Parkinson's disease

   1. General characteristics

   a. Idiopathic Parkinson's occurs in all ethnic groups, with an approximately equal sex distribution, and most often begins between 45 and 65 years of age.

   b. Parkinson's disease is characterized by degeneration of cells in the substantia nigra, causing a deficiency of the neurotransmitter dopamine and an imbalance of dopamine and acetylcholine.

   c. Patients generally complain of problems related to their slowed movements, difficulty arising from a seated position, difficulty ascending and descending stairs, trouble with getting dressed, and difficulty with handwriting (micrographia).

   2. Clinical features

   a. The essential features that establish a diagnosis of Parkinson's disease are resting tremor, bradykinesia, rigidity, and postural instability.

   b. The tremor is most noticeable at rest, at 4 to 6 cycles/sec, and may be only very slight with voluntary effort. It typically is described as "pill-rolling."

   c. Initially, the tremor is confined to one limb or the limbs on one side, but eventually it may be present in all the limbs and the lips and mouth.

   d. Bradykinesia, or a generalized slowness of voluntary movements, is evident in the slow, shuffling gait; reduced arm swing; slowed rapid alternating movements; infrequent blinking; and masklike facies.

   e. Rigidity is found on passive range of motion testing, and cogwheel rigidity may be noted.

   f. Postural instability is seen, including difficulty in standing from a seated position, unsteadiness on turning, difficulty in stopping, and a tendency to fall.

   g. Depression and cognitive impairment develop in more than 50% of patients over time.

   3. Laboratory studies

   a. Generally, no laboratory testing is needed or warranted.

   b. Blood tests and imaging studies can be done to rule out other causes.

   4. Treatment

   a. Treatment is designed to best restore the balance between dopamine and acetylcholine by blocking the effect of acetylcholine with anticholinergic drugs, administering levodopa (the precursor of dopamine), or a combination of both.

   b. Amantadine, a mild anticholinergic, often is helpful for patients with mild symptoms but no disability.

   c. Benztropine, trihexyphenidyl, and other anticholinergic drugs are particularly helpful in treating the tremor of Parkinson's disease and are less helpful for bradykinesia.

   d. Levodopa is converted to dopamine in the body and improves all symptoms of Parkinson's disease. Carbidopa, when added to levodopa in various combinations, allows lower doses of levodopa and reduced side effects.

   e. Dopamine agonists, such as bromocriptine, act directly on dopamine receptors and often are reserved for patients who become refractory to levodopa therapy.

   f. Selegiline, a monoamine oxidase B inhibitor, inhibits breakdown of dopamine, and studies indicate that it may arrest progression of the disease.

   g. Catecholamine-O-methyl-transferase (COMT) inhibitors reduce the metabolism of levodopa to 3-O-methyldopa and result in more stable plasma levels and more constant dopaminergic stimulation of the brain. Two COMT agents, tolcapone and entacapone, are available as adjuncts to levodopa/carbidopa therapy.

   h. Physical therapy may help some patients, and quality of life may be improved with household modifications or the availability of special utensils.

   i. Psychological support for both the patient and the family is helpful.

C. Huntington's disease

   1. General characteristics

   a. Huntington's disease is an inherited, autosomal dominant disorder that occurs throughout the world in all ethnic groups, with a prevalence of less than 5 per 100,000.

b. The gene responsible for Huntington's disease is on the short arm of chromosome 4.

c. Symptoms of the disease usually do not develop until after 30 years of age. By this time, those who are affected often have already had children who may be similarly affected.

2. Clinical features

   a. The disease is characterized by progressive chorea and dementia; it is usually fatal within 15 to 20 years.

   b. The earliest mental changes often are behavioral, with irritability, moodiness, and antisocial behavior that generally progress to an obvious dementia.

   c. The earliest physical signs may be a mere restlessness or fidgetiness, but, eventually, severe choreiform movements and dystonic posturing occur.

3. Laboratory studies: CT demonstrates cerebral atrophy as well as atrophy of the caudate nucleus. MRI and PET scans have shown decreased glucose metabolism in an anatomically normal caudate nucleus.

4. Treatment

   a. Huntington's disease has no cure, and progression of the disease cannot be halted.

   b. Symptomatic treatment for the disease may include phenothiazines to control dyskinesia, and haloperidol or clozapine to control any behavioral disturbances.

   c. Children of Huntington's patients should receive genetic counseling in conjunction with genetic testing, which now is available for making a definitive diagnosis even in the presymptomatic state.

D. Cerebral palsy

1. Cerebral palsy is a chronic impairment of muscle tone, strength, coordination, or movements. It is believed to result from cerebral injury before birth, during delivery, or in the perinatal period.

2. Clinical features are widely varied and include spasticity (75% of patients), ataxia, seizure disorders, and mental retardation as well as disorders of speech, hearing, vision, and sensory perception.

3. Physical examination may reveal hyperreflexia, microcephaly, limb length discrepancies, cataracts, retinopathy, and congenital heart defects.

4. Diagnostic testing is done to rule out other neurologic disorders. Depending on the presentation, MRI, immunoglobulin G, immunoglobulin M, urine acid tests, blood amino acids, lactate, pyruvate, and ammonia concentrations may aid in the diagnostic quest.

5. Treatment is supportive, with the goal of attaining maximum function and potential in physical, occupational, and speech ability. Pharmacologic treatment of spasticity and seizures often is required.

E. Restless leg syndrome (RLS)

1. RLS affects 3%-30% of the population. Women are affected more often then men.

2. Most cases are primary although it may occur secondary to peripheral neuropathy, uremia, pregnancy, or iron deficiency.

3. Patients feel a subjective need to move and abnormal sensations including tingling, creeping or crawling sensation, itching, heaviness, burning, coldness, or tension. Symptoms occur most commonly during periods of prolonged inactivity.

4. The majority of patients also demonstrate frequent myoclonus at rest.

5. Treatment

   a. Dopamine agonists or ropinirole are the drugs of choice.

   b. Opiate agonists and benzodiazepines may also be effective.

   c. Tolerance often develops.

   d. In patients with reduced ferritin levels, replacement of iron will help.

VII. DISEASES OF PERIPHERAL NERVES

A. Bell's palsy

1. General considerations

   a. Unilateral facial muscle weakness is noted without evidence of other neurologic disease and without apparent cause. More than 60% of cases occur on the right side.

   b. Although the cause of the weakness is unknown, it is seen more frequently in pregnant women and in people with diabetes. It often is associated with trauma, infection, neoplasia, or toxins.

   c. There can be a paralysis of all muscles supplied by the cranial nerve VII (complete palsy) or variable weakness in different muscles (incomplete palsy).

2. Clinical features

   a. Facial muscle weakness typically begins abruptly but may progress over a matter of hours to 2 days. Paralysis involves the forehead and lower face; patients cannot close the eye, raise the brow, or smile on the affected side.

   b. Pain about the ipsilateral ear often precedes the facial weakness or is noted concurrently with the weakness.

   c. Depending on the site of the nerve lesion, patients may demonstrate impairment of taste, lacrimation, or hyperacusis.

   d. Clinical evaluation reveals no abnormality beyond the motor function of cranial nerve VII.

3. Diagnostic studies

   a. Bell's palsy is a clinical diagnosis. Specific diagnostic confirmation with nerve conduction studies or electromyography (EMG) is only done in patients with atypical or prolonged Bell's palsy.

   b. Appropriate diagnostic procedures may be done to identify other conditions that may produce facial palsy including tumors, Lyme disease, AIDS, and sarcoidosis.

4. Treatment

   a. Approximately 60% of cases resolve spontaneously and require no treatment, although the course is varied and may extend from a few days to a few months.

   b. A poorer prognosis, with possible incomplete recovery, is associated with patients presenting with severe pain and complete palsy, hyperacusis, or advanced age.

   c. A course of oral prednisone, with or without acyclovir, if begun soon after the onset of symptoms, has been shown to increase the percentage of patients who completely recover and should be considered in those at risk of a poor prognosis.

B. Diabetic peripheral neuropathy

1. General considerations

   a. Peripheral nerve abnormalities in patients with diabetes are common and present as a mixed polyneuropathy (motor, sensory, and autonomic) in 70% of cases. The remainder of cases involve largely sensory neuropathies.

   b. Less commonly, patients may develop mononeuropathies involving specific peripheral or cranial nerves.

   c. Neuropathy generally is related to the duration and severity of hyperglycemia, but it may be the presenting symptom in occult diabetes. Neuropathy is the result of vascular insufficiency or nerve infarction.

2. Clinical features

   a. Symptoms are more common in the lower extremities than in the arms and consist of numbness, pain, dysesthesias (burning), or paresthesias.

   b. A distal symmetric polyneuropathy also can be diagnosed before the development of any symptoms in the form of reduced deep tendon reflexes or impaired vibratory sensation.

   c. Autonomic complications related to diabetes include postural hypotension, cardiac arrhythmias, impaired thermoregulatory sweating, and disturbances of bowel, bladder, gastric, and sexual function.

3. Diagnostic studies

   a. Serial nerve conduction studies can be completed to document the presence, severity, and course of the neuropathy.

   b. Additional diagnostic workup may be appropriate to rule out other causes of polyneuropathy, including uremia, alcohol abuse or nutritional deficiencies, connective tissue disease, vasculitis, vitamin B_{12} deficiency, hypothyroidism, or amyloidosis.

4. Treatment

   a. Tight control of hyperglycemia is vital to prevent or slow progression of the disease.

   b. There are no specific treatments for diabetic peripheral nerve complications, with the exception of an entrapment neuropathy that may respond to a decompression procedure.

   c. Phenytoin, mexiletine, or carbamazepine may be helpful in controlling the shooting or stabbing neuropathic pain.

   d. Amitriptyline, nortriptyline, desipramine, gabapentin, or fluphenazine may be useful in controlling deep, constant, aching pain.

   e. Duloxetine, a serotonin and norepinephrine reuptake inhibitor, has been approved for painful diabetic neuropathy.

   f. Postural hypotension may respond to salt supplementation, lower extremity pressure stockings, or medications such as fludrocortisone or midodrine.

C. Guillain–Barré syndrome (acute idiopathic polyneuropathy)

1. General considerations

a. Guillain–Barré syndrome is an idiopathic polyneuropathy often following minor infections, immunizations, or surgical procedures, but in many cases no cause is identified.

b. Clinical and epidemiologic evidence seems to indicate a relationship with a preceding infection of the lungs or gastrointestinal (GI) tract, in particular infection with *Campylobacter jejuni*. However, in about half of the cases, no preceding infection is confirmed.

2. Clinical features

a. Patients generally present with symmetrical extremity weakness that begins distally and ascends; proximal muscles tend to be affected more often than distal muscles. Deep tendon reflexes may be decreased or absent. Cranial nerves are affected in 45% to 75% of patients.

b. Sensory abnormalities are common but generally less marked than the motor symptoms.

c. Pain is present in more than 85% of cases and can be severe in a subset of patients.

d. Significant autonomic dysfunction may be noted, including tachycardia, cardiac irregularities, labile blood pressure, disturbed sweating, impaired pulmonary function, sphincter disturbances, or paralytic ileus.

e. Guillain–Barré syndrome can be life threatening if the muscles of respiration or swallowing are involved.

3. Diagnostic studies

a. Electrophysiologic studies may reveal marked slowing of nerve conduction velocities, both motor and sensory. These studies also may document denervation or axonal loss.

b. CSF evaluation typically yields an elevated protein, but the cell counts are normal.

4. Treatment

a. Patients should be hospitalized with close monitoring of respiratory status, because autonomic involvement may rapidly result in complications and death from orthostatic hypotension or arrhythmias.

b. Plasmapheresis, instituted as early as possible, is very effective in reducing the time required for recovery and may reduce the likelihood of residual neurologic deficits. In patients who are severely affected, plasmapheresis also may shorten the time on a respirator as well as the length of time it may take to resume walking independently.

c. IV immunoglobulin also is very effective and is used in preference to plasmapheresis in adults with cardiovascular instability and in children.

d. Patients will benefit from physical, occupational, and speech therapy during rehabilitation.

D. Myasthenia gravis

1. General characteristics

a. Myasthenia gravis involves muscle weakness and fatigability, which improve with rest.

b. The onset of myasthenia gravis usually is insidious, but the disorder sometimes is made evident by a coincidental infection that exacerbates the symptoms.

c. The disorder may occur at any age but is more common in young women and older men.

d. Antibodies directed against the acetylcholine receptor on the muscle surface cause an increased rate of receptor destruction, leading to weakness.

2. Clinical features

a. Typical presenting problems include ptosis, diplopia, difficulty in chewing or swallowing, respiratory difficulties, limb weakness, or a combination of any of these.

b. Symptoms may fluctuate in intensity during the day, and there is a tendency to have longer-term spontaneous relapses and remissions that may last for weeks.

c. Clinical examination confirms the weakness and fatigability of affected muscles, which improve after a short rest.

d. Sensation is normal, and there usually are no reflex changes.

e. The diagnosis may be confirmed if marked clinical improvement is achieved by administering a short-acting anticholinesterase (edrophonium).

3. Laboratory studies

a. Lateral and anteroposterior chest radiographs should be obtained to rule out a coexisting thymoma.

b. Electrophysiologic studies may show a decrementing muscle response.

c. Serum assay for elevated levels of circulating acetylcholine receptor antibodies is another way of establishing the diagnosis; this assay is positive in 80% to 90% of patients.

4. Treatment

   a. The mainstay of therapy is administration of a cholinesterase inhibitor, such as pyridostigmine, which produces a transient improvement in strength.

   b. Thymectomy often leads to improvement of symptoms.

   c. Corticosteroids, immunosuppressive agents, IV immunoglobulin, and plasmapheresis are effective in patients with refractory disease.

E. Lambert–Eaton syndrome (myasthenic syndrome)

  1. General characteristics

   a. The syndrome may be associated with small cell carcinoma and may surface prior to the tumor being diagnosed.

   b. There is defective release of acetylcholine in response to nerve impulse.

  2. Clinical features

   a. Unlike myasthenia gravis, power increases with sustained contraction.

   b. It is confirmed electrophysiologically, as the muscle response to repeated stimulation is increased significantly.

  3. Treatment

   a. Plasmapheresis and immunosuppressive therapy typically lead to both clinical as well as electrophysiologic improvement.

   b. Specific therapy on the tumor, when identified, is also indicated.

VIII. CNS INFECTION

A. Bacterial meningitis

  1. General characteristics

   a. Typical symptoms of meningitis are based on three processes: inflammation, increased intracranial pressure, or tissue necrosis.

   b. Causes of bacterial meningitis have changed over the past decades.

     (1) The primary causes today are *Streptococcus pneumoniae, Neisseria meningitidis,* and group B streptococci (especially in infants).

     (2) The rate of *Haemophilus influenzae* type b (Hib) meningitis has dramatically decreased since the widespread use of the Hib vaccine.

  2. Clinical features

   a. Fever, headache, vomiting, and a stiff neck are the typical signs and symptoms of meningitis, although all may not be present. A petechial rash is characteristic of *Neisseria meningitidis.*

   b. Symptoms typically are acute, with patients presenting within hours or 1 to 2 days of infection.

   c. Careful initial examination may reveal evidence of soft-tissue abscess, otitis, or other parameningeal infection.

   d. Meningeal signs may be absent or very subtle at the age extremes or be difficult to assess with impaired consciousness.

  3. Laboratory studies

   a. Prompt lumbar puncture and CSF analysis are essential. CT is performed before lumbar puncture to rule out evidence of a space-occupying lesion.

     (1) The CSF may be slightly turbid to grossly purulent.

     (2) CSF pressure is elevated in more than 90% of cases.

     (3) CSF white blood cell (WBC) count is elevated, ranging from 1,000 to as high as 10,000/μL with increased neutrophils.

     (4) CSF protein concentrations of 100 to 500 mg/dL are most common.

     (5) CSF glucose levels often are decreased and may be less than 40 mg/dL.

   b. Gram stain and culture of the CSF is diagnostic in more than 80% of cases.

  4. Treatment

   a. Antibiotic treatment is begun immediately if the CSF is not clear and colorless. The initial choice of antibiotic is based empirically on the patient's age and the most likely pathogen.

     (1) Neonates receive ampicillin and cefotaxime.

     (2) Infants up to 3 months of age receive the same combination, with higher doses of cefotaxime or ceftriaxone.

(3) Immunocompetent children older than 3 months and adults younger than 55 years receive cefotaxime or ceftriaxone plus vancomycin.

(4) Adults older than 55 and those of any age with alcoholism or debilitating illness receive ampicillin plus cefotaxime or ceftriaxone plus vancomycin.

(5) If it is a hospital-acquired, posttraumatic or postneurosurgery meningitis, or if the patient is immune compromised, the combination given is ampicillin plus ceftazidime plus vancomycin.

b. Repeat lumbar puncture and CSF analysis are crucial to assess response to treatment.

(1) The CSF should be sterile after 24 hours.

(2) A decrease in pleocytosis and the proportion of neutrophils should be seen within 3 days.

B. Viral (aseptic) meningitis and encephalitis

1. General considerations

a. Viral meningitis most frequently is associated with enteroviruses (coxsackievirus A or B, echoviruses), herpes simplex virus 2, and arthropod-borne viruses.

b. Aseptic meningitis also may reflect an inflammatory process in the parameningeal area (i.e., sinusitis, otitis, abscess).

c. Viral encephalitis may not have an identifiable cause in many cases but frequently is associated with childhood exanthems, arthropod-borne agents, and herpes simplex virus type 1.

2. Clinical features

a. Viral meningitis and encephalitis often present as an acute confusional state, especially in children and young adults.

b. Signs and symptoms generally are not as acute as in bacterial meningitis and may have persisted for several days.

c. Examination may reveal a number of systemic manifestations, suggesting a particular causal agent (e.g., rash, pharyngitis, adenopathy, pleuritis, carditis, jaundice, organomegaly, diarrhea).

d. In encephalitis, because it involves the brain directly, there may be markedly altered consciousness, seizures, personality changes, or other focal neurologic signs.

3. Laboratory studies

a. As with bacterial meningitis, prompt lumbar puncture and CSF analysis are crucial after assessing for evidence of increased intracranial pressure.

b. The CSF opening pressure generally is normal.

c. Cells present in the CSF are more likely to be lymphocytes or monocytes, and the WBC count generally is less than $1,000/\mu L$.

d. The CSF protein, glucose, and serum blood counts are more likely to be normal.

4. Treatment

a. With the exception of infection with herpes simplex virus, the course of aseptic meningitis generally is benign and self-limited, and no specific therapy is required. Suspected herpes virus infection is treated with acyclovir.

b. Mild headaches can be treated with acetaminophen.

c. Seizures can be suppressed with anticonvulsants.

d. Breathing should be supported, if necessary.

C. Granulomatous meningitis

1. General characteristics

a. Pathogens include *Mycobacterium tuberculosis*, fungi (*Cryptococcus*, *Coccidioides* sp., *Histoplasma*), and spirochetes (*Treponema pallidum*, *Borrelia burgdorferi*).

b. Incidence is highest in immunocompromised individuals.

c. Noninfectious causes include sarcoidosis and other granulomatous conditions.

2. Clinical features

a. Presentation is less acute; patients typically have symptoms for weeks to months.

b. Subtle mental status changes are common.

3. Laboratory

a. Culture is key but results may take weeks depending on etiology.

b. CSF shows high protein, low glucose, and a lymphocytosis.

c. CT or MRI will show marked enhancement of the meninges and, occasionally, hydrocephalus.

    d. Serologic studies may help to confirm suspected etiologies.

  4. Treatment is dependent on cause.

D. Brain abscess

  1. General characteristics

    a. Brain abscess typically results from direct spread of infection from sinus, ear, or soft tissue; hematogenous spread to the brain is rare.

    b. Abscesses may be localized to the extradural (epidural) space, subdural spaces, or the brain parenchyma.

  2. Clinical features

    a. Brain abscess presents as a space-occupying lesion; symptoms may include vomiting, fever, altered mental status, and focal neurologic signs.

    b. These signs and symptoms may have been preceded by previous evidence of otitis, sinusitis, or pharyngitis.

  3. Laboratory studies

    a. A lumbar puncture and CSF analysis should be performed following CT.

    b. CT or MRI is helpful in establishing the diagnosis, especially if performed using a contrast medium.

    c. The bacteriology of brain abscess usually is polymicrobial and may include both Gram-positive and Gram-negative organisms.

  4. Treatment

    a. Acute treatment may involve respiratory and circulatory support, airway management, and monitoring of other vital functions.

    b. Brain abscesses are treated with appropriate antibiotics that penetrate brain tissues well, including IV penicillin plus either chloramphenicol, metronidazole, or both. Nafcillin is added if *Staphylococcus aureus* infection is suspected.

    c. Surgical excision or decompression may be required in cases of very large lesions or a delayed response to therapy.

IX. CNS TRAUMA

A. Brain injury

  1. General characteristics

    a. Head injury accounts for nearly half of the trauma-related deaths in young people.

    b. Prognosis is directly related to the site and severity of brain damage.

    c. Loss of consciousness for more than 2 minutes implies a worse prognosis.

    d. The degree of retrograde and posttraumatic amnesia also is directly related to the severity of brain injury.

  2. Clinical features

    a. During the physical examination, special attention must be given to the level of consciousness and to the extent of any brain stem dysfunction.

    b. In concussion, there may be a brief loss of consciousness with bradycardia, hypotension, and respiratory arrest for a few seconds.

    c. In the setting of acute epidural hemorrhage, signs and symptoms may include headache, confusion, somnolence, seizures, and focal deficits occurring several hours after the injury.

    d. Bruising may be on the side of the injury (coup injury) or on the contralateral side (contracoup injury).

    e. The Glasgow Coma Scale assesses initial and ongoing consciousness by objectively scoring eye movement, verbal response, and motor response (Table 11-1).

  3. Laboratory studies

    a. Skull radiography or CT may detect skull fractures; further studies of the cervical spine should be done to look for related injuries.

    b. CT also is important to demonstrate intracranial hemorrhage, to show evidence of cerebral edema, and to identify displacement of midline structures.

  4. Treatment

    a. Surgical evacuation may be necessary after acute epidural, acute subdural, and cerebral hemorrhage.

    b. Increased intracranial pressure may be relieved by induced hyperventilation, IV mannitol infusion, and IV furosemide.

TABLE 11-1	**Glasgow Coma Scale**	
Eye opening	Spontaneous eye opening	4 points
	Eyes open to verbal command	3 points
	Eyes open to pain	2 points
	No eye opening	1 point
Verbal response	Alert and oriented	5 points
	Confused, yet coherent speech	4 points
	Inappropriate words and jumbled phrases	3 points
	Incomprehensible sounds	2 points
	No sounds	1 point
Motor response	Obeys commands	6 points
	Localizes to a noxious stimulus	5 points
	Withdraws from a noxious stimulus	4 points
	Abnormal flexion (decorticate posturing)	3 points
	Abnormal extensor response (decerebrate posturing)	2 points
	No response	1 point

Lowest possible score = 3 points; highest possible score = 15 points.
Minor brain injury, >13 points; moderate brain injury, 9–12 points; severe brain injury, <9 points (coma).

B. Spinal cord injury

1. General characteristics

   a. Whiplash injury may cause spinal cord damage, but severe injury typically relates to fracture or dislocation causing compression or angular deformity of the cord.

   b. Sites of injury may extend from the cervical to the upper lumbar region.

   c. Extreme hypotension after acute injury may result in cord infarction.

2. Clinical features

   a. Total cord transection

      (1) Total cord transection results in immediate, flaccid paralysis and loss of sensation below the level of the lesion.

      (2) Reflex activity is lost for a variable time, and there is urinary and fecal retention.

      (3) With the slow return of reflex function, spastic paraplegia or quadriplegia develops, with hyperreflexia and extensor plantar responses.

   b. Partial cord injury

      (1) Patients may be left with mild limb weakness or distal sensory disturbance.

      (2) Sphincter function impairment may lead to urinary urgency and incontinence.

   c. A unilateral cord lesion produces an ipsilateral motor disturbance with accompanying impairment of proprioception and contralateral loss of pain and temperature below the lesion (Brown–Séquard syndrome).

   d. A central cord syndrome may lead to a lower motor neuron deficit and loss of pain and temperature, with sparing of posterior column functions.

   e. A radicular deficit may occur at the level of the injury; if the cauda equina is involved, there may be dysfunction in several lumbosacral roots.

3. Laboratory studies

   a. No laboratory testing is needed or warranted.

   b. Imaging studies (plain-film radiography, CT, MRI) are indicated based on signs and symptoms.

4. Treatment

   a. Treatment of spinal cord injury involves immobilization as well as decompressive laminectomy and fusion if there is cord compression.

   b. Early treatment with high-dose corticosteroids has been shown to improve neurologic recovery if started within 8 hours of the injury.

    c. Anatomic realignment of the spinal cord by traction and other orthopaedic procedures is important.

    d. Subsequent care of residual neurologic deficit requires therapy for spasticity and care of the skin, bowel, and bladder.

X. PRIMARY CNS NEOPLASMS

A. General characteristics

    1. Approximately half of all primary intracranial neoplasms are gliomas; the remainder are meningiomas, pituitary adenomas, neurofibromas, and others.

    2. Approximately 10% of spinal tumors are intramedullary; ependymoma is the most common.

    3. Certain tumors, especially neurofibromas, hemangioblastomas, and retinoblastomas, may have a familial basis.

    4. The most common sources of intracranial metastasis are carcinoma of the lung, breast, kidney, and the GI tract.

B. Clinical features

    1. Spinal tumors may lead to spinal cord dysfunction by direct compression, by ischemia secondary to arterial or venous obstruction, or by invasive infiltration.

    2. Intracranial tumors may produce a generalized disturbance of cerebral function and lead to evidence of increased intracranial pressure (i.e., personality changes, intellectual decline, emotional lability, seizures, headaches, nausea, malaise).

    3. Intracranial tumors also may produce focal deficits, depending on their location.

        a. Frontal lobe lesions often produce progressive intellectual decline, slowing of mental activity, personality changes, contralateral grasp reflexes, and, possibly, expressive aphasia.

        b. Temporal lobe lesions may lead to seizures, olfactory or gustatory hallucinations, licking or smacking of the lips, depersonalization, emotional and behavioral changes, visual field defects, and auditory illusions.

        c. Parietal lobe lesions typically cause contralateral disturbances of sensation and may cause sensory seizures, a cortical sensory loss (impaired stereognosis) or inattention, or some combination of these.

        d. Occipital lobe lesions characteristically produce crossed homonymous hemianopia or a partial field defect, visual agnosia for objects and colors, or unformed visual hallucinations.

        e. Brain stem and cerebellar lesions produce cranial nerve palsies, ataxia, incoordination, nystagmus, and pyramidal and sensory deficits in the limbs on one or both sides.

    4. Symptoms of spinal tumors usually develop insidiously, with pain characteristically aggravated by coughing or straining and either localized to the back or felt diffusely in an extremity as motor defects, paresthesias, or numbness, especially in the legs.

    5. Physical examination of patients with spinal tumors may reveal localized spinal tenderness.

C. Laboratory studies

    1. CT or MRI performed with contrast medium may detect the lesion, define its location and size, evaluate the extent to which the normal anatomy is distorted, and the degree of any associated cerebral edema or mass effect.

    2. Arteriography may demonstrate stretching or displacement of normal cerebral vessels as well as the presence of tumor vascularity.

    3. EEG may demonstrate a focal disturbance resulting from the neoplasm or a more diffuse change reflecting altered mental status.

    4. CT myelography or MRI may be needed to identify and localize the site of spinal cord compression.

    5. CSF removed at myelography often is xanthochromic and contains greatly increased protein concentration, normal cell content, and normal glucose concentration.

D. Treatment

    1. Complete surgical removal of the tumor may be possible if it is extra-axial or not in a critical or inaccessible region of the brain.

    2. Surgical shunting of an obstructive hydrocephalus may dramatically reduce clinical deficits.

    3. Radiation, chemotherapy, or both increase median survival rates, regardless of any preceding surgery.

    4. Corticosteroids help to reduce cerebral edema and usually are started before surgery.

5. Anticonvulsants commonly are administered in standard doses.

6. Intramedullary cord lesions are treated by decompression and surgical excision and by irradiation.

7. Treatment of epidural spinal metastases consists of irradiation, irrespective of cell type.

XI. SLEEP DISORDERS

A. General chacteristics

1. Sleep consists of two distinct states: rapid eye movement (REM) and non-REM.

   a. REM sleep is predominant when dreaming takes place.

   b. Non-REM sleep is divided into four stages (1, 2, 3, and 4), with stages 3 and 4 termed *delta* sleep.

2. Dyssomnia (insomnia) complaints include difficulty getting to sleep or staying asleep, intermittent wakefulness during the night, early morning awakenings, or some combination of all these. Psychiatric disorders, including depression and manic disorders, often are associated with persistent insomnia.

   a. Depression is associated with fragmented sleep, decreased total sleep time, quicker onset of REM sleep, and a shift of REM to earlier in the night.

   b. In manic disorders, total sleep time is decreased with shortened REM latency and increased REM activity.

3. Hypersomnia (excessive daytime sleepiness) generally is a more severe problem and may manifest in patients with sleep apnea, narcolepsy, or those who demonstrate nocturnal myoclonus.

4. Parasomnias (abnormal behaviors during sleep) include sleep terrors, nightmares, sleepwalking, and enuresis.

   a. Nightmares occur during REM sleep.

   b. Sleep terrors occur during stage 3 and 4 delta sleep.

   c. Sleepwalking is associated with stage 3 or 4 sleep in the first third of the night and with REM sleep later in the night.

   d. Childhood enuresis typically takes place within 3 to 4 hours of bedtime but is not limited to particular stages of sleep.

B. Clinical features

1. Taking a careful history of those with insomnia may reveal depression, abuse of alcohol, heavy smoking (>1 pack/day), inappropriate use of sedatives/hypnotics, or a medical history of uremia, asthma, or hypothyroidism.

2. Sleep apnea often is seen in obese, middle-aged, and older men with hypertension and associated congestive heart failure.

3. Patients with narcolepsy experience sudden, brief sleep attacks; cataplexy; sleep paralysis; and hypnagogic hallucinations, which may precede sleep.

C. Laboratory studies

1. Polysomnography (sleep studies) assesses EEG activity, heart rate, respiratory movement, and oxygen saturation.

2. Thyroid studies may be helpful if hypothyroidism is suggested.

D. Treatment

1. Insomnia

   a. In transient insomnia, de-emphasis and reassurance are sufficient treatment.

   b. A variety of sleep hygiene rules should be discussed to remove numerous barriers to effective sleep. Sleep hygiene rules include avoidance of alcohol, caffeine, nicotine, or exercise prior to bedtime, establishment of regular sleep hours, relaxation techniques, etc.

   c. Medications should be avoided if possible. Antihistamines may be effective for milder problems, however, and rapidly acting hypnotics may be used for short periods if necessary.

2. Treatment of sleep apnea includes weight reduction (if appropriate) and administration of air under continuous pressure through the nasopharynx during sleep (continuous positive airway pressure [CPAP]).

3. Narcolepsy is managed by administration of stimulants including dextroamphetamine and modafinil.

4. Nocturnal myoclonus typically is treated with clonazepam.

5. Sleep terror and sleepwalking can be treated with benzodiazepines.

12 Psychiatry

Melanie Trecartin

I. DIAGNOSIS OF PSYCHIATRIC DISORDERS

A. Background

1. Psychiatric diagnoses conform to the *Diagnostic and Statistical Manual of Mental Disorders* (DSM) published and periodically updated by the American Psychiatric Association.

2. The DSM is widely accepted because professionals from a number of specialties within psychiatry were involved in its conception and development.

3. The *International Statistical Classification of Diseases and Related Health Problems* (ICD) is published by the World Health Organization. It is similar to the DSM and is used in most countries of the world, except the United States and Japan.

B. The DSM endorses a criteria-based diagnostic approach that requires the following three conditions be met:

1. The condition is not caused by the direct effects of any drug.

2. The psychiatric disorder is not caused by the effects of a medical condition.

3. There is significant impairment of social functioning, occupational functioning, or both.

C. If a patient's signs and symptoms result from a medical condition or substance abuse, the diagnosis should reflect this situation; in this case, the psychiatric symptoms take a secondary role. This relationship holds regardless of the behavior manifested by the patient.

D. The DSM contains a catchall category for each group, labeled "not otherwise specified" (NOS), which allows a diagnosis for patients with atypical symptoms.

1. NOS includes a mixed presentation, symptoms below the diagnostic threshold, or a presentation that does not meet the criteria for a specific disorder.

2. It allows a patient to be assigned to a diagnostic group while avoiding a forced classification based on incomplete or contradictory symptomatology.

E. The DSM employs a multiaxial system for reporting diagnoses.

1. Axis I: All mental disorders, including substance abuse and developmental disorders.

2. Axis II: Personality disorders and mental retardation.

3. Axis III: Any general medical condition or physical disorder.

4. Axis IV: Psychosocial and environmental situations that contribute to the disorder (e.g., homelessness, economic difficulties).

5. Axis V: The global assessment of function (GAF), a rating system designed to assess the level of daily functioning based on social, occupational, and psychological assessment.

II. SCHIZOPHRENIA AND OTHER PSYCHOTIC DISORDERS

A. Definition

1. Brief psychotic disorder, schizophreniform disorder, and schizophrenia present with common symptoms, which are differentiated by severity and duration.

2. Psychotic disorders

a. Patients exhibit disordered thought content and thought processes as well as perceptual disturbances, such as illusions or hallucinations, delusions, and impaired reality orientation.

b. Patients' social and occupational functions are disrupted by problems with affect, motivation, perception, and communication or disorganized speech; memory and consciousness are not impaired.

c. Symptoms are categorized as positive (hallucinations, bizarre behavior, delusions) or negative (flat affect, apathy, poor grooming, social withdrawal, anhedonia, poor eye contact, poverty of speech).

3. Subtypes of schizophrenia

a. Paranoid schizophrenia: The most common form; characterized by persecutory or grandiose delusions or auditory hallucinations.

b. Disorganized schizophrenia: Characterized by disorganized speech or behavior and flat or inappropriate affect.

c. Catatonic schizophrenia: A rare subtype; manifested by at least two of the following: motor immobility, excess motor activity that is without purpose, extreme negativism or mutism, peculiarly voluntary movement (bizarre postures, stereotyped movements, grimacing), and echolalia (mimicking sound) or echopraxia (mimicking behavior).

d. Undifferentiated schizophrenia: Delusions and hallucinations are prominent; paranoid, disorganized, and catatonic symptoms are absent.

e. Residual schizophrenia: Negative symptoms predominate, and there are only minimal positive symptoms.

B. Clinical features

1. Schizophrenia usually runs a chronic and debilitating course. Prognosis is more favorable with late onset, acute (vs. insidious) onset, obvious precipitating factor, and the presence of positive symptoms.

   a. An estimated 1% to 2% of the population is affected; it most commonly manifests in early adulthood. Onset before age 10 or after age 60 is rare.

   b. The prodromal phase, which precedes the first psychotic break, is manifested by functional decline, social withdrawal, and irritability. Onset of disease tends to be earlier for men (ages 10 to 25) than for women (ages 25 to 35).

   c. The psychotic phase consists of delusions, disorganized thought process and content, and perceptual disturbances.

   d. The residual phase generally occurs between psychotic episodes. It is characterized by blunted affect, odd thinking or behavior, and other negative symptoms.

2. At least two of the following symptoms must be present during a 1-month period (or less if successfully treated), and continuous signs of the disorder must persist for at least 6 months. The presence of hallucinations or delusions is not necessary for a diagnosis.

   a. Delusions: Erroneous beliefs based on a misinterpretation of reality, such as paranoia, ideas of reference, thought broadcasting, delusions of grandeur, or delusions of guilt.

   b. Hallucinations: False perceptions in any of the sensory modalities, such as auditory (most common), tactile, olfactory, and visual. To qualify for the diagnosis, the hallucination must not occur as an isolated experience, in a clouded sensorium, or as part of a religious or cultural experience.

   c. Disorganized speech: Used as a marker for disorganized thought processes.

      (1) The patient is unable to stay on a topic (loose associations), unable to provide an answer related to questions (tangential response), or both.

      (2) The symptoms need to be severe enough to impair an individual's ability to communicate effectively.

   d. Grossly disorganized behavior: May be exhibited as unpredictable agitation, inappropriate sexual behavior, childlike silliness, catatonic motor behavior, or a reduced level of self-care and hygiene.

   e. Negative symptoms: Manifested as blunted affect, poor posture, or lack of goal-directed activities or initiative.

3. Social functioning, occupational functioning, or both must be affected.

   a. This impairment may be manifested as an inability to hold a job for an extended period, inability to maintain relationships, or withdrawal from established friends and social relationships.

   b. The patient's educational progress may be disrupted or not completed.

C. Cause

1. The cause is unknown.

2. Theories consider neurotransmitter abnormalities, such as excess dopamine activity, elevated serotonin and norepinephrine, and decreased γ-aminobutyric acid (GABA). A dysfunctional limbic system is another potential site of pathology.

3. Enlarged ventricles and cortical atrophy on computed tomography (CT) are common in chronic disease.

D. Treatment

1. Hospitalization is recommended for patients who exhibit suicidal ideation or an inability to care for themselves or who pose a threat to self or others.

2. Pharmacotherapy

   a. No therapeutic intervention is totally effective in ameliorating all symptoms.

      (1) Patients with diagnostic subtypes react differently to the various neuroleptics available.

      (2) Combined use of antipsychotic drugs and psychosocial treatment is better than either treatment alone.

    b. Neuroleptic and antipsychotic medications

      (1) Typical neuroleptic and antipsychotic medications with dopamine antagonist activity (haloperidol, chlorpromazine, thioridazine, loxapine, fluphenazine) are best for decreasing positive symptoms (i.e., delusions).

      (2) Second-generation antipsychotics or atypical neuroleptics with serotonin and dopamine antagonist (SDA) activity (risperidone, olanzapine, aripiprazole, ziprasidone, quetiapine) generally are preferred for the management of negative symptoms (i.e., withdrawal) and have fewer side effects.

      (3) The SDAs are the drugs of first choice to treat schizophrenia. Clozapine is considered second line because of propensity to cause agranulocytosis. Conventional antipsychotics (i.e., haloperidol) are an alternative second line.

    c. Side effects, such as extrapyramidal symptoms, parkinsonian-like symptoms, neuroleptic malignant syndrome, and tardive dyskinesia, are more likely to be encountered with the typical neuroleptics.

    d. A 4- to 6-week medication trial is optimal before concluding nonresponse.

  3. Resistant cases may be treated with an antipsychotic medication combined with another drug, such as carbamazepine, valproate, lithium, or benzodiazepines.

  4. Behavior-oriented therapy targeted toward social skills training (as an adjunct to group and/or family therapy) may be helpful.

E. Other forms of psychoses

  1. Schizoaffective disorder

    a. This disorder meets the criteria for major depressive episode, manic episode, or mixed episode, during which criteria for schizophrenia also are met.

    b. Delusions or hallucinations lasting for 2 weeks without mood disorder symptoms help to differentiate schizoaffective disorder from mood disorder with psychotic features.

    c. It carries a better prognosis than schizophrenia but worse prognosis than a mood disorder.

  2. Delusional disorder

    a. This disorder is characterized by the presence of nonbizarre delusions (i.e., situations that occur in real life) for at least 1 month.

    b. The behavior is not obviously odd, and functioning is not significantly impaired.

    c. Subtypes include erotomanic (belief that another person is in love with the patient), somatic (delusions of a physical defect or medical condition), jealous (delusions of sexual partner's infidelity), and persecutory (delusion of mistreatment or persecution).

  3. Psychotic disorders may be caused by alcohol, illicit drug use, or medications (anticholinergics, antidepressants, hallucinogens, psychostimulants).

  4. Psychotic disorders can be caused by general medical conditions (central nervous system disease, endocrinopathies, vitamin deficiency states, HIV/AIDS, systemic lupus erythematosus).

  5. In brief psychotic disorder, symptoms are present for at least 1 day but for less than 1 month, and the patient returns to premorbid levels of functioning after the symptoms abate. This commonly is encountered after a catastrophic event.

  6. Schizophreniform disorder presents with the same symptoms as seen in schizophrenia; symptoms last between 1 and 6 months.

III. SOMATOFORM DISORDERS

A. Somatization disorder

  1. General characteristics

    a. Patients present with vague physical complaints involving many organ systems that cannot be explained by general medical condition or substance use. Visits to health care providers are numerous, although no medical disorder is found.

    b. Patients commonly complain of symptoms related to the gastrointestinal (GI) tract or to the reproductive or neurologic systems; they also may complain of pain. Periods of increased stress are associated with worsening of the somatic symptoms.

    c. This disorder occurs in females more often than in males and more often in low socioeconomic groups. Onset is before 30 years of age, most commonly during adolescence, and 50% of patients have a comorbid mental disorder. Lifetime prevalence is 0.2% to 2.0%. The course of illness is often chronic and debilitating.

2. Treatment
   a. Treatment is regularly (i.e., monthly) scheduled visits with a health care provider.
   b. Patients often are very resistant to seeing a mental health care provider. Group and individual psychotherapy is beneficial to develop coping strategies.
   c. Secondary gain should be minimized and medications avoided.

B. Body dysmorphic disorder
   1. General characteristics
      a. This disorder is characterized by a preoccupation with an imagined defect in physical appearance or an exaggerated distortion of a minor flaw. The most common concerns are facial flaws.
      b. Patients feel self-conscious and fear humiliation; they go to great lengths to hide or correct their perceived anomaly.
      c. Visits to a dermatologist and/or plastic surgeon are common, although the patient usually is still not satisfied with his or her appearance.
      d. Age of onset is 15 to 30 years; females are affected more often than males.
   2. Treatment
      a. Serotonin-modulating drugs (fluoxetine, clomipramine) are efficacious in a majority of patients.
      b. Coexistent psychiatric disorders should be treated appropriately. The most common coexisting disorder is a major depressive episode, followed by anxiety disorder.

C. Conversion disorder
   1. General characteristics
      a. This disorder is characterized by one or more neurologic complaints that cannot be explained clinically.
      b. Symptoms are not intentionally produced and may be motor (involuntary movements, tics, blepharospasm, weakness), sensory (paresthesia and/or anesthesia, tunnel vision, deafness), seizure activity, or mixed (psychogenic vomiting, syncope, globus hystericus). The most common symptoms are shifting paralysis, blindness, and mutism.
      c. Patients display an unexpected lack of concern and indifference to their symptoms (la belle indifference).
      d. Symptoms tend to be episodic, lasting for days to a month, and may remit for a period of time, only to recur during times of stress.
      e. Conversion disorder is common. There is a 20% to 25% incidence in general medical practice.
      f. It most commonly is diagnosed during adolescence and young adulthood and is two to five times more common in females than in males. With men, there often is an associated occupational or military accident.
   2. Treatment
      a. Psychotherapy, such as insight-oriented or behavioral therapy, is considered first-line treatment.
      b. Hypnosis, anxiolytics, and relaxation therapy may help.
      c. Some patients have responded to amobarbital interviews to uncover underlying psychological factors. Lorazepam, especially if a patient has experienced a traumatic event, may be beneficial.

D. Factitious disorder
   1. General characteristics
      a. Patients with this disorder intentionally fake signs and symptoms of medical or psychiatric symptoms, with the primary motivation being to assume the sick role.
      b. It usually begins in early adulthood and carries a poor prognosis.
      c. Often, patients will seek hospital admission under different names and by feigning different illnesses. When (or if) confronted with their ruse, they usually become angry and abruptly sign out.
      d. Obtaining a reliable past medical history is unlikely. Patients usually are familiar with the disease process that they are feigning; however, true disease processes must be ruled out.
      e. Related disorders include Munchausen syndrome and Munchausen syndrome by proxy, which is a form of child abuse. Munchausen syndrome is a factitious disorder with predominantly physical complaints.
   2. Treatment
      a. Early recognition is paramount in the management of this disorder so as to avoid unnecessary and/or potentially dangerous procedures.

   b. Once the diagnosis is confirmed, the patient should be confronted in a nonthreatening manner. No specific psychiatric intervention has been notably effective, but psychotherapy (individual, family) is suggested.

   c. Selective serotonin reuptake inhibitors (SSRIs) may be useful to reduce impulsive tendencies seen in acting-out factitious behavior.

E. Malingering

   1. Malingering involves the deliberate production of physical or psychological symptoms, motivated by external gain. Some of these obvious, definable goals are avoiding responsibility, police or legal action, punishment, or dangerous or difficult situations; receiving monetary compensation (e.g., in a lawsuit) or free hospital room and board; and obtaining drugs.

   2. Patients tend to express vague, poorly defined complaints and claim that these symptoms cause great distress and impaired functioning. Injuries often are found to be self-inflicted, and history reveals multiple, undiagnosed illnesses or previous injuries and even tampering with laboratory results.

   a. Patients are uncooperative and refuse to accept a clean bill of health.

   b. Their symptoms typically improve when the objective has been met or the ruse has been exposed.

F. Hypochondriasis

   1. General characteristics

   a. Hypochondriasis is a preoccupation with the belief of having or the fear of contracting a serious illness. This belief is not of delusional intensity; normal bodily sensations are misinterpreted as manifestations of disease.

   b. This condition commonly is coexistent with symptoms of anxiety and depression.

   c. The patient's fear persists even though medical investigation reveals no cause.

   d. The course, although generally chronic, is episodic and may be exacerbated after a major stressor.

   2. Treatment

   a. Group and insight-oriented psychotherapy can be helpful, but patients usually are resistant to psychiatric care. Discussing mechanisms for coping with stress without reinforcing their perceived illness behavior is important.

   b. Regularly scheduled appointments with a practitioner are recommended to provide reassurance.

   c. Pharmacotherapy can be used if the patient has a concurrent or underlying anxiety or major depressive disorder (MDD). Specifically, SSRIs can be useful in treating hypochondriasis.

G. Pain disorder

   1. General characteristics

   a. Pain is reported in one or more areas without any identifiable cause and results in significant distress and impairment in functioning.

   b. These patients may describe atypical facial pain, low back pain, headache, pelvic pain, and other types of chronic pain syndromes.

   (1) When a medical condition does coexist, the pain cannot be fully explained as a result of the condition.

   (2) Patients tend to view the pain as a cause of all their problems.

   c. Usually, there is an abrupt onset, and pain may increase in intensity over weeks or months. Acute pain disorder is defined as pain with duration of less than 6 months, and chronic pain disorder is defined as pain with duration of greater than 6 months.

   (1) A long history of medical and surgical attention is common, because this tends to be a chronic (and sometimes disabling) disorder.

   (2) Psychological factors, such as stress or loss of a loved one, are felt to have an important role in the pathogenesis.

   (3) Peak onset is 30 to 50 years of age; it is twice as common in women as in men.

   2. Treatment

   a. Psychotherapy, behavioral therapy (e.g., biofeedback and hypnosis), and pain control programs may be helpful. Pain reduction may not be feasible, so the treatment focus should be on rehabilitation.

   b. Analgesics and sedatives generally are not beneficial and may lead to abuse or dependence.

   c. SSRIs and tricyclic antidepressants (TCAs) have been used with some positive results and currently are the most effective drug therapies. Some patients benefit from amphetamines as an adjunct to SSRIs.

IV. MOOD DISORDERS

A. Definition

1. Mood disorders (affective disorders) are a group of clinically distinct entities identified by patterns of mood episodes, which are periods of time (weeks to months) in which some mood impairment is present. The defining feature is a change in mood from a premorbid state. Normally, people feel more or less in control of their moods; however, this sense of control is lost in mood disorders, resulting in a feeling of great turmoil.

2. Mood episodes include major depressive episodes, manic episodes, hypomanic episodes, and mixed episodes.

3. Mood disorders include MDD, bipolar I, bipolar II, dysthymia, and cyclothymia.

4. Cause: The cause is largely unknown; however, neurochemical (serotonin, norepinephrine, dopamine, growth hormone, cortisol), genetic, and psychosocial factors (life events) have been implicated.

B. Mood episodes

1. Major depressive episode

   a. Depressive signs and symptoms must be present for the better part of a 2-week period (Table 12-1).

   b. At least one of the symptoms must include depressed mood or anhedonia (loss of interest or pleasure in all activities).

   c. Patients should not exhibit manic signs or symptoms (Table 12-1).

   d. The mood episode is not the result of bereavement.

2. Manic episode

   a. Manic episode is characterized by an abnormally and persistently elevated, expansive, or irritable mood that lasts for at least 1 week.

   b. At least three manic symptoms (four if mood is irritable) are present (Table 12-1).

   c. Patients may exhibit psychotic features or require hospitalization to prevent harm to self or others.

   d. Mania results in severe social and/or occupational dysfunction.

TABLE 12-1 Symptoms of a Mood Episode
Depression
Depressed mood (either reported by the patient or observed by others)
Anhedonia
Excessive feelings of guilt
Indecisiveness
Lack of self-worth
Sleep problems such as insomnia or hypersomnia
Cognitive problems (difficulty with memory and concentration)
Psychomotor retardation or agitation
Either decreased or increased appetite or a 5% or greater unintentional change in body weight over a 1-month period
Decreased interest in sex
Either suicidal ideation or thoughts of death without suicidal ideation
Chronic fatigue or decreased energy
Mania
Inflated self-esteem or grandiosity
Irritability
Decreased need for sleep
Pressured speech
Flight of ideas
Distractibility
Impaired judgment, resulting in pursuit of pleasurable activities with a high probability of adverse outcomes
Psychomotor agitation

3. Hypomanic episode

   a. Hypomanic episode is characterized by at least four continuous days of an abnormally and persistently elevated, expansive, or irritable mood.

   b. At least three manic symptoms (four if the mood is irritable) must be present.

   c. Although the patient's mood and functioning are changed from premorbid functioning, social and occupational functioning is not significantly affected, and there are no psychotic features.

   d. Hypomanic episode does not require hospitalization.

4. Mixed episode

   a. Mixed episode is characterized by rapidly alternating moods, with symptoms of both a manic episode and a depressive episode, which lasts for at least 1 week.

   b. Symptoms typically are severe enough that there is marked impairment in occupational or social functioning.

C. Mood disorders

1. MDD

   a. General characteristics

      (1) MDD has a chronic course with relapses.

         (a) Premorbid functioning may return between episodes.

         (b) Between 5% and 10% of patients subsequently develop a manic episode.

         (c) MDD is two to three times more common in females than in males. The lifetime prevalence of depressive syndromes is 13% to 20%.

      (2) The suicide rate is estimated at 15%.

         (a) Patients may be at highest risk of suicide after initiating treatment; therapy may bring out the energy that the patient previously lacked to undertake a suicide attempt.

         (b) Higher suicide rates are associated with a previous attempt, white males older than 45 years, a detailed plan, a self-destructive pattern, a recent severe loss, poor support system, poor health, concurrent substance abuse, psychotic symptoms, and an inability to accept help.

   b. Subtypes

      (1) Seasonal affective disorder

         (a) Seasonal affective disorder is characterized by the predominance of fall or winter onset and likely is caused by the lessening daylight hours; it typically remits in the spring.

         (b) It is more common in colder climates and in young females; the average age at presentation is 40 years.

         (c) Light therapy and SSRIs have been used successfully.

      (2) Melancholia

         (a) Melancholia is characterized by anhedonia, psychomotor retardation or agitation, anorexia, weight loss, depressed mood (especially in the morning), feelings of guilt, and sleep disturbance (most often early morning awakening). Suicidal ideation may be present.

         (b) Melancholia characterizes about 50% of hospitalized patients with major depression.

         (c) Melancholic patients respond better to pharmacotherapy than nonmelancholic patients. Antidepressants or electroconvulsive therapy (ECT) is effective.

      (3) Atypical depression

         (a) Atypical depression is characterized by overeating and weight gain, oversleeping, reactive mood, leaden paralysis, and oversensitivity to interpersonal rejection.

         (b) Monoamine oxidase inhibitors (MAOIs) are useful in this group. SSRIs may also be effective.

      (4) Catatonic depression

         (a) Catatonic depression is characterized by motor immobility or stupor, blurred affect, purposeless motor activity, extreme withdrawal, negativism, bizarre mannerisms or posturing, echolalia, echopraxia, or "waxy flexibility."

         (b) It often is treated with antidepressants and antipsychotics simultaneously.

      (5) Psychotic depression is characterized by the presence of delusions or hallucinations.

      (6) Postpartum depression is characterized by the onset of symptoms within 4 weeks of delivery.

c. Pharmacotherapy

(1) If well tolerated, antidepressants should be continued for a minimum of 3 to 6 weeks to determine efficacy. Maintenance therapy should be continued long term (>6 months), both because of the high relapse rate and because future episodes may be more severe.

(2) SSRIs (fluoxetine, paroxetine, sertraline) are considered to be first-line therapy, because they have minimal adverse effects and are safer than other antidepressant classes.

(a) Selection of a particular SSRI should be based on side-effect profiles and the presenting problems.

(b) Side effects include GI upset, headache, and sexual dysfunction.

(3) Bupropion, venlafaxine, nefazodone, and mirtazapine also are very effective and have a safer side-effect profile than TCAs or MAOIs. Nefazodone and mirtazapine have not been associated with decreased libido, erectile dysfunction, or anorgasmia.

(4) TCAs and tetracyclics cause side effects such as weight gain, orthostatic hypotension, anticholinergic effects, and somnolence. Overdosage with these agents is more lethal than with other antidepressants.

(5) MAOIs require a tyramine-free diet (no wine, beer, nearly all cheeses, aged foods, smoked meats) to avoid side effects, such as hypertensive crisis.

(6) Precautions

(a) Use of MAOIs with SSRIs can result in serotonin syndrome, which causes acute mental status changes, restlessness, diaphoresis, tremor, hyperthermia, seizures, and, occasionally, coma and death.

(b) TCAs and MAOIs used concurrently can cause delirium and hypertension.

(c) The serious risks associated with MAOIs make this class of drugs the least likely to be used.

d. ECT

(1) ECT is effective in all types of MDD. Usually, however, it is reserved for severely depressed patients or patients who are unresponsive or intolerant of psychiatric medications or when the clinical picture is so debilitating that rapid improvement is warranted.

(2) ECT can safely be used in pregnant and elderly patients, produces a rapid response, and has very few relative contraindications. Maintenance antidepressant therapy is indicated after ECT is completed.

(3) Common adverse effects include postictal confusion and somatic complaints, such as headache, nausea, and muscle soreness.

(4) The greatest concern is memory loss, which often returns to baseline by 6 months after treatment.

e. Psychotherapy treatment for mood disorders: Most studies indicate that cognitive, interpersonal, and behavioral therapy is effective, especially in combination with pharmacotherapy.

2. Bipolar I disorder

a. General characteristics

(1) Bipolar I disorder is characterized by the occurrence of one or more manic or mixed episodes, which often cycle with depressive episodes, but the latter is not required for diagnosis. It commonly is known as manic depression.

(2) Manic episodes

(a) Episodes are characterized by a sudden escalation of mood, which is abnormally and persistently euphoric, expansive, or irritable.

(b) Patients may go for days without sleep; become excessively talkative or loud, socially outgoing, overly self-confident, hypersexual, or disinhibited; and display a flamboyant clothing style.

(3) Thought processes are difficult to follow because of racing thoughts, flights of ideas, and easy distraction. Judgment is quite impaired, resulting in spending sprees, promiscuity, or foolish business investments.

(4) Psychotic symptoms (e.g., hallucinations, paranoia, delusions) may be present.

(5) The course usually is chronic with relapses. In general, it carries a worse prognosis and a higher suicide rate than MDD.

(6) Epidemiology

(a) The lifetime prevalence is about 1%.

(b) The average age of diagnosis is 30 years, and early onset is correlated with a higher incidence of psychotic symptoms and a poorer prognosis.

(c) Diagnosis is often delayed as misdiagnosis is very common; the most common misdiagnoses are MDD and anxiety.

(d) First-degree relatives have an increased incidence of developing the disorder. Monozygotic twin concordance rates are about 75%.

b. Treatment

(1) Lithium, valproic acid, olanzapine, or carbamazepine is effective. Gabapentin, topiramate, and lamotrigine also show beneficial effects. Second-generation antipsychotics such as risperidone, aripiprazole, quetiapine, and ziprasidone are a good choice to treat acute mania.

(a) Lithium has a narrow therapeutic window, and plasma levels need to be monitored every 4 to 8 weeks.

(b) Although usually well tolerated, lithium has side effects, including weight gain, tremor, nausea, increased thirst and urination, drowsiness, hypothyroidism, arrhythmias, and seizures.

(2) Haloperidol or benzodiazepines (i.e., lorazepam or clonazepam) may be added if agitation or psychotic symptoms are present, especially at the initiation of treatment when acute manic episodes are likely.

(3) Acute depressive episodes can be treated with SSRIs or bupropion. *Caution*: Antidepressant medication may precipitate mania.

(4) Secondary treatment measures include ECT, MAOIs, and TCAs (caution must be exercised, because these drugs can result in rapid cycling between mood states).

(5) Family, group, supportive, interpersonal, and/or cognitive therapy may help.

3. Bipolar II disorder

a. General characteristics

(1) Bipolar II disorder is characterized by at least one or more major depressive episodes and at least one hypomanic episode. The patient has never experienced a manic episode or a mixed episode.

(2) Hypomanic symptoms are similar to manic symptoms but are less severe and cause less social impairment. Hypomania also usually does not present with psychotic symptoms, racing thoughts, or excess psychomotor agitation.

(3) Prevalence is estimated at 0.5%; it appears to be slightly more common in females than in males.

b. Treatment: Same as for bipolar I disorder.

4. Dysthymic disorder

a. General characteristics

(1) Dysthymic disorder is a chronic, persistent mild depression that is manifested by pessimism, brooding, generalized loss of interest, decreased productivity, feelings of inadequacy, and social withdrawal.

(2) There are no psychotic or manic/hypomanic features.

(3) MDD eventually will develop in 10% to 20% of patients. Bipolar disorder may develop in others, and 25% of patients will have lifelong dysthymic symptoms.

(4) It is two to three times more common in women than in men; onset is during young adulthood.

b. Diagnosis

(1) Patient is in depressed mood for most of the day, for more days than not, for at least 2 years (at least 1 year in children and adolescents).

(2) During the 2-year period, the person has not been without the symptoms for more than 2 months at a time, and no major depressive episode occurred during the first 2 years of symptoms.

(3) At least two of the following conditions are noted: poor concentration or indecisiveness, hopelessness, poor appetite or overeating, insomnia or hypersomnia, low energy or fatigue, and lack of self-esteem.

c. Treatment

(1) Antidepressants (SSRIs, bupropion, TCAs, or, occasionally, MAOIs) are effective.

(2) Insight-oriented behavior and cognitive therapies are beneficial, especially when combined with pharmacotherapy.

5. Cyclothymic disorder

a. General characteristics

(1) Patients are described as moody, erratic, impulsive, and somewhat volatile.

(2) This disorder (similar to bipolar II but less severe) is characterized by recurring periods of relatively less severe depressive episodes and hypomania over a 2-year period, with symptom-free periods lasting for no more than 2 months at any one time. The depressive episodes are not severe enough to be classified as a major depressive episode, and manic or mixed episodes have not occurred.

(3) It has a chronic course, and there is a 15% to 20% risk of bipolar disorder.

b. Treatment: similar to bipolar I disorder (mood stabilizers and antimanic drugs are first-line therapies).

6. Adjustment disorder

   a. General characteristics

     (1) This disorder is characterized by maladaptive behavioral or emotional symptoms that develop within 3 months after a stressful life event and end within 6 months of the event.

     (2) Among adolescents, precipitants include parental rejection and divorce, problems at school, and leaving home.

     (3) Among adults, stressors include marital discord, financial difficulties, or loss of a job, marriage, or parenthood. Also included are natural disasters and racial/religious persecution.

     (4) The symptoms cause significant impairment in functioning.

     (5) The symptoms are not caused by bereavement.

   b. Treatment

     (1) Adjustment disorder is treated with supportive psychotherapy or group therapy.

     (2) Short-term pharmacotherapy for associated insomnia, anxiety, or depression may be used but is not first-line treatment.

V. PERSONALITY DISORDERS

A. Definition

  1. Personality disorders are deeply ingrained, inflexible patterns of relating to others that are maladaptive and cause significant impairment in social or occupational functions.

  2. Patients are egosyntonic and lack insight regarding their problems. Personality disorders are axis II and are divided into three clusters.

   a. Cluster A (mad)

     (1) This cluster includes schizoid, schizotypal, and paranoid personality disorders.

     (2) Patients are viewed as weird or peculiar.

     (3) It is associated with psychotic disorders.

   b. Cluster B (bad)

     (1) This cluster includes antisocial, borderline, histrionic, and narcissistic personality disorders.

     (2) Patients are viewed as emotional and inconsistent.

     (3) It is associated with mood disorders.

   c. Cluster C (sad)

     (1) This cluster includes avoidant, dependent, and obsessive–compulsive personality disorders.

     (2) Patients are viewed as fearful or anxious.

     (3) It is associated with anxiety disorders.

B. Cluster A personality disorders

  1. Paranoid personality disorder

   a. General characteristics

     (1) Paranoid personality disorder is characterized by a pervasive distrust and suspicion of others, beginning by early adulthood. Patients blame their own problems on others and seem hostile and angry.

     (2) Males are more commonly affected than females.

   b. Clinical features

     (1) Suspicion (without evidence) that others are exploiting or deceiving him or her

     (2) Preoccupation with doubts regarding the loyalty or trustworthiness of acquaintances; doubts regarding fidelity

     (3) Reluctance to confide in others

     (4) Interpretation of benign remarks as threatening or demeaning

     (5) Persistence of grudges; quick to counterattack

   c. Treatment

     (1) Individual psychotherapy is the key.

     (2) Antianxiety medications or a short course of antipsychotics for transient psychosis may be needed.

2. Schizoid personality disorder
   a. General characteristics
      (1) This disorder is characterized by a lifelong pattern of voluntary social withdrawal, often perceived as eccentric and reclusive.
      (2) Patients are quiet and unsociable and have constricted affect. They have no desire for close relationships and prefer to be alone.
      (3) Males are affected twice as often as females.
   b. Clinical features
      (1) Patients neither enjoy nor desire close relationships (including family).
      (2) They generally choose solitary activities.
      (3) They show little (if any) interest in sexual activity with another person.
      (4) They are indifferent to praise or criticism.
      (5) An emotional coldness, detachment, or flattened affect is seen.
   c. Treatment
      (1) Group therapy and psychotherapy are recommended.
      (2) Low-dose, short-term antipsychotics or antidepressants can be given if indicated for comorbidity.
3. Schizotypal personality disorder
   a. General characteristics
      (1) This disorder is characterized by a pervasive pattern of eccentric behavior and peculiar thought patterns beginning in early adulthood.
      (2) The patient often is perceived as strange and eccentric.
   b. Clinical features
      (1) Patients have ideas of reference, which are beliefs or perceptions that irrelevant, unrelated, or innocuous things in the world are referring to them directly or have special personal significance. Ideas of reference are less firmly held or more disorganized beliefs than delusions of reference.
      (2) Patients display odd behaviors, thoughts, speech, beliefs, or magical thinking inconsistent with cultural norms; these may include belief in clairvoyance or telepathy, bizarre fantasies or preoccupations, and belief in superstitions.
      (3) Unusual perceptual experiences (e.g., bodily illusions) may be noted.
      (4) Patients show suspiciousness and excessive social anxiety.
      (5) Inappropriate or restricted affect is seen.
   c. Treatment
      (1) Psychotherapy (social skills training) is the treatment of choice.
      (2) A short course of low-dose antipsychotics (such as risperidone or olanzapine), antidepressants, or benzodiazepines to decrease anxiety can be used if necessary.
C. Cluster B personality disorders
   1. Antisocial personality disorder
      a. General characteristics
         (1) This disorder is characterized by an inability to conform to social norms.
         (2) A pervasive pattern of disregard for and violation of the rights and feelings of others is characteristic.
         (3) Patients are described as extremely manipulative, deceitful, impulsive, and totally lacking empathy or remorse. On interview, however, they can act exceedingly charming and seem normal.
         (4) It may begin in childhood as a conduct disorder.
            (a) These children may have a history of physical and/or sexual abuse.
            (b) Symptoms may decrease with age.
         (5) Multiple physical complaints, substance abuse, and depression are common.
         (6) An abnormal electroencephalogram (EEG) may be seen.
         (7) Males are affected three times more often than females. There is a familial pattern, and it is more common in urban areas and prison populations.

b. Clinical features

(1) Patients show deceitfulness, lying, and conning others for personal gain.

(2) Irritability and aggressiveness, manifested by repeated physical assaults, are noted, and patients have a reckless disregard for the safety of self or others.

(3) Patients are irresponsible and unable to sustain work.

c. Treatment

(1) Treatment is psychotherapy with socially based intervention.

(2) Pharmacotherapy with SSRIs, lithium, valproate, carbamazepine, and, possibly, propranolol may help to reduce anxiety, impulsivity, and aggression. Caution must be exercised, however, because of the high potential for abuse.

2. Borderline personality disorder

a. General characteristics

(1) This disorder is characterized by an unstable and unpredictable mood, affect, and behavior as well as a poorly established self-image. Mood swings and impulsivity are common, and the patient always appears to be in a state of crisis.

(2) Short and transient psychotic episodes, paranoid ideation, or dissociative symptoms may occur, especially during times of increased stress.

(3) Self-mutilation and manipulative suicide attempts are common.

(4) The patient desperately attempts to avoid abandonment.

(5) Patients cannot tolerate being alone yet can exhibit intense anger toward their friends.

(a) Splitting (i.e., seeing people as either all good or all bad) is common.

(b) Patients have unstable and intense relationships.

(c) Inappropriate anger or difficulty controlling anger is seen.

(6) There is a high incidence of MDD; suicide rates peak during early adulthood.

(7) Females are affected twice as often as males.

b. Treatment

(1) Treatment includes psychotherapy with social skills training, behavioral therapy, and individual and group therapy.

(2) Pharmacotherapy in addition to psychotherapy yields better results.

(a) Antipsychotics are used to control hostility and brief psychotic episodes.

(b) Antidepressants/SSRIs such as fluoxetine are used to improve mood.

(c) Benzodiazepines can help decrease anxiety, but should only be used short term (days to weeks).

(d) Anticonvulsants have been beneficial to improve global functioning.

3. Histrionic personality disorder

a. General characteristics

(1) Individuals with this disorder are overly emotional, dramatic, and seductive; they are excitable, with a high degree of attention-seeking behavior and a tendency to exaggerate their thoughts and feelings.

(a) Patients are flamboyant and extroverted, but their rapidly shifting emotions and superficiality renders them unable to maintain a deep, long-lasting relationship.

(b) They are easily influenced by others.

(c) They need to be the center of attention and may throw a temper tantrum if the attention shifts. They have a pattern of excessive emotionality and attention-seeking behavior and often are inappropriately seductive or provocative, with exaggerated expression and emotion.

(2) Somatization and substance use disorders are common.

(3) Speech can be excessively impressionistic and lacking in detail.

b. Treatment

(1) Treatment includes psychotherapy, either group or individual.

(2) Antidepressants and/or anxiolytics may be useful for specific symptoms.

4. Narcissistic personality disorder

a. General characteristics

(1) Patients have an inflated self-image, pattern of grandiosity, need for admiration, and lack of empathy. They consider themselves to be special and expect to be treated as such, and they may have an arrogant, haughty attitude.

(2) Although they have a sense of entitlement and grandiosity, their self-esteem is quite fragile. They have a need for excessive admiration, and they are prone to depression if criticized.

(3) They have a preoccupation with fantasies of unlimited success, beauty, brilliance, and so forth. Aging is difficult and makes them prone to midlife crisis.

(4) They may be exploitative and take advantage of others to meet their own needs.

  b. Treatment

(1) This disorder is difficult to treat.

(2) Psychotherapy is key.

(3) Lithium has been used if mood swings are present. Antidepressants (especially SSRIs) are a useful adjunct.

D. Cluster C personality disorders

  1. Avoidant personality disorder

    a. General characteristics

(1) These individuals have an extreme sensitivity to rejection (inferiority complex).

(2) Patients see themselves as unappealing.

(3) They have intense social anxiety and feelings of inadequacy, which may lead to interpersonal withdrawal and total avoidance of any situation in which they may be criticized.

(4) Although shy, they display a great desire for companionship, but with strong guarantees of unconditional acceptance. They may avoid occupational activities that involve interpersonal contact because of fear of rejection.

(5) They show great restraint with intimate relationships because of fear of rejection.

(6) Social phobia (fear of embarrassment or rejection in a particular setting) is common in this group.

    b. Treatment

(1) Psychotherapy, social skills training, group therapy, and assertiveness training may be beneficial.

(2) β-Blockers and SSRIs (especially paroxetine, sertraline, or escitalopram) are useful for managing anxiety and depression and may help to reduce the patient's sensitivity to rejection. Benzodiazepines can be used short term to decrease anxiety.

  2. Dependent personality disorder

    a. General characteristics

(1) These individuals have an enduring pattern of dependent, clinging, and submissive behavior; they cannot make their own decisions without help from others.

(2) Patients have difficulty disagreeing with others for fear of loss of support or approval.

(3) They lack self-confidence, avoid positions of responsibility, and have a dislike of being alone. They are passive, self-doubtful, and reliant on others to take care of them.

(4) Depression may ensue, especially if they experience loss of the person on whom they depend.

(5) They go to extreme lengths to seek another relationship.

(6) Social and occupational functioning is impaired; risk for depression is high. Some suffer physical or mental abuse because they fail to assert themselves.

(7) They feel uncomfortable when alone for fear of being unable to care for self.

    b. Treatment

(1) Psychotherapy, especially insight-oriented, behavioral, group, and family therapy, and assertiveness training may help.

(2) Anxiolytics and antidepressants may be useful to target symptoms; benzodiazepines and SSRIs are used.

  3. Obsessive–compulsive personality disorder

    a. General characteristics

(1) Obsessive–compulsive personality disorder is characterized by a pervasive pattern of orderliness (rules, lists, details), perfectionism, and inflexibility. Unlike other personality disorders, these patients often have an awareness of their disorder and seek treatment on their own.

(2) Patients tend to be rigid, stubborn, and emotionally constricted, and they insist that others submit to their ways, causing difficulty with interpersonal and occupational relationships.

(3) Perfectionism interferes with the ability to complete tasks or form relationships.

(4) A change in routine threatens to upset their perceived stability and can lead to extreme anxiety.

(5) The course of this disorder is variable. The disorder may remit, or obsessions and compulsions may develop. Schizophrenia and MDD may develop.

(6) Obsessive–compulsive personality disorder is egosyntonic (not distressing to the patient), whereas obsessive–compulsive disorder is egodystonic (distressing to the patient).

(7) Patients display excessive devotion to work and productivity to the exclusion of leisure activities; they have a reluctance to delegate tasks unless those tasks are done the way they want.

(8) Miserly spending or hoarding of money is seen.

b. Treatment

(1) Psychotherapy and group or behavioral therapy are recommended.

(2) Clomipramine, clonazepam, and SSRIs help manage obsessive–compulsive symptoms.

E. Personality disorder NOS

1. This category includes disorders that do not fit into any of the true personality disorders.

2. Passive–aggressive

a. Passive–aggressive is characterized by procrastination, irritability, stubbornness, negativistic attitudes, and passive resistance to demands for adequate performance. These patients are sullen, argumentative, and envious/resentful toward those who seem to be more fortunate.

b. Patients lack self-confidence, make excuses for delays, find fault with others, and are intentionally inefficient. They complain of being misunderstood and unappreciated.

c. Treatment is psychotherapy. Antidepressants and benzodiazepines can be used only when clinically indicated for depressive symptoms.

3. Depressive

a. The disorder is manifested by chronic unhappiness, very similar to dysthymic disorder.

b. Patients tend to be gloomy and pessimistic, have low self-esteem, and may be overly conscientious with work performance and critical of self and others.

c. Treatment includes psychotherapy (insight-oriented, group, or self-help) along with antidepressants (SSRIs).

4. Sadomasochistic

a. Sadism is the desire to cause pain to others by being sexually, physically, or mentally abusive; masochism generally is the seeking of humiliation rather than of physically inflicted pain.

b. Patients may exhibit sadism, masochism, or both.

5. Sadistic

a. This is characterized by a pervasive pattern of demeaning, humiliating, and cruel behavior toward others.

b. Patients may be fascinated with violence, torture, or weapons and are aggressive without gain (e.g., sexual, monetary).

c. Treatment is insight-oriented psychotherapy.

VI. ANXIETY DISORDERS

A. Definition

1. Anxiety disorders are characterized by excessive amounts of anxiety that impede performance.

2. These disorders can result in physiologic symptoms, such as dizziness, palpitations, perspiration, loss of appetite, nausea, trembling, and other symptoms that cause the patient distress.

B. Generalized anxiety disorder

1. General characteristics

a. Generalized anxiety disorder is characterized by persistent, excessive anxiety regarding general life events that lasts for 6 months or more.

b. The patient has difficulty coping with the anxiety, which usually is expressed as worry or apprehension.

c. There is a high (50% to 90%) comorbidity with other psychiatric disorders, such as MDD, specific and social phobias, and panic disorder.

    d. Diagnostic criteria include at least three of the following: restlessness or hypervigilance, easy fatigability, irritability, sleep disturbance, muscle tension, and difficulty concentrating. Medical disorders, such as thyroid dysfunction, stimulant abuse, alcohol withdrawal, caffeine intoxication, and cardiac arrhythmias, must be ruled out.

    e. Generalized anxiety disorder is very common, with lifetime prevalence estimated at 45%. It affects women twice as often as men. Age of diagnosis is around 20, although patients typically report feeling anxious for as long as they can remember.

  2. Treatment

    a. SSRIs and buspirone are effective; low-dose TCAs also may help but are not considered first line.

    b. Benzodiazepines can be used as an adjunct for short-term management of severe symptoms but are not recommended for monotherapy because of the risk of dependence or abuse.

    c. Behavioral and insight-oriented therapy also should be initiated.

C. Panic attacks and panic disorder

  1. Panic attacks

    a. Panic attack is defined as a period of extreme anxiety that peaks within 10 minutes, typically declines within 30 minutes, and rarely lasts for longer than 1 hour.

    b. Panic attacks may have a definable trigger or be totally unexpected.

    c. Patients may experience palpitations or tachycardia, sweating, trembling, dyspnea, sensation of choking, chest discomfort, nausea, depersonalization (feel estranged from self and/or the external world), derealization (people, events, and surroundings appear to be changed or unreal), fear of losing control, fear of dying, light-headedness, numbness or tingling, chills, or hot flashes.

  2. Panic disorder

    a. Panic disorder is characterized by recurrent, unexpected panic attacks that occur abruptly and are accompanied by debilitating fear of having additional attacks.

    b. The intense fear and physical symptoms may be accompanied by feelings of impending harm or death, fear of a heart attack or stroke, and/or fears of "going crazy."

    c. Panic disorder occurs in 1% to 5% of the population. It is two to three times more common in females than in males.

    d. Average age at onset is the mid-20s, but panic disorder can occur at any age, including childhood.

  3. Diagnosis should specify panic disorder with or without agoraphobia (extensive avoidance of settings in which panic attacks have occurred).

  4. Cause

    a. Evidence points toward a biologic cause, though genetics and psychosocial factors most likely contribute.

    b. Nervous system dysregulation and abnormal activity of norepinephrine, serotonin, and GABA have been implicated.

    c. Some substances (e.g., intravenous [IV] sodium lactate or inhalation of carbon dioxide) have panic-inducing effects on patients with panic disorder yet rarely have any effect on those without panic disorder.

  5. Treatment

    a. For acute management of anxiety, a short course of benzodiazepines (alprazolam or lorazepam) is beneficial.

    b. For maintenance, SSRIs should be instituted, as benzodiazepines are tapered. Paroxetine is beneficial, as are fluoxetine, venlafaxine, and sertraline.

    c. Treatment should continue for 8 to 12 months, because relapse rates are high after medication is discontinued.

    d. Mild cases may be managed with psychotherapy alone. Cognitive, insight-oriented, relaxation training, and behavioral therapies have been shown to be effective.

D. Obsessive–compulsive disorder

  1. General characteristics

    a. Obsessions refer to persistent and recurrent thoughts, images, or impulses that are intrusive and inappropriate and cause significant anxiety.

    b. Compulsions are the ritualistic or repetitive behaviors or thoughts that patients feel compelled to engage in to relieve the anxiety caused by the obsessions and to reduce distress. The behaviors or mental acts are excessive and have no realistic connection to the events the patient is trying to avoid.

    c. Patients typically have insight and realize that their thoughts and behaviors are irrational and causing distress.

d. This disorder is egodystonic as opposed to obsessive–compulsive personality disorder, which is egosyntonic (not distressing to the patient).

e. Two-thirds of patients are diagnosed before age 25 and one-third during adolescence.

f. Evidence indicates that neurotransmitter dysregulation, as well as genetic and psychosocial factors, contribute to the disorder.

g. Common types of obsessive compulsions, in order of frequency, are as follows:

(1) Contamination: Patients wash their hands excessively or compulsively avoid objects presumed to be contaminated.

(2) Pathologic doubt: Patients worry about such things as forgetting to lock the door or turn off the stove; these doubts result in repetitive checking.

(3) Intrusive thoughts: Patients have obsessive thoughts without a compulsion; these thoughts may be of a sexual or aggressive nature.

(4) Need for symmetry: Patients must order and arrange objects, leading to extreme precision and slowness.

(5) Other: Patients have religious obsessions, compulsive hoarding, nail biting, and trichotillomania (compulsively pulling out hair).

2. Treatment

a. SSRIs (sertraline, paroxetine, fluvoxamine, citalopram), in doses often higher than normally prescribed, are considered to be first-line therapy; the TCA clomipramine has shown efficacy, but has many side effects.

b. Patients who show only a partial remission of symptoms may undergo a trial of lithium, venlafaxine, buspirone, clonazepam, or an add-on antipsychotic with an SSRI.

c. Behavioral therapies should be initiated. Relaxation therapy may be beneficial.

E. Posttraumatic stress disorder (PTSD)

1. General characteristics

a. PTSD results from exposure to or witnessing a physiologically or psychologically traumatic event that is out of the range of normal human experience. Symptoms can develop in as little as 1 week or many years after the event and can fluctuate over time, becoming worse during stressful times.

b. PTSD is manifested by overwhelming sensations of helplessness, fear, and horror that impair occupational or social functioning.

c. A patient may have a sense of repeatedly reliving the event, have intrusive memories or disturbing dreams of the event, or experience distress when exposed to stimuli that trigger event review.

d. PTSD must be differentiated from brief psychotic, acute stress, adjustment, and borderline personality disorders. There is a high comorbidity with substance abuse and depression.

e. PTSD is most common in young adults because of the nature of the precipitating event. In men, it most often results from combat experience; in women, it most often results from assault or rape.

2. For diagnosis, three or more of the following should be present for more than 1 month:

a. Inability to recall an important aspect of the event

b. Avoidance of activities, places, or people that remind the patient of the event

c. Attempts to avoid thinking or talking about the event

d. Feelings of detachment or estrangement from others

e. Markedly decreased interest or anhedonia

f. Restricted range of affect

g. Belief that one's future has been foreshortened because of the event

h. An increased state of arousal characterized by at least two of the following: insomnia, irritability or angry outbursts, poor concentration, hypervigilance, or exaggerated startle response

3. Treatment

a. SSRIs (sertraline, paroxetine) are considered to be first-line treatment; TCAs (imipramine, doxepin, amitriptyline) may be effective. Buspirone, MAOIs, and anticonvulsants, such as carbamazepine and valproate, also may be effective.

b. Crisis counseling should be initiated as a preventive measure when feasible. Support groups, family therapy, and cognitive or behavioral therapies are recommended. Hypnosis, coping mechanisms, and relaxation techniques can be beneficial as well.

F. Acute stress disorder

1. General characteristics

   a. Symptoms of acute stress disorder occur within 1 month of the traumatic event and last from 2 days to 4 weeks, whereas symptoms of PTSD may develop any time after the event and last for more than 1 month.

   b. Common comorbidities include depression, anxiety, substance abuse, and cognitive difficulties (e.g., impaired concentration).

   c. It is most prevalent in younger ages.

2. Clinical features

   a. Either during or after the event, the person has three or more of the following: sense of numbing or detachment, reduced awareness of surroundings (in a daze), derealization, depersonalization, or dissociative amnesia (inability to recall an important component of the trauma).

   b. Patients experience excessive anxiety or arousal (e.g., insomnia, irritability, poor concentration, hypervigilance, exaggerated startle response).

   c. The distressing event is reexperienced in at least one of the following ways: recurrent dreams, images, or thoughts; flashback; sensation of reliving the event; or exposure to reminders of the trauma, causing distress.

   d. Patients avoid stimuli that remind them of the trauma (e.g., activities, places, people).

   e. Distress results in marked impairment in important areas of functioning.

3. Treatment

   a. Treatment includes cognitive and behavioral therapy and supportive counseling.

   b. Anxiolytics (lorazepam, clonazepam) can be used to decrease insomnia and irritability.

   c. Similar measures to treat PTSD also can be employed to treat acute stress disorder, including support groups, family therapy, SSRIs, TCAs, and anticonvulsants.

G. Phobias (specific and social)

1. General characteristics

   a. Phobias are considered to be the most common mental disorders in the United States.

   b. They are characterized by an irrational fear and persistent excessive anxiety when presented with an object or a situational event.

   c. Exposure results in an immediate increase in anxiety and can precipitate a panic attack.

   d. Because of the discomfort caused by the increased anxiety, the panic attack, or both, the situation or object is either feared and avoided or endured with considerable apprehension.

   e. Except for children, patients with this disorder know that their fear is excessive and unreasonable.

   f. Diagnosis of a phobia is made if the response to phobic stimuli interferes with the patient's daily routine, social, or occupational functioning.

   g. Common comorbidities are MDD, substance abuse, other anxiety disorders, and personality disorders.

2. Specific phobia

   a. Specific phobias are more common than social phobias.

   b. Specific phobia and agoraphobia are two to three times more common in women than in men; social phobia affects men and women equally.

   c. Many phobias can begin in childhood, and the majority of these are in place by early adulthood.

   d. Specific phobia refers to the fear of a specific object or situation. There are five types:

      (1) Animal: The fear is of animals or insects; onset generally is during childhood.

      (2) Natural environment: The fear is of natural phenomena (e.g., storms, heights, water, lightning).

      (3) Blood–injection–injury: The fear of invasive procedures is paramount; the phobic trigger may be the possibility of injury, the sight of blood, or fear of contamination by exposure to bodily fluids.

      (4) Situational: The fear of bridges, tall buildings, flying, driving, and confined spaces are examples of this type.

      (5) Other: This type includes fear of situations that may lead to choking, vomiting, or getting an illness; in children, the fear may be of loud noises or costumed characters.

3. Social phobia

   a. Social phobia is the fear of social situations in which embarrassment or humiliation in front of other people may occur.

   b. Common inciting events are public speaking, using public restrooms, and eating in public.

4. Agoraphobia

    a. Agoraphobia is an intense anxiety about placing oneself into a situation in which an incapacitating problem could occur and no help would be available. The event usually is viewed by the patient as extremely embarrassing or humiliating.

    b. Often, there is fear of being in public places where escape may be difficult in the event of a subsequent attack. Anxiety-producing situations may include riding on a train or bus; being in any crowded area, mall, supermarket, or theater; or just being alone outside the home.

    c. Agoraphobia may occur with or without a history of panic disorder, although 50% to 70% of patients with agoraphobia have coexisting panic disorder. If the feared incapacitating event is a panic attack, then agoraphobia is diagnosed as secondary to the panic disorder.

    d. Diagnostic criteria

        (1) Any of the symptoms that are characteristic of a panic attack may be present. In addition, the patient may have a potentially incapacitating or embarrassing medical condition, such as a heart condition or a lack of bowel or bladder control.

        (2) In extreme cases, symptoms may render the patient either unwilling or unable to leave home.

5. Treatment

    a. For social phobias and agoraphobia, SSRIs (particularly paroxetine, fluoxetine, sertraline, and venlafaxine) are considered to be first-line therapy. If SSRIs are not successful, benzodiazepines, buspirone, and, lastly, TCAs (imipramine) may be initiated but are less effective.

    b. β-Blockers, such as propranolol, have been used successfully to reduce autonomic hyperarousal symptoms and tremor associated with performance situations.

    c. Insight-oriented therapy should be initiated, and hypnosis may be helpful.

    d. Specific phobias can be treated with short-term benzodiazepines and β-blockers; however, systematic desensitization/exposure therapy, hypnosis, and supportive and insight-oriented psychotherapy probably are more useful.

VII. EATING DISORDERS

A. Anorexia nervosa

  1. General characteristics

    a. Patients have a distorted body image and an intense fear of becoming fat, even though they are underweight.

    b. This results in a self-imposed starvation, despite normal appetite and craving for food. Patients generally are less than 85% of expected weight for height.

    c. Patients often feel that losing weight is a desired achievement of self-control, whereas gaining weight is thought of as an unacceptable lack of discipline. Patients deny the seriousness of their low body weight.

    d. Patients may exercise excessively, and they commonly have food-related obsessions (e.g., hoarding food, collecting recipes).

    e. There are two types of anorexia:

        (1) Restricting: The patient eats very little and does not regularly engage in binge eating or purging behavior, such as induced vomiting, abusing laxatives or diuretics, or using enemas.

        (2) Binge eating and purging: The patient eats in binges followed by purging behavior.

    f. Physical signs include emaciation, orthostatic hypotension, bradycardia, hypothermia, dry skin, lanugo, peripheral edema, amenorrhea, salivary gland hypertrophy, dental erosion, calluses or abrasions on the back of the hand from induced vomiting, leukopenia, electrolyte abnormalities (hypochloremia, hypokalemia, elevated blood urea nitrogen, metabolic alkalosis), and arrhythmias.

    g. Approximately 90% of patients are female. Anorexia nervosa is more common in developed countries and in professions that require thinness (e.g., modeling, ballet). Peak onset is during early adolescence.

    h. Causes

        (1) Biologic, genetic, social, and psychological factors have been implicated.

        (2) The increased incidence of this disorder during the latter half of the 20th century may be the result of cultural and societal pressure on women to attain exceedingly thin physiques.

  2. Treatment

    a. Patients rarely seek treatment; family members usually are first to bring this disorder to attention. A multidisciplinary approach to treatment is essential.

b. The first goal of management is to restore the patient's nutritional state. Hospitalization often is indicated, especially if the patient is more than 20% below the expected body weight. There is a high (10%) mortality rate. Fluid and electrolyte abnormalities must be corrected, and weight restoration is crucial.

c. Outpatient management consists of behavioral therapy, family therapy, and supervised weight gain programs.

d. Certain antidepressants (amitriptyline, paroxetine, mirtazapine) can be used, especially when depression is present. Bupropion is contraindicated since it lowers the seizure threshold in patients with eating disorders.

e. An appetite stimulant may be of use, as might a drug that has weight gain as a side effect. Overall, medications do not play a major role in the treatment of this disorder.

B. Bulimia nervosa

1. General characteristics

a. Patients with bulimia employ binge eating as well as vomiting, use of laxatives and/or diuretics, excessive exercise, or other measures to avoid gaining weight.

b. The binge eating causes emotional distress and a feeling of loss of control.

c. Unlike patients with anorexia, those with bulimia commonly maintain a normal body weight, or they may even be overweight.

d. There are two types of bulimia:

(1) Purging: This involves self-induced vomiting as well as misuse of laxatives, diuretics, or enemas.

(2) Nonpurging: The patient uses other compensatory behaviors, such as excessive exercise or fasting.

e. Medical complications are seen more often in the purging type.

f. Physical findings include dental erosion, esophagitis, calloused or abraded knuckles, hypochloremic hypokalemic alkalosis, hypomagnesemia, and salivary gland hypertrophy.

g. Bulimia is significantly more common in females than in males. It is more prevalent than anorexia.

h. The behavior is quite common, affecting about 36% of young females; the disorder is present in 1% to 3% of these young women.

i. Patients with bulimia tend to be high achievers and respond to societal pressure to be thin.

j. There is an increased rate of anxiety and mood disorders, bipolar I disorders, impulse control disorders, and history of sexual abuse.

2. Treatment

a. The prognosis for patients with bulimia is better than that for patients with anorexia. They also are more likely to seek treatment, both because their uncontrolled eating is egodystonic and because there is less denial.

b. Antidepressants, such as SSRIs (fluoxetine), are useful. TCAs and MAOIs may be effective; however, their side-effect profile limits their use and so are not considered first line. Again, bupropion is avoided in these patients.

c. Behavioral psychotherapy should be used in conjunction with family therapy. Group therapy with others suffering from bulimia also should be considered.

d. Hospitalization usually is not necessary; exceptions are the presence of suicidal ideation or severe purging, resulting in significant metabolic or electrolyte disturbances.

C. Obesity (binge eating disorder)

1. General characteristics

a. Obesity is defined as 20% or more over ideal body weight or a body mass index (BMI) of greater than 30. The BMI is calculated by weight divided by height squared (kg/m^2).

b. Obesity affects more than half of the U.S. population and is more common in lower socioeconomic groups. Women are more likely than men to be obese.

c. Overeating; lack of exercise; and developmental, psychological, endocrine, and genetic reasons all contribute to the development of this disorder.

d. Obese patients often suffer emotional distress over their eating binges but do not purge or restrict eating in an attempt to control their weight. They admit to a loss of control over their eating behavior.

e. Diagnostic criteria

(1) Recurrent episodes of binge eating at least 2 days/week for 6 months, characterized by eating a larger amount of food in a 2-hour period than most average people would consume.

(2) The binge eating episodes are associated with three or more of the following: eating faster than normal; eating until feeling uncomfortably full; eating to excess, even though not hungry; eating alone out of embarrassment; and feeling disgusted, guilty, or depressed after the episode.

(3) Episodes are not associated with any inappropriate compensatory weight loss behaviors (vomiting, fasting, excess exercise, laxatives), and patients are not fixated on body image.

2. Treatment

a. Behavior modification therapy, food diaries, and development of new eating patterns (eating slowly, not eating between meals or when not seated) are beneficial. Implementation of a low-calorie, balanced diet and establishment of an exercise regimen are important. Group therapy helps to provide education and motivation.

b. Pharmacotherapy

(1) Sympathomimetics, such as amphetamine, dextroamphetamine, phentermine, phendimetrazine, and benzphetamine, can be used.

(2) Orlistat (Xenical), a lipase inhibitor, and sibutramine (Meridia), a mixed neurotransmitter reuptake inhibitor, also can be useful adjuncts.

c. Surgical methods (gastric bypass and gastroplasty) have been used for patients who are markedly obese.

VIII. SUBSTANCE ABUSE DISORDERS

A. General characteristics

1. The most commonly abused drugs are alcohol, nicotine, and caffeine; others include opiates, barbiturates, benzodiazepines, and over-the-counter medications.

2. Activation of the dopaminergic system has been implicated.

B. Types of abuse

1. *Addiction* is a nonscientific, nonmedical term denoting psychological and/or physical dependence that results in substance-seeking behavior that may or may not pose risks to the individual.

2. Physical dependence is the physiologic changes that occur with drug use and result in withdrawal symptoms on termination of use.

3. Psychological dependence refers to the craving or desire for the substance independent of the physiologic withdrawal symptoms.

4. Because both physiologic and psychological dependence occur together, a more appropriate term is *substance dependence*. This occurs when substance use results in impairment, as manifested by three of the following within a 12-month period:

a. Tolerance: There is either a decreased effect over time when the same amount of substance is used or a need for an increased amount of a substance over time to achieve a baseline.

b. Withdrawal: There is a need to use the substance to relieve or avoid physical symptoms associated with deprivation of it.

c. There is a use of increasingly larger amounts of a substance over a longer period than desired.

d. There are unsuccessful efforts to stop or decrease the amount of a substance used.

e. There are significantly larger amounts of time spent in attempts to acquire or use the substance or to recover from its effects.

f. There is social, occupational, or recreational impairment.

g. There is continued use of a substance despite the awareness that doing so has adverse consequences.

5. Substance abuse is substance use that has not met the criteria for dependence but has resulted in impairment, as manifested by at least one of the following within a 12-month period:

a. Patient fails to meet home, school, or work obligations.

b. Patient repeatedly uses the substance in hazardous situations (e.g., driving a car).

c. Patient has recurrent substance-related legal problems.

d. Patient continues to use the substance, even though he or she is experiencing interpersonal or social problems as a result.

6. Substance intoxication refers to maladaptive behavioral or psychological changes attributed to recent ingestion of a substance. Intoxication is reversible and is not caused by a mental disorder or medical condition.

C. Epidemiology

1. Lifetime prevalence of substance abuse or dependence is about 17%.

2. The most likely age group is 18- to 34-year-olds. Men are more commonly affected than women.

3. In the United States, substance abusers have a threefold risk of having a mental disorder (excluding those who use nicotine and caffeine).

TABLE 12-2	**CAGE Screening Test for Alcohol Abuse or Drug Use**
C (cut down)	Have you ever felt you should cut down on your drinking (or drug use)?
A (annoyed)	Have people annoyed you by criticizing your drinking (or drug use)?
G (guilty)	Have you felt bad or guilty about your drinking (or drug use)?
E (eye opener)	Have you ever had a drink (or used drugs) first thing in the morning to steady your nerves or to get rid of a hangover (eye opener)?

Reprinted with permission from Ewing JA. Detecting alcoholism: the CAGE questionnaire. *JAMA.* 1984;252:1905–1907. Copyright © 1984 American Medical Association. All rights reserved.

D. Treatment

1. Substance dependence is viewed as a chronic relapsing disease by the Substance Abuse and Mental Health Services Administration (SAMHSA). Relapses are not considered to be a failure in the treatment but, rather, a step toward what will, it is hoped, be a complete remission of all symptoms.

2. Risk factors can be assessed in an office setting through use of the CAGE screening test for alcohol abuse or drug use (Table 12-2).

3. Nonpharmacologic modalities include education, coping skills, relaxation therapy, family therapy, various kinds of psychotherapy (insight-oriented, group), health and nutritional counseling, lifestyle changes, and aftercare programs.

4. The 12-step program is a popular form of therapy for those with a number of different types of substance abuse (e.g., Alcoholics Anonymous, Narcotics Anonymous) as well as for family members (e.g., Al-Anon, Alateen).

5. Pharmacologic therapy

   a. Some forms of dependence require intensive detoxification, rehabilitation, and/or ongoing medication to keep the patient free of drugs (e.g., daily methadone as therapy for a patient with a dependence on opiates).

   b. Withdrawal symptoms may ensue on discontinuation of substance abuse, especially if the use was prolonged or heavy.

      (1) Withdrawal typically begins with tremulousness/shakes/jitters that start 6 to 8 hours after cessation of alcohol.

      (2) Additional manifestations include psychomotor symptoms and abnormal perception (8 to 12 hours after cessation), seizures, and delirium tremens (generally within 72 hours of cessation but can occur after 1 week).

   c. Alcohol withdrawal commonly requires the use of benzodiazepines, such as diazepam (Valium) or chlordiazepoxide (Librium), as well as thiamine, folic acid, and multivitamin administration.

   d. Disulfiram (Antabuse) is an alcohol-deterrent medication that causes nausea when alcohol is consumed.

   e. Withdrawal from other central nervous system depressants can be managed with phenobarbital. Anxiolytics or neuroleptics can be used for acute agitation seen in stimulant withdrawal.

   f. Naloxone is used to reverse the effects of any opioid. Opioid abuse and withdrawal also can be managed in several ways, including a slow taper of methadone or clonidine along with adjuncts, such as ibuprofen for muscle cramps, loperamide for diarrhea, and promethazine for nausea.

   g. Nicotine and tobacco cravings can be treated with nicotine transdermal patches, nasal spray, gum, lozenges, inhaler, and antidepressants, such as bupropion (Zyban) or varenicline (Chantix).

   h. Marijuana, phencyclidine (PCP), and hallucinogen withdrawal usually does not require medication; however, anxiolytics can be used. In the latter two, neuroleptics, such as haloperidol, can be used if acute psychotic symptoms are present.

IX. CHILDHOOD DISORDERS

A. Attention-deficit disorder (ADD) or attention-deficit hyperactivity disorder (ADHD)

1. General characteristics

   a. ADD and ADHD can manifest as hyperactivity and impulsivity or as inattentiveness. Most children manifest symptoms that result in a diagnosis emphasizing both attention deficits and hyperactivity.

   b. Secondary symptoms include emotional immaturity and lability, poor social skills, and, sometimes, motor incoordination. Disruptive behavior may result in peer rejection and deflated self-image. At home, these children often do not comply with parents' requests and can become explosive and irritable.

   c. Between 2% and 20% of school-age children may be affected. It is two to five times more frequent in boys than in girls and is most common in the firstborn son.

d. Approximately 50% of affected children continue to have dysfunctional symptoms into adulthood.

e. A multifactorial cause is likely, including prenatal exposure to infections and toxins, prenatal complications, familial or genetic factors, psychosocial factors, and neurochemical dysregulation.

f. Diagnosis

(1) The diagnosis generally is established through parental and teacher rating scales, such as the Connors' scales.

(2) Diagnostic criteria

(a) Symptoms of hyperactivity, impulsivity, or inattentiveness resulting in impairment must have been manifest before 7 years of age.

(b) Symptoms must occur in at least two settings (e.g., home, school).

(3) At least six symptoms of inattention, hyperactivity/impulsivity, or both, as listed in Table 12-3, are developmentally inappropriate and present for at least 6 months.

2. Treatment

a. Treatment involves central nervous system stimulants in combination with behavioral therapies; a multimodal approach is crucial for success. Remissions may occur, most often between 12 and 20 years of age.

b. Pharmacotherapeutic agents, such as methylphenidate (Ritalin, Concerta, Metadate), dexmethylphenidate (Focalin), and amphetamine/dextroamphetamine (Adderall, Dexedrine), have been used successfully and are considered to be first-line treatment.

c. Atomoxetine (Strattera) is a selective norepinephrine reuptake inhibitor (nonstimulant) approved for treatment of ADD and ADHD. Efficacy is equal to that of the stimulants, and side effects are similar but less frequent. It is *not* a controlled substance and, therefore, will add convenience to therapy.

d. Antidepressants, including bupropion, venlafaxine, clonidine, and imipramine, can be used as adjuncts. Guanfacine, a centrally acting antihypertensive, has also been approved for use in ADHD.

e. Therapy should include behavior modification, educational and classroom management, and family therapy. Group therapy can improve social skills and self-esteem.

B. Disruptive behavioral disorders

1. Conduct disorder

a. General characteristics

(1) This disorder affects boys more often than girls.

TABLE 12-3	**Symptoms of Attention-Deficit Disorder and Attention-Deficit Hyperactivity Disorder Used for Diagnostic Criteria**

Inattention symptoms

Makes careless mistakes and has trouble attending to details

Problems in sustaining attention; does not appear attentive when directly addressed

Does not follow through or complete assigned work

Forgetful

Easily distracted from activities by other things going on at the same time

Loses items critical to accomplishing assigned activities

Avoids activities requiring sustained mental effort

Has difficulty in organizing tasks

Hyperactivity and impulsivity symptoms

Fidgets or squirms

Leaves seat often

Restlessness

Difficulty playing quietly

Talking excessively

Blurting out

Difficulty awaiting turn

Interrupts or intrudes on others

    (2) There is a 40% risk of antisocial personality disorder in adulthood.

    (3) There is a high comorbidity with ADD and ADHD, learning disability, mood disorders, and substance abuse disorder.

    (4) Diagnostic criteria: The diagnosis is established on the basis of a pattern of behavior that involves violation of the basic rights of others or of social norms, with at least three acts of the following types: aggression toward people and animals, destruction of property, deceitfulness, and serious violations of rules.

  b. Treatment

    (1) A multimodal approach is used, involving environmental and behavioral modifications and psychotherapy, with the use of pharmacotherapy for specific behaviors.

    (2) Haloperidol, lithium, risperidone, and olanzapine can be used to treat aggressive/assaultive behaviors.

    (3) The SSRIs may aid to reduce impulsivity and mood lability/irritability.

2. Oppositional defiant disorder

  a. General characteristics

    (1) This disorder affects 16% to 22% of children. It will remit in 25%, but it also may progress to conduct disorder.

    (2) There is a high comorbidity with substance abuse disorders, mood disorders, and ADD and ADHD.

    (3) Diagnostic criteria: The diagnosis includes at least 6 months of negativistic, hostile, and defiant behavior, including at least four of the following: frequent loss of temper, arguments with adults, defying adults' rules, deliberately annoying others, easily annoyed, anger and resentment, spitefulness, and blaming others for mistakes or misbehaviors.

  b. Treatment

    (1) Family intervention using training skills in child management for the parents/caregivers is crucial.

    (2) Individual psychotherapy, focusing on behavioral modification and problem-solving skills, is recommended. Treat comorbid psychiatric disorders with medications as needed.

C. Pervasive developmental disorders

  1. Autistic disorder is characterized by impaired social interaction, impaired communication, and repetitive stereotyped patterns of behavior and activities.

  2. Asperger's disorder is characterized by impaired social interaction and restricted or stereotyped behavior, interests, or activities.

  3. Rett's disorder is characterized by decreasing head circumference per height and weight advances as well as loss of previously learned behaviors, social interactions, and motor and language development. It is almost exclusively seen in girls.

  4. Treatment: These disorders require supportive treatment.

X. ABUSE AND NEGLECT

A. Child abuse

  1. Definition

    a. In most states, health care providers are required to alert the appropriate authorities if abuse or neglect of a child is suspected.

    b. When a young patient presents with any condition that appears questionable for physical, emotional, or sexual abuse or neglect, it is best to consult with a mental health professional or family social services.

    c. The child must be protected from further abuse as well as treated for current injuries.

  2. Physical signs of abuse

    a. Any injury that cannot be adequately explained or is not consistent with the history given has the potential of being abuse.

    b. Bruises, lacerations, soft-tissue swelling, dislocations, or fractures and spiral fractures are common.

    c. Burns that are doughnut shaped, in a stocking-glove distribution, or symmetrically round (e.g., caused by a lit cigarette) are other signs.

    d. Bruises or injuries that form regular patterns on the face, back, buttocks, or thighs may be the result of abuse.

    e. Retinal hemorrhages or hyphema should alert suspicion of shaken baby syndrome.

    f. Other physical signs are internal hemorrhages, abdominal injuries, bite marks, and injuries that have the shape of the instrument used to make them (e.g., belt, cord, hand).

3. General characteristics ·
   a. Psychiatric disturbances as a result of abuse are common and include anxiety, aggressive or violent behavior, PTSD, depression, suicide, substance abuse, poor self-esteem, dissociative disorders, and paranoid ideation.
   b. Abuse or neglect also can be manifested in subtle ways, such as failure to thrive.
   c. Munchausen syndrome by proxy
      (1) This is a form of abuse usually perpetrated by the mother. Symptoms are fabricated or clinical signs are induced in a child, resulting in repeated visits to a health care provider for relief.
      (2) The perpetrator induces the various signs and symptoms to receive attention as being either an attentive or a suffering parent.
   d. Corporal punishment within reason is not normally considered to be abuse; it becomes abuse if the parent indicates receiving gratification while administering the punishment.
   e. Neglect also can be considered when a client allows a minor to engage in potentially harmful behavior (e.g., alcohol consumption) or remain unattended. In some states, leaving a child younger than 13 years of age at home alone is considered to be neglect.

B. Sexual abuse
   1. General characteristics
      a. Approximately 25% of women and 12% of men report histories of being sexually abused as children.
      b. Common ages of abuse are between 9 and 12 years. Such abuse often involves a male who is known by the child.
   2. Any of the following should raise the suspicion of sexual abuse in a child:
      a. Evidence of a sexually transmitted disease
      b. Bruises, pain, itching, or any trauma of the anal or genital area
      c. Detailed knowledge about sexual acts that are inappropriate for age
      d. Child initiates sexual acts with others, especially peers
      e. Child exhibits sexual knowledge through play

C. Intimate partner abuse (Spousal abuse, Domestic abuse)
   1. General information
      a. When confronted with a patient who may be a victim of intimate partner abuse, the following actions are needed:
         (1) There should be immediate medical attention to address the physical sequelae.
         (2) There should be recognition of suspected abuse and engagement of the patient, with nonthreatening questioning to confirm whether abuse has occurred. If abuse has occurred, it must be emphasized to the abused patient that someone does care and that there are alternatives.
      b. There should be provision of contact numbers for referral agencies (e.g., legal recourse, local emergency shelters, support groups). The decision to accept a referral ultimately is the patient's, but if help is offered and accepted, one must ensure that a referral can be made immediately.
   2. Precautions
      a. Caution is required in dealing with cases of intimate partner abuse.
         (1) The patient should be presented with options and allowed to decide which path to take.
         (2) The abused may close ranks with the abuser and confront the clinician for attempting to break up the family.
         (3) It is estimated that a woman who leaves an abusive partner has a 70% greater risk of being killed by the batterer than a woman who stays.
      b. Battered victims have suffered a blow to their ego defenses and may not be assertive enough to believe that their rights have been violated.
      c. It is not uncommon to find battered women who believe that they either deserved the beating or must accept the beatings as the price for a roof over their head and food on the table.

D. Elder abuse
   1. General characteristics
      a. Elder abuse affects 10% of the population older than 65 years. Most victims are very old, frail, and vulnerable.
      b. Abuse can be physical, sexual, psychological, emotional, or financial, or it can be in the form of neglect.
   2. Forms of abuse
      a. Physical or sexual abuse is suspected in the presence of bruises, puncture wounds, fractures, cuts, burns, poor hygiene, soiled clothing, hair loss in clumps, weight loss or poor nutrition, dehydration, lack of eyeglasses or

hearing aids, injuries from use of restraints, genital or rectal injuries or bleeding, evidence of excessive drugging, or a lack of or delay in seeking medical attention.

  b. Psychological abuse can be manifested by threats, insults, or verbal abuse, or refusal to allow travel, church attendance, or family visits.

  c. Financial abuse may come in the form of misuse of the patient's funds.

  d. Neglect includes the withholding of food, medicine, clothing, routine health care, or other basic necessities.

  3. Clinicians should be aware of the following:

  a. Previous history of abuse by the caregiver

  b. Conflicting accounts of accidents by caregiver

  c. Unwillingness of a caregiver to agree to implementation of treatment plans

  d. Inappropriate defensiveness by the caregiver

  e. A caregiver who will not allow, or who limits, the patient's responses to questions

  f. Some states have the same reporting requirements for suspected elder abuse as for child abuse

XI. RAPE CRISIS

A. Definition

  1. Rape is an act of aggression that may be perpetrated on a spouse, a known partner, or a stranger.

  2. Forced acts of fellatio and anal penetration are considered to be sodomy.

  3. Forced participation in any sexual acts can result in psychological sequelae.

  4. A patient who has been raped or sodomized may experience depression; lack of appetite; sleep disturbances; rage and anger; feelings of worthlessness; enduring patterns of sexual dysfunction; agoraphobia; fear of future violence, death, or contracting a sexually transmitted disease; feelings of being used or dirty; and anxiety attacks.

B. Approach to the patient

  1. History and physical examination, including genital and rectal examinations

  a. Rape constitutes both a psychiatric emergency and a legal situation; all procedures should be documented, clothing saved, and samples taken.

  b. A rape kit, which has instructions on questions to include in the history, on how specimen samples are to be collected and under what conditions, and on how samples should be handled after collection, is valuable and ensures that the proper evidence is secured.

  c. Explain to the patient the purpose of all procedures, and inform him or her of what is being done before doing it. This provides the patient with a feeling of some control.

  2. Prevention of sexually transmitted diseases and pregnancy: Prophylactic antibiotic therapy should be initiated; the patient should be given the option of emergency contraception.

  3. Counseling: As soon as possible after the event, and preferably before leaving the emergency department, the patient should talk to a mental health professional, and follow-up counseling should be scheduled.

XII. UNCOMPLICATED BEREAVEMENT

A. Definition

  1. Uncomplicated bereavement is defined as a normal response to a major loss.

  2. Duration of the reaction depends on the suddenness of the loss, the relationship of the survivor to the deceased, and the age or physical condition of the person who has died.

  3. Normal grief symptoms resolve within 1 year; the most severe symptoms occur within the first 2 months.

  4. Some patients do develop MDD. This diagnosis is not made until grief symptoms fail to resolve.

B. General characteristics

  1. The mourner experiences shock, confusion, sadness, numbness, or guilt. Symptoms of depression may be seen.

  2. Mourners sometimes report illusions, such as briefly seeing or hearing the deceased, or they may deny certain aspects of the death. These are considered to be normal reactions; however, hallucinations that are persistent and/or intrusive, or the belief that the deceased is still alive, are not.

  3. Treatment

  a. Treatment consists of social contact and reassurance.

  b. Patients probably are not helped by antidepressant medications. Benzodiazepines, in short courses only, may alleviate insomnia.

Dermatology

Edward D. Huechtker

13

I. DIAGNOSIS

A. History and physical examination

   1. History

      a. A thorough history is the first step in accurate diagnosis of skin diseases.

      b. Past medical history, medication history, family history, psychosocial factors, recreational and employment risk, and diet and environmental/travel exposures should be investigated.

   2. Physical examination

      a. A general physical examination, paying particular attention to the skin, hair, nails, and mucocutaneous surfaces, should be carried out under natural or bright light.

      b. A magnifying glass may be useful.

      c. Describe lesions using the **MAD** criteria:

         (1) **M**orphology: Shape or type of lesion(s), color, elevation, margination, and other descriptive terms

         (2) **A**rrangement: Single, grouped, arciform, annular, serpiginous, and other patterns

         (3) **D**istribution: Localized, disseminated, and other patterns

   3. Special signs and tests

      a. Darier's sign: Rubbing a lesion causes urticarial flare.

      b. Auspitz's sign: Pinpoint bleeding after scale is removed.

      c. Nikolsky's sign: Pushing a blister causes further separation of the dermis.

      d. Photopatch test: Documents photoallergy.

      e. Patch test: Demonstrates hypersensitivity reaction.

      f. Koebner's phenomenon: Minor trauma leads to new lesions at site of trauma.

      g. Shagreen skin: An oval-shaped nevoid plaque. Skin is colored or pigmented on the trunk or back and is associated with tuberous sclerosis.

   4. Diagnostic techniques

      a. Diascopy

         (1) A glass slide or diascope is pressed against the skin.

         (2) Blanching indicates intact capillaries; extravasated blood (purpura) does not blanch.

      b. Potassium hydroxide preparation (KOH prep)

         (1) Microscopic examination of skin scrapings mounted in KOH, which dissolves keratin and cellular material but does not affect fungi, is performed.

         (2) This method readily identifies dermatophytes.

      c. Scrapings and smears

         (1) Blunt and sharp instruments facilitate specimen collections.

         (2) Various staining techniques and visualization methods (e.g., Tzanck's smear, dark-field microscopy) bring out certain characteristics of the lesion or responsible pathogen.

      d. Wood's light examination is used to assess changes in pigment or to fluoresce infectious lesions.

      e. Acetowhitening, using acetic acid, is used to facilitate examination of warts.

      f. Biopsy (excisional, incisional, shave, punch) is indicated if pathologic confirmation is necessary.

B. Common dermatologic terminology

   1. Common skin lesions are defined in Table 13-1.

   2. The following descriptive terms also are useful:

      a. Telangiectasia: Dilated, superficial blood vessel

      b. Lichenification: Thickened skin with distinct borders

TABLE 13-1	**Common Skin Lesions**
Papule	Solid, palpable lesion <10 mm in diameter
Nodule	Solid, palpable lesion >10 mm in diameter
Macule	Flat, nonpalpable lesion <10 mm in diameter
Patch	Flat, nonpalpable lesion >10 mm in diameter
Plaque	Plateau-like lesion >10 mm in diameter, may be a group of confluent papules
Vesicle	Circumscribed, elevated lesion containing serous fluid <5 mm in diameter
Bulla	Circumscribed, elevated lesion containing serous fluid >5 mm in diameter
Wheal	Transient, elevated lesion caused by local edema
Petechiae	Minute hemorrhagic spots that cannot be blanched by diascopy
Crust	Hard, rough surface formed by dried sebum, exudate, blood, or necrotic skin
Scale	Heaped-up piles of horny epithelium with a dry appearance
Pustule	Vesicle or bulla containing purulent material
Erosion	Defect of the epidermis; heals without a scar
Ulcer	Defect that extends into the dermis or deeper; heals with a scar

    c. Macerated: Swollen and softened by an increase in water content; the appearance that skin gets when left in water too long

    d. Verrucous: Irregular, rough, and convoluted surfaces

II. MACULOPAPULAR AND PLAQUE DISORDERS

A. Eczematous disorders

    1. The terms *eczema* and *dermatitis* are used interchangeably. Eczema more commonly denotes endogenous disorders, and dermatitis denotes exogenous disorders.

    2. There are many eczematous disorders, encompassing a wide range of polymorphic inflammatory reaction patterns.

    3. Contact dermatitis

        a. General characteristics

           (1) Irritant contact dermatitis is caused by chemical irritants, such as cleaners, solvents, and detergents, in contact with the skin.

           (2) Irritant contact diaper dermatitis, also known as diaper rash, is usually due to prolonged contact with urine, feces, or detergents from washable diapers.

           (3) Allergic contact dermatitis denotes an allergic type IV cell-mediated hypersensitivity reaction. Occupational or personal contact with irritants, such as cleaning supplies, solvents, oils, abrasives, oxidizing or reducing agents, dust, nickel, enzymes, and plants (poison ivy, others), are common causes of dermatitis.

        b. Clinical features

           (1) Patients complain of itching and burning in the affected areas. In diaper rash the lesions are within the borders of the diaper.

           (2) Acute lesions typically are well-demarcated areas of erythema and, possibly, exudative lesions; vesicles, erosions, and crusts may develop.

           (3) Chronic lesions show plaques and scaling with lichenification. Satellite papules and excoriations are common.

        c. Laboratory studies

           (1) Patch tests that result in similar reactions support the diagnosis.

           (2) Gram stains or cultures should be done if secondary infection is suspected.

        d. Treatment

           (1) Avoid or remove the offending agent. Wet dressings with Burrow's solution (aluminum acetate in water) and topical corticosteroids are sufficient in most cases. For diaper rash, a barrier of petrolatum or zinc oxide is helpful. Keep the area clean and dry with frequent diaper changes and use of disposable diapers.

           (2) Severe cases may necessitate systemic steroids.

           (3) Chronic lesions can be treated with topical steroids.

      (4) Supportive measures include cleaning with mild soaps or oatmeal preparations and antihistamines to help alleviate itching.

4. Atopic dermatitis

  a. General characteristics

      (1) This is a chronic relapsing skin disorder that begins in childhood.

      (2) It is a type I immunoglobulin E–mediated hypersensitivity reaction.

      (3) Many patients also have asthma or allergic rhinitis (atopy).

  b. Clinical features

      (1) Papules and plaques, with or without scales, are noted and may be associated with edema, erosion, and crusts.

      (2) Patients complain of pruritus and dry, scaly skin. Scratching leads to lichenification, fissures, and worsening rash; secondary infections most commonly are caused by *Staphylococcus aureus*.

      (3) The rash is most common on the flexural surfaces, neck, eyelids, forehead, face, and dorsum of the hands and feet.

      (4) Dermatographism is characteristic.

  c. Laboratory studies: These are not routinely done, although cultures for suspected secondary infection may help to guide treatment.

  d. Treatment

      (1) Antihistamines help to reduce itching.

      (2) Topical corticosteroids are the mainstay of the treatment; systemic corticosteroids should be avoided.

      (3) Tacrolimus and pimecrolimus are topical calcineurin inhibitors (immunomodulators) approved for moderate to severe atopic dermatitis. There is less atrophy with prolonged use when compared to topical corticosteroids; however, they may carry a potential to cause malignancy.

      (4) Hydration and topical emollients are key to management. Soaps, vigorous rubbing, and irritant clothing such as wool should be avoided.

      (5) Ultraviolet B (UVB) phototherapy is effective.

      (6) Severe systemic cases may necessitate cyclosporine.

5. Nummular dermatitis

  a. General characteristics

      (1) This is a pruritic inflammatory disorder that typically affects young adults and the elderly.

      (2) It typically occurs during the fall and winter.

  b. Clinical features

      (1) Small, grouped vesicles coalesce to form coin-shaped plaques with an erythematous base and clearly demarcated borders.

      (2) Crusting and excoriations occur.

  c. Treatment

      (1) This is a chronic disorder that responds to moisturizers or topical steroids.

      (2) Tar baths or UVB phototherapy is helpful for refractory cases.

6. Seborrheic dermatitis

  a. General characteristics

      (1) Seborrheic dermatitis is common during infancy and puberty and in young to middle-aged adults.

      (2) It occurs where sebaceous glands are most active (body folds, face, scalp, genitalia).

  b. Clinical features

      (1) Scattered yellowish or gray, scaly macules and papules with a greasy look are noted.

      (2) Sticky crusts and fissures are found behind the ears, especially in infants. On the scalp, it manifests as cradle cap in infants and dandruff in adults.

  c. Treatment

      (1) Ultraviolet radiation is helpful; lesions improve during the summer and flare during the fall and winter.

      (2) Cradle cap: Treat with olive oil compresses and baby shampoo or ketoconazole shampoo or cream or with hydrocortisone.

       (3) Dandruff: Use shampoos containing selenium or zinc and ketoconazole shampoo for acute flare-ups; tar shampoos or topical steroids can be used for severe cases.

       (4) Other areas: Use ketoconazole shampoo or topical steroids. Blepharitis is treated with gentle scrubs using baby shampoo; follow with a suspension of sulfa and/or steroid preparation or ketoconazole cream, if needed.

  7. Perioral dermatitis

    a. General characteristics: This typically occurs in young women.

    b. Clinical features: Papulopustules form on erythematous bases and may become confluent with plaques and scales; vermilion border is spared; and satellite lesions are common.

    c. Laboratory studies: Culture to rule out staphylococcal infection.

    d. Treatment

       (1) Avoid topical steroids because they will aggravate the lesions.

       (2) Use topical metronidazole or erythromycin or oral minocycline, doxycycline, or tetracycline.

       (3) Untreated lesions will fluctuate over time, similar to rosacea.

  8. Stasis dermatitis

    a. General characteristics

       (1) Chronic venous insufficiency leads to edema, stasis dermatitis, hyperpigmentation, fibrosis, and ulceration.

       (2) Varicose veins, superficial phlebitis, and venous thrombosis commonly occur before skin changes.

       (3) Women are affected three times more often than men. Pregnancy will exacerbate both venous insufficiency and stasis dermatitis.

    b. Clinical features

       (1) Patients complain of heaviness or aching in the legs, which is aggravated by standing and relieved with walking.

       (2) Dermatitis of the lower legs and feet manifests with inflammatory papules, scales, and crusts. Stippled pigmentation develops, and excoriations are common.

       (3) Ulcerations will occur in 30% of patients.

    c. Laboratory studies

       (1) Doppler studies, sonography, or venography will confirm chronic insufficiency.

       (2) Biopsy of lesions shows dilated vessels, tortuous veins, edema, and fibrin deposition.

    d. Treatment

       (1) Chronic venous insufficiency is treated with compression stockings. Sclerosis of varicose veins helps to prevent further dermatitis, but recurrence is common.

       (2) Vascular bypass or angioplasty may benefit severely compromised areas, but results are only fair.

       (3) Ulcers demand chronic treatment.

B. Lichen simplex chronicus

  1. General characteristics

    a. Lichenification is a long-term manifestation of atopic dermatitis due to repetitive scratching and rubbing.

    b. The skin of patients with atopic dermatitis is sensitive to minor trauma, including touch, rubbing, or scratching.

    c. Lichenification develops as well-circumscribed plaques that are highly pruritic. This sets up a cycle of itch–scratch lesions.

  2. Clinical features

    a. Solid, firm, thick plaques with little to no scaling are seen.

    b. Light touch precipitates a strong desire to scratch.

    c. Lesions can be single or multiple. Common areas include the nuchal area, scalp, ankles, lower legs, upper thighs, exterior forearms, or genital areas.

    d. Black skin more typically shows a follicular pattern of smaller papules rather than larger plaques.

  3. Laboratory studies

    a. A KOH prep is done to rule out fungal infection.

    b. Biopsy shows hyperplasia and hyperkeratosis.

    4. Treatment

        a. Key to management is stopping the itch–scratch cycle.

        b. Occlusive dressing with or without topical steroids or tar preparations can be used.

        c. Antihistamines will reduce itching.

C. Pityriasis rosea

    1. General characteristics

        a. Pityriasis rosea is characterized by a herald patch, which precedes a widespread symmetrical papular eruption.

        b. The cause is unknown but is thought to be viral (human herpes virus 7).

        c. It is most common in teenagers and young adults.

    2. Clinical features

        a. There may be a mild upper respiratory tract infection–like prodrome before the onset of the rash.

        b. The herald patch is a solitary round or oval pink plaque with a raised border and fine adherent scales in the margin. It typically precedes the rash by a week or so.

        c. The rash begins to appear on the trunk as round or oval, salmon-colored, slightly raised papular and macular lesions usually 1 cm in diameter.

        d. The long axis of each lesion usually follows the natural skin folds, giving a Christmas tree–like distribution. It is usually confined to the trunk.

        e. In the beginning, the lesions are covered with a fine scale that desquamates, leaving an inverse collarette scale around each lesion.

        f. Pityriasis rosea usually lasts for 3 to 8 weeks and disappears spontaneously.

    3. Treatment

        a. No treatment is indicated other than lotions or emollients for the scales.

        b. UVB phototherapy may be helpful if started during the first week of eruption.

        c. Lotions, antipruritics, or oral antihistamines may help if itching is bothersome.

D. Molluscum contagiosum

    1. General characteristics

        a. This is a common viral disease of the skin and mucous membranes caused by a poxvirus. It is common in children but can affect adults.

        b. In adults, the lesions are commonly in the groin areas and on the lower abdomen.

        c. The virus can be transmitted during sexual activity.

        d. In immunocompromised patients (such as HIV), lesions can be larger and more widespread, including predominance on the head and neck.

    2. Clinical features

        a. Lesions manifest as discrete, flesh-colored, waxy, dome-shaped, umbilicated papules over the face, trunk, and extremities.

        b. They range in size from 3 to 6 mm and appear in groups.

        c. A white, curd-like material can be expressed from under the depression of the lesion.

    3. Laboratory studies: Biopsy may be needed in immunocompromised patients to rule out fungal dissemination.

    4. Treatment

        a. Treatment usually is not necessary, because the disease is self-limited.

        b. If therapy is indicated, it consists of local destruction of individual lesions either by curettage (first-line), cryotherapy, electrodessication, or an acid or exfoliative peel (e.g., tretinoin, imiquimod [Aldara]). These treatments can be painful.

E. Lichen planus

    1. General characteristics

        a. This is an acute or chronic inflammatory dermatitis that occurs in adults. Females are more commonly affected than males.

        b. Lichen planus–like eruptions may occur in graft-versus-host disease, malignant lymphoma, and drug reactions.

    2. Clinical features

        a. Lichen planus is designated as the 4 Ps: purple, polygonal, pruritic, papule.

    b. Lesions are flat-topped, shiny, violaceous papules with fine white lines on the surface (Wickham's striae). They typically are grouped and most commonly occur on the flexor aspect of the wrists, lumbar area, eyelids, shins, and scalp. Koebner's phenomenon is seen.

    c. Mucosal lesions occur on the vaginal mucosa, glans and penis, and in the mouth. They usually are very painful and often ulcerate.

    d. Variants include follicular, vesicular, actinic, and ulcerative lesions.

    e. Lesions may affect hair (scarring alopecia) or nails (destruction of nail fold and nail bed with longitudinal splintering).

  3. Laboratory studies

    a. Biopsy and immunofluorescence confirm the diagnosis.

    b. Screening for hepatitis C should be considered due to the higher prevalence of anti-hepatitis C virus antibodies in patients with lichen planus.

  4. Treatment

    a. Topical steroids with occlusive dressings are used.

    b. Intralesional steroids or topical tretinoin is used for severe localized lesions.

    c. Cyclosporine mouthwash is used for oral lesions.

    d. Systemic therapy (cyclosporine, corticosteroids, or retinoids) may be needed in severe, painful cases.

    e. Psoralens plus ultraviolet A (PUVA) radiation therapy is helpful in generalized eruptions.

F. Dyshidrosis

  1. General characteristics

    a. This dermatitis generally develops in people younger than 40 years. Half of those affected have an atopic background.

    b. Eruptions follow stress or occur in hot, humid weather.

  2. Clinical features

    a. Early disease

      (1) Pruritus is common; pain develops if secondarily infected.

      (2) Small vesicles in clusters (tapioca appearance) are seen, and occasionally bullae form.

    b. Late disease

      (1) Papules, scaling, lichenification, and erosions from ruptured vesicles are seen.

      (2) Painful fissures may develop.

    c. There is a predilection for the hands and feet.

  3. Laboratory studies

    a. Culture is done to rule out secondary infection.

    b. KOH prep will rule out dermatophytosis.

  4. Treatment

    a. Use wet dressings with Burrow's solution. Large bullae should be drained but kept intact.

    b. Fissures are treated with topical collodion.

    c. Topical steroids are used for localized lesions and systemic steroids for severe cases.

    d. PUVA is recommended in generalized disease.

    e. Treat secondary infection with systemic antimicrobials.

G. Psoriasis

  1. General characteristics

    a. Psoriasis affects 2% of the population (3 to 5 million people).

    b. Most patients have localized psoriasis, but more severe forms exist.

    c. A genetic predisposition exists, although only about one-third of the patients have family members with the condition.

    d. Psoriasis is a chronic, inflammatory, scaling condition of the skin that also may involve the mucous membranes. It seems that the earlier the onset of the disease, the more severe it will be. Psoriasis in HIV-positive patients can be very severe and resistant to treatment.

    e. The basic pathology is a greatly enhanced epidermal cell turnover (to a rate 28 times normal).

2. Clinical features

    a. Psoriasis patches usually are raised, pink to red papules and plaques with distinct margins and loosely adherent silvery scales. Peeling away a scale produces specks of bleeding from the capillaries (Auspitz's sign).

    b. Patches most often are found on the scalp and the extensor surfaces of the elbows and knees but can be found anywhere on the body.

    c. Pruritus is common. Scratching leads to more lesions (Koebner's phenomenon).

    d. Patients with extensive disease also have nail involvement. The nails have tiny pits and ridges, are separated from the nail bed (onycholysis), and have oil spots.

    e. Psoriatic arthritis occurs in 5% to 10% of patients. It involves the distal joints of the hands and feet, typically is asymmetric, and may be present without skin lesions.

    f. Diagnosis is made by history and appearance. The symptoms usually are mild, but the lesions are unsightly and interfere with business and social activities.

    g. Variants

        (1) Psoriasis vulgaris is the most common type and involves chronic recurring scaling papules and plaques.

        (2) In psoriatic erythroderma, lesions involve the entire skin surface; this variant is exfoliative and serious.

        (3) Guttate psoriasis is characterized by acute eruption of typical and atypical lesions in a disseminated pattern; it spares the palms and soles and often appears after streptococcal pharyngitis.

        (4) Pustular psoriasis (von Zumbusch's syndrome) is an abrupt, life-threatening condition characterized by widespread pustules that coalesce to form lakes of pus; fever, malaise, and leukocytosis are seen.

3. Treatment

    a. In mild cases, treatment consists of topical corticosteroids and topical vitamin D preparations (calcipotriene).

    b. Systemic steroids help, but the disease often will flare after withdrawal.

    c. Coal tar or salicylic acid preparations and occlusive dressings are effective in controlling or removing scales.

    d. Moderate psoriasis may respond to tazarotene gel (topical retinoid).

    e. For more serious cases, UVB phototherapy, PUVA, and methotrexate have been effective but carry risks of skin cancer, cataracts, and hepatotoxicity. Avoid methotrexate in immunocompromised patients, as it is a potent immune suppressant.

    f. Pustular psoriasis may respond to acitretin, a synthetic retinoid, with or without ultraviolet treatment. This also is helpful in erythroderma and psoriatic arthritis but is teratogenic.

    g. Cyclosporine may be effective in severe recalcitrant disease, but recurrence after cessation is common.

III.   VESICULOBULLOUS DISORDERS

  A. Pemphigus vulgaris

    1. General characteristics

      a. This is a serious bullous autoimmune disease; immunoglobulin G antibodies induce acantholysis, resulting in a loss of cell-to-cell adhesion.

      b. The disorder occurs in middle-aged adults. It is more common in people of Jewish or Mediterranean ancestry.

    2. Clinical features

      a. Lesions usually begin in the oral mucosa; skin lesions occur 6 to 12 months later. There may be pain or burning, but not pruritus. Weakness and malaise are common.

      b. Lesions are round vesicles or bullae that contain clear liquid and easily rupture. Nikolsky's sign occurs (lateral extension of the lesions when pushed). The lesions are discrete and randomly scattered. Erosions and crusts occur because of the fragility of the blisters.

      c. Secondary infection as well as fluid and electrolyte imbalance are common causes of morbidity and mortality.

      d. Variants include pemphigus vegetans, pemphigus foliaceous, Brazilian pemphigus (fogo selvagem), pemphigus erythematosus, drug-induced pemphigus, and paraneoplastic pemphigus.

    3. Laboratory studies

      a. Immunofluorescence of serum or blister material highlights immunoglobulin G.

      b. Biopsy proves acantholysis.

    4. Treatment

      a. Systemic therapy is required. Start with prednisone, and then add immunosuppressive agents, azathioprine, and/or methotrexate as needed.

      b. Dapsone, gold, or cyclophosphamide may help in refractory cases.

      c. Supportive therapies include fluid and electrolyte replacement, cleansing baths, wet dressings, topical steroids, and antibiotics as needed.

B. Bullous pemphigoid

  1. General characteristics

      a. This autoimmune disorder occurs typically in patients in their sixth decade of life.

      b. Autoantibodies, complement fixation, neutrophil, and eosinophils cause bullous formation.

  2. Clinical features

      a. There may be a prodrome of urticarial or papular lesions.

      b. Bullae are large, tense, oval, or round and contain serous or hemorrhagic fluid. They rupture less easily than in pemphigus.

      c. Typically, bullae collapse and crust; at times, bleeding erosions occur.

      d. Axillae, thighs, groin, and abdomen commonly are affected. Mucous membrane lesions are less severe and less painful than in pemphigus vulgaris.

  3. Laboratory studies: Biopsy and immunofluorescence will confirm the diagnosis.

  4. Treatment

      a. Systemic prednisone may be given at high doses until remission, and then at a lower dose for maintenance.

      b. Azathioprine may be added.

      c. Mild cases or localized recurrences are treated with topical steroids.

IV. PAPULOPUSTULAR INFLAMMATORY DISORDERS

A. Acne vulgaris

  1. General characteristics

      a. Acne affects all age groups, from neonates to older adults. It is most prevalent in adolescents and more severe in males.

      b. Pathology includes plugged follicles, retained sebum, bacterial overgrowth, and release of fatty acids. Androgens stimulate sebum production.

  2. Clinical features

      a. Acne is an inflammatory follicular, papular, and pustular eruption involving the pilosebaceous apparatus.

      b. Acne lesions can be open comedones or closed, noninflammatory comedones.

        (1) Open comedones often are referred to as "blackheads" because of melanin depositions on a keratin plug.

        (2) Closed comedones, often called "whiteheads," are flesh-colored 1-mm papules.

        (3) Open or closed comedones can become erythematous papules, pustules, nodules, or cysts, ranging in size from 1 to 5 mm.

      c. Sinus tracts occur with nodular acne. Inflammatory lesions can lead to hyperpigmentation and scarring.

  3. Laboratory studies: Testosterone, follicle-stimulating hormone, luteinizing hormone, or dehydroepiandrosterone 5 levels can be measured if an endocrine disorder is suggested; however, the majority of acne cases are not endocrine based.

  4. Treatment

      a. Treatment for mild acne can be accomplished by keeping the affected areas clean and applying topical preparations, such as retinoids, azelaic acid, and salicylic acid.

      b. If inflammatory lesions are present, topical benzoyl peroxide, tretinoin, erythromycin, clindamycin, or sodium sulfacetamide can be used.

      c. In more serious or cystic acne, oral antibiotics should be used in conjunction with the topical preparations.

        (1) Tetracyclines were the drug of choice early on and are still effective. Erythromycin, doxycycline, minocycline, trimethoprim/sulfamethoxazole, and clindamycin also frequently are used.

        (2) The bacterium that is involved in acne is becoming resistant to some medications. It is best to treat as conservatively as possible and only for as long as necessary.

        (3) Recurrence after cessation of treatment is common.

      d. Accutane (oral isotretinoin)

        (1) This medication can be prescribed only by a dermatologic provider approved by Roche.

(2) Side effects can be very serious, ranging from dry eyes, nose, and lips to epistaxis, joint pains, mood swings, and suicidal thoughts.

(3) Premature closure of the long bones, visual changes, hepatic enzyme elevation, leukopenia, triglyceridemia, and teratogenicity also occur.

B. Acne rosacea

1. General characteristics

a. Acne rosacea is a chronic acneiform disorder mainly affecting females between 30 and 50 years of age.

b. It is a disease of the pilosebaceous units associated with increased activity of capillaries, which leads to flushing and telangiectasias.

c. The outbreaks are episodic and typically occur in response to heat, alcohol, sun, or hot, spicy foods. Coffee and tea stimulate outbreaks because of the heat, not the caffeine content.

2. Clinical features

a. It is characterized by the insidious onset of scattered, small papulopustules and sometimes nodules; comedones do not occur. The face appears red or flushed.

b. There is a symmetric distribution on the face (cheeks, chin, forehead, glabella, nose). Sometimes, lesions appear on the neck, chest, back, or scalp.

c. Later telangiectasia, hyperplasia, and lymphedema develop.

d. Patients often complain of disfiguring appearance.

e. When describing effects, the suffix -phyma, meaning "enlarged," is used: rhinophyma (nose), blepharophyma (eyelid), metophyma (forehead), otophyma (ear), or gnathophyma (mouth).

3. Treatment

a. Reduce triggers such as alcohol or hot beverages.

b. Topical metronidazole (most effective), sodium sulfacetamide, or erythromycin often is sufficient.

c. If topical treatment fails, systemic antibiotics, such as tetracycline, minocycline, or doxycycline, are tried until remission and then continued at lower doses for maintenance.

d. Very severe cases may need oral isotretinoin under the care of a dermatologic specialist.

C. Folliculitis

1. General characteristics

a. Folliculitis is an inflammation of the hair follicles.

b. It most commonly is caused by *Staphylococcus aureus* but can be caused by other organisms. Pseudomonal folliculitis is found in hot tub users.

c. Noninfectious folliculitis is common among people working in hot, oily environments, such as engine workers on ships, machinists, or anyone working in a hot, dirty environment.

d. Occlusion, perspiration, and rubbing from tight clothes also may cause folliculitis.

e. Pseudofolliculitis is defined as ingrown hairs occurring in the beard area.

2. Clinical features

a. The lesions are erythematous papules or pustules. They usually are not painful but may burn.

b. Sycosis is severe, deep-seated, recalcitrant folliculitis with surrounding eczema and crusting.

c. Abscesses may form at the site of folliculitis.

3. Treatment

a. Gentle cleansing and mild compresses help. Protection from offending substances and use of drying agents also help.

b. Topical application of clindamycin or erythromycin works well on mild cases. Mupirocin (Bactroban) ointment also may be used.

c. In more extensive cases, oral antibiotics may be necessary.

d. Hot tub folliculitis usually resolves without treatment; severe or recalcitrant cases may be treated with a fluoroquinolone.

D. Erythema multiforme (EM)

1. General characteristics

a. EM can be induced by drugs (sulfonamides, phenytoin, barbiturates, penicillin, allopurinol) and infections (herpes simplex virus, *Mycoplasma* sp.), or be idiopathic (50% of cases).

b. Half of all cases occur in patients younger than 20 years.

     c. Previous history of EM is a strong risk factor for subsequent cases.

  2. Clinical features

     a. Lesions begin as macules and become papular, and then vesicles and bullae form in the center of the papules. Target or iris lesions are characteristic.

     b. Lesions can be localized to the hands and feet or become generalized.

     c. Mucosal lesions (hallmark of EM major) are painful and erode.

     d. Patients complain of fever, weakness, and malaise. Lungs and eyes may be affected.

  3. Treatment

     a. Avoid precipitating substances, and control herpes outbreaks with acyclovir.

     b. Severely ill patients are treated with systemic steroids.

E. Stevens–Johnson syndrome (SJS) and toxic erythema necrolysis (TEN)

  1. General characteristics

     a. These are mucocutaneous blistering reactions most often caused by a drug reaction. Drugs associated with SJS or TEN include sulfonamides, aminopenicillins, quinolones, cephalosporins, tetracyclines, phenobarbital, carbamazepine, phenytoin, valproic acid, oxicam, allopurinol, and corticosteroids.

     b. SJS is thought to be a severe variant of EM, and TEN is thought to be a severe variant of SJS.

     c. SJS or TEN may occur in patients of any age or gender.

     d. The pathogenesis is unknown, but it is thought to be an immunologic response.

     e. The dangers are secondary infection, fluid loss, and electrolyte imbalance. TEN can be life threatening.

  2. Clinical features

     a. Patients present with fever, photophobia, sore throat, mucosal inflammation, and sore mouth. The cutaneous lesions tend to be concentrated more on the trunk at first. The lesions may be painful or may sting.

     b. Progression occurs over 4 days: diffuse erythema, morbilliform lesions, necrotic epidermis, wrinkled surfaces, sheetlike loss of epidermis, and raised, flaccid blisters (Nikolsky's sign).

     c. TEN exhibits higher fever and more severe epidermal separation and loss compared with SJS.

     d. Regrowth of skin takes 3 weeks; it is delayed in pressure-point areas.

     e. About 90% of patients have mucosal lesions that are painful and eroding.

     f. Other complications include acute tubular necrosis, erosion in the lungs and gut, and bronchitis.

  3. Laboratory studies

     a. Patients have anemia and lymphopenia.

     b. Biopsy is diagnostic.

  4. Treatment

     a. There should be prompt withdrawal of the offending or causative agent.

     b. Patients with extensive necrolysis should be transferred to a burn unit for care.

     c. Treat patients for fluid and electrolyte imbalance and any complications or infections.

     d. Treatment debate

       (1) Corticosteroid treatment is being debated. Some feel massive doses are appropriate, while others feel steroids may exacerbate the disease. If corticosteroids have to be given, they should be started early in the course of the disease.

       (2) The same controversy applies to antibiotic therapy, because antibiotics may be the causative agent.

       (3) Intravenous immunoglobulin (IVIG) is commonly used, but data do not show any improvement in mortality.

F. Hidradenitis suppurativa

  1. General characteristics

     a. Hidradenitis suppurativa is a disease of the apocrine gland areas (axilla, anogenital, and scalp).

     b. It affects females between puberty and menopause (axillary disease) more often than males (anogenital disease).

     c. Predisposing factors include obesity, history of acne, apocrine duct obstruction, and bacterial infection. There appears to be a genetic tendency.

  2. Clinical features

     a. Tender inflammatory nodules or abscesses form. Lesions are not related to hair follicles.

     b. Open comedones and sinus tracts form and may drain purulent material.

    c. Fibrosis, scarring, and contractures may occur. Severity is variable.

  3. Laboratory studies include culture for secondary bacterial infection.

  4. Treatment

    a. Lesions are treated with intralesional triamcinolone, incision and drainage of abscesses, and excision of sinus tracts.

    b. Oral antibiotics are given until lesions resolve; prednisone is added if the lesions are severe and should be tapered over 2 weeks.

    c. Severe cases, especially in the anogenital area, may benefit from psychological support.

V. LOCALIZED SKIN INFECTIONS

A. Furuncles and carbuncles

  1. General characteristics

    a. Furuncles sometimes are referred to as "boils" or "risens." These lesions are deep-seated infections of the hair follicles; *Staphylococcus aureus* is the most common pathogen.

    b. A furuncle is an infection of a single follicle; a carbuncle includes more than one infected follicle as a conglomerate mass.

  2. Clinical features

    a. Furuncles and carbuncles present as red, hard, tender lesions in the hair-bearing areas of the head, neck, or body.

    b. Lesions progress to become fluctuant and rupture spontaneously, draining pus and necrotic tissue.

  3. Treatment

    a. Treatment should be started with warm, moist compresses.

    b. Antibiotic therapy as well as incision and drainage are added as appropriate once the lesion is mature.

    c. Cloths used for warm compresses and/or towels used to clean or dry these lesions should be handled with care to prevent additional infection.

B. Cellulitis

  1. General characteristics

    a. Cellulitis is an acute, spreading inflammation of the dermis and subcutaneous tissue.

    b. Although the causative organism can be identified by culturing any drainage or discharge or by needle aspiration, it probably is best to begin treatment with antibiotics that will cover *Haemophilus influenzae*, *Streptococcus* sp., and *Staphylococcus* sp.

  2. Clinical features

    a. The area involved is swollen, red, hot, and tender.

    b. The patient may have lymphadenopathy, fever, chills, and malaise.

  3. Treatment

    a. Mild or early infections may be treated with oral penicillinase-resistant penicillin, such as dicloxacillin or a cephalosporin. For patients who are allergic to penicillin, erythromycin is appropriate.

    b. In severe infections, first-generation cephalosporins are given intravenously (IV). Patients started on parenteral therapy may be switched to oral therapy when the fever, chills, and malaise subside.

    c. It may be appropriate to mark the margins of involvement before treatment to follow the progression or regression of the area.

    d. If there is poor response to antimicrobial therapy or a necrotizing, soft-tissue infection is suspected, surgical intervention is mandatory.

C. Abscess

  1. General characteristics

    a. An abscess is a localized infection characterized by a collection of purulent material in a cavity formed by necrosis or disintegration of tissue.

    b. A sterile abscess is one formed without a bacterial pathogen.

  2. Clinical features

    a. Abscess presents as a tender, erythematous, and often fluctuant area, indicating the formation of pus.

    b. The most common locations are axillary and perirectal regions, buttocks, perirectal, and the head and neck.

    c. Discharge or drainage can be cultured; however, more than one causative organism is the norm.

    d. An abscess may develop at the site of therapeutic or drug-use injection.

  3. Treatment

    a. Early abscess should be treated with hot soaks for 20 minutes four times daily to bring it to a head. Once the lesion is fluctuant, it can be incised and drained and an iodoform gauze wick can be placed in the wound to facilitate drainage.

    b. Alternatively, hot soaks can be followed by a dressing saturated with a drawing salve.

    c. Oral antibiotics, such as dicloxacillin, a cephalosporin, or erythromycin, should be started if the patient has a fever or cellulitis surrounding the abscess.

VI. DERMATOPHYTOSIS

A. General characteristics

  1. Dermatophytosis is a superficial fungal infection that can affect the hair, nails, and skin.

  2. The three most common dermatophytes affecting humans are *Trichophyton*, *Microsporum*, and *Epidermophyton* spp.; *Trichophyton rubrum* is the most common dermatophyte in the industrialized world.

  3. When describing the area of infection, the word tinea (meaning "fungal infection") is followed by the affected part of the body: tinea pedis (foot), tinea cruris (groin), tinea corporis (trunk, legs, arms, or neck), tinea barbae (beard area), tinea unguium (nails), tinea manuum (hand), tinea facialis (face), and tinea capitis (head).

B. Clinical features

  1. Generally, dermatophytosis presents as an erythematous, annular patch with distinct borders and a central clearing. A fine scale usually covers the patch.

  2. Symptoms include itching, stinging, and/or burning. Maceration or peeling fissures are common between the digits.

  3. The nails present with a thickening discoloration and onychomycosis of the nail bed and nail plate.

  4. In tinea capitis, broken hair shafts are seen as black dots.

  5. A kerion (indurated, boggy, inflammatory plaque studded with pustules) can appear with any of these infections but most commonly is found with tinea capitis. It represents an intense inflammatory reaction to superficial dermatophytes.

C. Laboratory studies: A KOH prep should be done to confirm the presence of fungus.

D. Treatment

  1. There is a wide selection of topical creams, ointments, lotions, powders, and sprays to treat dermatophytosis. They should be used twice daily for 4 weeks or more. If vesicles are present, powders help to dry the area and to prevent maceration.

  2. Chronic or resistant infections or nail infection may require oral griseofulvin, itraconazole, terbinafine, or ketoconazole. Treatment may take 3 months.

  3. Kerions are treated with fluconazole or griseofulvin.

  4. Compliance and monitoring are very important in treating these infections.

    a. It is important to advise patients taking griseofulvin not to use alcohol in any form, because it may cause a reaction similar to that with disulfiram (Antabuse), including flushing, headache, nausea, vomiting, sweating, weakness, vertigo, chest pain, dyspnea, and confusion.

    b. Patients with hepatic disorders should be monitored closely when using oral antifungal medications.

    c. If the patient will be on these medications for a long period, such as when treating tinea unguium for several months, he or she should have liver enzymes monitored, starting with a baseline.

  5. Steroids should be avoided. Long-term use will exacerbate the condition and increase the risk of side effects.

  6. Local measures include keeping the skin clean and dry and wearing cotton socks and loose-fitting underclothes.

E. Tinea versicolor (pityriasis versicolor)

  1. Tinea versicolor is caused by *Malassezia furfur*, a yeast found on the skin of humans. It is not understood why this yeast manifests in the spore and hyphal form in some patients, causing disease.

  2. Clinical features

    a. Tinea versicolor consists of hypo- or hyperpigmented macules that do not tan. Most patients are asymptomatic and notice the infection only during the summer, when their tan is spotted due to localized areas of yeast overgrowth. The disease does not appear to be contagious.

    b. The upper trunk is the most common area involved.

3. Laboratory studies: KOH prep of scrapings will show hyphae and spores (spaghetti and meatballs).

4. Treatment

   a. Treatment consists of daily applications of selenium sulfide shampoo from the neck to the waist; the shampoo is left on for up to 15 minutes for seven consecutive days. This can be repeated monthly for maintenance therapy as necessary.

   b. There are other less popular topical methods of treatment as well as oral treatment with ketoconazole. Patients should not shower for 18 hours after taking oral ketoconazole, because it works by being delivered to the skin surface through the patient's sweat.

   c. Newer imidazole creams, lotions, and solutions are effective, but the expense is prohibitive.

VII. PARASITIC INFESTATIONS

A. Scabies

1. General characteristics

   a. Scabies is infestation with *Sarcoptes scabiei,* an eight-legged mite.

   b. Scabies can be found in patients of any age but rarely in infants younger than 3 months.

2. Clinical features

   a. Distribution is most common on the hands, genitalia, and axillary areas. Lesions often are seen in the web spaces between the fingers and toes, around the belt line, or at the edges of socks.

   b. The lesions are pruritic burrows, vesicles, or nodules with excoriations and crusting.

   c. Secondary infections typically are caused by group A streptococci.

3. Laboratory studies

   a. Look for mites, eggs, or feces in a scraping. A drop of mineral oil before scraping facilitates yield.

   b. Positive microscopy is confirmative but not always successful.

4. Treatment

   a. Use 1% lindane or 5% permethrin in a lotion or cream. It is applied to the skin from the chin to the bottom of the feet and is left on overnight (8 hours), and then washed off in the morning. The treatment should be repeated in 7 days.

   b. Antihistamines or topical steroids may help relieve the itching.

   c. Lindane is more toxic and should be avoided in children younger than 2 years, people with extensive dermatitis, and those who are pregnant or lactating.

   d. All bedclothes and clothing of infected patients and household contacts should be washed.

B. Spider bites

1. General characteristics

   a. Although all spiders in the United States are venomous, only a few can puncture the human skin. The most important is the brown recluse (*Loxosceles reclusa*).

   b. Most spider bites occur while the patient is sleeping or dressing in the morning after the spider had crawled into the clothing during the night.

2. Clinical features

   a. Generally, the patient will begin to feel pain 3 hours after a bite; systemic symptoms begin 4 to 6 hours after the bite.

   b. An acute necrotic injury to the skin lasts 10 to 15 days.

   c. Black widows can cause a neurologic overstimulation (e.g., muscle aches, spasms, rigidity). These spiders are not prevalent today.

   d. The brown recluse can cause a significant reaction.

      (1) The single bite is accompanied by an infarct of skin caused by rapid blood coagulation within the vessels.

      (2) The lesion is a sinking macule, pale gray in color, slightly eroded in the center, and has a halo of very tender inflammation and hemorrhage.

      (3) The lesion can extend to the muscle and be as large as the palm of the hand.

3. Treatment

   a. Most spider bites can be managed with local care and analgesics.

   b. Neurologic manifestations of black widow bites are treated with diazepam and calcium gluconate.

    c. Brown recluse bites may be treated locally with wound cleansing and analgesia. Extensive debridement has not proven to be beneficial. Usually, the wound decreases significantly in 5 to 10 days.

    d. Antivenin rarely is indicated and not readily available.

C. Pediculosis

  1. General characteristics

    a. Lice are 1- to 3-mm flat creatures with three pairs of legs. Females lay 300 nits during a lifetime. Nits are opalescent, found on hair shafts, and hatch in about 1 week.

    b. *Pediculus humanus* var. *capitis* infects the scalp (head lice), and *P. humanus* var. *corporis* infects the body. *Phthirus pubis* infects the pubic area (crabs).

    c. Transmission is from person to person.

  2. Clinical features

    a. Pruritus is variable in severity. Excoriations may become secondarily infected.

    b. Lice are visible but often difficult to find. Nits are more readily seen on the hair shafts.

  3. Laboratory studies: Specimens can be viewed under the microscope to confirm the diagnosis.

  4. Treatment

    a. Prevention is key; avoid sharing contact items, such as hats, hairbrushes, and so forth. All contacts should be examined.

    b. Topical insecticides are effective. Permethrin, pyrethrins, and malathion are considered to be first-line treatments; lindane or ivermectin is an alternative.

    c. Special combs help to remove nits; petroleum jelly or other occlusive materials may help to suffocate the lice.

    d. Reapplication in 7 to 10 days is recommended to kill any newly hatched lice.

VIII. WARTS (VERRUCAE)

A. General characteristics

  1. Warts are caused by the human papilloma virus (HPV). There are greater than 100 known serotypes.

  2. HPV replicates in cutaneous and mucosal epithelium. Growths remain local and regress spontaneously.

  3. Common warts can arise on any skin surface. Genital warts (condylomata) are spread through sexual contact.

B. Clinical features

  1. Skin warts can be flat or superficial. Plantar warts are deeper. The surface is rough, resembling tiny heads of cauliflower.

  2. Warts of the oral cavity or larynx can be life threatening if they block the airway.

  3. Anogenital warts occur almost exclusively on the squamous epithelial of the external genitalia and perianal area.

  4. Cervical warts, especially HPV types 16 and 18, are a risk factor for dysplasia, which may progress to cervical cancer.

C. Laboratory studies

  1. Microscopic study shows characteristic hyperplasia and hyperkeratosis. Koilocytotic squamous cells are present.

  2. The presence of HPV is confirmed by immunofluorescence. Molecular probes can detect HPV in cervical tissue.

D. Treatment

  1. Spontaneous regression is typical over time.

  2. Type, location, and age of the patient dictate treatment. The extent of the lesions, the patient's motivation, and the patient's immunologic status also affect treatment choice.

  3. Salicylic acid plasters can be effective for common warts. Cryosurgery or electrodessication can be effective but risks scarring.

  4. Imiquod (Aldara) is a topical therapy that patients can apply at home, but compliance is a problem.

  5. Intralesional interferon also may be effective if other treatments fail.

  6. Anogenital warts can be treated with trichloroacetic acid or topical podophyllin, but this may require many applications.

  7. Surgical excision is successful, but recurrence is common.

  8. A vaccine that is effective against four of the strains of HPV (two associated with cervical cancer [16 and 18] and two associated with warts [6 and 11]) has been developed and is effective for at least 4 to 5 years. It is approved for females aged 9 to 26 years.

IX. TUMORS

A. Benign neoplasm

1. A keratoderma is a generalized thickening of the horny layer of the epidermis.

   a. Types of keratoderma

   (1) Punctate keratodermas (found on the palms of the hands and the soles of the feet) and keratodermas on the digits are more prevalent in African American patients. The lesions develop central plugs.

   (2) Solar keratoderma (actinic keratosis) is a premalignant condition caused by cumulative exposure to the sun and is more prevalent in fair-skinned people. The thickened lesions progress very slowly to squamous cell carcinomas; they also can progress to a cutaneous horn.

   (3) Actinic cheilitis is actinic dermatosis of the lip.

   (4) Seborrheic keratosis is a benign plaque, beige to brown or black, with a velvety, warty surface that appears "stuck on." Lesions are more common in older persons.

   b. Treatment

   (1) Liquid nitrogen can be used successfully to treat keratodermas.

   (2) Electrodessication and curettage also are effective.

   (3) Mild acid treatments and the application of Monsel's solution (ferric subsulfate solution) have been used.

   (4) 5-Fluorouracil (applied topically twice daily for 2 to 4 weeks) is effective, but patients must be warned that their lesions will look worse before they look better.

2. Lipomas (adipose tumors) are benign neoplasms of mature fat cells that pose no harm to the patient. Surgical excision may be appropriate for cosmetic reasons or if the lipoma is located where it is constantly irritated.

3. Pyogenic granulomas (capillary hemangiomas): This term is a misnomer, because the lesion does not have an infectious cause.

   a. Clinical features

   (1) These bright red, raspberry-like nodules usually present on exposed parts of the body, such as the arms, hands, fingers, or legs.

   (2) They often appear after an injury or surgery but also can appear spontaneously.

   b. Treatment: Electrodessication and curettage or excision is used. Cauterization with silver nitrate and cryosurgery has not proved to be curative.

B. Malignant neoplasms

1. Melanoma

   a. General characteristics

   (1) Although only approximately 3% of skin cancers are melanomas, they cause 66% of skin cancer deaths.

   (2) Melanomas frequently metastasize widely to regional lymph nodes, skin, liver, lungs, or brain.

   b. Clinical features

   (1) Melanomas usually are black or dark brown but can be flesh colored. They sometimes have blue, pink, or red components.

   (2) The lesions have an irregular border, with an outward spreading of pigment. If the lesion changes in size over a relatively short period, malignant degeneration should be considered.

   (3) Although most commonly seen on the skin, a melanoma can occur anywhere on the body, including the eye and mucous membranes of the genitalia, anus, or oral cavity, subungual areas, and soles of the feet.

   (4) Lesions can be macular to nodular, and four types exist: lentigo maligna melanoma, superficial spreading malignant melanoma (most common), nodular malignant melanoma, and acral lentiginous melanomas (palms, soles, nail beds).

   c. Prognosis is strongly related to the depth of the lesion.

   (1) A melanoma entirely within the epidermis carries a very good prognosis.

   (2) As the thickness progresses beyond the epidermis, the prognosis diminishes.

   (3) The likelihood of survival is further diminished if the melanoma is on the upper back, upper arm, neck, or scalp.

   d. Treatment

   (1) Early detection is the key to successful treatment.

    (2) Since the 1970s, the 5-year survival rate has increased from 25% to 40% to more than 80%. However, the incidence of melanoma is on the rise and is occurring in younger individuals.

    (3) Patients with melanoma need to be referred to a dermatologist or surgeon for complete excision and follow-up.

2. Squamous and basal cell carcinomas are the most common neoplasms of the skin. Metastasis is rare.

  a. Clinical features

    (1) The lesions are asymptomatic but may itch or bleed. The patient seeks treatment because the nodules do not heal.

    (2) Lesions most commonly present on areas that usually are exposed to the sun (face, head, neck).

    (3) There are several types of basal cell lesions:

      (a) Nodular: Translucent or pearly papule or nodule

      (b) Ulcerating: Ulcer with a rolled border, often covered with a crust

      (c) Sclerosing: Infiltrating carcinoma; white sclerotic patch with ill-defined borders

      (d) Superficial: Erythematous, slightly scaly, thin plaques, often with a fine rolled or pearly border

      (e) Pigmented: Thick, hard area of variegated pigmentation

    (4) Squamous cell lesions typically appear as sharply demarcated, scaling, or hyperkeratotic macule, papule, or plaque. Erythema, scaling, erosions, and crusts may occur.

  b. Treatment

    (1) Complete eradication of the lesion is recommended.

    (2) Options include excision with clear margins, electrodessication with curettage, 5-fluorouracil, cryosurgery, radiation therapy, Mohs' micrographic surgery, and laser vaporization.

X.   ULCERS, BURNS, AND WOUNDS

A. Ulcers

  1. General characteristics

    a. Diabetic ulcers, stasis ulcers, and arterial leg ulcers are common in the lower limbs.

    b. Decubitus ulcers occur in areas of pressure in patients with limited mobility.

  2. Clinical features

    a. Diabetic ulcers tend to be deep, punched-out lesions over the malleoli, the plantar surfaces of the feet, or the toes. They usually are painless because of associated neuropathies.

    b. Stasis ulcers are a result of chronic venous stasis. Stasis dermatitis develops initially, and then ulcers that are wide but not deep develop, with irregular, undulating edges and a clean base. Elevation of the affected limb eases any pain.

    c. Arterial ulcers usually do not become as large as venous ulcers and are not preceded by dermatitis. Arterial ulcers are painful, pulses are diminished or absent, and the distal area is cold.

    d. Decubitus ulcers are a result of impaired blood supply caused by localized pressure. The sacrum and hip areas most commonly are affected. Complications include osteomyelitis, bacteremia, and sepsis.

    e. There are four stages of decubiti:

      (1) Stage I: Nonblanching erythema of intact skin

      (2) Stage II: Necrosis, superficial, or partial thickness involving the epidermis and/or dermis; shallow ulcer

      (3) Stage III: Deep necrosis; crater ulcers with full-thickness skin loss; damage or necrosis can extend down to, but not through, fascia

      (4) Stage IV: Full-thickness ulceration with extensive damage and necrosis to muscle, bone, or supporting structures

  3. Treatment

    a. All limb ulcers can be difficult to treat.

    b. Diabetic and arterial ulcers are treated similarly.

      (1) Lifestyle changes include smoking cessation and moderate exercise to enhance blood flow.

      (2) Debridement is necessary if the wound is necrotic.

(3) Wet-to-dry dressings or hydrogels are standard treatment, because wounds heal better in a moist environment. Hydrocolloids (e.g., DuoDERM) and enzymatic preparations maintain moisture, enhance granulation, promote debridement, and improve rates of epithelialization.

   c. Stasis ulcers are treated with elevation and compression to enhance venous return.

     (1) The affected limb should be whirlpooled, the lesion painted with gentian violet, and an Unna boot applied weekly.

     (2) Wraps or support hose also may be used for compression; they should be applied while the leg is elevated and before the veins fill again.

   d. Prevention is the key to managing decubitus ulcers.

     (1) Repositioning, massaging prone areas, and frequent monitoring are essential.

     (2) Efforts to minimize friction, use of an air mattress to reduce compression, meticulous hygiene, and good nutrition help.

     (3) If an ulcer develops, moist sterile gauze (e.g., Gelfoam), hydrocolloid, and/or surgical debridement may be necessary.

   e. Topical and/or systemic antibiotics are indicated for any signs of infections.

B. Open wounds

  1. Tetanus status should be assessed with any open wound.

   a. If the last tetanus booster was more than 10 years ago, an update is needed; if the wound is particularly dirty, a tetanus booster may be given sooner.

   b. If the tetanus status is unknown, the patient should receive tetanus immunoglobulin as well as the vaccine.

  2. Wounds should be cleansed well, irrigated, and closed unless they are more than 8 hours old or signs of infection exist. Dirty wounds may need antibiotic coverage.

C. Burns (see Chapter 15)

XI. HAIR AND NAILS

A. Alopecia (loss of hair)

  1. Androgenetic alopecia (male pattern baldness)

   a. Male pattern baldness has a genetic component.

   b. Its extent is variable and unpredictable.

   c. Minoxidil solutions are most effective in persons with recent onset and smaller areas of hair loss.

   d. Finasteride may also be effective. Side effects include loss of libido and erectile dysfunction.

  2. Alopecia areata is of unknown cause.

   a. It may be seen in thyroiditis, pernicious anemia, systemic lupus erythematosus (SLE), or Addison's disease.

   b. Tiny hairs typically are found. Loss can be patchy, involve only the scalp (alopecia totalis), or include the entire body (alopecia universalis).

   c. It may respond to systemic steroids, but relapse is common.

  3. Drug-induced alopecia may occur with thallium, vitamin A, retinoids, antimitotic agents, anticoagulants, oral contraceptives, and others.

B. Nails

  1. Onycholysis is distal separation of the nail plate from the nail bed.

   a. Common causes include excessive exposure to water, soaps, detergents, or alkalis; psoriasis; drugs; or thyroid disease.

   b. Onychomycosis indicates infection with fungi or yeast.

  2. Discolorations and crumbly nails are seen in dermatophytosis and psoriasis.

  3. Paronychia is an inflammation of the nail fold. Erythema, swelling, and throbbing pain may extend into the proximal nail fold and eponychium.

  4. Felon is a subcutaneous infection of the pulp space. This is a closed infection that may rupture or cause osteitis or osteomyelitis; the abscess should be drained.

  5. Congenital nail disorders include nail atrophy and clubbed fingers.

  6. Systemic disease may cause Beau's lines (transverse furrows), atrophy, clubbed fingers, spoon nails, stippling or pitting, and hyperpigmentation.

XII. PIGMENTATION DISORDERS

A. Acanthosis nigricans
   1. General characteristics
      a. This hyperpigmentation disorder can be hereditary or acquired.
      b. It commonly is associated with obesity, endocrine disorders (most notably insulin resistance), and paraneoplastic syndromes, or it may be drug induced.
   2. Clinical features: Acanthosis nigricans develops insidiously. Initially, the skin darkens and appears dirty; later the skin is thick and velvety, with accentuated skin lines.
   3. Laboratory studies: If the disorder is thought to be associated with an underlying disorder, further investigation is needed.
   4. Treatment: There is no treatment except for that of addressing any underlying disorder.

B. Melasma (also known as chloasma)
   1. Melasma means "a black spot"; it is an acquired hyperpigmentation disorder of sun-exposed areas and may be associated with pregnancy or with oral contraceptives or other medications.
   2. Clinical features
      a. Young females are more commonly affected.
      b. Hyperpigmented macular areas evolve rapidly over weeks. The color usually is uniform.
   3. Laboratory studies: Wood's lamp examination accentuates the hyperpigmented macules.
   4. Treatment
      a. Treatment includes 3% hydroquinone solution in combination with 0.025% tretinoin gel. Alternatively, 4% hydroquinone and glycolic acid in a cream base may be used.
      b. Sunblock is essential.

C. Vitiligo
   1. General characteristics
      a. Destruction of melanocytes can be associated with thyroid disease, pernicious anemia, diabetes mellitus, and Addison's disease, or it may be idiopathic.
      b. Vitiligo occurs at any age, in every race, and in males and females equally. About 30% of patients report a family history.
      c. Macules of hypopigmentation may occur focally, segmentally, or in a generalized pattern.
   2. Treatment: Sunscreens, cosmetic cover-up products, or repigmentation therapies under the direction of an experienced dermatologist may be used.
   3. Vitiligo can be very psychologically distressing, especially in dark-skinned patients.

XIII. ANGIOEDEMA AND URTICARIA

A. General characteristics
   1. Urticaria is a group of disorders that can have many causes, most commonly food or drug allergies, heat or cold, and stress or infection.
   2. Urticaria affects 15% to 20% of the population.
   3. Hives or wheals are raised red areas on the skin or mucous membranes caused by the release of histamines, bradykinin, kallikrein, and other vasoactive substances from mast cells and basophils in the skin, causing small blood vessels to leak and resulting in intradermal edema.
   4. The wheals may be the size of a pencil eraser up to the size of a dinner plate, and they may coalesce into even larger areas.
   5. The lesions most commonly are pruritic but may sting or burn.

B. Acute urticaria may be self-limiting, lasting from a few minutes to hours.
   1. Most often, acute urticaria is an allergic reaction to food or drugs. Immunoglobulin E attaches itself to a receptor on the mast cell and causes a chemical release.
   2. Common causes of acute urticaria are things that are ingested, such as drugs like penicillin or other antibiotics, sulfa drugs and other medications, shellfish, peanuts, and food preservatives in processed and canned foodstuffs.
   3. Other less common causes include things the skin may contact (e.g., laundry detergents, shampoos, perfumes, and cleaning solvents) or things the patient may breathe (e.g., fabric softeners).

C. Chronic urticaria lasts more than 6 weeks. Typically, the lesions wax and wane.

   1. Chronic urticaria is idiopathic; exacerbations can be precipitated by stress.

   2. Females are affected twice as often as males.

D. Physical urticaria can be caused by reaction to heat or cold, water, infection, exercise, or sun exposure. Dermatographism is caused by pressure.

E. Treatment

   1. Any known causes should be eliminated, but it is estimated that the cause is not found in up to 80% of cases.

   2. For acute or idiopathic urticaria, an H_1 antihistamine, such as diphenhydramine (Benadryl), hydroxyzine (Vistaril), fexofenadine (Allegra), or cetirizine (Zyrtec), may be used orally.

   3. In chronic urticaria or in acute urticaria that does not respond initially, an H_2 antihistamine, such as famotidine (Pepcid) or ranitidine (Zantac), may be added to the H_1 regimen.

   4. Recurring urticaria or chronic urticaria may require steroids.

   5. If there is a concern that urticaria may progress to anaphylaxis, a prescription for an EpiPen should be given to the patient along with education regarding how to use it.

14 Infectious Disease

Claire Babcock O'Connell

I. FEVER

A. General information

1. The normal range of body temperature is 97°F to 99.5°F (36.0°C to 37.4°C), averaging 98.6°F (36.7°C). There is a normal diurnal variation of 1.25°F to 2.5°F (0.5°C to 1.0°C).

   a. Stimulation of monocyte–macrophage cells elaborates pyogenic cytokines, which cause an elevation of the set point of the body temperature (i.e., fever). Increased heat production causes shivering; reduction causes peripheral vasoconstriction.

   b. A body temperature of greater than 106.8°F (41.1°C) risks irreversible brain damage.

2. Elevated temperature and the symptoms caused by change in body temperature are fairly well correlated with illness, particularly infection.

   a. The degree of elevation does not correlate with severity of illness.

   b. Children typically mount high fevers; the elderly and people on chronic medications (e.g., nonsteroidal anti-inflammatory drugs (NSAIDs), steroids) may not mount a fever at all.

B. Fever of unknown origin (FUO) is defined as a temperature of greater than 101.8°F (38.3°C) for 3 weeks with no discernible cause despite at least 1 week of diagnostic workup.

1. The most common causes of FUO are infections and multisystem disease (e.g., autoimmune disorders, neoplasms).

2. No diagnosis is found in 25% of FUO cases.

C. Treatment of fever is mainly for patient comfort. Reduction in temperature is not part of the therapy for the underlying cause.

1. Fevers can be reduced by supportive measures, such as alcohol or cold sponge baths, ice bags, or ice water enemas, or through administration of antipyretics, such as aspirin or acetaminophen. Aspirin products should be avoided in children because of the risk of Reye's syndrome.

2. Empiric broad-spectrum antibiotics often are begun when infection is suspected.

II. BACTERIAL INFECTIONS

A. *Streptococcus* sp.

1. General characteristics

   a. Streptococci are a group of Gram-positive, catalase-producing cocci that appear in chains. They can be aerobic, anaerobic, or facultative and are cultured on blood agar media: complete hemolysis is identified as α-hemolytic, incomplete hemolysis as β-hemolytic, and no hemolysis as γ-hemolytic streptococci.

   b. The β-hemolytic streptococci are the most common pathogenic type.

   (1) Lancefield classified the β-hemolytic streptococci into groups, labeled A through O.

   (2) The group A β-hemolytic streptococci are the most common of all pathogenic streptococci.

   c. Humans are the only reservoir of group A β-hemolytic streptococci.

   (1) Asymptomatic carriers are frequent. The highest incidence of infection with group A β-hemolytic streptococci is in patients younger than 10 years.

   (2) Crowded conditions and person-to-person transmission are responsible for its perpetuity.

2. Clinical manifestations

   a. Pharyngitis

   (1) An abrupt onset of sore throat and painful swallowing with fever and chills herald infection.

   (2) There is enlargement of the cervical lymph nodes, edema and hypertrophy of pharyngeal mucosa, and erythema and exudates that may be punctate or confluent.

   (3) The disease usually is self-limited and typically resolves in 3 to 4 days, even without specific treatment. Untreated infections may lead to nonsuppurative complications.

b. Scarlet fever is characterized as strep throat with a rash.

(1) The rash is a diffuse erythema that blanches; superimposed fine red papules may be appreciated only by touch (sandpaper rash). It is described as a sunburn with goose bumps.

(2) The face typically is flushed, with circumoral pallor and a strawberry tongue.

(3) The rash fades in 2 to 5 days, with fine desquamation.

c. Erysipelas is a painful macular rash with well-defined margins; it is characterized by an abrupt onset and rapid progression.

(1) The rash typically is confined to the face, which becomes fiery red, but it may progress to the extremities. Flaccid bullae may develop.

(2) The rash desquamates in 5 to 10 days.

d. Impetigo (*Streptococcus pyoderma*) is characterized by thick, crusted, golden "honey" yellow lesions.

(1) There is a higher prevalence with poor hygiene and malnutrition.

(2) The bacteria colonize unbroken skin and, with abrasions or bites, inoculate the intradermal space, where lesions develop.

(3) Impetigo also can be caused by staphylococci (bullous impetigo).

e. Cellulitis manifests with local swelling, erythema, and pain.

(1) The skin is pinkish and indurated.

(2) Group A streptococci are the most common cause of cellulitis in the United States; they are common in patients with lymphedema, chronic stasis, or venous grafts.

(3) Surgical debridement may be necessary if there is poor response to medical treatment.

f. Necrotizing fasciitis (flesh-eating bacteria) is a deep subcutaneous infection that results in destruction of fascia and fat.

(1) Swelling, heat, erythema, and pain spread proximally and distally.

(2) The skin darkens, and blisters and bullae with clear yellow fluid form.

(3) Development of gangrene and necrosis is associated with mental status changes and delirium; mortality is high.

g. Toxic shock syndrome is a bacteremia with susceptible strains of streptococci following deep soft-tissue infection.

(1) A viral-like prodrome and history of minor trauma, surgery, or varicella may be found.

(2) Onset is abrupt with severe pain, typically in an extremity; abdominal infection may mimic peritonitis, pelvic inflammatory disease, myocardial infarction, or pericarditis.

(3) Fever or hypothermia, confusion, combativeness, and coma develop. Patients develop shock and multiorgan failure. A violaceous or blue vesicular or bullous rash is an ominous sign. Mortality is 30% despite treatment.

(4) Complications include endophthalmitis, myositis, peritonitis, septic arthritis, myocarditis, perihepatitis, meningitis, and sepsis.

(5) Common laboratory findings include hemoglobinuria, elevated serum creatinine, low albumin, low calcium, mild leukocytosis and a severe left shift, and low platelets.

(6) Management includes intravenous (IV) fluids (colloids and crystalloids) and antibiotics as well as pressors, mechanical ventilation, and surgical intervention, as needed.

h. Nonsuppurative complications of group A β-hemolytic streptococcal infections

(1) Acute glomerulonephritis (see Chapter 6)

(2) Acute rheumatic fever (ARF) is a systemic immune process occurring 15 to 20 days after exposure to streptococcal pharyngitis.

(a) Once rare, it has become more prevalent since the 1980s. Peak age is 5 to 15 years, and mortality is 1% to 2% despite treatment.

(b) Jones' criteria for ARF diagnosis (Table 14-1): The presence of two major criteria or one major and two minor criteria *plus* evidence of recent β-hemolytic streptococci (culture or antistreptolysin O [ASO] titer) makes the diagnosis.

(c) Complications of ARF

(i) Congestive heart failure, rheumatic pneumonitis, and rheumatic heart disease (RHD) are possible complications. RHD most commonly results in valvular defects but also may cause arrhythmias, pericarditis, or effusions.

TABLE 14-1	Jones' Criteria for Diagnosis of Acute Rheumatic Fever
Major Criteria	**Minor Criteria**
Carditis	Fever
Erythema marginatum	Polyarthralgias
Subcutaneous nodules	Reversible prolongation of the PR interval
Sydenham's chorea	Rapid erythrocyte sedimentation rate
Arthritis	Elevated C-reactive protein
	Leukocytosis
	History of rheumatic fever

(ii) The 2007 American Heart Association Revised Guidelines no longer recommend prophylactic antibiotics before invasive procedures to prevent endocarditis in patients with a history of RHD.

(iii) Prophylaxis is recommended if a patient has a prosthetic cardiac valve, previous endocarditis, or specific forms of congenital heart disease.

(d) Early treatment of streptococcal infection is imperative to reduce risk of ARF and RHD. Recurrence is common; those at high risk are given prophylactic antibiotics (penicillin, sulfadiazine, or erythromycin) during outbreaks of streptococcal pharyngitis.

(e) Patients with carditis have the poorest prognosis: 30% of patients will die within 10 years, two-thirds will develop detectable valvular abnormalities, and 10% will have permanent significant heart disease or cardiomyopathy.

3. Laboratory findings

   a. The diagnosis of streptococcal infection is established by a combination of clinical manifestations, rapid reagent tests, and identification of the bacteria through Gram staining or culture.

   b. The Centor criteria will aid in proper diagnosis of streptococcal pharyngitis.

     (1) There are four possible criteria: tonsillar exudates, absence of a cough, tender anterior lymphadenopathy, and history of fever.

     (2) Presence of three out of the four criteria suggests a 40% to 60% chance that the sore throat is caused by group A β-hemolytic streptococcus. Further consideration or testing is warranted in patients with score lower than three.

   c. An elevated white blood cell (WBC) count, erythrocyte sedimentation rate, and other markers of infection may be found in severe infections or sepsis.

4. Treatment

   a. For the most part, group A β-hemolytic streptococci remain susceptible to penicillins; cephalosporins are also effective.

   b. For patients who are allergic to penicillins, macrolides are recommended.

   c. Supportive care (i.e., fluids, analgesics, antipyretics) should be encouraged as needed.

B. Botulism

1. General characteristics

   a. *Clostridium botulinum,* a strictly anaerobic, spore-forming bacillus found in the soil, may inadvertently be packed in food (home canned, smoked, or commercial), where toxin is produced and stored until ingested. Botulinum toxin inhibits the release of acetylcholine at the neuromuscular junction.

   b. Infant and wound botulism result from exposure to the bacteria or spores and elaboration of the toxin in vivo. Injection drug users are at increased risk of wound botulism. Infants should not be fed honey because of the increased risk of botulism.

2. Clinical findings

   a. The initial clinical symptom is visual changes, including diplopia and loss of accommodation. Manifestations typically appear 12 to 36 hours after ingestion.

   b. Additional manifestations include ptosis, impaired extraocular muscle movements, and fixed, dilated pupils. Other manifestations include cranial nerve palsies, dysphonia, dry mouth, dysphagia, nausea, and vomiting.

   c. Mental status changes or sensory deficits do not occur.

   d. Respiratory paralysis ensues and, unless mechanic assistance is provided, death results.

3. Laboratory findings: The toxin can be identified using specific antiserum after mouse inoculation with the patient's serum.

4. Treatment

    a. Botulinum antitoxin is available through the Centers for Disease Control and Prevention (CDC); the CDC also will assist with obtaining assays of serum, stool, or suspect food.

    b. Respiratory failure necessitates intubation and mechanical ventilation. If dysphagia persists, IV nutritional support and hyperalimentation are required.

C. Anthrax

1. General characteristics

    a. *Bacillus anthracis* is a spore-forming, Gram-positive aerobic rod found in sheep, cattle, horses, goats, and swine.

    b. It is transmitted to humans via inoculation of broken skin or mucous membranes or via inhalation. Farmers, veterinarians, and tannery and wool workers are at high risk.

    c. The organism is a likely candidate for biologic warfare.

2. Clinical findings

    a. Dermatologic

        (1) Approximately 2 weeks after exposure to spores, anthrax causes an erythematous papule at the site of inoculation that becomes vesicular with a purple-to-black center, which in turn ulcerates, becomes necrotic (eschar), and eventually sloughs. Surrounding skin is edematous and vesicular. The lesion is painless unless secondarily infected with staphylococci or streptococci.

        (2) Regional adenopathy, fever, malaise, headache, and nausea and vomiting may occur. The infection usually is self-limited.

        (3) Hematogenous spread results in sepsis and hemorrhagic meningitis. This can occur anywhere between 10 days and 6 weeks after exposure.

    b. Pulmonary

        (1) Initially, fever, malaise, headache, dyspnea, cough, and congestion of the nose, throat, and larynx are seen.

        (2) Hours to days later, a fulminating pneumonia or mediastinitis may occur.

    c. Gastrointestinal (GI)

        (1) Ingestion of contaminated meat may lead to fever, diffuse abdominal pain, rebound tenderness, vomiting, and change in bowel habits, which may range from bloody diarrhea to constipation. Ulcerations may lead to bowel perforation, dysphagia, or obstruction.

        (2) Although less common, an overwhelming sepsis may develop, causing delirium, obtundation, meningeal irritation, and hemorrhagic meningitis.

        (3) GI anthrax and its complications have not been reported in the United States.

3. Laboratory studies

    a. Skin lesions yield Gram-positive, encapsulated, box-shaped rods in chains; sputum, blood, cerebrospinal fluid (CSF), or skin lesion cultures are positive for *Bacillus anthracis*.

    b. Chest radiography in cases of inhalation anthrax will reveal mediastinal widening secondary to hemorrhagic lymphadenitis.

    c. Any suspected case of anthrax should be reported to the CDC, which can perform immunohistologic testing or polymerase chain reaction (PCR) to confirm.

4. Treatment

    a. Combination therapy is recommended for inhalation anthrax or disseminated disease or cutaneous infection that involves the head or neck.

    b. Ciprofloxacin or another fluoroquinolone is the treatment of choice; doxycycline is the alternative.

    c. An attenuated vaccine is available for persons with a high likelihood of exposure (e.g., laboratory workers).

    d. Prognosis is excellent in cutaneous anthrax. Prognosis for inhalation or GI anthrax is poor (85% mortality) despite treatment; results are best if treatment is begun early.

D. Cholera

1. General characteristics

    a. *Vibrio cholerae* produces a toxin that activates adenylyl cyclase in intestinal epithelial cells of the small intestine. This results in hypersecretion of water and chloride ion and a massive diarrhea. Death results from hypovolemia.

    b. Epidemics of cholera occur in times of war, overcrowding, and famine, and where sanitation is inadequate. Infection results from ingestion of contaminated food or water.

2. Clinical findings: A sudden onset of severe, frequent, "rice water" diarrhea (gray, turbid, and without odor, blood, or pus); dehydration; hypotension; and electrolyte imbalance develop rapidly.

3. Laboratory studies: Stool cultures are positive for *Vibrio cholerae;* serum agglutination tests are available.

4. Treatment

    a. Replacement of fluids and electrolytes is essential. Oral rehydration with water containing salt and sugar is adequate for mild or moderate cases (1 tsp salt, 4 tsp sugar, 1 cup water). Severe cases require IV replacement.

    b. Antibiotics will shorten duration and reduce severity of symptoms, but rehydration is vital to survival.

    c. Tetracycline, ampicillin, chloramphenicol, trimethoprim/sulfamethoxazole (TMP/SMX), and fluoroquinolones are effective. Resistance exists, so susceptibility testing is encouraged.

    d. The key to prevention is clean water and food sources as well as proper waste disposal. A vaccine is available, but protection is temporary, with boosters needed every 6 months.

E. Tetanus

  1. General characteristics

    a. *Clostridium tetani* spores are ubiquitous in soil. The spores germinate in wounds where the bacteria produce a neurotoxin (tetanospasmin), which interferes with neurotransmission at spinal synapses of inhibitory neurons. The result is uncontrolled spasm and exaggerated reflexes.

    b. Puncture wounds are most susceptible. The elderly, migrant workers, newborns, and injection drug users are at particular risk. The incubation period is from 5 days to 15 weeks.

  2. Clinical findings

    a. Pain and tingling at the site of inoculation is followed by spasticity of the muscles nearby.

    b. Jaw and neck stiffness, dysphagia, and irritability are common. Hyperreflexia and muscle spasms develop, especially in the jaw (trismus) and face.

    c. Painful tonic convulsions, spasm of the glottis and respiratory muscles, and asphyxia develop if the patient is untreated.

    d. The patient typically is alert throughout the course.

  3. Treatment

    a. Tetanus immune globulin should be given intramuscularly (IM). A full course of tetanus toxoid should be administered once the patient recovers. Bed rest, sedation, and mechanical ventilation often are necessary to control tetanic spasms. Penicillin is given to all patients to eradicate toxin-producing organisms. Mortality is high.

    b. Active immunization is recommended starting in childhood. Three to four initial doses are followed by boosters every 10 years. An additional booster is recommended if a major injury occurs and if it has been more than 5 years since the last booster. Passive immunization with tetanus toxoid in addition to vaccine is recommended for patients with major wounds and uncertain tetanus status.

F. Salmonellosis

  1. General characteristics: There are more than 2,000 serotypes of salmonellae, all of which are members of the species *Salmonella enterica* and are transmitted by ingestion of contaminated food or water.

  2. Clinical features

    a. Three patterns are recognized.

    b. Enteric fever (typhoid fever)

      (1) The incubation period is 5 to 14 days. Organisms enter the mucosal epithelium of the intestines and invade and replicate within macrophages in Peyer's patches, mesenteric lymph nodes, and the spleen; bacteremia accompanies infection.

      (2) Onset is insidious, with a prodrome of malaise, headache, cough, and sore throat. Abdominal pain, distention, and constipation and/or diarrhea ("pea soup") develop as the fever increases. Fever reaches a peak on days 7 to 10, and the patient appears toxic and then generally improves over the next 7 to 10 days. Relapses are common (15% of cases). Children commonly have an abrupt onset.

      (3) Physical findings include splenomegaly, abdominal distention and tenderness, and bradycardia. A rash develops during the second week; it appears as pink papules, primarily on the trunk, that fade on pressure.

      (4) The organism can be isolated from blood during the first week of the illness; later, the blood cultures will likely be negative. Stool culture is not reliable.

      (5) Complications occur in 30% of untreated cases. Intestinal hemorrhage can be fatal. Other complications include urinary retention, pneumonia, thrombophlebitis, myocarditis, psychosis, cholecystitis, nephritis, osteomyelitis, and meningitis.

(6) Treatment: Resistance to ampicillin, chloramphenicol, and TMP/SMX is increasing. Resistant strains may be susceptible to ceftriaxone or fluoroquinolones (contraindicated in children and pregnancy). Treatment should be done for 2 weeks.

(7) Prevention: Treatment of carriers often is not effective. Immunization may be provided for household contacts of carriers, travelers to endemic areas, or during epidemics, but it is not always effective. Protection of the food and water supplies as well as proper waste disposal are key to control of the disease.

c. Gastroenteritis

(1) This is the most common form of *Salmonella* infection. The incubation period is 8 to 48 hours after ingestion of contaminated food or drink. Fever, nausea and vomiting, crampy abdominal pain, and bloody diarrhea last 3 to 5 days. Diagnosis is made through stool culture.

(2) Illness is self-limited, and treatment is symptomatic. Specific treatment with TMP/SMX, ampicillin, or ciprofloxacin is required for severely ill or malnourished patients, sickle cell disease, or patients who develop bacteremia.

d. Bacteremia

(1) This is characterized by prolonged or recurrent fevers, with bacteremia and local infection in bone, joints, pleura, pericardium, lungs, or other sites.

(2) It is most common in immunosuppressed persons.

(3) Treatment is the same as that for typhoid fever; any abscesses should be drained.

(4) Immunosuppressed patients may benefit from therapy with ciprofloxacin.

G. Shigellosis

1. General characteristics: *Shigella sonnei*, *Shigella flexneri*, and *Shigella dysenteriae* are the most common species that cause dysentery.

2. Clinical findings

a. Illness starts abruptly with diarrhea, lower abdominal cramps, and tenesmus accompanied by fever, chills, anorexia, headache, and malaise.

b. Stools are loose and mixed with blood and mucus. Abdomen is tender; dehydration is common.

c. HLA-B27 individuals may mount a reactive arthritis because of temporary disaccharidase deficiency.

3. Laboratory studies

a. Stool is positive for leukocytes and red blood cells; culture yields *Shigella* spp.

b. Sigmoidoscopy will reveal inflamed engorged mucosa, punctate lesions, or ulcers.

4. Treatment

a. Replacement of fluid volume is essential.

b. Antibiotics: TMP/SMX is the antibiotic of choice, although ciprofloxacin or a fluoroquinolone may be substituted; amoxicillin is not effective.

H. Diphtheria

1. General characteristics

a. *Corynebacterium diphtheriae* is transmitted via respiratory secretions. The organism has a propensity for mucous membranes, especially the respiratory tract.

b. It produces an exotoxin that causes myocarditis and neuropathy.

2. Clinical findings

a. Nasal infection produces few symptoms other than nasal discharge.

b. Laryngeal infection causes upper airway and bronchial obstruction.

c. Pharyngeal infection is the most common form. A tenacious gray membrane covers the tonsils and pharynx, and patients complain of mild sore throat, fever, and malaise.

d. Myocarditis and neuropathy involving the cranial nerves may develop; untreated cases exhibit toxemia and prostration.

3. Diagnosis is clinical; culture will confirm.

4. Treatment

a. A horse serum antitoxin must be given in all cases of diphtheria. It is obtained from the CDC.

b. Airway obstruction may necessitate removal of the membrane via laryngoscopy.

c. Penicillin or erythromycin is effective. Azithromycin or clarithromycin is an effective alternative.

d. Patients should be isolated until three negative pharyngeal cultures are documented.

e. Contacts should be treated with erythromycin to eradicate carrier states.

5. Diphtheria toxoid is available as a vaccine (diphtheria, tetanus, and acellular pertussis [DtaP]; tetanus and diphtheria toxoid [Td]). Unimmunized persons who are exposed to diphtheria should receive active immunization and antibiotic therapy.

I. Pertussis

1. General characteristics

   a. *Bordetella pertussis* is a Gram-negative pleomorphic bacillus. Humans are the sole reservoir.

   b. Since the advent of immunization, the United States has seen 99% reduction in cases; however, pertussis remains a disease of importance globally. Vaccination is not lifelong.

   c. Infection is highest in premature infants and in those with cardiac, pulmonary, or neuromuscular disorders.

   d. Older children and adults tend to have milder disease.

2. Clinical findings

   a. Clinical manifestations occur in three stages:

      (1) The catarrhal stage: Insidious onset of sneezing, coryza, loss of appetite, and malaise along with a hacking cough most prominent at night. This stage is often misdiagnosed as an upper respiratory viral illness. This is the most infectious stage.

      (2) The paroxysmal stage: Spasms of rapid coughing fits followed by deep, high-pitched inspiration (the whoop). Paroxysms may last several minutes. Infants are at risk for apnea.

      (3) The convalescent stage: Decrease in frequency and severity of paroxysms; this stage is usually 4 weeks after onset of the cough and may last for an additional several weeks.

   b. Adults are often misdiagnosed; any cough persisting for greater than 2 weeks with no other cause should be questioned.

   c. Physical exam is generally unremarkable. Fever is rare.

3. Laboratory

   a. Diagnosis is made by culture using a special media.

   b. PCR assays may be available through some health departments.

   c. WBC count is usually mildly elevated; a lymphocytosis is characteristic.

4. Treatment

   a. Erythromycin is the medication of choice. Treatment is aimed at stopping transmission, although it may also aid in reducing severity of paroxysms.

   b. Alternative therapies include azithromycin, clarithromycin, and TMP/SMX.

   c. Supportive therapy is essential.

   d. Close contacts should also be treated with antibiotics (erythromycin).

5. Prevention

   a. Acellular pertussis vaccine is recommended, beginning in infancy. It is given in combination with diphtheria and tetanus toxoids.

   b. Vaccination of adults is now recommended. Tdap (tetanus toxoid, reduced diphtheria toxoid, and acellular pertussis) is the vaccine of choice.

III. VIRAL INFECTIONS

A. Epstein–Barr virus (EBV)

1. General characteristics

   a. EBV is human herpes virus 4, a universal virus transmitted via saliva.

   b. The most characteristic disease is mononucleosis (the "kissing disease"). EBV has also been implicated in Burkitt's lymphoma, nasopharyngeal carcinoma, pediatric leiomyomas, collagen vascular diseases, and other disorders.

2. Clinical findings

   a. After an incubation period of several weeks, patients develop fever and sore throat. Oral lesions include exudative pharyngitis, tonsillitis, gingivitis, and soft palate petechiae. Severe infections also exhibit malaise, anorexia, and myalgias.

   b. Lymph nodes, typically the posterior cervical nodes, are enlarged, discrete, and nonsuppurative, with minimal pain.

    c. Splenomegaly is present in 50% of cases.

    d. A maculopapular and, occasionally, petechial rash develops in 15% of cases; administration of amoxicillin raises the incidence of rash to 90%.

    e. Less common manifestations are hepatitis, mononeuropathy, aseptic meningitis, myositis, gallbladder disease, renal failure because of interstitial nephritis, and dyspnea and cough ("pseudocroup").

    f. Complications are many; the most common include secondary bacterial pharyngitis (most commonly strep), splenic rupture, pericarditis, myocarditis, aseptic meningitis, transverse myelitis, and encephalitis.

3. Laboratory studies

    a. An early granulocytopenia is followed by a lymphocytic leukocytosis. Atypical lymphocytes appear as larger cells that stain darker and are frequently vacuolated.

    b. Hemolytic anemia and thrombocytopenia may develop.

    c. Heterophile antibodies and screening mononucleosis tests usually are positive within 4 weeks. A false-positive syphilis test (Venereal Disease Research Laboratory [VDRL] or rapid plasma reagent [RPR]) occurs in 10% of infected patients.

    d. Increased hepatic aminotransferases, increased bilirubin, and decreased cryoglobulins also may be found.

4. Treatment

    a. Treatment is symptomatic, with nonaspirin antipyretics and anti-inflammatories. Antivirals will decrease viral shedding but do not affect the course of the illness.

    b. Patients with splenomegaly should avoid contact sports.

    c. Steroids are indicated for thrombocytopenia, hemolytic anemia, or airway obstruction secondary to enlarged lymph nodes.

    d. Prognosis is good. Although full recovery may take months, 95% recover without specific treatment.

B. Human papillomavirus (HPV)

1. General characteristics

    a. HPV is a group of nonenveloped icosahedral virions. There are 77 known types based on DNA sequence.

    b. They invade the cutaneous and mucosal epithelium, proliferate, and cause warts. The local growths commonly regress, but the virus persists, and lesions frequently recur.

2. Clinical findings

    a. Common skin warts are ubiquitous and most commonly occur in children and young adults.

      (1) Most are caused by HPV types 1 to 4 and typically are asymptomatic.

      (2) Hands and feet most commonly are affected. Plantar warts may cause pain with pressure.

      (3) Warts vary in size, shape, and appearance; they may be flat and superficial or plantar and deep.

    b. Laryngeal warts are caused by serotype 11.

      (1) They are the most common benign epithelial tumors of the larynx.

      (2) In children, they may be life threatening if they obstruct the airway and must be removed surgically.

    c. Anogenital warts (condyloma acuminata) occur in the squamous epithelium of the external genitalia and perianal area.

      (1) They most commonly are caused by HPV types 6 and 11 and are sexually transmitted. Condoms reduce transmission of the virus.

      (2) They rarely turn cancerous, unless the patient is immunosuppressed.

    d. Cervical warts are found in 5% of females and may be visible only by colposcopy.

      (1) Between 40% and 70% will regress.

      (2) HPV types 16, 18, and others have been implicated in intraepithelial cervical dysplasia, neoplasia, and invasive carcinoma.

      (3) A vaccine against HPV types 6, 11, 16, and 18 is available. The vaccine is given as a series of three shots. It is recommended for females ages 11 to 12 years and approved for females ages 9 through 26 years. It is effective against the four most common disease-causing HPV.

3. Laboratory findings

    a. The diagnosis is established by histologic sampling. Hyperplastic prickle cells with excess keratin are found in skin warts. Koilocytotic or vacuolated squamous epithelial cells in clumps on a Pap smear are typical of cervical warts.

    b. Molecular probes have been developed to detect HPV DNA in cervical swabs.

4. Treatment
   a. Spontaneous remission in months to years is typical of skin warts.
   b. The goal of treatment is to reduce the number and frequency of lesions, especially in immunocompromised hosts.
   c. Persistent lesions or cosmetically bothersome lesions may be treated medically or surgically.
      (1) Medical options include liquid nitrogen, salicylic acid, podophyllum, or topical interferon (imiquimod [Aldara]).
      (2) Surgical options include blunt dissection, electrocautery, or carbon dioxide laser.
   d. Recurrence is common.

C. Herpes simplex virus (HSV)
   1. General characteristics
      a. Humans are the only reservoir of HSV. Transmission is via close contact and inoculation of virus into the mucosal surface or through cracks in the skin. The virus is inactivated at room temperature or by drying.
      b. HSV type 1
         (1) More than 85% of the U.S. population has evidence of infection with HSV type 1. Transmission is via infected saliva.
         (2) Primary infection can be asymptomatic or produce severe disease.
         (3) Recurrent, self-limited attacks are common. Precipitating factors include sun exposure, surgery, stress, fever, and viral infection.
      c. HSV type 2
         (1) About 25% of the U.S. population is infected with HSV type 2. Transmission is via sexual contact or from the mother's genital tract during delivery.
         (2) This virus typically causes genital lesions (vulva, vagina, cervix, glans, prepuce, and penile shaft).
         (3) Asymptomatic shedding and painful eruptions can be frequent.
      d. HSV remains latent within the dorsal root ganglia (HSV-1 has a predilection for the trigeminal nerve and HSV-2 for the sacral root ganglia). Reactivation may be precipitated by fever, stress, menses, trauma, ultraviolet light, weight gain or loss, immunosuppression, or other factors. Reactivation is more frequent and more severe in those who are immunocompromised.

   2. Clinical findings
      a. Initial infection has a higher rate of systemic signs, longer duration of herpetic symptoms, and a higher rate of complications.
         (1) Acute herpetic gingivostomatitis (HSV-1)
            (a) This typically occurs in those from 6 months to 5 years of age.
            (b) The incubation period is 3 to 6 days; acute symptoms last 5 to 7 days. Lesions heal in about 2 weeks, although shedding may continue.
            (c) Patients present with abrupt onset, fever, anorexia, listlessness, and gingivitis. Mucosa is red, swollen, and friable. Vesicles appear on the oral mucosa, tongue, and lips; these vesicles may rupture and coalesce to form ulcers and plaques. Regional lymphadenopathy is common.
         (2) Acute herpetic pharyngotonsillitis
            (a) This is common in adults manifesting initial HSV-1 disease and less common in those manifesting HSV-2 disease.
            (b) Patients present with fever, malaise, headache, and sore throat. Vesicles form on the posterior pharynx and tonsils; these vesicles rupture and form shallow ulcers. A grayish exudate may be present over the posterior mucosa.
         (3) Primary genital herpes (invariably HSV-2)
            (a) The initial episode may be asymptomatic or severe, with a prodrome of systemic and local symptoms.
            (b) Preexisting antibodies to HSV-1 may have an ameliorating effect on the severity of primary HSV-2 infection.
            (c) Fever, headache, malaise, and myalgias are common. Vesicles develop on the external genitalia, labia, vaginal mucosa, glans, penis, prepuce, shaft, or perianal area. Nearby cutaneous lesions also may occur.
            (d) Vesicles rupture and form tender ulcers, which crust over. Mucosa may be red and edematous.
            (e) Females tend to have more severe disease and higher rates of complications. The cervix is involved in more than 70% of female patients, manifesting as ulcerative or necrotic mucosa.

b. Recurrence of HSV lesions is heralded by burning or stinging. Neuralgia also may occur, but constitutional symptoms are unlikely.

    (1) Lesions begin as erythematous papules that rapidly develop into tiny, thin-walled, grouped vesicles, which continue to erupt over 1 to 2 weeks.

    (2) Typical locations are the vermillion border (type 1) and the genital area, including the penile shaft, labia, perianal area, and buttocks (type 2).

    (3) On average, HSV-1 infections tend to recur twice per year; maximum shedding is during the first 24 hours. The number of episodes tends to decrease with time.

    (4) In 90% of cases, HSV-2 can reactivate within 12 months. More than 30% of patients have six episodes per year, and about 20% have more than 10 episodes per year. Reactivation can be subclinical; however, viral shedding leads to further transmission of the virus.

c. Complications of HSV infection

    (1) Complications include pyoderma; eczema herpeticum; herpetic whitlow (grouped vesicles on the fingers, common in health care workers); herpes gladiatorum (disseminated cutaneous infections, common in wrestlers); esophagitis; keratoconjunctivitis (dendritic corneal ulcers, may cause blindness); and disseminated neonatal infection. Viremia may result in visceral infection with multiple organ involvement, leukopenia, thrombocytopenia, and disseminated intravascular coagulation (DIC).

    (2) Herpes simplex infection of the central nervous system (CNS) may cause aseptic meningitis, ganglionitis, myelitis, or encephalitis. HSV accounts for 10% to 20% of all encephalitides in the United States. Patients develop headache, meningeal irritation, change in mental status, seizures, and focal necrosis syndromes (temporal cortex, limbic system). CSF shows a moderate pleocytosis of mixed cells, mildly elevated protein, and normal glucose. HSV DNA by PCR or magnetic resonance imaging (MRI) will confirm infection. The mortality rate is greater than 70% without treatment; neurologic sequelae are typical even with treatment.

    (3) Genital herpes in pregnancy is dangerous to both the mother and the infant. First infection during pregnancy has a high risk of disseminated infection and maternal mortality. Infants exposed to herpes in utero or during delivery have a high rate of visceral and CNS infection. Mortality and sequelae rates are high. Cesarean section is recommended for women with active infection.

3. Laboratory studies

    a. The diagnosis usually is established clinically.

    b. Vesicular fluid may be cultured or stained (Tzanck smear), revealing multinucleated giant cells.

    c. Antibodies can be identified in the serum by PCR techniques.

4. Treatment

    a. Local wound care and supportive therapy are recommended.

    b. Treatment is with antivirals (e.g., acyclovir, valacyclovir).

    c. Patients with frequent outbreaks may benefit from suppressive therapy. Foscarnet is beneficial in immunocompromised patients with resistant infections.

    d. Keratitis is treated with trifluridine.

D. Influenza

1. General characteristics

    a. Influenza is caused by an orthomyxovirus. It is readily transmitted through droplet nuclei and occurs in epidemics and pandemics during the fall or winter.

    b. Three strains exist (A, B, and C) and are typed based on the surface antigens hemagglutinin (H) and neuraminidase (N). Influenza A is more pathogenic. Major mutations cause antigenic shifts; minor mutations cause antigenic drifts. Public health authorities follow changes in strains to predict new virus.

    c. An avian influenza A subtype (H5N1) has caused epidemic infection in birds and has been transmitted from birds to humans. If a mutation occurs to allow human-to-human transmission, this highly virulent and lethal subtype could become responsible for widespread disease.

    d. In 2009, a new highly transmissible H1N1 variant emerged with potential to become a severe pandemic.

2. Clinical findings

    a. After an incubation period of 18 to 72 hours, patients exhibit an abrupt fever, chills, malaise, muscle aches, substernal chest pain, headache, nasal stuffiness, and, occasionally, nausea. The fever lasts for 1 to 7 days and is accompanied by coryza, nonproductive cough, photophobia, eye pain, sore throat, pharyngeal injection, and flushed facies. Wheezes and rhonchi may be heard, and children often develop diarrhea.

    b. Primary influenza pneumonia may develop in the elderly or those with chronic cardiovascular disease. Patients exhibit progressive cough, dyspnea, and cyanosis.

    c. Complications are especially common in the elderly and the chronically ill. Necrosis of respiratory epithelium results in secondary bacterial infection (*Staphylococcus*, *Streptococcus*, or *Haemophilus* sp.), acute sinusitis, otitis media, and purulent bronchitis.

    d. Reye's syndrome

      (1) Reye's syndrome is defined as a fatty liver with encephalopathy.

      (2) It is rapidly progressive, has a 30% fatality rate, and may develop 2 to 3 weeks after onset of influenza A or varicella infection, especially if aspirin is ingested. Peak age is 5–14 years; it rarely occurs in patients over age 18 years.

      (3) Clinical manifestations include vomiting, lethargy, jaundice, seizures, hypoglycemia, increased liver enzymes and ammonia levels, prolonged prothrombin time, and changes in mental status.

      (4) Treatment is supportive.

      (5) The mortality rate is approximately 30%.

3. Laboratory studies

    a. Leukopenia and proteinuria may be found.

    b. The virus can be isolated from the throat or nasal mucosa. Viral cultures take 3 to 7 days to return. Direct immunofluorescent tests are labor intensive and less sensitive, but recently developed rapid serology tests are proving to be helpful. Sensitivities range from 50%–70%; specificities 90%–95%. Results are most accurate during the first few days of illness.

    c. Chest radiography in primary influenza pneumonia will show bilateral diffuse infiltrates.

4. Treatment

    a. All patients require supportive care with rest, analgesics, and cough suppressants as needed.

    b. Amantadine and rimantadine are no longer recommended as single therapy agents because of resistance.

    c. Neuraminidase inhibitors (zanamivir inhalation [Relenza] or oral oseltamivir [Tamiflu]) will significantly reduce severity if given within 48 hours of the onset of symptoms. They are effective against both influenza A and influenza B and have fewer side effects than amantadine and rimantadine. They are recommended for patients with influenza requiring hospitalization or in those with high risk of morbidity and mortality.

      (1) The prevalence of resistance to oseltamivir is on the rise. The 2009 recommendation from the CDC is to use zanamivir or a combination of oseltamivir and ramanditine if influenza A is suspected or confirmed. Local surveillance monitoring will provide direction for choice of therapy.

      (2) Neuraminidase inhibitors are contraindicated in patients younger than 12 years. Emergency use with half strength dosing also may be effective in preventing influenza during times of high transmission.

    d. Prognosis in uncomplicated cases is very good; patients generally recover in 1 to 7 days. Morbidity and mortality is highest in the very young and the very old. Pneumonia is the cause of most influenza fatalities.

5. Prevention of influenza is through a trivalent influenza virus vaccine.

    a. Its configuration is based on the strains isolated during the preceding year. The vaccine should be given to all patients yearly in October or November and is especially recommended for all people older than 65 years (some sources suggest all people older than 50 years), children or adolescents on chronic aspirin therapy, nursing home residents, patients with chronic lung or heart disease, and all health care workers.

    b. The vaccine is contraindicated in patients with hypersensitivity to eggs or other components of the vaccine, during acute febrile illness, or in cases of thrombocytopenia.

    c. Tenderness, redness, and induration at the injection site may occur; myalgias and fever are rare. It also is available as a nasal spray (FluMist) for those from 5 to 49 years of age.

    d. Immunity is set within 2 weeks of the vaccination. Antibodies wane quickly in the elderly and the sick, but the vaccine has been proven to decrease mortality and morbidity from the flu.

E. Varicella-zoster

1. General characteristics

    a. Varicella virus is highly contagious, especially the day before the rash appears.

    b. The incubation period is 10 to 20 days. A single attack confers lifelong immunity.

    c. Most cases occur in late winter or spring.

    d. It typically is a benign illness in childhood, but it can be life threatening, especially in adults or the immunocompromised.

    e. Zoster represents reactivation of varicella virus that has been dormant in ganglionic satellite cells.

    f. Outbreaks may be precipitated by illness, stress, or advancing age.

2. Clinical findings

    a. Varicella is characterized by a generalized eruption that follows a centripetal pattern.

         (1) Lesions begin as erythematous macules and papules, form superficial vesicles, and later crust over.

         (2) Lesions appear in "crops," so at any given time, several morphologies can be identified.

         (3) The mucous membranes also may be involved.

    b. Systemic symptoms are highly variable and include low-grade fever, malaise, muscles aches, arthralgias, and headache. Severe, progressive infections manifest with deeper lesions of the lung, liver, pancreas, or brain; the mortality rate approaches 10%.

    c. Complications are varied, including secondary bacterial infection of excoriated lesions, varicella embryopathy, and Reye's syndrome.

    d. Zoster is characterized by a painful eruption, usually following a dermatomal pattern. The thoracic and lumbar areas are the most common sites. Trigeminal eruptions that include the tip of the nose (Hutchinson's sign) risk corneal involvement.

3. Laboratory findings

    a. The diagnosis is established clinically.

    b. Confirmatory laboratory studies rarely are done, but, if necessary, serology and fluorescent microscopy will confirm the diagnosis.

4. Treatment

    a. Treatment generally is supportive.

    b. Prevention

         (1) Prevention of bacterial superinfection involves good hygiene and trimming of fingernails.

         (2) Immunocompromised patients exposed to varicella should receive acyclovir and varicella-zoster immunoglobulin.

         (3) Anecdotal evidence suggests that steroids may prevent postherpetic neuralgia in some patients. Postherpetic neuralgia rates are higher in the elderly and in patients with trigeminal lesions and can be quite debilitating. Treatment is difficult; choices include tricyclic antidepressants, capsaicin cream, narcotic analgesics, or corticosteroids.

         (4) Prevention of varicella is through a live attenuated vaccine given at 1 to 2 years of age. Older patients without evidence of immunity should receive two doses, given 2 months apart. Avoid giving the vaccine during pregnancy.

         (5) Zostavax vaccine was licensed in 2006. A single dose is indicated in patients aged 60 years or older. It has been shown effective in cutting the incidence of shingles by 50% and substantially reducing the risk of postherpetic neuralgia. It is contraindicated in patients who are allergic to gelatin or neomycin, are immunocompromised, have untreated tuberculosis, or are pregnant.

F. Rabies

1. General characteristics

    a. Rhabdovirus is transmitted via infected saliva from an animal bite or an open wound.

    b. Vectors include dogs, bats, skunks, foxes, raccoons, and coyotes; rodents and lagomorphs do not transmit rabies.

    c. Incubation period between the bite and the onset of symptoms is from 10 days to years (typically 3 to 7 weeks). A correlation exists between the length of incubation and the distance of the wound from the brain.

2. Clinical findings

    a. A history of an animal bite may not be apparent.

    b. There typically is pain and paresthesias at the site; the skin is sensitive to changes in temperature and wind.

    c. Patients are restless, with muscle spasms and extreme excitability. They exhibit bizarre behavior, convulsions, and paralysis. Thick, tenacious saliva is produced.

    d. Hydrophobia is defined as painful spasms caused by drinking water.

    e. Less commonly, patients may exhibit an ascending paralysis.

3. Laboratory studies

    a. Suspect animals should be sacrificed so that their brains can be tested for the virus using fluorescent antibody markers.

    b. Domestic animals may be quarantined and observed for bizarre behavior.

    c. PCR tests and genetic probes for use in humans are expensive and often negative early in the disease.

    d. CSF may show rabies reverse transcriptase by PCR. MRI may reveal nonenhancing, ill-defined changes in the brain stem, hypothalamus, or subcortical matter.

4. Treatment
   a. No specific treatment against rabies disease is available. Mechanical ventilation and oxygen therapy should be started. Rabies vaccine immunoglobulin is given along with monoclonal antibodies, ribaviron, interferon-α, and ketamine. It is almost universally fatal within 7 days, most likely from respiratory failure.
   b. Prevention is key.
      (1) Control of bat populations is helpful in preventing spread.
      (2) All household pets should be immunized. Persons who are exposed regularly (vets, park rangers) also should receive active immunization.
   c. After an animal bite, local care with cleansing, debridement, and flushing is recommended. Wounds should not be sutured.
   d. Postexposure immunization includes rabies immunoglobulin (in the wound and IM at a distant site) and human diploid cell vaccine (HDCV). Five injections of 1 mL IM are given on days 0, 3, 7, 14, and 28. The vaccine may cause pruritus, erythema, and tenderness in 25% of cases, and 20% also develop myalgias, headache, and nausea.
   e. If the patient has received active immunization in the past, immunoglobulin is not given; HDCV doses are given on days 0 and 3 only.
   f. Preexposure vaccination of persons at high risk (vets, animal handlers, Peace Corps volunteers, travelers) is accomplished with IM HDCV doses on days 0, 7, and either 21 or 28. HDCV also can be administered intradermally on days 0, 7, and 28. Rabies antibody titers should be checked every 2 years; boosters are given to persons who become seronegative.

G. HIV and AIDS
   1. General characteristics
      a. HIV was first recognized when a cluster of patients with opportunistic infections was identified in 1981. A human retrovirus that requires reverse transcriptase for replication was later identified as the cause.
      b. Currently, more than 40 million people worldwide are infected with the virus. The highest prevalence is in Central and East Subsaharan Africa, where approximately one-third of all adults are infected. An estimated 5 million new cases and 3 million deaths occur per year worldwide.
      c. HIV infects all cells containing the T4 antigen, primarily the CD4 helper inducer lymphocytes.
         (1) The result is a disordered function of the immune system.
         (2) HIV attaches to the T4 antigen, replicates, and causes cell fusion or cell death.
         (3) Macrophages serve as a reservoir of virus and promote its dissemination to other organs.
      d. HIV is transmitted through bodily fluids. Risk includes sexual contact, parenteral exposure (blood or blood products, including injection drug use and occupational exposure), and perinatal exposure.
   2. Clinical features
      a. The acute HIV syndrome is infrequently identified. It is a cluster of nonspecific findings similar to EBV infection. Some patients may develop persistent generalized lymphadenopathy without symptomatic HIV disease.
      b. HIV disease is a syndrome of nonspecific and specific diagnoses. It can be progressive and insidious, or it can be rapidly fatal. The time from infection to symptomatic disease averages 10 years but is quite variable.
      c. Systemic manifestations include fever, night sweats, and weight loss. The wasting syndrome is a result of increased metabolic rate and decreased protein synthesis. There is disproportionate loss of muscle mass.
      d. Immunodeficiency causes infections and malignant diseases at any site; common sites include the lungs, upper respiratory system, lymph system, CNS, peripheral nervous system (PNS), mouth, GI tract, eyes, and skin.
      e. AIDS is defined by the CDC as a CD4 count below 200 cells/μL or the development of an AIDS indicator disease (Table 14-2). A diagnosis of AIDS can be made with or without laboratory evidence of HIV infection.
      f. Opportunistic infections and malignancies develop as the CD4 count drops (Table 14-3). Few patients in the United States develop opportunistic infections or malignancies because of the successes of highly active antiretroviral therapy.
      g. The current World Health Organization HIV/AIDS Classification System is based on symptoms: stage I, asymptomatic disease; stage II, minor symptoms; stage III, moderate symptoms; stage IV, AIDS. In general, as the CD4 count decreases, the viral load increases, and symptoms of infections and malignancies become more frequent and severe.
   3. Laboratory studies
      a. Screening for HIV infection detects antibodies. Two enzyme-linked immunosorbent assay (ELISA) tests followed by a confirmatory Western blot analysis confirm HIV infection with a sensitivity of greater than 95%; most patients develop antibodies within 6 months of exposure.

TABLE 14-2 **AIDS Indicator Diseases**
Bacterial infections, multiple or recurrent
Candidiasis
Bronchi, trachea, or lungs
Esophageal
Cervical cancer, invasive
Coccidioidomycosis, disseminated or extrapulmonary
Cryptococcosis, extrapulmonary
Cryptosporidiosis, chronic intestinal (>1 month)
Cytomegalovirus disease (other than liver, spleen, or nodes)
Encephalopathy, HIV related
Herpes simplex
Chronic ulcer(s) (>1 month)
Bronchitis, pneumonitis, or esophagitis
Histoplasmosis, disseminated or extrapulmonary
Isosporiasis, chronic intestinal (>1 month)
Kaposi's sarcoma
Lymphoid interstitial pneumonia and/or pulmonary lymphoid hyperplasia
Lymphoma
Burkitt's (or equivalent term)
Immunoblastic (or equivalent term)
Primary, of brain
Mycobacterium sp.
Mycobacterium avium complex or *Mycobacterium kansasii*, disseminated or any site
Mycobacterium tuberculosis, any site
Mycobacterium, other species or unidentified species, disseminated or extrapulmonary
Pneumocystis jiroveci (nee *carinii*) pneumonia
Pneumonia, recurrent
Progressive multifocal leukoencephalopathy
Salmonella septicemia, recurrent
Toxoplasmosis of brain
Wasting syndrome, HIV related

(1) Persons at high risk for infection, patients in all health care settings and all pregnant women should be tested for HIV.

(2) Testing is recommended after notifying the patient that it will be done unless the patient opts out.

(3) Written separate consent is no longer recommended by the CDC.

b. Other laboratory findings may include anemia, leukopenia, thrombocytopenia, polyclonal hypergammaglobulinemia, hypercholesterolemia, and cutaneous anergy.

c. The CD4 count typically decreases as the illness progresses. For best accuracy, it should be measured at the same time of day and by the same laboratory. Patients with a CD4 count of greater than 350 cells/μL can have levels measured every 6 months; otherwise, it should be measured every 3 months or with any change in patient status. Risk of disease progression increases with a CD4 count of less than 200 cells/μL or CD4 lymphocyte percentage of less than 20%.

d. The viral load is a measure of actively replicating virus, which correlates with disease progression. Changing viral loads also may support treatment response.

4. Treatment

a. Prevention is essential if the HIV epidemic is to end. Primary prevention efforts include safer sex with barrier methods (latex only), harm reduction programs, drug rehabilitation, screening of all blood products, and universal precautions in health care delivery. Development of a vaccine against HIV has been unsuccessful.

TABLE 14-3	HIV-related Illnesses by Usual CD4 Count
CD4 Count	**Illness**
Any time; generally <500	*Salmonella*, recurrent or septicemia
	Clostridium difficile colitis
	Kaposi's sarcoma
	Mycobacterium tuberculosis, pulmonary, extrapulmonary, or disseminated
	Herpes simplex; herpes zoster
<200	*Candida*, esophagus, bronchi, trachea, lungs
	HIV encephalopathy; AIDS dementia syndrome
	Pneumocystis jiroveci (nee *carinii*) pneumonia
<100	B-cell lymphoma (non-Hodgkin's)
	Toxoplasmosis
	Isospora; *Microsporidia*
	Histoplasmosis
	Cryptococcosis
	Coccidioidomycosis
	Cryptosporidia
<50	PML
	MAC
	Cytomegalovirus
	CNS lymphoma

PML, progressive multifocal leukoencephalopathy; MAC, *Mycobacterium avium* complex; CNS, central nervous system.

b. Secondary prevention efforts include antiretrovirals (Table 14-4) and chemoprophylaxis. Patients should be screened for diseases such as tuberculosis and other infections, and they must be counseled on ways to maintain health and prevent spread of the virus.

c. Postexposure prophylaxis (PEP) may be offered to individuals with a high probability of exposure, including health care workers who sustain occupational injuries. PEP should be started within 72 hours of exposure.

(1) The chance of contracting HIV from a needlestick injury involving a patient with known HIV disease is 0.3%.

(2) Health care workers who sustain an injury must be counseled. Testing should be done on the health care worker and the patient; retesting is recommended in 6 weeks, 3 months, and 6 months.

(3) Antiretroviral therapy is an option; the decision to begin therapy should be made by the patient. Combination therapy with drugs from different classes should be continued for at least 4 weeks. Full-course PEP reduces the chance of HIV transmission by up to 70%.

d. Pregnant women with HIV disease should be counseled on the risk to the fetus. Antiretroviral therapy to the mother during pregnancy, labor, and delivery and to the newborn reduces the chance of transmission significantly. HIV also can be transmitted through breast milk.

e. Drug treatment of HIV disease includes antiretroviral therapy and treatment of or prophylaxis against opportunistic infections and malignancies.

(1) The patient must be counseled and made to understand the complexity of treatment. Combination antiretroviral therapy is based on CD4 count, viral load, and overall patient status (nutrition, compliance, access, and acceptance of therapy). Treatment may be aggressive, complex, and toxic.

(2) Patients must be monitored closely for adherence, effectiveness, adverse effects, and resistance.

(3) The goal is suppression of the viral load. A rising or persistently high viral load, clinical progression, or continued immunologic deterioration signals treatment failure.

(4) Prophylaxis against opportunistic infections and malignancies is based on the likelihood of developing disease as judged by the CD4 count and viral load. Discontinuation of prophylaxis after a sustained response to highly active antiretroviral therapy may be considered.

TABLE 14-4 Antiretroviral Medications

Drug Category	Drug	Common Adverse Effects
NRTIs	Zidovudine (AZT; Retrovir)	Anemia, neutropenia, nausea, malaise, headache, insomnia, myopathy
	Didanosine (ddI; Videx)	Pancreatitis, peripheral neuropathy, hepatitis
	Zalcitabine (ddC; Hivid)	Pancreatitis, peripheral neuropathy, hepatitis
	Stavudine (d4; Zerit)	Peripheral neuropathy, hepatitis, pancreatitis
	Lamivudine (3TC; Epivir)	Peripheral neuropathy, rash
	Emtricitabine (Emtriva)	Dyspigmentation, especially palms and soles
	Abacavir (Ziagen)	Rash, fever
NNRTIs	Nevirapine (Viramune)	Rash
	Delavirdine (Rescriptor)	Rash
	Efavirenz (Sustiva)	Neurologic manifestations
Protease inhibitors	Saquinavir (Fortovase, Invirase)	Headache, GI dysfunction
	Ritonavir (Norvir)	Peripheral paresthesias, GI dysfunction
	Indinavir (Crixivan)	Renal calculi
	Nelfinavir (Viracept)	Diarrhea
	Amprenavir (Invirase)	Rash, GI dysfunction
	Lopinavir/ritonavir (Kaletra)	Diarrhea
	Fosamprenavir (Lexiva)	GI symptoms, rash
	Atazanavir (Reyatez)	Hyperbilirubinemia
Nucleotide reverse transcriptase inhibitors	Tenofovir (Viread)	GI distress, renal insufficiency
Entry inhibitors	Enfuvirtide (Fuzeon)	Injection site pain, allergic reactions

NRTI, nucleoside reverse transcriptase inhibitor; AZT, zidovudine, azidothymidine; NNRTI, nonnucleoside reverse transcriptase inhibitor; GI, gastrointestinal.

H. Cytomegalovirus (CMV; human herpes virus type 5)

1. General characteristics

   a. Most infections with CMV are asymptomatic.

   b. Illness occurs in the immunocompromised, especially patients with HIV disease or posttransplant.

2. Clinical findings

   a. Perinatal infection and CMV inclusion disease occur in 10% of babies born to mothers with primary CMV infection during pregnancy.

   (1) The infant may be asymptomatic until later in life.

   (2) Clinical findings include jaundice, hepatosplenomegaly, thrombocytopenia, periventricular CNS calcifications, mental retardation, motor disability, and purpura.

   b. Acute acquired CMV can be transmitted through sexual contact, breast milk, blood transfusion, or respiratory droplets. Patients develop fever, malaise, myalgias, arthralgias, splenomegaly, abnormal liver enzymes, leukopenia, and atypical lymphocytes. It is similar to EBV infection but without pharyngitis, respiratory symptoms, or heterophil antibodies.

   c. Posttransplant patients and those who are otherwise immunocompromised are at risk for myriad clinical manifestations.

   (1) Retinitis occurs with a CD4 count of less than 50 cells/μL. Examination reveals neovascularization and proliferative lesions, commonly referred to as "pizza pie." With aggressive treatment of HIV disease, the frequency of retinitis can be reduced.

   (2) GI manifestations include esophagitis and odynophagia, small bowel inflammatory ulcers, diarrhea, hematochezia, abdominal pain, weight loss, and cholangiopathy. Diagnosis may require biopsy.

   (3) Pulmonary manifestations occur in 15% of bone marrow transplant patients; 80% to 90% of these are fatal.

   (4) Neurologic manifestations include polyradiculopathy, transverse myelitis, and encephalitis.

   (5) CMV infection is theorized to play a role in the pathogenesis of inflammatory bowel disease, atherosclerosis, and breast cancer.

3. Laboratory studies
   a. Patients may exhibit lymphocytosis or leukopenia.
   b. Culture is very difficult; antigens can be detected in blood, urine, or CSF via PCR.
   c. Tissue biopsy looks for intracytoplasmic inclusions ("owls' eyes").
4. Treatment
   a. Measures to prevent CMV infection include limiting blood transfusions, filtering to remove leukocytes, and restricting the organ donor pool to seronegative donors. CMV immunoglobulin and IV ganciclovir reduce the risk of pneumonia in bone marrow transplant recipients.
   b. Ganciclovir, valganciclovir, foscarnet, and cidofovir are effective against CMV.
      (1) Initial IV loading therapy is followed by maintenance therapy.
      (2) Sustained-release ganciclovir implants for suppression of retinal infections are effective.

IV. FUNGAL INFECTIONS

A. Candidiasis
   1. General characteristics
      a. *Candida albicans* is the most common form of pathogenic *Candida* sp. It is part of the normal flora of human hosts and is an opportunistic pathogen.
      b. Risk factors for disease include neutropenia, recent surgery, chronic illness (especially diabetes mellitus), broad-spectrum antibiotic therapy, IV catheterization (especially total parenteral nutrition), chemotherapy or corticosteroids, injection drug use, and cellular immunodeficiency, as in HIV disease.
   2. Clinical findings and treatment
      a. Cutaneous disease
         (1) Diaper dermatitis commonly is caused by *Candida* sp. and does not indicate immune deficiency in newborns. The diaper area is red, with defined margins. Pustules, vesicles, papules, or scales may be seen, and satellite lesions are characteristic.
         (2) Children and adults (particularly adults with diabetes) may develop candidal dermatitis in dark, moist areas, such as axillae or under the breasts or large pannus, especially if the immune system is stressed. Lesions have distinct borders, and satellite lesions are common.
         (3) Treatment is with topical antifungal creams.
      b. Mucosal disease of the mouth and esophagus
         (1) Oral mucosal candidiasis (thrush) causes white plaques that can be scraped off, revealing reddened mucosa. In denture wearers, infection may manifest as a painful red palate.
         (2) Esophagitis is heralded by odynophagia and pain on swallowing. Symptoms resemble gastroesophageal reflux.
         (3) Treatment is with oral fluconazole, itraconazole, or amphotericin B if recurrent or recalcitrant.
      c. Vulvovaginal disease occurs in 75% of females at least once during their lifetime.
         (1) Risk factors include age extremes, pregnancy, uncontrolled diabetes mellitus, corticosteroids, and HIV disease.
         (2) Symptoms include pruritus, burning, dyspareunia, and a white, cottage cheese or curd-like discharge. Physical examination reveals white plaques on vaginal walls.
         (3) Treatment is with topical azoles or oral fluconazole.
      d. Candidal fungemia can be life threatening.
         (1) It occurs in very ill patients with indwelling instrumentation. Any suspect catheters should be removed.
         (2) IV amphotericin B is recommended. The mortality rate is greater than 40%.
         (3) If disseminated disease develops (positive blood cultures; retinal lesions; infection of skin, brain, meninges, or myocardium), flucytosine should be added; alternatively, fluconazole can be tried.
      e. Hepatosplenic candidiasis occurs in patients with very low WBC counts, such as those with leukemia.
         (1) With aggressive chemotherapy, the WBC count begins to rise, and the patient develops fever, right upper quadrant pain and tenderness, and nausea.
         (2) An increase in alkaline phosphatase and multiple low-density defects in the liver, spleen, and kidneys develop. The diagnosis is confirmed with biopsy.
         (3) Treatment is amphotericin B; once the patient is responding, he or she can be switched to fluconazole.

f. Endocarditis occurs through direct inoculation at surgery, in injection drug users, or in late-stage HIV disease.

   (1) Approximately 50% of cases involve nonalbicans *Candida* sp. and are resistant to treatment. These organisms cause large vegetations.

   (2) Splenomegaly, petechiae, murmur, and large vessel embolization are common.

   (3) Treatment is amphotericin B, but infected valves must be surgically replaced. Once the patient has recovered, he or she typically will receive lifelong fluconazole.

B. Histoplasmosis

1. General characteristics

   a. *Histoplasma capsulatum* is a dimorphic fungus found in soil infested with bird or bat droppings.

   b. It is endemic to many areas and is transmitted by inhalation.

2. Clinical findings

   a. Most infections are asymptomatic or mild and unrecognized. Patients with cellular immunodeficiency are at risk for symptomatic infections.

   b. Acute histoplasmosis occurs in epidemics when soil is disturbed. Patients are prostrate and febrile, with few pulmonary complaints.

   c. Progressive disseminated histoplasmosis may be fatal within 6 weeks. Patients complain of fever, dyspnea, cough, weight loss, and prostration; ulcers may develop in the mouth, pharynx, liver, spleen, adrenals, and elsewhere.

   d. Chronic progressive pulmonary histoplasmosis occurs in older patients, especially those with chronic obstructive pulmonary disease (COPD). It manifests as chronic progressive pulmonary changes with calcified nodes and pericarditis.

   e. Disseminated disease occurs in immunocompromised patients, especially those with late-stage HIV disease. It more likely represents reactivation rather than a new acute infection.

   (1) Highest risk is with a CD4 count of less than 100 cells/μL. Patients develop fever and multiorgan failure; fulminant disease, septic shock, and death are common.

   (2) Chest radiography shows miliary infiltrates.

3. Laboratory studies

   a. Anemia of chronic disease and increased alkaline phosphatase, lactate dehydrogenase (LDH), and ferritin are seen in the severely ill. A pancytopenia also may develop.

   b. A urine antigen assay can confirm the presence of disseminated disease; bronchoalveolar lavage may be done with chronic pulmonary disease.

4. Treatment

   a. Itraconazole orally for weeks to months is recommended.

   b. Amphotericin B is recommended for patients who cannot tolerate or fail itraconazole therapy or in patients with meningitis or severe disease.

   c. Lifelong suppressive therapy with itraconazole is recommended for the immunocompromised.

C. *Cryptococcus* sp.

1. General characteristics

   a. *Cryptococcus neoforms* is an encapsulated, budding yeast found in soil contaminated with dried pigeon dung.

   b. It is transmitted through inhalation and causes illness in patients with cellular immune deficiency, such as HIV, cancer, or long-term corticosteroid therapy.

2. Clinical findings

   a. Pulmonary disease may develop in patients with chronic obstructive pulmonary disease, chronic steroid use, or post transplant. Fever, cough, and dyspnea occur; chest radiography reveals nodules or pneumonitis.

   b. Cryptococcal CNS disease causes headache and meningeal signs. It occurs with a CD4 count of less than 50 cells/μL. Patients exhibit mental status changes and cranial nerve or visual abnormalities.

   c. Cryptococcoma is a rare, intracerebral mass lesion that causes obstructive hydrocephalus.

   d. Disseminated disease, although rare, may affect the skin, prostate, osteoarticular surfaces, eye, lymph tissue, or other sites.

3. Laboratory studies

   a. CSF shows variable pleocytosis (predominantly lymphocytes), increased opening pressure, increased protein, and decreased glucose.

    b. Budding, encapsulated fungus may be isolated on culture.

    c. Cryptococcal antigen can be detected in CSF and serum. India ink stain or serology with latex agglutination assay or cryptococcal antigen assay (CRAG) is helpful.

    d. Computed tomography (CT) or MRI is indicated if cryptococcoma is suspected.

4. Treatment

    a. In patients with HIV disease, oral fluconazole is continued for 10 weeks. In severe infections, amphotericin B can be given for the first 2 weeks, followed by oral fluconazole. Flucytosine may be added in severe disease. Lifelong fluconazole therapy is recommended.

    b. In non-HIV immunocompromised patients, the mortality rate is much higher. Treatment is amphotericin B.

D. *Pneumocystis jiroveci* pneumonia (PCJ; formerly known as *Pneumocystis carinii* pneumonia [PCP])

1. General characteristics

    a. PJP is caused by a fungus found in the lungs of humans and many animals. Evidence of infection can be found in almost all persons by a young age. It probably is transmitted through the air and lies latent in alveoli.

    b. Premature or debilitated infants in underdeveloped areas are infected during epidemics. Sporadic cases are found in patients with abnormal cellular immunity, which is caused by factors such as cancer, severe malnutrition, immunosuppressive drugs, irradiation, or in those with HIV/AIDS and a CD4 count of less than 200 cells/μL.

    c. PJP is the most common opportunistic infection in HIV disease.

2. Clinical findings

    a. Typically, PJP disease presents with fever, shortness of breath, and a nonproductive cough. Physical examination findings are disproportionate to imaging results, which show diffuse interstitial infiltrates that may be heterogeneous, miliary, or patchy. Between 5% and 10% of patients have a normal chest radiograph.

    b. Less commonly, patients may present with spontaneous pneumothorax. Recurrent pneumothorax is related to previous pentamidine use.

    c. Patients also may develop fatigue, weakness, and weight loss. Infection is likely to recur without treatment of the underlying disease or chemoprophylaxis.

3. Laboratory studies

    a. Blood gas reveals hypoxia, hypocapnia, and reduced carbon dioxide diffusion. LDH typically is increased, and the WBC count usually is low.

    b. The organism can be demonstrated with specific stains of induced sputum or via bronchoalveolar lavage.

4. Treatment

    a. Empiric treatment is recommended for immunocompromised patients presenting with cough or dyspnea. The drug of choice is TMP/SMX.

        (1) Patients often get worse at the start of treatment. Steroids are added if the partial pressure of oxygen in arterial blood (PaO$_2$) is less than 70 mm Hg to prevent deterioration and promote oxygenation.

        (2) Hypersensitivity reactions to TMP/SMX (likely because of the sulfa component) manifest with fever, rash, malaise, neutropenia, hepatitis, nephritis, thrombocytopenia, and hyperbilirubinemia. Systematic desensitization often is successful.

    b. Dapsone is an alternative treatment and is as effective as TMP/SMX. It is more expensive than TMP/SMX, but it is a good choice for patients who are sensitive to sulfa. Side effects include anemia, rash, and fever. It should not be taken with didanoside.

    c. Alternatively, pentamidine can be used either IV or IM. Nebulized pentamide can be used to prevent PJP. Side effects include rash, neutropenia, abnormal liver function, serum folate deficiency, calcium imbalance, hypoglycemia or hyperglycemia, hyponatremia, and nephrotoxicity. Rarely, fatal pancreatitis occurs.

    d. Atovaquone is reserved for patients who cannot tolerate TMP/SMX or pentamidine. It must be taken with a fatty meal and causes mild to minimal side effects.

    e. Once a patient is successfully treated for PJP, prophylaxis is continued. All patients with a CD4 count of less than 200 cells/μL also should receive prophylactic treatment. TMP/SMX is the drug of choice.

V. PARASITIC INFECTIONS

A. Amebiasis

1. General characteristics

    a. Cysts of *Entamoeba histolytica* are viable in the soil and water for weeks to months. Transmission to humans, the only host, occurs through fecally contaminated food or water, fly droppings, or human-to-human contact.

b. Once ingested, cysts pass through to the intestines where they hatch. Trophozoites invade the mucosa and induce necrosis. Amebic ulcers typically are flask shaped and occur anywhere in the large bowel or terminal ileum. They usually are limited to the muscularis, but if they penetrate the serosa, they may cause perforation, abscess, or peritonitis.

2. Clinical findings

  a. Intestinal disease often is asymptomatic.

  b. Colitis can be mild to moderate (few semiformed stools without blood) or severe dysentery (greater number of liquid stools streaked with blood or bits of necrotic tissue).

   (1) Patients may have cramps, fatigue, weight loss, and increased flatulence. Cycles of remission and recurrence are typical.

   (2) Physical examination may reveal distention, hyperperistalsis, and generalized abdominal tenderness during recurrences.

   (3) Patients with severe disease become prostrate and toxic with fever, colic, tenesmus, and vomiting.

   (4) Complications include appendicitis, bowel perforation, fulminant colitis, massive mucosal sloughing, and hemorrhage.

   (5) Localized ulcerative lesions of the colon and localized granulomatous lesions of the colon (ameboma) result in pain, intestinal obstruction, and hemorrhage.

   (6) Amebomas may be single or multiple and must be differentiated from colon cancer, tuberculosis, or lymphogranuloma venereum. Biopsy reveals granulation tissue.

  c. Extraintestinal disease

   (1) Hepatic amebiasis and amebic liver abscess can be asymptomatic or result in symptoms either suddenly or gradually, over days to months.

   (2) Findings include fever, pain, tender hepatomegaly, malaise, prostration, sweating, chills, anorexia, and weight loss.

   (3) Pulmonary symptoms (coughing, right lower lung findings) may occur if the abscess is in the superior liver.

   (4) Abscesses may rupture and spill into the pleural, peritoneal, or pericardial space; this can be fatal.

   (5) Less commonly, amebiasis may metastasize to the lungs, brain, or genitalia.

3. Laboratory studies

  a. Stool specimens reveal cysts or trophozoites. Sigmoidoscopy, colonoscopy, or rectal biopsy shows ulcers; collection of exudates should be examined for trophozoites.

  b. Serology can detect antibodies up to 10 years after infection and, therefore, cannot be used to differentiate past from present infection. Serology will be positive, but stool examination frequently is negative.

  c. WBC count is moderately elevated but without eosinophilia. There will be minimal changes, if any, to liver enzymes.

  d. Ultrasonography, CT, MRI, or radioisotope scanning reveals the size and location of hepatic abscesses.

4. Treatment

  a. Asymptomatic infection should be treated with a luminal amebicide (diloxanide furoate, iodoquinol, or paromomycin).

  b. Mild to moderate infections should be treated with tinidazole or metronidazole plus a luminal amebicide. Alternatives include tetracycline and a luminal amebicide followed by chloroquine.

  c. Severe infection also should be supported with fluids, electrolyte replacement, and opioids to control bowel motility and decrease the risk of toxic megacolon.

  d. Hepatic abscess is treated with tinidazole or metronidazole plus a luminal amebicide, followed by chloroquine. If there is no response within 3 days of initial treatment, the abscess should be drained. Complications include bacterial infection, bleeding, and peritoneal spillage.

  e. Follow up with at least three stool examinations at 2- to 3-day intervals starting 2 to 4 weeks after the end of treatment.

   (1) Colonoscopy also may be used to confirm treatment success.

   (2) Postdysenteric colitis after severe infection usually is self-limited but may be a trigger for ulcerative colitis.

  f. Prognosis with treatment is very good. Without treatment, mortality can be high.

  g. Prevention is through adequate control of the food and water supply, proper sanitation, and personal hygiene.

B. Hookworms

  1. General characteristics

    a. Hookworm is endemic to the moist tropics and subtropics.

      (1) Sporadic cases occur in the southeastern United States; 25% of the world's population is infected.

      (2) Humans are the only host.

    b. Eggs are passed in the stool and hatch in moist soil.

      (1) The larvae last for hours to weeks. They penetrate the skin and migrate in the bloodstream to the pulmonary capillaries, where they destroy alveoli and are carried by cilia to the mouth. Once swallowed, the larvae attach to the small bowel mucosa and suck blood. Once mature, they release eggs to continue the cycle.

      (2) A light infection is defined as 1,000 eggs/g feces and moderate infection as 2,000 to 8,000 eggs/g feces.

  2. Clinical findings

    a. The site of penetration is pruritic. An erythematous dermatitis with maculopapular or vesicular eruption follows; scratching can cause secondary bacterial infections.

    b. The pulmonary stage may cause cough, wheeze, blood-tinged sputum, and low-grade fever.

    c. With a light infection and adequate iron intake, the patient may remain asymptomatic during the intestinal stage. Heavy infection leads to anorexia, diarrhea, vague pain, and ulcer-like epigastric symptoms. Severe infection causes anemia, protein loss, and malabsorption.

  3. Laboratory studies

    a. The eggs can be demonstrated in feces.

    b. Stool is positive for occult blood. Hypochromic microcytic anemia and eosinophilia may be found.

  4. Treatment

    a. Mebendazole (twice per day for 3 days) or either pyrantel or albendazole (once daily for 2 to 3 days) is effective.

    b. Pyrantel cannot be used in children younger than 5 years; none of the treatments are recommended in pregnancy.

    c. Supportive treatment includes a high-protein diet, vitamins, and ferrous sulfate.

C. Pinworms (enterobiasis)

  1. General characteristics

    a. Humans are the only host for *Enterobius vermicularis.* There is a worldwide distribution, and children are infected more often than adults.

    b. Adult worms are loosely attached to the mucosa, primarily in the cecum. Gravid females pass through the anus to lay eggs on the perianal skin. Each female is capable of producing a large number of eggs. The eggs are viable for 2 to 3 weeks outside the host and are infective within a few hours.

    c. Infection is easily passed through hands, food, drink, and fomites. The eggs are swallowed and hatch in the duodenum; larvae pass to the cecum and mature in 3 to 4 weeks. The lifespan is 30 to 45 days.

  2. Clinical findings

    a. Many patients are asymptomatic.

    b. Characteristic symptoms include perianal pruritus (crawling sensation that is worse at night), insomnia, weight loss, enuresis, and irritability. Examination at night may reveal worms in the anus or in the stool. Scratching causes excoriations and impetigo.

    c. Migration can cause vulvovaginitis, diverticulitis, appendicitis, cystitis, and granulomatous reactions.

  3. Laboratory studies: Eggs can be captured on a piece of cellophane tape over the perianal skin; three tries over three consecutive nights are 90% successful.

  4. Treatment

    a. All members of the household should be treated concurrently.

    b. Albendazole, mebendazole, or pyrantel is given in a single dose and then repeated 2 to 4 weeks later.

    c. Hand washing after defecation and before meals must be stressed. Linens should be washed thoroughly.

D. Malaria

  1. General characteristics

    a. *Plasmodium vivax, Plasmodium malariae, Plasmodium ovale,* and *Plasmodium falciparum* are endemic to the tropics and subtropics.

    b. There are 300 to 500 million cases per year worldwide, with 1 million deaths. There are 800 cases per year in the United States; almost all are imported.

   c. Transmission is through the bite of the *Anopheles* mosquito.

     (1) The mosquito ingests the parasite, and sporozoites mature and get transferred to humans via saliva. Incubation period ranges between 8 and 60 days.

     (2) The sporozoites invade hepatocytes and mature as tissue schizonts. The schizonts escape the liver and invade red blood cells, where they multiply and cause rupture of the cell within 48 hours.

     (3) The cycle of invasion, multiplication, and red blood cell rupture continues.

2. Clinical findings

   a. The typical malarial attack starts with shaking chills (the cold stage), followed by fever (the hot stage), and, finally, diaphoresis (the sweating stage).

     (1) Patients are fatigued between attacks.

     (2) Release of tissue necrosis factors and cytokines contributes to fatigue, headache, dizziness, GI complaints, myalgias, arthralgias, backache, and dry cough.

     (3) There may be liver and spleen enlargement if symptoms continue for more than 4 days.

   b. Infection with *Plasmodium falciparum* can be much more severe and can manifest as cerebral malaria, hyperpyrexia, hemolytic anemia, noncardiogenic pulmonary edema, acute tubular necrosis, adrenal insufficiency, cardiac dysrhythmias, and other complications.

3. Laboratory studies

   a. Blood films are stained with Giemsa or Wright stain and examined at 8-hour intervals for 3 days during and between attacks. The percentage of infected red blood cells ranges from 5% to 20%.

   b. During attacks, leukocytosis or leukopenia may develop.

   c. Severe infections cause hepatic changes, hemolytic jaundice, thrombocytopenia, marked anemia, and reticulocytosis.

   d. Antibodies appear 8 to 10 days later, which is too late for diagnostic benefit in most cases. Antibodies also persist for 10 years, making the distinction between old and new infection difficult.

4. Treatment

   a. Prevention is key to the control of malaria. Evaluation and reduction of risk of exposure, prevention of mosquito bites through proper clothing, mosquito repellant, insect spraying programs, and barriers (mosquito netting and screens) is the first step.

   b. Chemoprophylaxis is recommended for patients traveling to areas of endemicity. Resistance is increasing; travelers should check with the local health authorities. In areas of chloroquine resistance, mefloquine is recommended.

     (1) Chloroquine is the drug of choice for both prophylaxis and treatment. It generally is well tolerated and is safe in pregnancy.

     (2) Transient GI symptoms, headache, pruritus, dizziness, blurred vision, malaise, and urticaria can be reduced if taken with meals or given in divided doses twice per week rather than daily.

   c. Severely ill patients can be treated with parenteral quinine, quinidine, or chloroquine plus either doxycycline, clindamyin, or a tetracycline.

   d. Alternative drugs include malarone, mefloquine, hydroxychloroquine, atovaquone/doxycycline, or other combinations, especially if resistance to chloroquine is suspect.

   e. Prognosis is good if treated except for cases involving *Plasmodium falciparum*, which has a mortality rate of 14% to 17% despite treatment.

VI. SEXUALLY TRANSMITTED DISEASES

A. Syphilis

1. General characteristics

   a. *Treponema pallidum* is a spirochete that can affect almost any organ or tissue. Transmission occurs most frequently during sexual contact. There has been a rising incidence of the disease in urban areas, particularly among adolescents and young adults as well as injection drug users.

   b. Congenital syphilis is transmitted via the placenta from the mother to the fetus and can result in severe defects.

2. Clinical findings

   a. Early infectious (primary and secondary) and late (tertiary) syphilis are separated by a symptom-free latent phase, during which the infectious stage may recur.

   b. Primary syphilis is characterized by chancre, which is a painless ulcer with a clean base and firm, indurated margins. It develops at the site of inoculation, most commonly the genital area. It is associated with regional lymphadenopathy (rubbery, discrete, nontender).

    c. Secondary lesions may involve skin, mucous membrane, eye, bone, kidneys, CNS, or liver. There may be relapsing lesions during early latency.

    d. Late (tertiary) syphilis includes gummatous lesions involving skin, bones, and viscera; cardiovascular disease; and nervous system and ophthalmic lesions.

        (1) Neurosyphilis can result in asymptomatic disease, meningovascular syphilis (chronic meningitis), generalized paresis, or tabes dorsalis (chronic progressive degeneration of parenchyma).

        (2) Tabes dorsalis manifests with impaired proprioception, loss of vibratory sense, Argyll Robertson pupil (reacts to light but does not accommodate), or tabes dorsalis crises.

    e. Congenital syphilis leads to abnormalities in the skin or mucous membranes, nasal discharge (snuffles), hepatosplenomegaly, anemia, and osteochondritis. If infants are not treated, they may develop interstitial keratitis, Hutchinson's teeth, saddle nose, deafness, and CNS abnormalities.

3. Laboratory studies

    a. *Treponema pallidum* may be identified on dark-field microscopy, but the technique is difficult. Immunofluorescent staining techniques are somewhat more reliable. The organism cannot be cultured. Serologic testing is the recommended method for diagnosis.

    b. Nontreponemal antigen tests detect nonspecific antibodies to lipoidal antigens.

        (1) The VDRL and RPR tests become positive 4 to 6 weeks after infection. These tests are positive in 99% of cases during primary and secondary syphilis but may be negative during late forms of syphilis. False-positive results occur, especially in patients with autoimmune disorders.

        (2) The nontreponemal tests also are used to assess the effectiveness of treatment.

    c. Treponemal antibody tests use live or killed *Treponema pallidum* as antigen to detect specific antibodies.

        (1) The fluorescent treponemal antibody absorption (FTA-ABS) test is the most widely used. It is useful in determining whether a positive nontreponemal antigen test is a true positive.

        (2) The test is accurate in most patients with primary syphilis and in virtually all patients with secondary syphilis, but it may be falsely positive in patients with Lyme disease, systemic lupus erythematosus, malaria, or leprosy.

    d. Specific testing for tertiary syphilis includes lumbar puncture, joint fluid analysis, and biopsy as indicated.

4. Treatment

    a. Benzathine penicillin G, 2.4 million U IM in a single dose, is the treatment of choice. Late latent and tertiary syphilis require three weekly injections.

    b. Neurosyphilis is treated with aqueous penicillin every 4 hours for 10 to 14 days. This may be followed with three weekly doses of benzathine penicillin G as mentioned earlier.

    c. The Jarisch–Herxheimer reaction (fever, toxic state) occurs when there is a sudden massive destruction of spirochetes. To prevent this, patients should be given antipyretics during the first 24 hours of treatment.

    d. All cases of syphilis must be reported to the appropriate public health agency for contact tracing. All sexual partners who may have been exposed should be treated.

    e. Careful follow-up is essential to monitor the effectiveness of treatment and to identify treatment failures. HIV testing and screening as well as treatment of concurrent sexually transmitted diseases should be done.

B. Gonorrhea

1. General characteristics

    a. *Neisseria gonorrhoeae* is a Gram-negative intracellular diplococcus that is transmitted during sexual activity.

    b. The highest incidence is found in 15- to 29-year-olds.

2. Clinical findings

    a. The incubation period is 2 to 8 days after exposure.

    b. Men

        (1) Men complain of burning on urination and a serous or milky discharge. Then, 1 to 3 days later, the urethral pain is more pronounced, and the discharge becomes yellow, creamy, profuse, and, occasionally, tinged with blood.

        (2) Without treatment, the infection may regress and become chronic or progress to involve the prostate, epididymis, and periurethral glands with acute, painful inflammation. This may progress to chronic infection, resulting in prostatitis and urethral strictures.

    c. Women

      (1) Women often remain asymptomatic or may develop dysuria, urinary frequency and urgency, and a purulent urethral discharge. Vaginitis and cervicitis are common.

      (2) Asymptomatic gonorrhea is a cause of pelvic inflammatory disease and infertility as well as perpetual transmission of the pathogen.

    d. Gonococcal bacteremia is associated with peripheral skin lesions or septic arthritis of the knee, ankle, or wrist.

    e. Conjunctivitis is caused by direct inoculation. Patients present with copious purulent discharge, which usually is unilateral. Global rupture is a risk if the patient is not treated adequately.

3. Laboratory studies

    a. Gram stain of urethral discharge typically shows Gram-negative intracellular diplococci. Smears are less often positive in women.

    b. Cultures are essential in all cases.

4. Treatment

    a. Resistance to penicillin, tetracyclines, and fluoroquinolones is widespread. Currently, the treatment of choice is IM ceftriaxone or oral cefixime.

    b. All partners must be treated. Concurrent treatment against *Chlamydia* sp. is recommended.

    c. Infection is reportable in most states.

C. *Chlamydia* sp.

1. General characteristics: Chlamydiae are a large group of obligate intracellular parasites, including *Chlamydia psittaci* (psittacosis), *Chlamydia pneumoniae* (respiratory infections), and *Chlamydia trachomatis* (trachoma, inclusion conjunctivitis, pneumonia, and genital infections).

2. Clinical findings

    a. Lymphogranuloma venereum starts with a vesicular or ulcerative lesion, which may go unnoticed.

      (1) The infection spreads to the lymph nodes, causing inguinal buboes. These may fuse and break down, resulting in multiple draining sinuses and scarring.

      (2) Anorectal disease causes tenesmus, discharge, and fistulae.

    b. Urethritis and cervicitis

      (1) In males, infection with *Chlamydia* sp. is the most common cause of nongonoccal urethritis. Discharge is less painful than with gonococcal urethritis and usually is watery.

      (2) Females typically are asymptomatic or may develop cervicitis, salpingitis, or pelvic inflammatory disease. Infection with *Chlamydia* sp. is a leading cause of infertility.

3. Laboratory studies

    a. The diagnosis typically is established clinically and is presumptive. Gram stain is negative.

    b. Complement fixation test or immunofluorescence, ELISA, or DNA probes (nucleic acid amplification) may help to confirm the presence of the disease.

4. Treatment

    a. Azithromycin, doxycycline, and erythromycin are effective. Erythromycin is the drug of choice in pregnant women.

    b. All partners should be treated.

D. *Trichomonas* sp.

1. General characteristics

    a. *Trichomonas* is a flagellated protozoan.

    b. It infects the vagina, Skene's gland, and lower urinary tract of females and the genitourinary tract of males.

2. Clinical findings

    a. There is pruritus and a malodorous, frothy, yellow-green discharge.

    b. Diffuse vaginal erythema and red macular lesions may be visible on the cervix.

3. Laboratory studies: Wet mount reveals motile flagellates.

4. Treatment

    a. Metronidazole in a single 2-g dose; it may need to be repeated if infection does not clear.

    b. All partners should be treated.

VII. SPIROCHETAL INFECTIONS

A. Lyme disease

1. General characteristics

   a. *Borrelia burgdorferi* is transmitted to humans by *Ixodides*, a small tick that often goes unnoticed. The tick must feed for more than 24 to 36 hours to transmit the spirochete.

   b. Lyme disease is the most common vector-borne disease in the United States.

   c. Up to 75% do not recall having been bitten by a tick.

2. Clinical findings

   a. Stage 1: Early localized infection (7 to 10 days after bite)

      (1) Erythema migrans, a flat or slightly raised red lesion that expands over several days, typically with central clearing ("bull's eye"). Most common sites are the groin, thigh, or axilla, and it typically resolves in 3 to 4 weeks without treatment.

      (2) About 25% of patients either do not exhibit erythema migrans or do not recall having a rash. Up to 20% of patients have multiple lesions.

      (3) Flu-like illness occurs in 50% of patients.

   b. Stage 2: Early disseminated infection (days to weeks later)

      (1) Manifestations typically involve the skin, CNS, and musculoskeletal system.

      (2) Headache, stiff neck, fatigue, malaise, and intermittent musculoskeletal symptoms are common.

      (3) Cardiac (pericarditis, arrhythmias, heart block) or neurologic (aseptic meningitis, Bell's palsy, encephalitis) manifestations occur in up to 20% of cases.

   c. Stage 3: Late persistent infection (months to years later)

      (1) Musculoskeletal disease includes joint pain without objective findings, frank arthritis (typically large joints), and chronic synovitis. This most likely is an immunologic rather than an infectious phenomenon.

      (2) CNS and PNS manifestations include subacute encephalopathy (memory loss, mood changes), axonal polyneuropathy (paresthesias, encephalopathy), and leukoencephalitis (cognitive change, paraparesis, ataxia, bladder dysfunction).

      (3) Acrodermatitis chronicum atrophicans, a bluish-red discoloration of distal extremities with atrophy, is seen in Europe but not in the United States.

3. Laboratory findings

   a. Antibodies can be detected by immunofluorescent assay or ELISA techniques. A Western blot assay is used as a confirmatory test. Immunoglobulin M wanes after 6 to 8 weeks; immunoglobulin G may persist indefinitely.

   b. Up to 50% of patients with early disease can be antibody negative during the first few weeks. Acute and convalescent titers can be compared for support of the suspected diagnosis.

   c. The tests lack sensitivity; the probability of a false-positive test may be greater than that of a true-positive test. False-positive tests are common in patients with rheumatoid arthritis, systemic lupus erythematosus, mononucleosis, endocarditis, and other infections. Therefore, diagnosis of early Lyme disease should be based on clinical findings. Late disease is diagnosed by objective evidence of clinical manifestations and laboratory evidence of disease.

   d. Other laboratory tests, such as CSF, synovial fluid analysis, aspirations, or biopsy, may be helpful in patients with discrete manifestations.

4. Treatment

   a. Doxycycline is the drug of choice in patients with erythema migrans or a suspicion of Lyme disease based on clinical findings (neurologic, cardiac, musculoskeletal) and a history of tick bite. Alternatives include amoxicillin, cefuroxime, ceftriaxone, or cefotaxime.

   b. Symptomatic treatment with analgesics, such as nonsteroidal anti-inflammatory drugs, may be beneficial in patients with musculoskeletal complaints.

   c. Prevention is important. Proper clothing, tick repellent, and a thorough search for ticks after outdoor exposure are essential. Prophylactic antibiotic therapy after tick bite is not recommended.

   d. The LYMErix vaccine is no longer being manufactured. The vaccine was associated with painful and debilitating side effects in some patients.

B. Rocky Mountain spotted fever

1. General characteristics

   a. *Rickettsia rickettsii* is transmitted by the wood tick. Transmission is highest during the late spring and summer.

   b. It most commonly occurs in the eastern United States.

2. Clinical findings

   a. Fever, chills, headache, nausea, vomiting, myalgias, restlessness, insomnia, and irritability develop 2 to 14 days after exposure. Less common manifestations include cough, pneumonitis, delirium, seizures, stupor, and coma.

   b. The face typically is flushed and the conjunctiva injected. Faint macules to maculopapules to petechiae develop first on the wrists and ankles and then spread to the extremities and trunk. About 10% of patients do not exhibit a rash.

   c. Less common findings include splenomegaly, hepatomegaly, jaundice, myocarditis, uremia, acute respiratory distress syndrome (ARDS), and necrotizing vasculitis.

3. Laboratory studies

   a. Leukocytosis, thrombocytopenia, hyponatremia, proteinuria, and hematuria are common. A transient rise in aminotransferases or bilirubin is possible.

   b. CSF reveals pleocytosis and hypoglycorrhachia.

   c. A rise in antibody titers appears during the second week of illness.

4. Treatment

   a. Mild, untreated cases wane during the second week.

   b. Prompt treatment with doxycycline or chloramphenicol hastens recovery.

   c. Poor outcomes occur in advanced age and in patients with atypical features. Death is caused by pneumonitis or respiratory or cardiac failure.

   d. Sequelae of disease may include seizures, encephalopathy, peripheral neuropathy, paraparesis, bowel or bladder incontinence, cerebellar dysfunction, vestibular dysfunction, hearing loss, or motor deficits.

   e. Prevention is key. Protective clothing, tick repellant, and prompt tick removal reduce the incidence of disease.

15 Surgery

Frank Acevedo

I. PATIENT HISTORY

A. A comprehensive patient history should be performed whenever possible. In emergent situations, the mnemonic **AMPLE** should be followed:

Allergies

Medications

Past medical history

Last meal

Events preceding the emergency

When time and the patient's condition permit, every effort should be made to complete the history.

B. Allergy history should include not only food and medication reactions but also any history of problems with anesthesia and anesthetic agents. Specific allergies to latex, tape, or surgical appliances should be sought. Patient's responses may reveal a difficult intubation history, malignant hyperthermia, previous reaction to an anesthetic agent, or other important information.

C. Medications should be reviewed for any that cause increased bleeding tendencies: aspirin, warfarin, alcohol, nonsteroidal anti-inflammatory drugs (NSAIDs), chemotherapeutic agents, and antibiotics are the most likely culprits. At particular risk are patients undergoing procedures on the central nervous system or those undergoing spinal anesthesia. Risk must be reevaluated in the presence of these medications. Herbal medications in particular should be specifically asked for, as many can interfere with normal coagulation and cause an increase in bleeding. These herbal supplements include feverfew, garlic, ginger, gingko biloba, ginseng, and vitamin E. The mnemonic DRUGS encourages better drug history taking and may help to prevent morbidity and mortality associated with medications (Table 15-1).

D. Conditions in the medical history that significantly alter the surgical risk should be explored. These include significant cardiopulmonary disease, endocrine disorders, cirrhosis, renal disease, immunosuppression, and previous surgical procedures. Assessment of preoperative surgical risk in elective patient populations may require ancillary diagnostic tests, such as stress testing, coronary angiography, carotid artery duplex B-mode scanning, and pulmonary function tests.

E. Events leading up to the current presentation should be documented. Focus on the seven cardinal signs of the symptom: location of the complaint, quality of the symptom, quantity or severity, timing, setting, alleviating or aggravating factors, and any associated complaints. Determine if the complaint is acute, subacute, or chronic.

II. PREOPERATIVE EVALUATION

A. Routine laboratory assessment

1. No documentation exists linking a reduction in mortality and morbidity to routine laboratory testing in otherwise healthy patients undergoing elective surgical procedures.

2. The history and physical examination are the *most* important preoperative evaluations that can be performed by the surgical team.

B. Selective diagnostic tests

1. The utilization of ancillary tests for further delineation of pre- and perioperative risk should only be guided by a thorough history and physical examination tempered by prudent clinical suspicion. About 5% of healthy individuals will have abnormal test results.

2. Complete blood count (CBC): Consider performing if the patient has signs and symptoms compatible with anemia or if the loss of blood during the procedure is anticipated to be significant.

3. Serum electrolytes

   a. Not indicated for patients without medical problems

   b. Should be considered in patients taking certain medications (e.g., warfarin, digoxin) because of the association with potassium abnormalities and toxicity

   c. More useful as a postoperative laboratory evaluation

TABLE 15-1	DRUGS Mnemonic for Taking a Drug History
	DRUGS
D	**Dispensed:** by doctor or other medical or dental provider
R	**Recreational:** alcohol, tobacco, street drugs, anabolic steroids
U	**User:** over-the-counter preparations, herbal supplements
G	**Gynecologic:** birth control preparations, hormone replacement therapy
S	**Sensitivities:** focus is on drug sensitivities rather than on allergies

Adapted with permission from Hocking G, deMello WF. Taking a DRUGS history. *Anaesthesia.* 1997;52:904–905. Published by Wiley-Blackwell.

4. Serum creatinine
   a. This is a convenient and inexpensive marker for renal function; creatinine levels decrease with age and decreased muscle mass.
   b. Preoperative creatinine levels generally should be obtained in all patients older than 40 years.
   c. Consider following creatinine levels if the patient is going to receive nephrotoxic medications or agents as part of the preoperative workup (i.e., radiologic dyes), if intraoperative hypotension is anticipated, or if cross-clamping of the aorta will be performed.

5. Blood glucose: Obtain in patients with a personal or family history of diabetes or those who will undergo bypass grafting for peripheral vascular disease, abdominal aortic aneurysm repair, or coronary artery bypass grafting.

6. Hepatic enzymes
   a. Not indicated routinely in healthy patients
   b. Order if clinical signs and symptoms indicate hepatic dysfunction

7. Coagulation studies
   a. The best determinant of bleeding tendencies during surgery is an accurate history detailing coagulation response to minor traumas.
   b. Bleeding time, activated partial thromboplastin time (PTT), and prothrombin (PT) time do not reveal a risk of perioperative bleeding in healthy patients.
   c. Results of coagulation studies should be documented in patients taking anticoagulants.

8. Urinalysis
   a. The incidence of asymptomatic urinary tract infections (UTIs) is 2% to 7%. Asymptomatic UTIs are a concern to the surgical team whenever a prosthetic device is to be used.
   b. Transient bacteremia during vascular procedures can infect the pseudointimal layer of the bladder and may seed an orthopaedic prosthetic device.
   c. There is no consensus on the routine use of urinalysis in healthy patients.

9. Electrocardiography
   a. This is generally recommended in all patients older than 40 years. The rationale is that preoperative myocardial infarction and arrhythmias are associated with higher morbidity and mortality.
   b. Silent myocardial infarctions are more common in elderly patients and in those with diabetes.

10. Chest radiography
    a. Little evidence supports or refutes routine chest radiography in patients without significant risk.
    b. Chest radiography may be indicated in patients older than 60 years, and it should be performed in all patients, regardless of age, who have any history of significant pulmonary or cardiac disease.

11. Spirometry
    a. The American College of Physicians recommends preoperative spirometry for patients being evaluated for thoracic and upper abdominal surgery and for patients who have a history of smoking or dyspnea.
    b. It is indicated in abdominal surgery if pulmonary disease is poorly controlled or if the extent of the disease is not clear.

12. Arterial blood gas

    a. Not routinely indicated for preoperative evaluation. Perform if there is any indication of severe underlying cardiopulmonary disease or to confirm acid–base disturbance.

    b. Pulse oximetry should be used before considering an arterial blood gas; often, the oxygen saturation information is enough in the preoperative patient.

    c. Arterial puncture carries the risk of bleeding from the site during the postoperative period.

13. Pregnancy test: Indicated in all women of childbearing age who are undergoing surgery.

C. Risk assessment for postoperative complications: The goal of this crucial assessment is to identify factors that increase morbidity and mortality.

    1. General history and physical examination

        a. Determine previous myocardial infarction, heart failure, chronic pulmonary disease, diabetes mellitus, peripheral vascular disorders, and hepatic or renal impairment.

        b. Look for jugular venous distention, cardiac murmurs, irregular pulses, pulmonary rales, abnormal aortic pulsations, and peripheral edema.

        c. Many rating systems have been developed to stratify patients into risk categories, particularly with regard to cardiac disease (Table 15-2).

TABLE 15-2	**Detsky's Modified Cardiac Risk Index**	
Risk	**Points**	
Age older than 70 yr	5	
Myocardial infarction		
Within 6 months	10	
After 6 months	5	
Canadian Cardiovascular Society Angina Classification[a]		
Class III	10	
Class IV	20	
Unstable angina within 6 months	10	
Alveolar pulmonary edema		
Within 1 week	10	
Ever	5	
Suspected critical aortic stenosis	20	
Arrhythmia		
Rhythm other than sinus or sinus plus atrial premature beats	5	
More than five premature ventricular beats	5	
Emergency operation	10	
Poor general medical status[b]	5	
Class	**Points**	**Cardiac Risk**
I	0–15	Low
II	20–30	Intermediate
III	31+	High

[a]Canadian Cardiovascular Society Classification of Angina: 0 = asymptomatic; I = angina with strenuous exercise; II = angina with moderate exertion; III = angina with walking one- to two-level blocks or climbing one flight of stairs or less at a normal pace; IV = inability to perform any physical activity without development of angina.

[b]As defined by Goldman risk index.

Data from Goldman L, Caldera DL, Nussbaum SR. Multifactorial index of cardiac risk in noncardiac surgical procedures. *N Engl J Med.* 1977;297:845–850; Detsky AS, Abrams HB, McLaughlin JR, et al. Predicting cardiac complications in patients undergoing non-cardiac surgery. *J Gen Intern Med.* 1986;1:213; Karnath BM. Preoperative cardiac risk assessment. *Am Fam Physician.* 2002;10:1889–1896.

2. Cardiac complications

    a. Cardiac complications, particularly perioperative myocardial infarction, occur with alarming frequency in certain surgical patients. Over 1.5 million patients suffer some perioperative cardiovascular morbidity.

    b. Clinical predictors of significant cardiac risk include recent myocardial infarction (MI) (within 30 days), unstable or severe angina, active heart failure, high-grade atrioventricular block, symptomatic ventricular arrhythmias with underlying cardiac disease, supraventricular arrhythmias with an uncontrolled rate, and severe valvular disease. Predicting major cardiac events in noncardiac surgery should be attempted in appropriate patient populations. Lee's Revised Cardiac Risk Index has been validated as a good tool to perform this very task (Table 15-3).

3. American Society of Anesthesiologists (ASA) classification (Table 15-4): Although performed by anesthesiologists since 1941, the ASA classification does *not* predict operative risk; instead, it was developed as an aid to assess the physical status of the patient before a surgical procedure and help make the choice of the anesthetic used.

D. Deep vein thrombosis (DVT) prophylaxis

    1. General characteristics

        a. Classically, the triad of stasis, intimal damage, and hypercoagulability described by Rudolph Virchow has been used to identify patients at risk.

        b. DVT is thought to start at the induction of anesthesia in elective surgical cases, so any attempts at prophylaxis should be started preoperatively.

        c. Specific surgical populations are at varying risk (Table 15-5).

            (1) Those patients identified as being at high risk should have preoperative prophylaxis against DVT.

            (2) High-risk populations include patients older than 70 years, those undergoing a surgical procedure anticipated to last longer than 2 hours, and those listed in Table 15.5.

        d. Prophylaxis using agents that alter blood coagulability should *not* be considered for procedures within the central nervous system.

TABLE 15-3   Lee's Revised Cardiac Risk Index

Criterion	Point Value
High-risk surgery	1
Coronary artery disease	1
Congestive heart failure	1
Cerebrovascular disease	1
Insulin-dependent diabetes mellitus	1
Elevated serum creatinine >2 mg/dL	1

Interpretation: Scoring

1. Points 0: Class I, very low (0.4% complications)
2. Points 1: Class II, low (0.9% complications)
3. Points 2: Class III, moderate (6.6% complications)
4. Points 3: Class IV, high (>11% complications)

Reprinted with permission from Lee TH, Marcantonio ER, Mangione CM, et al. Derivation and prospective validation of a simple index for prediction of cardiac risk of major noncardiac surgery. *Circulation.* 1999;100:1043–1049.

TABLE 15-4   Classification by the American Society of Anesthesiologists[a]

Class 1	Healthy patient, no medical problems
Class 2	Mild systemic disease
Class 3	Severe systemic disease, but not incapacitating
Class 4	Severe systemic disease that is a constant threat to life
Class 5	Moribund, not expected to live 24 hr regardless of operation

[a]The letter *e* is sometimes added to the class designation to designate an emergency operation.

TABLE 15-5	Classification of Risk for Deep Vein Thrombosis
Low risk	Minor surgery, no risk factor other than age
	Minor surgery, age <40 yr, no other risk factor
	Minor trauma or medical illness
Moderate risk	Major general, urologic, gynecologic, cardiothoracic, vascular, or neurologic surgery; age >40 yr; or other risk factor
	Major medical illness, heart or lung disease, malignancy
	Major trauma or thermal injury
	Minor surgery, trauma in patients with thromboembolism history
High risk	Fracture or orthopaedic procedure of pelvis, hip, or lower extremity
	Pelvic or abdominal surgery for malignancy
	Major surgery or trauma in patients with thromboembolism history
	Lower limb paralysis
	Major lower limb amputation

    e. Some high-risk patient populations (orthopaedics, obesity surgery) may require DVT prophylaxis for up to 30 days after discharge.

  2. Prophylaxis options

    a. Unfractionated heparin, 5,000 U subcutaneously every 8 or 12 hours, should be started preoperatively and continued until the patient is fully ambulatory.

       (1) The every-8-hour dose is associated with a higher incidence of wound complications, such as hematoma formation.

       (2) Heparin therapy is a cost-effective and efficacious method of prophylaxis.

    b. Enoxaparin (a low molecular weight heparin), 40 mg subcutaneously daily, should be started 12 hours before or after the procedure and continued until the patient is fully ambulatory or up to 14 days following surgery.

       (1) Enoxaparin is more expensive per dose than unfractionated heparin, but it may be cost-effective when factoring in other requirements of dosing with low-molecular-weight heparin.

       (2) The dosage may need to be adjusted in cases of renal impairment.

    c. Warfarin has been used primarily in orthopaedic patient populations after initial use of heparin.

       (1) The dosing is usually begun the night before or the day following surgery and is usually 5 or 10 mg.

       (2) Dosing is complicated and a PT level must be checked periodically. Warfarin is also associated with a higher incidence of bleeding complications.

    d. Fondaparinux is associated with a lower incidence of DVT in hip surgery.

       (1) It works by blocking activated factor X. The dose is 2.5 mg subcutaneously daily, starting 6 hours postoperatively.

       (2) Adjustment is necessary in patients with renal insufficiency.

    e. Nonfitted thromboembolic stockings are not recommended.

       (1) The elastic band at the top of the stocking can actually promote a tourniquet effect and stimulate the development of DVT.

       (2) Only fitted stockings should be used, if at all; their benefit for preventing thromboembolism in surgical patients is questionable.

    f. Sequential compression devices are beneficial in all patient populations.

       (1) Application usually is to both lower extremities on call to the operating room, and they are continued until the patient is fully ambulatory. In lieu of bilateral lower extremity application, they may be used on one lower and one upper extremity.

       (2) They are the prophylactic measure of choice for patients in whom anticoagulation is contraindicated.

    g. Greenfield filter insertion

      (1) This is an invasive procedure that allows prophylaxis only from clots that form in the lower extremities.

      (2) A filter is indicated in some trauma patients, those who have bled while on anticoagulation, those in whom anticoagulation is contraindicated because of procedure or adverse reaction, those in whom a thromboembolic event has developed while on prophylaxis or full anticoagulation, and those undergoing central nervous system procedures. After Greenfield filter insertion, anticoagulation should be continued if there are no compelling contraindications due to the risk of inferior vena cava (IVC) thrombosis and insertion site thrombosis.

    h. Dextran

      (1) Dextran has been used by some as a prophylactic measure against DVT.

      (2) Its use is not associated with significant decreases in the incidence of DVT but is associated with the development of heart failure, renal failure, and difficulties in cross-matching blood.

E. Surgical nutrition

  1. General characteristics

    a. A malnourished patient is defined as someone who has lost more than 10% of his or her lean body mass and/or has not had adequate nutritional intake for more than 7 days.

    b. Expected risks of malnutrition include greater incidence of infection, immune dysfunction, wound complications, and operative morbidity and mortality.

    c. Increased nutritional requirements will be present because of the hypermetabolic hypercatabolic response seen in the systemic inflammatory response syndrome. Tumor necrosis factor-α has been shown to enhance muscle catabolism and promote patient cachexia in metabolic stress.

  2. Clinical features

    a. Weight loss, reduction of subcutaneous fat stores, and wasting may be apparent.

    b. Decreased cognitive function may be associated with severe malnourishment.

    c. Subtle changes in skin and hair occur, especially with essential fatty acid deficiency syndromes.

  3. Physiologic impact

    a. Cardiovascular system will develop decreased myocardial mass, stroke volume, and cardiac output.

    b. Respiratory system will undergo catabolism of major muscles of respiration, with decreased vital capacity and difficulty in extubation of patients.

    c. Gastrointestinal (GI) tract will develop atrophy of villi, with overgrowth of bacteria. Overgrowth of bacteria plus mucosal dysfunction may result in bacterial translocation and subsequent multisystem organ dysfunction. Depletion of the amino acid glutamine has been linked with the occurrence of bacterial translocation from the gut.

    d. Immune system will develop both impaired cell-mediated and humoral immunity.

    e. Ultimately, poor wound healing will develop, with an increased incidence of wound infection, dehiscence, and evisceration.

    f. In severe malnutrition, marasmus or kwashiorkor may develop.

  4. Diagnostic studies

    a. Serum creatinine, creatinine height index, total lymphocyte count, albumin, prealbumin, and/or transferrin may be abnormal.

    b. Body mass index, arm circumference, and nitrogen balance are useful parameters to measure overall status.

  5. Treatment

    a. Treatment aims at replacement of caloric and nitrogen requirements necessary to maintain nutritional homeostasis or at prevention of catabolism and promotion of anabolism.

    b. Basal energy expenditure is calculated using the Harris–Benedict equation (Table 15-6). Stress factors can then be used to increase the kcal calculations depending upon the severity of the underlying condition.

TABLE 15-6   **Calculation of Basal Energy Expenditure (kcal/day)**[a]
Men = 66.5 + 13.6(weight) + 5.0(height) − 6.8(age)
Women = 655.1 + 9.6(weight) + 1.9(height) − 4.7(age)

[a]Height and weight measurements are in centimeters and kilograms, respectively. Age is measured in years.

c. Preferred nutritional replacement is always via the enteral route to maintain GI viability and aid in the prevention of multisystem organ dysfunction. Another option includes the use of peripheral or central catheters and the infusion of intravenous (IV) hyperalimentation.

d. Overfeeding of the surgical patient should be avoided as it can result in increased oxygen consumption, increased production of carbon dioxide, fatty liver infiltration, depressed leukocyte function, and an increased incidence of infections.

6. Complications

a. Aspiration

(1) Enteral feedings should be used in alert patients to avoid the major complication of aspiration pneumonitis.

(2) Gastrostomy tube feedings are better than nasoenteric tube feedings but are still associated with aspiration.

(3) Jejunostomy tube feedings are a preferred nonenteral alternative to prevent this complication, especially in patients with pancreatitis.

b. Diarrhea

(1) Diarrhea caused by osmotic loading is a common complication and can be controlled by limiting the concentration or rate of infusion.

(2) Never assume that diarrhea is solely from enteral feedings, and always consider *Clostridium difficile* pseudomembranous enterocolitis as a potential etiology.

c. Hyperalimentation complications can be broken down into those related to catheter insertion and those related to the infusion of the solution.

(1) Catheter-related problems include air embolus, sepsis, pneumothorax, hemothorax, hydrothorax, and cardiac rupture.

(2) Infusion complications include severe hyperglycemia (including nonketotic hyperosmolar coma), hepatic steatosis, electrolyte abnormalities, and trace element and vitamin deficiencies.

III. TRAUMA

A. General characteristics

1. Traumatic injuries are the leading cause of death between the ages of 1 and 44 years.

2. Motor vehicle accidents are the leading cause of accidental deaths in the United States. Alcohol is linked to at least half of all fatal motor vehicle incidents.

3. In-field emergency medical services, rapid transport to trauma centers, and application of Advanced Trauma Life Support guidelines generate the best results. There is some evidence supporting rapid transport without aggressive field resuscitation as a means to utilize permissive hypotension. Permissive hypotension prevents the dislodgment of "fresh clot" and further exsanguination.

B. Primary survey: ABC (airway, breathing, circulation)

1. Assuring a patent and functioning airway is the first priority.

a. Cervical spine stabilization should be provided by a hard (Philadelphia) collar.

b. Altered mental status is the most common indication for intubation.

c. Orotracheal intubation is the preferred modality.

d. Nasotracheal intubation requires that the patient be awake.

e. Cricothyroidotomy can be performed in emergent situations but only by experienced operators and not in patients under the age of 12 because of the risk of developing subglottic stenosis.

2. Breathing is the next priority in the trauma patient.

a. Caregivers should look for the presence of tension pneumothorax, open chest wounds, or flail chest.

b. Tension pneumothorax is associated with hypotension, tracheal deviation away from the side of injury, jugular venous distention, lack of or decreased breath sounds on the affected side, hyperresonance on the affected side, and subcutaneous emphysema.

3. Open chest wounds should never be completely occluded with dressings, because this may convert the wound into a tension pneumothorax.

4. Flail chest is characterized by paradoxical breathing.

a. Segmental rib fractures cause free-floating segments that move opposite to normal respiratory patterns.

b. The major problem is not the fractures but, rather, the underlying pulmonary contusion.

5. Circulatory status should be assessed after the above have been secured.

    a. Cardiopulmonary resuscitation may be necessary.

    b. IV access with at least two angiocatheters ($\geq$16 gauge) should be established.

    c. Initial infusion of balanced solutions, such as Ringer's lactate or normal saline, should be started (fluids should be warmed if large quantities are to be infused). Resuscitation with Ringer's lactate needs to be undertaken with care particularly in the patient with marginal renal function or unknown renal status, as each liter of Ringer's lactate solution contains 4 mEq of potassium. Use of multiple liters may result in unrecognized hyperkalemia.

    d. Persistent hypotension requires the exclusion of tension pneumothorax, myocardial contusion or infarction, or cardiac tamponade. Beck's triad (jugular venous distention, hypotension, and muffled heart sounds) characterizes cardiac tamponade.

C. Secondary survey

    1. After completion of the primary survey and assurance of ABCs, a secondary survey should be performed. The focus during this survey is to identify any occult injuries the patient may have sustained.

    2. Thoracic or abdominal injuries, neurologic deficits, lacerations or hematomas, or musculoskeletal injuries must be identified.

    3. Progressive changes or additional clinical manifestations are important indicators of ongoing pathology.

        a. Some major injuries may not be apparent at first inspection.

        b. Continued monitoring of the trauma patient is essential.

    4. Digital rectal examination may detect a high riding prostate and, in association with blood in the urinary meatus, may imply a pelvic fracture. A trauma evaluation is not complete until a finger or tube has been inserted in every orifice. Caution must be exercised with cerebrospinal fluid (CSF) rhinorrhea or suspected cribriform plate fractures and the insertion of nasogastric tubes.

D. Penetrating chest trauma

    1. Most cases of penetrating chest trauma (95%) can be managed by tube thoracostomy alone.

    2. The remaining cases (5%) must be evaluated regarding clinical indications for operative intervention (Table 15-7).

E. Blunt abdominal trauma

    1. The **F**ocused **A**ssessment with **S**onography for **T**rauma (FAST) examination has largely replaced diagnostic peritoneal lavage as the diagnostic test of choice for detecting intra-abdominal injury.

    2. FAST examination evaluates the abdominal cavity for air or fluid collection in the perihepatic, perisplenic, pericardial, and pelvic regions.

        a. A specific diagnosis of an injured organ does *not* have to be made.

        b. Computerized tomography (CT) may be added as needed to clarify the FAST results.

        c. CT, or any other diagnostic study that involves the transport of a trauma patient, should only be undertaken in patients who are hemodynamically stable and *must* be performed under constant hemodynamic and clinical monitoring. CT scans ordered for the initial evaluation of head trauma do not need to be performed with contrast agents, as blood is self-enhancing.

F. Penetrating abdominal trauma

    1. Immediate laparotomy is indicated if a patient exhibits any signs of shock, peritoneal irritation, or evisceration.

    2. Selective laparotomy can be done in the hemodynamically stable patient without any of the above signs after performance of a FAST examination. If the FAST examination reveals intraperitoneal air, laparotomy is indicated.

TABLE 15-7   **Indications for Thoracostomy in Penetrating Trauma**
Caked hemothorax unable to drain via thoracostomy tube
Evacuation of 1,500 mL of blood in an injury <3 hr old
Evacuation via tube thoracostomy of 200 mL of blood for three consecutive hours
Signs of cardiac tamponade
Signs of esophageal perforation
Bowel sounds in the chest, indicating diaphragmatic injury
Persistent leakage of air
Development of a bronchopleural fistula

G. Penetrating flank trauma

1. Workup in the stable patient includes CT with oral and IV contrast. Penetrating flank trauma is difficult to assess, because many injuries in this region may be retroperitoneal.

2. Wherever sequential clinical examinations are required, a team approach that utilizes practitioners who are involved with the initial care of the patient is best. Analgesia use should be considered in every patient with opioid or NSAIDs tailored to the diagnosis. Withholding appropriate analgesia for fear of changing the findings during sequential clinical examination is unfounded and can cause severe physiologic and psychological consequences in patients.

H. Vascular trauma

1. Look for signs of arterial injury, such as a pulsatile mass or hemorrhage, expanding hematoma, significant hemorrhage, presence of a thrill or bruit, or acute ischemia to the involved extremity.

2. The presence of a pulse distal to the injury does *not* rule out significant vascular injury.

3. Arteriography and the ankle–brachial index are useful diagnostic tests for determining arterial injury.

I. Head trauma

1. Glasgow Coma Scale (Table 15-8)

   a. The Glasgow Coma Scale score should be calculated in all trauma patients.

   b. It is useful for triage and prognosis.

   c. The initial Glasgow Coma Scale correlates to the severity of brain injury. Those patients with a score of 3 have an extremely poor prognosis for significant recovery. The avoidance of secondary insults to the brain as caused by hypotension and hypoxemia is paramount in determining the outcome and reducing the severity of the injury.

2. Basilar skull fractures

   a. Basilar skull fractures may be associated with rhinorrhea, otorrhea, or ecchymosis of lids (raccoon eyes).

   b. Also be vigilant for ecchymosis behind the ear (Battle's sign).

TABLE 15-8	Glasgow Coma Scale[a]
Points	**Adults**
Eye opening	
4	Spontaneous
3	To voice
2	To pain
1	None
Verbal	
5	Oriented
4	Confused
3	Inappropriate words
2	Incomprehensible words
1	None
Motor	
6	Obeys commands
5	Localizes pain
4	Withdraws
3	Abnormal flexion
2	Abnormal extension
1	None

[a]A score of 15 is normal. A score of 13 to 15 indicates mild head injury, 9 to 12 moderate head injury, and less than 9 severe head injury.

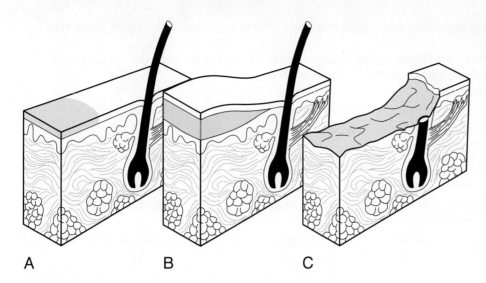

3. Epidural hematomas
    a. Epidural hematomas usually are caused by injuries to the middle meningeal artery.
    b. A brief period of unconsciousness is followed by a lucid interval.
    c. Herniation may develop and is heralded by a triad of coma, fixed and dilated pupils, and decerebrate posturing.
    d. Diagnosis is established by CT and requires emergent craniotomy.
4. Subdural hematomas
    a. Subdural hematomas usually result from injuries to bridging veins.
    b. They are associated with severe head injuries and can result in significant axonal injury even after evacuation.
    c. Chronic subdural hematoma is more common in alcoholics and elderly patients.
    d. It can occur after apparently minor trauma and is associated with mental status changes or focal neurologic signs.
    e. CT is diagnostic, and once the diagnosis has been established, burr holes over the hematoma are indicated to evacuate the clot.

IV. BURNS

A. General characteristics: Burns generally are classified as first, second, third, or fourth degree (Fig. 15-1). The classification of burns into a fourth degree is controversial, and many utilize only a three-tiered classification schema.
    1. First-degree burns involve minor damage to the epidermis.
    2. Second-degree burns are subdivided into superficial partial-thickness burns that extend to the papillary dermis and deep superficial burns that extend into the reticular dermis.
    3. Third-degree, or full-thickness, burns involve and destroy the epidermis and the dermis.
    4. Fourth-degree burns destroy the skin and subcutaneous tissue, with further involvement of fascia, muscle, bone, or other structures.
B. Incidence
    1. The American Burn Association estimates that more than 500,000 burn injuries are treated each year.
    2. Approximately 5,000 deaths per year occur among the approximately 40,000 patients who are hospitalized for burn injuries.
    3. Scald burns are the most common type of burn.
C. Clinical features
    1. First-degree burns are characterized by erythema, tenderness, and the absence of blisters.
    2. Second-degree burns (partial thickness)

    a. Superficial second-degree burns have thin-walled, fluid-filled blisters; are moist; blanche with pressure; and are painful.

    b. Deep second-degree burns have thicker-walled blisters, many of which are ruptured, exhibit a mixture of erythema and pallor, and are painful with application of pressure.

  3. Third-degree burns (full thickness)

    a. Third-degree burns give the skin a white, leathery, or charred appearance.

    b. The skin is characteristically dry and without the presence of sensation.

  4. Fourth-degree burns

    a. Fourth-degree burns are characterized by significant charring and exposure of muscle or bone.

    b. The extensive damage to nerves results in little to no sensation of pain.

  5. Any burn that occurs on the face, on the upper torso, or in an unconscious patient should raise the suspicion of associated upper airway involvement.

  6. In cases where burns are caused by electrical energy, the findings on the skin do not correlate with the extent of the clinical injury.

D. Laboratory studies

  1. In patients with moderate to severe or extensive burns, required laboratory studies include hematocrit, electrolytes, blood urea nitrogen (BUN) and creatinine, urinalysis, and chest radiography. Depending on the extent of the injuries and patient status, also consider obtaining an arterial blood gas, electrocardiography, carboxyhemoglobin, or glucose levels, contingent on the history obtained.

  2. Direct further laboratory and diagnostic studies once the secondary survey has been performed. Remember that burn patients may have significant associated trauma from falls or blunt injuries.

E. Treatment

  1. Maintain ABCs (see above).

  2. Estimate the percentage of burn.

    a. Many formulas are available: Rule of 9s, Lund and Broder, and Berkow. (Tidbit: The palm of the victim's hand is roughly equal to a 1% burn.)

    b. Rule of 9s (Fig. 15-2)

      (1) The major body areas are divided so that each area is a multiple of 9.

        (a) The head represents 9% of the body surface, and each arm is 9%.

        (b) The front of each leg (extending to the groin) is 9%, and the back is 9%.

        (c) The front of the torso is 18%, and the back of the torso is 18%.

      (2) This formula is accurate for adults only because of the larger head size and smaller thighs in children.

  3. Stop the burning process.

    a. Sterile water usually is sufficient, but first look for powders if dealing with a chemical substance, as pouring water on a chemical may activate it and cause further burn damage.

    b. If dealing with a chemical substance, first identify the substance in question, because specific neutralization measures may be required.

    c. Burns that are caused by white phosphorus may require neutralization with 1% copper sulfate solution and administration of calcium gluconate to address concomitant hypocalcemia.

    d. Hydrofluoric acid burns will require copious lavage for at least 30 minutes, with concomitant application of calcium gluconate gel to the affected area.

  4. Manage shock by aggressive fluid resuscitation.

    a. Many formulas exist; choose one and become familiar with it.

    b. Parkland formula: Percentage of burn area × body weight (kg) × 4 mL/hr equals total amount of fluid needed in next 24 hours.

      (1) Half the calculated fluid is given during the first 8 hours, with the rest over the remaining 16 hours.

      (2) Ringer's lactate solution is recommended.

      (3) Colloids can be introduced during the second 24 hours. However, their use remains controversial because thermal injury of capillaries may make them particularly prone to leakage. Administration of colloids with leaky capillaries may cause fluid loss from, rather than retention within, the intravascular space.

      (4) Monitor urine output as a measure of adequate circulation and hemodynamic stability.

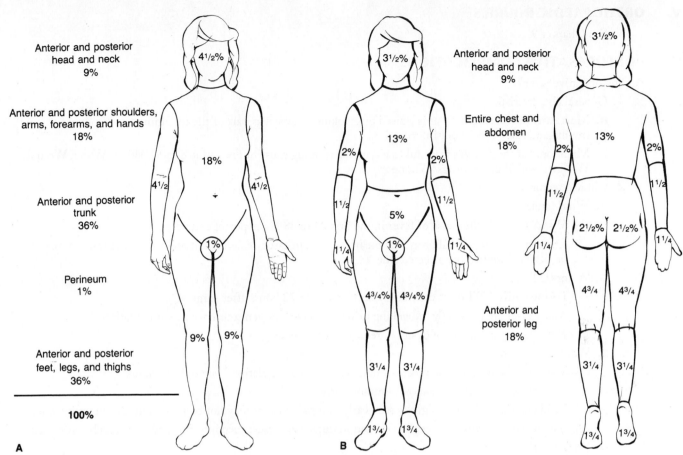

FIGURE 15-2 Rule of nines. From Harwood-Nuss AL, Wolfson AB, Linden C, et al. *The Clinical Practice of Emergency Medicine.* 3rd ed. Philadelphia: Lippincott Williams & Wilkins; 2001.

5. Insert a nasogastric tube because gastric distention can be problematic and, in severe cases, may cause non-fluid respondent hypotension because of mediastinal shift from an overly distended stomach.

6. A Foley catheter should be inserted early and used for monitoring urine output.

   a. Maintain a urine output of at least 0.5 mL/kg/hr in an adult.

   b. Maintain a urine output of at least 1 mL/kg/hr in a child.

7. Address the need for escharotomy in circumferential burns of extremities or the anterior trunk, as they can cause a compartment syndrome and make ventilation difficult.

8. Sulfadiazine (Silvadene) is the most commonly used topical burn ointment.

   a. Other preparations, such as mafenide (Sulfamylon), may be used.

   b. Care must be taken when using mafenide, because in large amounts, it can block the action of carbonic anhydrase and lead to severe metabolic alkalosis.

9. Deep dermal burns and full-thickness burns typically are excised on or about day 3.

   a. Coverage is attained by numerous methods.

   b. Autograph is the best method, but allographing of skin is acceptable.

   c. Other alternatives include epidermal cell culture, artificial skin, and porcine xenograph.

10. Complications

   a. Common complications of severe burns include inhalation injury, hypovolemic shock, neurogenic shock secondary to pain, renal failure, multiorgan system dysfunction, and gastric or duodenal ulcerations (termed Curling's ulcers).

   b. The most common complication associated with all burns is infection of the burn wound, which has the potential for hematogenous spread.

   c. Chronic healing burn wounds can undergo malignant transformation into a squamous cell carcinoma (Marjolin's ulcer).

V. ORTHOPAEDIC INJURIES

See Chapter 9.

VI. POSTOPERATIVE COMPLICATIONS

A. Postoperative fever

1. General characteristics

a. Most early postoperative fever is caused by cytokines released as part of the inflammatory response to tissue trauma and resolves without intervention.

b. Mnemonic of the five Ws is useful to aid in determining cause of fever (Table 15-9): **W**ind, **W**ater, **W**ound, **W**alking, and **W**onder drugs/**W**hopper.

2. Clinical features

a. Wind (atelectasis)

(1) Wind usually is the cause of fever in the first 24 to 48 hours postoperatively.

(2) Examination may reveal bronchial breathing, and in cases of significant atelectasis, the trachea may be deviated toward the affected side.

b. Water (UTIs)

(1) Postoperative UTI most commonly develops 48 to 72 hours after surgery.

(2) Many cases are caused by indwelling urinary catheters or genitourinary instrumentation.

(3) Patients may complain of dysuria, frequency, or urgency.

c. Wound infections

(1) Wound infections are the most common cause of postoperative fever after 72 hours.

(2) *Staphylococcus aureus* is the most common pathogen.

(3) Mild change in the vital signs is seen early, and pain may or may not be present at the site of infection.

(4) Superficial infections involve the skin and subcutaneous tissue; deep infections involve areas below the fascia.

d. Walking (thrombophlebitis)

(1) Superficial thrombophlebitis most commonly is associated with intravascular catheters. Purulent drainage around an indwelling catheter with induration of the vein may be detected on physical examination.

(2) Deep thrombophlebitis can be associated with indwelling central lines or DVT.

(3) Thrombophlebitis of the lower extremity may be associated with Homans' sign; however, this is nonspecific. Unilateral edema of an extremity is a more specific indicator of deep vein thrombophlebitis.

TABLE 15-9	Mnemonic of the Five Ws	
	Timing	**Findings**
Wind (atelectasis)	First 24–48 hr postoperatively	Bronchial breathing
		Shift of trachea toward affected side
Water (urinary tract infection)	48–72 hr postoperatively	Indwelling Foley catheter
		Genitourinary instrumentation
		Cloudy urine
		Positive urine cultures
Wound (wound infection)	After 72 hr postoperatively	Early on, possibly just mild elevation in vitals
	Most common cause of fever during this time period is wound infection	Undue pain at wound site with erythema and/or drainage
Walking (thrombophlebitis)	After 72 hr postoperatively	Indwelling catheters
		Cellulitic streaking indicates streptococcal infections; local abscess formation indicates staphylococcal infections
Wonder drugs/**W**hopper (drug fever/abscess)	Fever after 1 week is a serious complication unless caused by drug allergies	Persistent fever with negative cultures should raise index of suspicion for drug fever
		Intra-abdominal abscesses may present with blood cultures that are polymicrobial

    e. Wonder drugs

        (1) Wonder drugs, such as anesthetics, sulfa-containing antibiotics, and others, often are implicated in drug fever that develops 1 week postoperatively.

        (2) This is a diagnosis of exclusion and should be considered when faced with a negative sepsis workup in a postoperative patient with fever.

    f. Whopper

        (1) Whopper refers to the presence of a postoperative abscess.

        (2) In the case of intra-abdominal fluid collections, an ileus may develop as a sequela of an occult abscess.

        (3) Blood cultures may be polymicrobial, indicating anastomotic leakage.

3. Imaging studies

    a. A directed workup may include CBC, wound cultures, sputum cultures, blood cultures, chest radiography, and abdominal CT. Intra-abdominal abscesses, if intraloop (i.e., situated between two loops of the small bowel), can be associated with a 25% to 33% false-positive rate when performing CT.

    b. Chest radiography in patients with atelectasis may reveal shifting of the mediastinum toward the affected side, with evidence of loss of lung volume.

    c. When deep vein thrombophlebitis is suspected, B-mode real-time ultrasonography can be used to reveal clots. Venography is still the gold standard for DVT but is invasive and, in some patients, can cause inflammation because of intimal injury.

4. Treatment

    a. Atelectasis

        (1) Atelectasis is best treated by prevention.

            (a) Patients should be instructed to stop smoking at least 2 weeks before any thoracic or abdominal procedure.

            (b) Instruction in using an incentive spirometer should be given and its use encouraged as a preventive measure.

        (2) When atelectasis develops postoperatively, incentive spirometry, mucolytics, expectorants, and inhaled β-agonists are beneficial.

    b. Urinary tract infections

        (1) UTIs are the most common nosocomially acquired infection.

        (2) UTIs should be treated based on culture and sensitivity reports.

        (3) Antibiotics chosen should be based on urinalysis and Gram stain results. Where feasible the indwelling catheter should be removed.

        (4) In critically ill patients already on multiple antibiotics, a UTI with *Candida* sp. may be suspected.

    c. Superficial thrombophlebitis

        (1) Superficial thrombophlebitis requires termination of the IV line at the site of infection and use of warm compresses.

        (2) If systemic signs and symptoms are present or if the patient is immunocompromised or diabetic, antibiotics that cover both *Staphylococcus* sp. and *Streptococcus* sp. should be started.

    d. Septic thrombophlebitis requires a vein stripping of the affected site, because it will behave like an abscess and make antibiotic penetration difficult.

    e. DVT

        (1) DVT should be treated with anticoagulation, using either heparin or low-molecular-weight heparin.

        (2) For patients in whom anticoagulation is contraindicated, vena caval interruption with a Greenfield filter should be considered.

    f. Intra-abdominal abscesses

        (1) Intra-abdominal abscesses require either surgical debridement or percutaneous drainage, both in combination with appropriate antibiotics.

        (2) Percutaneous drainage by an interventional radiologist can be performed as either a CT- or an ultrasound-guided procedure.

        (3) Abscesses must be uniloculated to be amenable to percutaneous drainage.

B. Keloids and hypertrophic scars

   1. General characteristics

      a. Both keloids and hypertrophic scars represent abnormal healing and an imbalance between collagen deposition and degradation.

      b. Keloids are more common in African Americans and Asians.

   2. Clinical features

      a. Keloids tend to extend beyond the original wound or trauma, whereas hypertrophic scars usually are limited to their original boundaries.

      b. Hypertrophic tissue usually regresses without intervention, whereas keloid tissue will require intervention.

      c. Diagnosis is established based on clinical findings.

   3. Treatment

      a. No single treatment modality has been shown to be effective across the board in all patients.

      b. Topical triamcinolone (Kenalog), 40 mg/mL in a dosage of 2 mL every 6 to 8 weeks, has been shown to be effective. It can cause dermal atrophy, telangiectasia, and hypopigmentation.

      c. Excisional surgery also can be used but is associated with a very high recurrence rate unless combined with other treatment modalities.

C. Decubitus ulcers (pressure ulcers)

   1. General characteristics

      a. Decubitus ulcers are linked to pressure and shear forces over bony prominences.

      b. Most patients who develop this complication have an inability to change position and, thus, sustain long periods of uninterrupted pressure, with subsequent tissue ischemia.

      c. Patients with spinal cord injury are at the greatest risk of developing these types of ulcerations.

   2. Clinical characteristics: Follow the National Pressure Ulcer Advisory Panel (Table 15-10).

   3. Diagnostic procedures: Quantitative wound culture is essential to differentiate between colonization and true infection.

   4. Treatment

      a. Treatment should encompass a multimodal approach that includes removal of the pressure source, supplemental nutritional support, and surgical intervention.

      b. Reconstructive procedures are performed only after tissue cultures show that there is no evidence of infection.

      c. Treatment can include skin grafts or rotational flaps.

      d. Antibiotics should be reserved for those patients who manifest clinical signs of septicemia.

D. Necrotizing fasciitis

   1. General characteristics

      a. Although necrotizing fasciitis is a rare complication, it is more common in patients with diabetes, alcoholics, and IV drug abusers. Some case series have identified those with diabetes as accounting for 20% to 30% of identified cases.

      b. It is associated with mortality rates ranging from 25% to 70% in some studies.

      c. It can be polymicrobial or caused by group A streptococci or clostridial infections. Saltwater necrotizing fasciitis is caused by *Vibrio* sp.

TABLE 15-10	**Classification of Pressure Ulcers**
Stage I	Intact skin with erythema that blanches
Stage II	Partial-thickness skin loss; may present as abrasion, blister, or shallow crater
Stage III	Full-thickness skin loss extending to the subcutaneous tissue but not beyond the fascia; crater with or without undermining of adjacent tissue
Stage IV	Full-thickness skin and subcutaneous tissue loss with extension into muscle, tendons, bone, or joint capsule

2. Clinical characteristics: Patients can present with a multitude of symptoms, including rapidly progressing erythema, tissue crepitus, marked tissue tenderness, high temperatures, tachycardia, hypotension, and an altered mental status.

3. Diagnostic procedures

   a. Look for the triad: elevated white blood cell (WBC) (>14,000 cells/μL), elevated BUN (>15 mg/mL), and hyponatremia (<135 mmol/L).

      (1) This triad is not present in all patients.

      (2) If this triad is present, it should prompt a heightened index of suspicion.

   b. Ultrasonography, CT, and magnetic resonance imaging (MRI) have been used to demarcate the affected regions before surgical intervention.

   c. Plain-film radiographs are of use only if gas is present within the affected tissues.

4. Treatment

   a. Aggressive surgical debridement is the mainstay of therapy.

   b. Antibiotic therapy should cover all possible pathogens.

      (1) An initial therapeutic choice of penicillin G, 24 million units per day IV, divided into doses administered every 4 to 6 hours; clindamycin, 900 mg IV every 8 hours; and gentamicin, 1 mg/kg IV every 8 hours, is acceptable.

      (2) It is important to monitor renal function and adjust dosages accordingly, because renal impairment is a major hallmark of this disease.

Geriatrics

Kathy Kemle

I. BACKGROUND

A. Life expectancy

1. The number of years that an individual can expect to live at birth is increasing in all industrialized and many developing countries; it is approaching 80 years for both sexes.

2. Life tables predict that persons living until age 65 can expect to live 18 additional years, and those living until age 75 can expect to live 12 additional years.

B. Coupled with a declining birth rate, the result is an overall aging of the population; the number of persons older than 65 years is estimated to grow to 70 million by the year 2030.

C. This aging phenomenon brings with it higher burdens of chronic disease and greater use of health care resources.

II. PATIENT CARE

A. Normal changes of aging

1. Individuals and their organ systems age at varying rates, making the elderly the most heterogeneous group in the population.

2. Clinically significant aging changes by system are listed in Table 16-1.

B. Comprehensive geriatric assessment

1. Assessment has been shown to improve patients' placement and functional status, and it provides a baseline for comparison of future status changes. Despite the greater number of diagnoses discovered, fewer medications are used in patients who are followed by a comprehensive geriatric team.

2. Assessment encompasses cognitive status, physical evaluation, functional status, psychological status, nutritional status, and socioeconomic status. Table 16-2 lists some commonly used assessment instruments.

3. Functional status includes activities of daily living and instrumental activities of daily living (Table 16-3).

4. Assessment of driving skills is difficult because of the multidimensional nature of the tasks involved and the lack of easily administered standardized assessment tools.

C. Prevention

1. The efficacy of many preventive services in the elderly is uncertain.

2. Recommendations should be tailored to the individual and based on expected survival, functional status, and personal choice.

3. Table 16-4 lists routine tests recommended for the elderly as well as screening procedures that generally are not appropriate.

4. Tetanus boosters, the pneumococcal vaccine, and yearly influenza vaccines should be strongly encouraged in the elderly, because these patients are at greater risk for poor outcomes from these diseases. The herpes zoster vaccine is indicated once for those older than 60.

D. Pharmacology

1. The elderly are particularly vulnerable to adverse effects of medication.

2. Pharmacokinetics (absorption, distribution, metabolism, and excretion) is altered during the aging process, which results in higher frequency of drug-related adverse events.

   a. Altered absorption from the gastrointestinal (GI) tract is not a certainty of aging; however, a decline in gastric acid may affect absorption of those drugs that require a low pH for full absorption.

   b. Interstitial and skin perfusion declines, resulting in slower absorption of topical preparations and subcutaneous or intramuscular injections.

   c. Metabolism of drugs (biomedical modification and degradation mostly as a result of enzymatic processes) is not changed significantly by aging.

   d. Moderate reductions in free water and serum proteins occur with aging, resulting in higher active drug concentrations. Malnutrition adds to the decline in serum proteins, magnifying this effect.

   e. Decline in liver mass and hepatic blood flow as well as declines in renal clearance affect drug clearance. Dosages of many agents should be reduced. Renal insufficiency may be present even in persons with normal

TABLE 16-1	**Common Changes in Aging**
Dermatologic	Loss of rete pegs; thinning skin; loss of subcutaneous fat; fragile skin; decrease in collagen and elastin; increased photoaging
Pulmonary	Decline in forced vital capacity; less effective cough; decline in forced expiratory volume; increased fibrosis; less elastin; decreased chest wall compliance
Immune system	Decline in B- and T-cell function (most changes result from decreased nutrition rather than aging alone)
Cardiovascular	Decline in compliance; increased wall thickness; decreased maximal heart rate; decreased cardiac output; increased systemic vascular resistance; increased reliance on atrial contraction for ventricular filling; baroreceptor dysfunction
Endocrine	Impaired glucose tolerance; decreased testosterone and estrogen
Gastrointestinal	Impaired swallowing; slower transit time; decreased gastric acid; slight gallbladder duct dilation
Renal	Slow decline, but effect is variable; prostatic hypertrophy
Musculoskeletal	Loss of fluid in collagen; decreased elasticity; decrease in myocytes
Neurologic	Slower response times; decline in vibratory and proprioceptive senses; decline in righting reflexes
Vision	Increased lens opacity; decreased peripheral vision; decreased accommodation
Hearing	Loss of cochlear cells; increased and stickier cerumen

TABLE 16-2	**Instruments for Geriatric Assessments**
Cognition	Mini-Mental Status Exam
	Clock Drawing Test
	Geriatric Depression Scale
	Yesavage Geriatric Depression Scale
	Blessed Dementia Rating
	Categorical Word Fluency
	Short Portable Mental Status Questionnaire
	Montreal Cognition Scale
Function	Physical Self-Maintenance Rating Scale
	Lawton-Brody Function Scales (ADLs, IADLs)
	Performance of Activities of Daily Living
Nutrition	Mini-Nutritional Assessment Tool and Short Form
Mobility	Tinetti Get-Up-and-Go Test

ADLs: activities of daily living; IADLs: instrumental activities of daily living.

serum creatinine levels, so doses should be based on known or estimated creatinine clearance. Glomerular filtration rate (GFR) is a more sensitive indicator of renal function.

3. Pharmacodynamics (the effect of medication on targeted tissue) is difficult to measure in the elderly because of altered pharmacokinetics. The elderly are more sensitive to the effects of some drugs, such as warfarin, and centrally acting drugs, such as benzodiazepines.

4. Adverse drug events are the most common medical errors, with rates as high as 74% during stays in long-term care.

   a. Drugs and drug combinations with high risk of adverse consequences should be used with caution and very rarely in the elderly (Tables 16-5 and 16-6).

   b. Any drug with anticholinergic properties is likely to produce confusion in the elderly, and effects of multiple drugs are cumulative. Many commonly prescribed agents have anticholinergic effects (Table 16-7).

   c. Side effects and drug interactions may be readily apparent (rash, vomiting) or more subtle (change in personality, somnolence, delirium).

TABLE 16-3	Activities of Daily Living and Instrumental Activities of Daily Living
Activities of daily living	Bathing
	Grooming
	Dressing
	Mobility
	Toileting
	Eating
	Transferring
Instrumental activities of daily living	Telephoning
	Meal preparation
	Shopping
	Finances
	Stairs
	Reading
	Laundry
	Housework
	Transportation
	Medications
	Employment

5. About 30% of the elderly in the community use some form of alternative therapy, such as saw palmetto for prostatism, glucosamine/chondroitin for osteoarthritis, and melatonin for insomnia.

E. Assessment and management of the hospitalized older adult

1. Old age itself is not a contraindication to surgical procedures, but mortality/morbidity rates are higher for those with comorbidities.

2. Iatrogenic problems, especially delirium, are more common in older adults.

a. Delirium is characterized by alteration of consciousness, waxing and waning of symptoms, psychomotor retardation or agitation, and decreased attention span.

b. Delirium is a medical emergency and should be evaluated promptly. It is associated with poorer outcomes and higher mortality.

c. Delirium is most common with surgical admissions, especially orthopaedic and urologic procedures.

d. Evaluation and management of delirium include the following requirements:

(1) To maintain a high index of suspicion

(2) To perform a complete physical examination, including neurologic and rectal exam

(3) To identify and treat reversible factors (unnecessary medications, infection, anemia, dehydration, congestive heart failure, electrolyte imbalance, central nervous system oxygenation, sensory deprivation, fecal impaction, urinary retention); these are often additive, so all must be considered and addressed

(4) To encourage family visitation, remove/avoid restraints when possible, mobilize the patient, assist with feeding, reduce noise, and provide familiar surroundings

(5) To recommend lorazepam or haloperidol in small doses if medication is necessary

F. Rehabilitation

1. Sites of care include rehabilitation hospitals, subacute placements in long-term care facilities, outpatient facilities, and the home.

2. Premorbid function is the best predictor of outcome after stroke or serious fracture.

3. Mobility aids, such as canes and walkers, as well as functional assistive devices are helpful, especially if used in conjunction with education on their use by a physical or occupational therapist.

G. Palliative care

1. As it becomes clear that a disease process is not amenable to further treatment or cure, focus needs to shift to more intense concern with symptom amelioration.

TABLE 16-4	Recommended and Inappropriate Screening Procedures for Older Adults
Recommended Screening Procedures	
Height/weight	At least annually
Blood pressure	At least annually
Vision	Annually
Hearing	Annually
Depression	Uncertain
Alcohol questionnaire	Uncertain; base frequency on patient history
Lipids	Annually
Bone density	Uncertain
Glucose	Uncertain
Mammography	Every 2–3 yrs
Pap smear	Every 3 yrs; may cease if all Pap smears have been normal until age 65; if never tested, stop after two negative annual smears
Stool hemoccult	Every 3–5 yrs
Colonoscopy	At least once
Smoking cessation	Every visit
Dental care	At least annually
Calcium intake	At least annually
Exercise	Each visit
Safety counseling	At least annually
Immunizations	Pneumococcal—at least once; influenza yearly; zoster 60 and above
Aspirin	81 mg by mouth daily unless contraindicated
Inappropriate Screening Procedures	
Screens for pancreatic cancer, lung cancer, ovarian cancer, and bladder cancer	
Annual blood chemistry panel	
Annual complete blood count	
Annual electrocardiography	
Annual chest radiography	

2. Older adults and demented persons experience pain just as younger individuals do but may have more difficulty in expressing their sensations or describing them as painful. For example, chest pain due to myocardial infarction may be felt as tightness.

a. Nociceptive pain arises in somatic or visceral tissues and usually is described as aching, stabbing, or intense pressure and pain.

b. Neuropathic pain originates in disordered central or peripheral nerves and is described as electrical, burning, shooting, or stinging.

c. Pain management involves pharmacologic and nonpharmacologic modalities.

(1) Pharmacologic

(a) Dosing of pain medication must be titrated in the elderly, because these patients often are very susceptible to side effects and interactions.

(b) Pain is best managed by constant dosing of small amounts rather than less frequent larger doses. This produces better control of discomfort while minimizing side effects.

(c) Nociceptive pain

(i) Mild pain should be managed with acetaminophen or tramadol unless treating bony metastases; avoid nonsteroidal anti-inflammatory drugs (NSAIDs) because of the risk for GI bleeding and renal toxicity.

TABLE 16-5	Drugs Commonly Implicated in Adverse Drug Events
α-Methyldopa	Ciproheptadine
Reserpine	Cyclobenzaprine (and other relaxants)
Propoxyphene	Flurazepam
Diphenhydramine	Indomethacin (all NSAIDs)
Ticlodipine	Pentazocine
Doxepin	Dicyclomine
Diazepam	Chlorpropamide
Amitriptyline	Chlorpheneramine
Meperidine	Meprobamate
Minoxidil	Belladonna
Trazadone	Metoclopramide
Digoxin	

NSAIDs, nonsteroidal anti-inflammatory drugs.

TABLE 16-6	Drug Combinations Commonly Involved in Adverse Interactions	
Medication		**Risk**
ACE inhibitor + potassium		Hyperkalemia
ACE inhibitor + potassium-sparing diuretics		Hyperkalemia
ACE inhibitor + salt substitute		Hyperkalemia
Antiarrhythmic + diuretic		Arrhythmias
Benzodiazepine + other sedative		Sedation, confusion, falls
Calcium channel blocker + nitrate		Hypotension, falls
Digoxin + verapamil		Elevated digoxin levels
Digoxin + quinidine		Elevated digoxin levels
Nitrate + vasodilator		Hypotension
Theophylline + other xanthines		Tachyarrhythmias, anxiety
Warfarin + sulfa, quinolones, macrolides, NSAIDs		Increased effect
Digoxin + amiodarone		Increased digitalis level

ACE, angiotensin-converting enzyme; NSAIDs, nonsteroidal anti-inflammatory drugs.

TABLE 16-7	Medications with Anticholinergic Effects	
Furosemide (all loop diuretics)		Digitalis
H_2-blockers		NSAIDs
Clonidine		Amantadine
Opioids		Some antiarrhythmics
SSRIs		β-Blockers, especially propranolol
Benzodiazepines		Some antipsychotics
Tricyclic antidepressants		Fluoroquinolones
Antituberculin drugs, especially isoniazid and rifampin		

NSAIDs, nonsteroidal anti-inflammatory drugs; SSRIs, selective serotonin reuptake inhibitors.

   (ii) Moderate to severe pain should be managed with hydrocodone/acetaminophen, oxycodone, morphine, transdermal fentanyl, or methadone.

   (iii) Opioid-induced nausea can be minimized by avoiding rapid infusion of large doses. It will resolve predictably in 48 hours. If medication is needed, compazine, ondansetron, or haloperidol is preferable, as this type of nausea is mediated in the chemoreceptor trigger zone via dopamine and serotonin systems.

   (iv) Sedation will occur but fades with time.

   (v) Respiratory depression can be avoided by starting at low doses with slow titration. It does not occur until sedation, loss of reflexes, and lack of pupillary response develop sequentially.

   (vi) Unlike the other side effects, constipation will not decrease with time. It must be treated by initiation of stimulant laxatives when the opioid is started. Methylnaltrexone bromide (Relistor) is a narcotic preparation designed to reduce constipation induced by opioids. It has been approved for patients with advanced disease who require continuous opioid treatment to manage pain.

   (vii) A rare but frightening side effect is a fine red pruritic rash, which is caused by histamine release and is often mistaken for allergy. The rash will rapidly dissipate without treatment, but pruritus may be relieved by antihistamines.

  (d) Neuropathic pain

   (i) Neuropathic pain should be managed with anticonvulsant medication (especially the pentin agents, such as gabapentin, or pregabalin), duloxetine, or lidocaine topical patch. Avoid older anticonvulsants if possible because of sedation and other toxicities.

   (ii) Methadone is also highly effective for this type of pain but must be dosed very carefully, as its metabolism is highly variable and overdose is more likely with this agent. Its use should be limited to those with experience in palliative care.

   (iii) Avoid tricyclic antidepressants because of their potential for delirium and other anticholinergic effects.

 (2) Nonpharmacologic control of pain can be achieved through distraction (music, relaxation techniques, aromatherapy, massage), cold/warm applications, positioning, splinting, electrical stimulation, hypnosis, or biofeedback.

3. Nonpain symptoms of chronic disease may be just as distressing as pain.

 a. Nausea, dyspnea, fatigue, and anxiety are common.

 b. Treatment of underlying cause and supportive measures are key to management.

 c. Dyspnea is the subjective sensation of breathlessness and does not always correlate with pulse oximetry.

 d. Fatigue is common in the dying and is managed by advising rest and occasionally using steroids and stimulants.

H. Geriatric syndromes

1. Syndromes are multifactorial and require aggressive, multifaceted investigation.

2. Immobility is the great disabler.

 a. Encouraging the elderly to be active in even a limited exercise program is imperative. Exercise improves balance, has cognitive and physical benefits, and preserves functional capacity.

 b. Table 16-8 lists the most common consequences of immobility.

3. Accidents are the sixth leading cause of death in the elderly, and two-thirds of these are falls. Community dwellers should be asked yearly about any falls. If a fall is reported, further evaluation should be completed, including physical examination and medication review. A simple method to evaluate for fall risk is to ask the patient to arise from a chair without using his or her arms. Ability to complete this maneuver indicates adequate proximal muscle strength and balance.

 a. Falls are the result of disordered interaction between the individuals and their environment.

 b. Falls may be a sign of acute illness, most often urinary tract infection (UTI), exacerbation of congestive heart failure, or pneumonia.

 c. Changes in gait, balance, vision, and hearing as well as disease predispose older adults to falling.

 d. Evaluation of a fall should include a full history, physical examination including orthostatic blood pressure measurements, assessment and management of any injuries, and a search for the factors that may have precipitated the fall. Many medications are associated with falls (Table 16-9).

4. Urinary incontinence (see Chapter 6)

 a. Incontinence is *not* a normal part of aging; new onset requires evaluation and may indicate infection.

 b. Falls often are the result of an overactive bladder.

TABLE 16-8	**Consequences of Immobility**	
Deconditioning	Depression
Cardiac deconditioning	Mislabeling (dementia)
Renal lithiasis	Delirium
Pressure wounds	Hyperglycemia
Deep venous thrombosis	Worsened chronic disease
Pulmonary embolism	Constipation
Urinary retention, urinary tract infection	Fecal impaction
Atelectasis	Pneumonia
Reflux disease	Osteoporosis

TABLE 16-9	**Common Drug Classes Frequently Associated with Falls**
Anticonvulsants	
Antihypertensives (especially central acting)	
Benzodiazepines (especially long acting)	
Tricyclic and other antidepressants	
Hypnotics	
Diuretics	
Vasodilators	
Opioids (if oversedating)	

    c. Medications used for urge pattern incontinence are anticholinergic and, therefore, of limited utility in the elderly population.

    d. Diuretics and drugs such as caffeine and other xanthine derivatives may exacerbate incontinence.

5. Cognitive impairment

    a. Impairment of cognition is *not* a normal part of aging.

    b. Mild cognitive impairment

      (1) Mild cognitive impairment is characterized by deficits in cognition, especially memory, without deficiencies in activities of daily living.

      (2) It may progress to dementia in susceptible individuals, especially those with other risk factors such as lower educational level, history of head trauma, sedentary lifestyle, lack of cognitive or social stimulation, or history of diabetes/metabolic syndrome or hypertension.

      (3) Treatment with acetylcholinesterase inhibitors has not been shown to retard progression to dementia.

    c. Dementia (see Chapter 11)

      (1) Dementia is a progressive decline in cognitive function. Unlike delirium, dementia generally is irreversible.

      (2) Many causes of dementia are recognized, but all result in loss of intellectual capacity, eventually involving all activities of daily living.

      (3) Chronic dementia progresses to a terminal phase that is characterized by immobility, eating difficulties, and frequent infections.

    d. Behavioral complications of dementia

      (1) Troubling behaviors are common in dementia and cause a great burden for caregivers and safety issues for patients.

      (2) Medications do not remove target behaviors and are associated with undesirable side effects.

      (3) Behaviors are managed best by environmental manipulation.

      (4) Antipsychotic medications are *not* approved by the U.S. Food and Drug Administration for this purpose.

      (5) No drug therapy works well.

        (a) Acetylcholinesterase inhibitors and memantine as well as anticonvulsants and β-blockers may be helpful, but studies on efficacy for behavior are conflicting.

(b) Benzodiazepines, especially lorazepam in small doses, are the recommended agents for sedation if drugs must be used.

(6) Table 16-10 describes common behaviors seen in dementia and their management.

e. Dizziness

(1) One of the three most common complaints in primary care, dizziness is a sensation of light-headedness, spinning, or impending syncope. It is encountered frequently in older adults because age-related changes in balance predispose them to this disorder. Older adults rely on vision more than younger people and invariably have loss of proprioception and vestibular function.

(2) Dizziness is classified as vertigo (the sensation of rotational movement of self or surroundings) or nonvertigo (presyncope, disequilibrium, unsteadiness, floating, or light-headedness).

(3) Historical accuracy is the key to successfully establishing the diagnosis.

(4) Examination should include orthostatics, observation of gait, a check for nystagmus, as well as cardiac and neurologic examinations.

(5) Treatment varies with the cause.

(6) Prognosis for recovery is good in three-fourths of patients.

(7) Nonvertiginous

(a) Disequilibrium is a sensation of unsteadiness and is caused by vestibulopathies, visual and musculoskeletal disorders, and neuropathies or anxiety/depression disorders. Canes or walkers often are useful.

(b) Presyncope is the sensation that a faint is imminent and is caused by decreased cerebral perfusion, usually because of orthostatic hypotension or vagally mediated cardiac events. Advise the patient to arise slowly, and correct reversible causes.

(c) Light-headedness is a more vague sensation and often is psychiatric in origin. A trial of antidepressants may be warranted.

6. Syncope

a. A sudden, transient loss of consciousness not resulting from trauma, syncope increases in occurrence with age.

b. Common causes include arrhythmias, aortic stenosis, carotid sinus hypersensitivity, myocardial infarction, hypoglycemia, orthostatic hypotension, postprandial hypotension, psychogenic disorders, pulmonary embolus, and vagal faint.

c. History and physical examination are key to diagnosis.

d. Diagnostic tests should be chosen based on the history and physical examination.

e. Tests include electrocardiography, ambulatory monitoring (Holter), echocardiography, tilt-table test, electrophysiologic studies, and possibly computed tomography (CT) or magnetic resonance imaging (MRI) of the brain.

f. Treatment varies with the cause.

TABLE 16-10	Behaviors Seen in Chronic Dementia and Their Management
Behavior	**Management**
Wandering	Provide safe place to wander
	Patient identification system (bracelets, MedAlert)
	Identify and avoid precipitants
	Sedatives (last resort)
Screaming	Search for source and remove or ameliorate
	Distraction
Aggression	Identify and avoid precipitants
	Sedatives
Restlessness/agitation	Consider depression
Hallucinations	If bothersome, use atypical antipsychotics
	If Parkinson's or Lewy body disease, use quetiapine or benzodiazepine

7. Sensory impairment

    a. Vision

        (1) Declines in accommodation and peripheral vision occur with aging.

        (2) Clouding of the lens occurs even without disease.

        (3) See Chapter 1 for specific conditions.

    b. Hearing

        (1) Cerumen impaction and presbycusis are common causes of hearing loss in the elderly.

        (2) See Chapter 1 for specific conditions.

8. Malnutrition

    a. Undernutrition is the most common disorder, but overweight and obesity also are problematic.

    b. Undernutrition (macronutrients)

        (1) The cause is most often "pre-mouth" (i.e., problems with inability to shop for or prepare meals or inadequate assistance with feeding).

        (2) Other causes include mouth disorders such as edentulous state or oral candidiasis, dysgeusia (loss of or abnormal taste), dysphagia, mesenteric ischemia, gastritis, generalized fatigue, endocarditis, malignancy, depression, and pain.

        (3) Water deficit is common, because the elderly lack a thirst response and often are on diuretics, increasing water loss.

        (4) Evaluation should include a complete history, especially regarding medications, food availability and preferences, and pain referable to the GI tract, as well as a search for other medical causes.

        (5) Laboratory studies that may be useful include complete blood count (CBC), electrolytes, renal and liver function, thyroid-stimulating hormone, erythrocyte sedimentation rate, and urinalysis; chest radiography may be useful as well. Other studies may be needed as suggested by the evaluation.

        (6) Treatment is geared toward the cause.

    c. Undernutrition (micronutrients)

        (1) Vitamins C, D, B_{12}, and the other B vitamin deficiencies are the most common deficiencies in older adults.

        (2) Vitamin D deficiency is a frequently underrecognized cause of myalgias, arthralgias, and sarcopenia in older adults. Supplementation has been shown to reduce fall risk and improve quality of life. Obtain a serum 25-OH vitamin D level, and if severely reduced, prescribe 2,000 IU daily; moderate deficiencies can be treated with 800 IU/day. As more data are generated, these dose recommendations will probably be higher. Toxicity is extremely rare even at much higher doses.

        (3) For most, undernutrition results from reduced intake, but declines in gastric acid and intrinsic factor render the elderly especially vulnerable to vitamin B_{12} deficiency. It is important to recognize that serum levels are not necessarily coincident with central nervous system levels. Oral replacement with 1,000 mg daily is preferred to parenteral.

9. Pressure wounds (see Chapter 13)

    a. Predisposing factors in elderly skin consist of loss of subcutaneous fat, loss of the rete pegs (projections of dermis into the epidermis that help to prevent shearing off of the epidermis), and a decline in elasticity.

    b. Predisposing factors in general include diseases that reduce perfusion or delivery of nutrients to tissue, increased shearing force, moisture (such as fecal or urinary incontinence), dehydration, and immobility.

    c. Treatment primarily consists of paying attention to systemic factors, including hydration, nutrition, adequate oxygenation and carrying capacity, frequent turning, pressure-relieving devices, optimal management of related diseases, and pain relief.

10. Vertebral compression fractures

    a. Associated with osteoporosis, fractures usually are in the thoracic or lumbar spine and present as deep pain over the site of the fracture, sometimes radiating in the appropriate nerve root distribution.

    b. Trauma may be minimal or absent.

    c. Diagnosis is established by radiography or, occasionally, by MRI.

    d. Treatment is symptomatic, with analgesics and vertebroplasty or kyphoplasty.

    e. Complications include kyphosis, with possible restrictive lung disease as a result; immobility; chronic pain; and even death.

   I. Psychiatric disorders

      1. General characteristics

         a. Older adults tend to be self-reliant and satisfied with life.

         b. Stoicism and present focus are typical.

         c. They often deny mental illness.

      2. Common disorders

         a. Depression is characterized by sadness, withdrawal from previously enjoyed activities, and anhedonia, but the elderly concentrate on somatic complaints more than on mood. Typical presentations also include memory impairment, agitation, anxiety, or displaced anger.

            (1) Diagnosis is established by clinical suspicion and completion of a screen, such as the Yesavage Geriatric Depression Scale. One also must rule out depression induced by medical disease, such as an indolent cancer, or medication.

            (2) Although effective, older adults may be reluctant to participate in psychotherapy, so pharmaceuticals may be the usual therapy.

               (a) Lower side effects make selective serotonin reuptake inhibitors and agents like mirtazapine the drugs of choice.

               (b) Occasionally, stimulants in low doses, such as methylphenidate, are useful for a short time, especially in patients with psychomotor retardation.

               (c) Avoid tricyclic antidepressants.

            (3) Some patients are resistant to medications. Electroconvulsant therapy has been shown to be very effective and safe even in frail elderly patients.

         b. Anxiety

            (1) Avoid benzodiazepines if possible; if they must be used, shorter-acting agents are preferable. Although both long-acting and short-acting agents are associated with increased fall risk, long-acting ones are more often implicated.

            (2) Avoid antihistamines and use buspirone and antidepressants.

         c. Psychosis

            (1) Senile psychosis is characterized by hallucinations and delusions.

            (2) It is associated with isolation, sensory impairment, and dementia.

            (3) It should not be treated unless it is bothersome to the patient or prohibits the caregivers from providing care.

            (4) Newer antipsychotics in low doses are the agents of choice; however, some dispute their risk–benefit ratio because of higher risk of cardiovascular disease, diabetes, and falls.

         d. Substance abuse

            (1) Tobacco use is common and should be discouraged even in the very old, because cessation may be beneficial even at the extremes of age.

            (2) Ethanol produces intoxication with ingestion of lesser amounts.

               (a) Hidden sources, such as household cleaners, tonics, and personal hygiene products, are common.

               (b) Withdrawal is more lethal in the elderly.

            (3) Other agents, including prescription drugs, often are misused unintentionally but rarely are directly abused in the elderly population.

III. SELECTED COMMON DISEASES AND DISORDERS WITH UNIQUE FEATURES IN THE ELDERLY

   A. Xerosis

      1. Xerosis is characterized by dry skin, pruritus, and cracking skin.

      2. Treatment consists of decreasing the frequency of bathing and using tepid or cool water followed by emollients.

   B. Oral disorders

      1. Oral disorders frequently result in weight loss.

      2. Dysgeusia may be related to dental disease or sinusitis, but it often is secondary to drugs. Common drugs that cause taste disturbances include any anticholinergic agent, digitalis, and angiotensin-converting enzyme inhibitors.

      3. Toothlessness commonly reduces mastication. Dentures may contribute to decreased taste and lead to denture ulcers.

    4. Oral candidiasis is common and should be considered in any elderly patient who decreases oral intake, especially if dentures are used, which may harbor organisms, the patient is on steroids or antibiotics, or has diabetes or another immunodeficiency disorder.

        a. White patches are common, but red mucosa or angular chelitis may be the only sign.

        b. Treatment is with topical or oral antifungal agents.

C. Infectious diseases

    1. Decline in B- and T-cell immunity related to aging increases vulnerability to infection.

    2. Fever typically indicates bacterial infection but sometimes is the result of malignancy or medication intake. Elderly often do not mount a fever even with serious infections.

    3. Pneumonia

        a. Predisposing factors include decreased ciliary activity, less effective cough, and decreased vital capacity.

        b. Presentation may be atypical, with less cough, absent fever, and absent or unimpressive leukocytosis. Often, only confusion and tachypnea are seen. Chest x-ray (CXR) does not always show typical infiltrates, particularly early in the course of illness.

        c. Aspiration pneumonia is more common in the elderly but usually is not successfully treated by antibiotics. It is not reduced by use of a percutaneous endoscopic gastrostomy (PEG) tube; in fact, it is increased.

    4. Urinary tract infection

        a. UTI often presents with vague symptoms or confusion.

        b. It is difficult to distinguish from asymptomatic bacteriuria, which is common and should not be treated, because inappropriate antibiotic use leads to resistance and exposes patients to unnecessary risk.

        c. Diagnosis of a UTI requires urinalysis and culture and correlation with signs and symptoms.

        d. Treatment consists of appropriate antibiotics, increased fluids, and attention to hygiene.

        e. While UTI may cause delirium, it should not be assumed to be the etiology until other potential causes are ruled out.

D. Respiratory diseases

    1. Pulmonary fibrosis

        a. There is increased incidence with aging; limited fibrosis is a part of normal aging.

        b. Fibrosis is characterized by shortness of breath and bibasilar rales.

        c. Treatment is largely symptomatic, including supplemental oxygen.

    2. Chronic obstructive pulmonary disease (see Chapter 2): Avoid theophylline because of the high risk of side effects and interactions.

    3. Pulmonary embolus (see Chapter 2)

        a. Presentation often is less specific, with confusion or arrhythmia or fever.

        b. Diagnosis and treatment are the same as those in younger adults. Spiral CT may not be appropriate, however, because many elderly suffer from chronic renal insufficiency, limiting the use of contrast material.

E. Cardiovascular disease

    1. Ischemic heart disease

        a. Ischemic heart disease is very common in the elderly but frequently presents atypically, often with shortness of breath or fatigue, weakness, or confusion rather than with chest pain or tightness.

        b. Elderly patients are more likely to have severe or three-vessel coronary disease.

        c. Cardiac enzymes may not rise as much or may be difficult to interpret secondary to renal disease.

        d. Elderly patients who present with myocardial infarction are more likely to die than younger individuals.

        e. Treatment is the same as in younger adults; be mindful of comorbidities that may affect treatment options.

        f. Age alone is not a contraindication to invasive or surgical therapies.

    2. Hypertension

        a. Hypertension is very common in older adults.

        b. It should be treated aggressively unless side effects (e.g., falls secondary to orthostatic hypotension) preclude lowering the systolic pressure to recommended levels.

        c. Diagnosis and treatment are the same as in younger individuals.

        d. Renal artery stenosis, contributing to secondary hypertension, is more common in the elderly.

e. Systolic hypertension should be treated, because it is more highly associated with stroke than diastolic hypertension. Thiazide diuretics are the first choice for systolic hypertension.

f. Avoid centrally acting agents because of the high risk of sedation, dry mouth, and depression.

3. Valvular disease

a. Aortic sclerosis

(1) Aortic sclerosis results from thickening of the aortic leaflets.

(2) It causes a systolic murmur similar to that of aortic stenosis, from which it cannot be distinguished on physical examination.

b. Aortic stenosis: Elderly patients may not exhibit the classic pulsus parvus et tardus (slow, late pulse indicative of valvular disease) or the typical radiation pattern to the carotids and axillae. Presentation is more likely to be syncope, congestive heart failure, or fatigue.

c. Mitral regurgitation may cause heart failure or death. Treatment is surgical.

4. Congestive heart failure (see Chapter 3)

a. Diastolic dysfunction is more common and results in poor compliance and poor filling, leading to heart failure.

b. Presentation often is sudden shortness of breath and pulmonary edema.

c. Diagnosis is established clinically and supported with echocardiography.

d. Treatment is with angiotensin-converting enzyme (ACE) inhibitors, β-blockers, and calcium channel blockers.

e. Diuretics should be used judiciously because of the high probability of renal insufficiency and risk of dehydration.

f. Systolic heart failure is treated as in younger individuals.

F. Endocrine disorders

1. Hypothyroidism

a. Hypothyroidism is a very common problem, especially in elderly women, and may present in typical fashion or quite atypically.

b. Thyroid dysfunction often mimics changes associated with aging itself. These symptoms include a general slowing of mental and physical function, tendency to low body temperatures and cold intolerance, weight gain, constipation, hardening of the arteries, hearing loss, elevation of serum lipids (cholesterol), elevation of blood pressure, and anemia.

c. Evaluation is via thyroid function testing (thyroid-stimulating hormone typically is elevated).

d. Treatment

(1) Treatment is with levothyroxine, with a goal of restoring the thyroid-stimulating hormone to high normal or just above normal.

(2) Dosage should be very low, 12.5 to 25 g/day and increased at 4- to 6-week intervals, because the half-life of levothyroxine in the elderly is variable. Assessing levels at less frequent intervals may lead to overdose.

2. Hyperthyroidism

a. Hyperthyroidism may present as hypothyroidism (apathetic hyperthyroidism), atrial fibrillation with a rapid ventricular response, or dementia.

b. Evaluation is via thyroid function testing.

c. Treatment is the same as in younger patients.

G. GI disorders

1. Reflux disease is evaluated and treated as in younger adults; however, prokinetic agents, such as metoclopramide, should be avoided, if possible.

2. Peptic ulcer disease is more likely to present with failure to thrive, nausea, or melena rather than with dyspepsia or pain.

3. Constipation

a. Aged individuals are predisposed to bowel dysfunction due to changes of aging, immobility, inadequate hydration, and medications.

b. Diagnosis is established by history and physical examination and, occasionally, by abdominal flat plate.

    c. Treatment is increasing fluids and activity, improving mastication, increasing dietary fiber, and using stool softeners and laxatives/enemas if necessary. Avoid anticholinergic drugs as much as possible. Aggressively manage opioid-related constipation with stimulant laxatives or with methylnaltrexone in the terminal patient.

    d. If unrelieved, complications may ensue: impaction, stercoral ulcers (ulcerations of the colon because of pressure and irritation from retained feces), obstruction, and death.

H. Neurologic disorders

  1. Subdural hematoma

    a. Subdural hematomas may be chronic or acute.

    b. Chronic subdural hematomas are common and may arise with little or no trauma.

    c. Presentation usually is confusion, decreased level of consciousness, and perhaps focal findings, but may appear to be dementia.

    d. Diagnosis is established via CT.

    e. Treatment may be surgical (burr holes) or, if the hematoma is small and not progressing, watchful waiting.

    f. Chronic subdural hematomas frequently recur even after surgery.

  2. Cerebrovascular disease: See chapter 11.

IV. LEGAL AND ETHICAL ISSUES

A. Competence is a legal term and is determined by a judge.

B. Decisional capacity is determined by a physician and may change depending on circumstances and cognitive ability.

C. Elder mistreatment

  1. Suspicion of abuse requires a report to legal authorities.

  2. Abuse may take many forms, including neglect, exploitation, and verbal, psychological, or physical mistreatment.

  3. Abuse often is associated with caregiver stress, especially if the caregiver is financially dependent on the elder and has psychological or substance abuse problems.

  4. Patterns of injury that are not consistent with the history should raise suspicion.

TABLE 16-11	Medicare Coverage	
Plan	**Eligibility**	**Coverage**
	TRADITIONAL MEDICARE	
Part A	Social security eligible	Hospitalization
		Subacute nursing home
		Hospice care
		Home care
		Durable medical equipment
Part B	Social security eligible + premium	Physician, PA/NP visits
		Laboratory tests
		OT/PT outpatient care
		Emergency care
		Ambulance
		Outpatient mental health
		Does not cover eyeglasses or hearing aids
Part D	Social security + premium + co-pay	Prescription drugs
		Beneficiary chooses plan
		Formularies vary
	NONTRADITIONAL MEDICARE	
Medicare advantage	Health maintenance organization	Usually 100% coverage, but varies

PA/NP, physician assistant/nurse practitioner; OT/PT, occupational therapy/physical therapy.

D. Financing and costs

1. Elderly patients account for about one-third of U.S. health care dollars. Medicare pays for most of these expenditures.

2. Eligibility for Medicare depends on social security status, which is determined by enrollment in the system, aging and/or disease (end-stage renal disease [ESRD] confers automatic status), or disability. Table 16-11 describes Medicare coverage.

3. Hospice is covered under Medicare Part A and is accessed when the enrollee chooses comfort care and a physician certifies a life expectancy of 6 months or less.

4. Nursing home care for subacute rehabilitation is covered for up to 100 days after a 3-day qualifying hospital stay (20 days fully and 80 days with a co-pay).

5. Informal caregivers, usually family members, provide the majority of daily care for those in the community who require assistance.

17 Pediatrics

Patti Pagels

I. EXAMINATION OF THE NEWBORN

A. Examination at birth

1. Begin with observation, auscultation of the heart and lungs, and inspection for birth trauma/deformities.

2. Apgar score is assessed at 1, 5, and 10 minutes (see Table 8-9). Apgar scoring is completed in the delivery room; low serial scores alert the clinician to the need for resuscitation efforts.

3. The New Ballard Score is a more complex assessment of activity, position, and tone, which is used to evaluate for neuromuscular and physical maturity. This rubric estimates gestational age. Growth charts plot the number of weeks to birth weight to help determine if the newborn is small for gestational age, large for gestational age, or of normal weight.

   a. The causes of an infant's being small for gestational age may be maternal drug use, chromosomal abnormalities, exposure to intrauterine viral infection, multiple gestation, advanced maternal age (>35 years), placental insufficiency, or lack of maternal weight gain.

   b. Most often the cause of an infant's being large for gestational age is maternal diabetes.

B. Nursery examination

1. A complete newborn examination should be completed within 24 hours of birth.

2. Skin: Check for color, temperature, rashes or lesions, edema, and hair distribution.

   a. Erythema toxicum

      (1) Common; first appears 3 to 5 days after birth as small pustules on erythematous bases

      (2) Spontaneous resolution within 1 to 2 weeks is the norm

   b. Milia

      (1) Very small, white papules concentrated on nose, cheeks, forehead, and chin

      (2) Resolve without intervention in 1 to 2 months

   c. Miliaria

      (1) Caused by blockage of eccrine sweat glands, resulting in a flushed macular appearance frequently involving neck, face, scalp, and diaper area

      (2) Light clothing and decreased humidity speed resolution of the "heat rash"

   d. Mongolian spots

      (1) Common in dark-skinned infants and involve small to large, blue-black macules concentrated on the back and buttocks; these macules frequently are misdiagnosed as bruising.

      (2) Most will resolve spontaneously within 4 years, although they may persist for life.

   e. Nevus simplex (stork bite)

      (1) Occur secondary to areas of surface capillary dilation and are frequently found on the eyelids, nape of the neck, and forehead.

      (2) These almost always resolve spontaneously by age 2, although some may persist into adolescence, at which time they may be treated with laser therapy.

   f. Vernix caseosa (greasy covering) and lanugo (fine hairs)

      (1) This is more abundant in preterm infants.

      (2) Dry, cracked, and peeling skin is more likely in postterm infants.

3. Head/face

   a. Craniosynostosis

      (1) This refers to premature fusion of one or more sutures.

      (2) Referral to neurology is necessary.

   b. Fontanelles

      (1) Anterior: 1 to 4 cm in size in either direction; closes around 4 to 26 months of age

      (2) Posterior: 1 cm in size on average; closes around 1 to 3 months

(3) A third fontanelle along the sagittal suture may be present and may be associated with trisomy 21

c. Hematomas and hemorrhages

   (1) Caput succedaneum is fluid accumulation under the scalp secondary to birth trauma. Swelling is palpable crossing the midline.

   (2) Hematomas frequently appear contained within suture lines (cephalhematoma).

   (3) Subgaleal hemorrhages occur beneath the scalp; they are uncommon but may result in enough blood loss to cause hemorrhagic shock.

d. Odd facies beyond the edema and bruising secondary to delivery may represent an underlying syndrome.

4. Ears

   a. Oddly rotated or low-set ears should prompt suspicion of other congenital anomalies.

   b. Preauricular pits and tags are common and usually are benign when they appear in isolation. Infants with hereditary preauricular pits associated with deafness should be followed serially for hearing loss. Other auricular malformations may be linked to underlying genitourinary anomalies, and these infants should be screened with renal ultrasonography.

   c. Hearing is best assessed during the newborn period by auditory brain stem response or evoked otoacoustic emission testing. All infants should be screened regularly during development.

5. Eyes

   a. Abnormalities or asymmetry of red reflex warrants immediate referral to a pediatric ophthalmologist. Congenital cataracts, glaucoma, or retinoblastomas present as absent red reflex in the infant.

   b. Brushfield's spots (gray or pale yellow spots at periphery of the iris) are associated with Down syndrome.

   c. Subconjunctival hemorrhages are common benign findings associated with the trauma of delivery. They generally resolve with time.

   d. Strabismus, or crossing of the eyes, almost always is present during the newborn period and does not represent pathology unless it is fixed or persists past 4 months of age.

6. Nose and mouth

   a. Nose

      (1) Nasal patency is best assessed by testing the nares individually. This may be accomplished by placing a cold metal object below the nose to check for fogging or using a cotton wisp to look for air movement.

      (2) Choanal atresia or stenosis presents with unilateral or bilateral obstruction. Inability to pass a small caliber catheter may be helpful in establishing the obstruction, which is then confirmed with axial computed tomography (CT). Bilateral obstruction results in respiratory distress, because infants are obligate nasal breathers.

   b. Mouth

      (1) Esophageal atresia presents as excessive drooling.

      (2) Epstein pearls appear as small, pearly nodules along the midline of the hard palate and are benign retention cysts.

      (3) Cleft lip/palate deformities are easily identified via inspection. A bifid uvula indicates a submucosal cleft.

      (4) Pierre–Robin syndrome may first be recognized by observation of a small mandible and tongue as well as a clefted soft palate. Prone positioning often will control respiratory difficulties caused by the tongue occluding the airway.

      (5) Infants with trisomy 21 frequently have large tongues that often seem to be larger than the mouth.

      (6) Natal teeth may need to be extracted, if loose, to eliminate the possibility of aspiration.

      (7) Short frenulum may present with difficulty feeding. Lactation consult is the first step in evaluation of this condition.

7. Neck

   a. Webbed or redundant skin of neck may suggest Turner's syndrome.

   b. Masses

      (1) Midline: thyroid. Thyromegaly is associated with congenital hypothyroidism and requires immediate attention to prevent growth failure/cretinism

      (2) Anterior to sternocleidomastoid: brachial cleft (also may see sinus tract remnants)

      (3) Posterior to sternocleidomastoid: cystic hygroma

      (4) Within sternocleidomastoid: torticollis, hematoma

8. Lungs and chest

    a. Fractures resulting from birth trauma may be palpated in the clavicles; examine for tenderness, crepitus, or bruising. Treatment usually is not necessary.

    b. Decreased, asymmetric, or abnormal breath sounds

        (1) Grunting, intercostal retractions, tachypnea (>60 bpm), and cyanosis are all signs of respiratory distress. The etiology of these symptoms may include anything from hyaline membrane disease to sepsis.

        (2) Unilaterally decreased breath sounds may indicate pneumothorax or diaphragmatic hernia. A mediastinal shift supports pneumothorax.

        (3) The most common causes of infant respiratory distress are aspiration, congenital pneumonia, and transient tachypnea.

9. Heart

    a. Heart rate is rapid (average, 140 bpm). See Tables 17-1 and 17-2 for age-specific heart and respiratory rates.

    b. Murmurs are common and not always associated with pathology.

    c. Cyanosis, congestive heart failure, and diminished peripheral pulses are the most common serious presentations of heart disease in the infant.

10. Abdomen

    a. Prune belly or absence of abdominal musculature may be associated with renal anomalies.

    b. Severely scaphoid belly plus respiratory distress suggest diaphragmatic hernia.

    c. Prominent kidneys are suggestive of hydronephrosis or cystic kidney disease.

    d. The liver may be found up to 1 cm below the right costal margin. If larger, evaluation should be initiated.

11. Genitalia and anus

    a. Anus

        (1) Inspect the gluteal cleft for pits, birthmarks, or tufts of hair, as these findings may represent an underlying neurotubular defect or spina bifida. Follow up with x-rays and appropriate referral.

        (2) Anal patency is easily verified with the use of a lubricated thermometer.

    b. Male genitalia

        (1) Hypospadias

            (a) Hypospadias refers to abnormal placement of the urethra where the meatus is proximal and ventral to its normal or anterior location. Epispadias, dorsal displacement, is less common.

            (b) Do not circumcise; bilateral renal ultrasonography is warranted to rule out ascending pathology.

            (c) Refer to a pediatric urologist.

        (2) Empty scrotal sac

            (a) Testes usually descend by the third month of life; more than 80% descend by 1 year of age. If not descended by age 1, refer to a pediatric urologist for surgical intervention.

            (b) Testicular cancer and infertility are real concerns for these children. Bilateral absence of testes should raise suspicion of an infant not fully virilized. A referral to a pediatric endocrinologist is warranted.

        (3) Inguinal hernias

            (a) Inguinal hernias are more common in premature male infants.

            (b) Observe and palpate for an extra full scrotal sac after an episode of crying.

TABLE 17-1	**Age-specific Heart Rates**	
Age	**Average Rate (bpm)**	**Range (bpm)**
Birth	140	90–190
1–6 months	130	80–180
7–12 months	116	75–155
1–2 yr	110	70–150
2–6 yr	102	68–138
6–10 yr	94	65–125
10–14 yr	84	55–115

TABLE 17-2	**Age-specific Respiratory Rates**
Age	**Rate (bpm)**
Birth	30–60
2–12 months	40–50
1–8 yr	20–40
8–15 yr	15–25

(4) Hydrocele

    (a) Observed in about 80% of newborn males, hydrocele refers to a collection of fluid in the scrotum due to patency of the process vaginalis.

    (b) The majority will close within 18 months.

  c. Female genitalia

    (1) Vaginal leucorrhea or bloody discharge along with edematous labia is the result of maternal estrogens. These features usually resolve in 7 to 10 days, but they may resolve more slowly in the breast-fed infant.

    (2) Vaginal adhesions (fused introitus): Application of estrogen or beclomethasone cream for 5 to 10 days usually will resolve the problem; if not, refer to a pediatric urologist.

  d. Ambiguous genitalia most often are associated with rare conditions, such as chromosomal anomalies and adrenal hyperplasia, affecting the action of testosterone.

12. Skeletal

  a. Developmental hip dislocation

    (1) Occurs as frequently as 1 in 500 infants and at higher rates for infants delivered from the breech presentation

    (2) Examination techniques

      (a) The Barlow's maneuver is performed with the infant fully relaxed; it attempts to dislocate the hip via posterior pressure. The examiner adducts the fully flexed hips while pushing the thighs posteriorly. If during this maneuver the femoral head is felt to dislocate or leave the acetabulum, it is considered a positive Barlow's maneuver.

      (b) The Ortolani's maneuver attempts to identify the hip that is dislocated or subluxed. Grasp the medial aspect of the flexed knee with the thumb and fully abduct the hips. Feel for spasm or a clunk (not a click sound) as the hips are brought to full abduction.

      (c) Positive Barlow's and/or Ortolani's maneuvers require bilateral ultrasonography of hips and referral to a pediatric orthopaedic surgeon to prevent a lifelong disability.

  b. Extremities

    (1) Inspect for skin tags at the lateral borders of hands and feet, which represent rudimentary digits (polydactyly). Suspect other malformations when these are present.

    (2) Clubfoot, or talipes equinovarus, is a fixed, severe eversion of the plantar surface and warrants immediate orthopaedic referral.

  c. Spinal deformities, such as tufts of hair or hemangiomas that cross the midline as well as deep sinus tracts in the gluteal cleft, may represent spina bifida occulta, or a tethered spinal cord.

13. Neurologic (reflexes)

  a. Sucking and rooting

    (1) These two are the earliest reflexes.

    (2) Stroking the face elicits turning of the head toward the stimulus; when offered a nipple or the examiner's finger, the infant will instinctively suckle.

  b. Moro or startle reflex

    (1) Allow the infant's head to suddenly drop 1 to 2 cm, and observe for abduction at the shoulders and elbows along with spreading and extending of the fingers, followed by adduction and flexion of the same.

    (2) This reflex disappears by 3 to 4 months of age.

c. Palmar and plantar grasp: Placement of the examiner's finger in the infant's palm or sole should elicit the grasping reflex, which disappears by 4 months of age.

d. Traction response: Pull the infant by the arms to the sitting position, and observe the head lag initially, finally coming briefly to midline before falling forward.

e. Placing reflex

(1) This reflex is noted when the infant is dangled above the bed, allowing the toe to have minimal contact with the surface.

(2) The extremity will respond with flexion or a stepping response.

f. Deep tendon reflexes

(1) These reflexes are brisk; clonus may be noted.

(2) A Babinski (upgoing plantar) is normal and may be noted as late as 2 years of age.

II. PROBLEMS COMMON TO THE TERM NEWBORN

A. Hypoglycemia

1. General characteristics

a. Hypoglycemia is defined as blood glucose level of less than 40 to 45 mg/dL.

b. It is most commonly found in infants born to diabetic mothers and in those who are intrauterine growth restricted.

2. Physical examination

a. Infant may be asymptomatic or present with poor feeding, lethargy, jitteriness, tremulousness, irritability, apnea, or seizures.

b. In cases associated with hyperinsulinemia, cardiac failure may develop.

3. Laboratory testing

a. Heel blood and bedside glucometer readings are adequate for screening.

b. Abnormal results should be confirmed with whole-blood testing.

c. Normal glucose level is 50 to 80 mg/dL at 3 hours of age; an abnormal level is anything less than 40 to 45 mg/dL.

4. Treatment

a. Hypoglycemia is treated with a bolus of dextrose and water ($D_{10}W$) and intravenous (IV) glucose as needed.

b. Continue to monitor; resolution usually occurs by the fifth day of life.

c. Failure to resolve should prompt investigation for less likely causes.

B. Neonatal jaundice

1. General considerations (Table 17-3)

a. More than 65% of infants experience a bilirubin level of greater than 5 mg/dL in the first week of life.

b. Most common causes of unconjugated hyperbilirubinemia are physiologic jaundice, prematurity, and breast-feeding jaundice.

c. Common etiologies are divided into two categories: overproduction of bilirubin or decreased rate of conjugation.

(1) Excess production of bilirubin may result from hemolysis secondary to blood group sensitizations (Coombs' test–positive incompatibilities such as Rh and ABO) or hereditary spherocytosis or glucose-6-phosphate dehydrogenase (G6PD) deficiency (Coombs' test negative). Sepsis and nonhemolytic anemia (extravascular hemorrhage) are other possible causes. Reticulocyte counts are elevated.

(2) Decreased rate of conjugation with normal reticulocyte counts commonly results from physiologic jaundice and uncommonly from Gilbert's or Crigler–Najjar syndrome. Reticulocyte counts remain normal.

d. Kernicterus results from toxic bilirubin levels of greater than 20 to 25 mg/dL and is associated with encephalopathy.

e. Hyperbilirubinemia in the first 24 hours of life must be evaluated immediately.

2. Physical examination

a. Jaundice begins at the head and extends to the chest and extremities as bilirubin levels rise.

b. Scleral icterus and jaundiced oral mucosa help distinguish this in the darkly pigmented infant.

c. Splenomegaly may be present in hereditary spherocytosis.

3. Laboratory tests

a. Laboratory tests should include prenatal maternal blood type, Rh, and antibody testing. Baby's blood type should be done if the mother is type O or Rh negative with direct antibody testing.

TABLE 17-3	Characteristics and Management of Neonatal Jaundice		
Type	**Onset**	**Laboratory Tests**	**Treatment**
ABO incompatibility	First 24 hr after birth	Coombs (+)	Transfusion
		Reticulocytes ↑	Phototherapy
		Hct/Hgb ↓	
Rh isoimmunization	First 24 hr after birth	Coombs (+)	Transfusion
		Reticulocytes	Phototherapy
		Hct/Hgb ↓	
Hereditary spherocytosis	First 24 hr after birth	Coombs (−)	Transfusion if severe
		Reticulocytes ↑	Phototherapy
		Spherocytes on peripheral smear	
G6PD deficiency	First 24 hr after birth	Coombs (−)	Phototherapy
		Specific test for G6PD	
Physiologic jaundice	Appears after 24 hr Peaks at 3–5 days	Bilirubin increases by <5 mg/dL/day	Phototherapy when bilirubin is >15 mg/dL or not descending
Breast-feeding jaundice	Second to third day of life	Bilirubin ↑ and may persist for 6–8 weeks	Supplement breast milk with formula; feed or pump breast milk every 2 hr until an adequate supply is established
			Phototherapy when bilirubin is >15 mg/dL

Hct/Hgb, hematocrit/hemoglobin; G6PD, glucose-6-phosphate dehydrogenase.

  b. Direct and indirect bilirubin levels should be obtained. Complete blood count (CBC), reticulocyte count, and blood smear should also be considered.

  c. Conjugated hyperbilirubinemia (direct bilirubin >2 mg/dL and >10% of the total) may be caused by biliary obstruction/atresia, choledochal cyst, hyperalimentation, α_1-antitrypsin deficiency, hepatitis, sepsis, infections (especially urinary tract infections), hypothyroidism, inborn errors of metabolism, cystic fibrosis, and red blood cell abnormalities.

  d. Monitor hematocrit and hemoglobin in cases of hemolysis or hemorrhage.

  e. Septic workup as indicated.

 4. Management and treatment

  a. Transfusion is necessary if the cause is ABO incompatibility, Rh isoimmunization, or nonimmune hemolysis (Coombs' test negative).

  b. Phototherapy benefits all types of jaundice.

   (1) Phototherapy may be started as early as 12 hours of age. In term babies, bilirubin levels fall up to 1 to 2 mg/dL in 4 to 6 hours and should be monitored regularly using total serum bilirubin levels.

   (2) Decision to begin phototherapy depends on the baby's weight and the level of bilirubin (Table 17-4).

 C. Respiratory distress in the newborn

 1. General considerations: Respiratory distress may be due to pulmonary, cardiovascular, or other causes (Table 17-5).

 2. Physical examination

  a. The infant typically appears cyanotic on room air.

  b. Respiratory rate is greater than 60 bpm.

  c. Grunting as well as intercostal and sternal retractions are common.

  d. Cyanosis resolving with supplemental oxygen supports either a pulmonary or a noncardiovascular cause. This is known as the hyperoxia challenge test.

 3. Laboratory studies

  a. Chest radiography, pulse oximetry, and arterial blood gases provide the basic information.

TABLE 17-4	Guidelines for Phototherapy in Neonatal Jaundice
Weight (g)	**Bilirubin Level (mg/dL)**
500–1,000	12–15
1,000–1,500	15–18
1,500–2,500	18–20
>2,500	>20

b. CBC and blood cultures should be monitored if appropriate.

c. A complete metabolic profile typically is done on all cyanotic infants.

d. Echocardiography or CT of the head and chest may be warranted by the suspected cause.

4. Management

a. Provide immediate supplemental oxygen with close monitoring.

b. Begin IV fluids (glucose or saline, as the situation warrants).

c. Provide intubation if true respiratory failure is present.

d. Determine the underlying cause and manage appropriately.

III. DEVELOPMENTAL MILESTONES AND DISORDERS

A. Developmental milestones

1. General considerations

a. Typically, developmental surveys are done at each well-child examination; these examinations usually correspond to the typical vaccination schedule.

TABLE 17-5	Common Causes of Respiratory Distress Syndrome
Pulmonary causes	Unilateral or bilateral choanal atresia
	Transient tachypnea of the newborn (resolves in 24 hr)
	Fluid aspiration (blood or meconium)
	Hyaline membrane disease (especially in premature infants)
	Congenital pneumonia (rectal flora pathogens)
Cardiovascular causes	
1. Cyanotic lesions	Valvular pulmonary stenosis (only when severe)
	Pulmonary atresia with ventricular septal defect (the most extreme form of tetralogy of Fallot)
	Tricuspid atresia
	Transposition of the great arteries
	Total anomalous pulmonary venous return
	Truncus arteriosus (<1% of cases)
2. Mild cyanosis resulting from left-sided outflow tract obstruction	Hypoplastic left heart syndrome (usually involving atresia of mitral valve, aortic valve, or both)
	Aortic stenosis
	Coarctation of the aorta
Other causes	Hyperthermia or hypothermia (hypothermia is especially troublesome for the preterm infant)
	Intrauterine exposure to cocaine
	Metabolic acidosis
	Hemorrhage or asphyxia resulting in damage to the CNS (can occur as a result of traumatic delivery)

CNS, central nervous system.

b. Developmental screenings are done frequently between birth and 3 years of age and then each year thereafter.

c. Parents and caregivers are important sources of information regarding the child's abilities.

d. It is important to distinguish between a child whose pattern of development has slowed or regressed and a child who has always been developmentally slow, because the causes generally are quite different.

2. From birth to 5 years of age, the areas that typically are surveyed are gross and fine motor skills, personal and social behaviors, and language; assessment of older children shifts to higher cognitive functions and sexual maturation.

   a. Table 17-6 highlights milestones for children from birth to 5 years of age.

   b. Table 17-7 highlights milestones for children from 6 to 10 years of age.

   c. Between 10 and 19 years of age, the focus shifts from developmental milestones to physical maturation and psychological development. The classical and most efficient way to gauge sexual maturation in males and females is by using Tanner stages (Table 17-8).

TABLE 17-6	**Typical Developmental Milestones from Birth to 5 Years of Age**			
Age/Skill	**Gross Motor**	**Fine Motor**	**Personal/Social**	**Language**
0–2 months	Turns head side to side	Clenched fist Eye contact	Recognizes human face	Cries Startles at loud noise
2–3 months	Lifts head	Tracks object past midline Hands open	Smiles responsively	Vocalizes in play
4–5 months	Head steady in supported position	Hands together	Shows displeasure through vocalization	Looks for source of sound
6–8 months	Rolls over Sits leaning forward on arms	Reaches for objects Raking grasp	Responds to own name Holds own bottle	Imitates speech sounds Vocal imitation
9–11 months	Stands while holding on	Passes object from hand to hand	Feeds self Imitates waving	Understands *no* May say *mama*
12–14 months	Stands alone for 2 sec	Bangs two objects together Places pellet in bottle	Hugs dolls or stuffed animals Routinely gestures to meet needs	Uses one or two words with meaning
15–17 months	Stoops and recovers Walks well	Builds tower of two or three cubes	Attempts use of spoon	Waves bye-bye Uses four or five words
18–21 months	Runs well Kicks large ball Walks backward	Scribbles Turns pages of book	Drinks well from a cup Feeds self Uses a spoon well	Follows simple commands (e.g., *give me*) 20–50 words
24 months	Throws ball overhead Jumps	Turns doorknobs Builds towers of six to seven blocks	Washes and dries hands Little spilling during self-feeding	Two or three words combined Points to body parts
36 months	Stands on one foot at least 2 sec	Copies circle	Takes turns Toilet trained	Uses pronouns (*I, me, you*) Gives name
48 months	Hops on one foot	Wiggles thumb Copies cross	Dresses self	Knows colors Asks questions
5 yr	Skips using alternate feet	Holds a pencil correctly	Brushes teeth without help	Easily carries on a conversation May count or recite part of the alphabet

TABLE 17-7	Typical Developmental Milestones from 6 to 10 Years of Age				
Skill/Age	**6 yr (Grade 1)**	**7 yr (Grade 2)**	**8 yr (Grade 3)**	**9 yr (Grade 4)**	**10 yr (Grade 5)**
Language	Speaks using correct sentence structure	Defines words Compares and contrasts Speech reaches adult proficiency	Defines more words Recites days of week	Comprehends absurdities in sentences	Understands abstract words
Hand–eye coordination	Draws more precisely	Legible printing Ties own shoe laces	Begins to learn cursive writing	Draws people, with detail	Draws people, with great detail
Calculation and reading	Reads one-syllable words Counts to 20 Later reads simple sentence, adds and subtracts primary numbers	Reads two-syllable words Counts to 100 Adds and subtracts two-digit numbers	Reads many more two-syllable words Performs simple multiplication	Reads three- and four-syllable words Alphabetizes Does simple division Comprehends fractions	Able to read more complex words Easily uses addition, subtraction, fractions, division, multiplication, and estimation

B. Development disorders

1. General considerations

   a. Disorders of development often are first noted by parents or caregivers when a child fails to meet one or more milestones in development. Areas of concern include motor, visual–spatial, verbal, attention, behavioral, and social abilities.

   b. The most common neurodevelopmental disorder is attention-deficit hyperactivity disorder (ADHD); the most severe (in terms of affecting all areas of development) is mental retardation.

2. Evaluation of developmental disorders

   a. A comprehensive history should include a detailed prenatal history, labor and delivery, complications during pregnancy as well as the immediate postnatal period, major illness/hospitalizations, history of metabolic disease, and family history.

   b. A complete physical examination is essential, especially the neurologic examination and careful inspection for dysmorphic features.

   c. Referral to appropriate specialists, including speech and occupational therapists, psychologists, and educational specialists, should be made as dictated by the child's needs.

TABLE 17-8	Typical Tanner Stages for Males and Females from 11 to 17 Years of Age			
Tanner Stage	**2** **Age 11–12**	**3** **Age 13**	**4** **Age 14–15**	**5** **Age 16–17**
Males	Straight hair at base of penis	Coarse, dark, and curly pubic hair	Hair is almost completely full	Pubic hair achieves adult appearance
	Age 11	**Age 12**	**Age 13**	**Age 14–15**
Females	Minimal, straight pubic hair	Increased pubic hair that is dark and coarse	Hair approaches normal adult appearance	Pubic hair reaches adult appearance and forms inverted triangle

3. Speech and/or language delay

   a. Causes are many, with the most common being conductive hearing loss secondary to chronic middle ear effusion. Others causes include prematurity, neglect, autism, and congenital syndromes.

   b. Language delay may be characterized by omitted sounds, difficulty pronouncing certain letters, dysfluency, or failure to have appropriate language skills by 2 or 3 years of age. Language should be assessed as expressive language and receptive language.

   c. Hearing should be carefully assessed, especially when speech delay appears to be the only impairment.

   d. Management includes referral to speech and language specialists for specific diagnosis, development of a treatment plan, and monitoring during development.

4. Attention-deficit hyperactivity disorder (see Chapter 12)

5. Pervasive developmental disorders (see Chapter 12)

6. Mental retardation

   a. Mental retardation is defined as an IQ of less than 70, with disturbances in adaptive behavior.

   b. Physical examination

     (1) Abnormal muscle tone is seen at 6 months.

     (2) Motor delay is apparent by 1 year.

     (3) All spheres of development are affected to some degree by 2 years.

   c. Laboratory testing is carried out to uncover possible causes and includes CBC to rule out anemia; lead screen; chromosomal studies, especially if the child is dysmorphic; metabolic testing; thyroid studies; electroencephalography (EEG); and magnetic resonance imaging (MRI) as appropriate.

   d. Treatment includes referral to special programs for social, occupational, and cognitive support.

7. Spina bifida (myelomeningocele)

   a. Two forms exist.

     (1) Aperta is when the neural tube defect involves the overlying skin.

     (2) Occulta appears as hairy tufts, dimples, or dermal sinus noted in the lumbosacral region.

   b. Risks factors include insufficient intake of folic acid during pregnancy and maternal use of valproate.

   c. Characteristic findings

     (1) Neurologic: hypotonia, sensory deficits, paralysis, hydrocephalus, or macrocephaly

     (2) Extremities: contractures, tethered cord, which may cause back pain, clubfeet, scoliosis, or hip dislocations

     (3) Urinary: frequent urosepsis, incontinence

   d. Treatment includes prompt intervention for hydrocephalus through shunting and referral for supportive services.

8. Cerebral palsy (see Chapter 11)

IV. INBORN ERRORS OF METABOLISM, CHROMOSOMAL ABNORMALITIES, AND COMMON DYSMORPHIC SYNDROMES

A. Inborn errors of metabolism

1. General considerations

   a. All states screen infants for phenylketonuria, congenital adrenal hyperplasia, galactosemia, and hypothyroidism. These disorders are treatable, and testing generally is inexpensive.

   b. In general, more expansive and/or selective screening should be considered under the following conditions:

     (1) Acutely ill infant or neonate

     (2) Developmental delay (index of suspicion should be higher with regression of development)

     (3) Failure to thrive

     (4) Mental retardation

     (5) Organomegaly

2. Management and treatment

   a. Better outcomes are associated with early identification and when families both understand and can adhere to treatment regimens.

TABLE 17-9	Common Inborn Errors of Metabolism: Epidemiology, Signs, Symptoms, Testing, and Management		
Condition	**Signs and Symptoms**	**Specific Evaluations**	**Treatments**
Hypothyroidism (1:4,500 live births)	Lethargy, mental retardation, eczema, failure to thrive; rarely goiter, thick tongue; up to 75% of newborns are asymptomatic during the first 2 months of life	Serial TSH, free T_4	Replacement therapy with L-thyroxine
Congenital adrenal hyperplasia (1:5,000 live births)	Virilized female; males may have ambiguous genitalia; infants may present early in life with salt-wasting, adrenal crisis	17-Hydroxyprogesterone	Corticosteroid replacement
Phenylketonuria (1:12,000 live births)	Moderate to severe mental retardation, hyperactivity, seizures, autism, and hypopigmentation	Test after 24 hr of protein intake, then quantitative serum phenylalanine determination	Lifetime of low-protein diet; avoid products with phenylalanine
Galactosemia (1:60,000 live births)	Neonatal nausea and vomiting, jaundice, hepatic dysfunction and liver enlargement, mental retardation, cataracts, and death	Galactose-1-phosphate uridyltransferase electrophoresis after galactose intake	Lactose- and galactose-free diet

TSH, thyroid-stimulating hormone; T_4, thyroxine.

b. Table 17-9 describes the specific characteristics, special tests, and management principles for phenylketonuria, congenital adrenal hyperplasia, galactosemia, and hypothyroidism.

B. Chromosomal abnormalities

1. General considerations

    a. Chromosomal abnormalities are found in 1 in 200 live births and approximately 7% of aborted concepti.

    b. Occurrence of one or more of the following should prompt further evaluation: certain dysmorphology, metabolic disorder, degenerative disorders, ambiguous genitalia, multiple congenital anomalies, retinoblastoma, Wilms' tumor, developmental delay, abnormal stature, and primary amenorrhea.

    c. Types of chromosomal anomalies

        (1) Structural: deletions, duplications, translocations, inversions

        (2) Numeric: triploidy and tetraploidy (both lethal), trisomy, monosomy, aneuploidy of sex chromosomes, and mosaicism

    d. Initial evaluation when chromosomal abnormalities are suspected should include karyotype and fluorescence in situ hybridization (FISH). Evaluation is based on clinical suspicion, DNA analysis and BAC-CGH arrays.

    e. Management is specific to the disorder and may include supportive care, environmental and educational supports, physical therapy, and other modalities.

2. Common chromosomal abnormalities

    a. Trisomy 21 (Down syndrome)

        (1) Incidence is 1 in 750 live births.

        (2) It is frequently associated with advanced maternal age.

        (3) Common characteristics:

            (a) Diagnosis is made if any six of the following characteristics are seen: hypotonia, poor Moro reflex, hypermobility of joints, flattened facies and occiput, excess skin on the posterior neck, anomalous auricles, upward-slanting palpebral fissures, pelvic dysplasia, dysplasia of the middle-phalanx of the fifth finger, and a single transverse palmar crease (simian crease).

            (b) Other features may include macrosomia, mental retardation, hearing loss, Brushfield's spots in the eyes, thyroid disease, gastrointestinal atresia, and atlantoaxial instability.

            (c) Congenital heart disease is present in up to 40% of cases; atrioventricular septal defects are most common.

    b. Klinefelter's syndrome (XXY)

        (1) Incidence is 1 in 800 live births.

        (2) Common characteristics

(a) Initially tall, thin, and long limbed; become obese in the adult years. Scoliosis is frequent.

(b) Ataxia, expressive language disorders, and usually mild developmental delay

(c) Males: small penis, hypogonadism, scant pubic and facial hair, and gynecomastia

(d) Females: eunuchoid habitus

c. Turner syndrome (monosomy X)

(1) Incidence is 1 in 2,000 female live births.

(2) Common characteristics

(a) These include short stature, webbed neck, prominent ears and low posterior hairline, broad chest with widely spaced nipples, increased carrying angle, congential lymphedema.

(b) Other features may include hearing impairment as well as visual and spatial perceptive disabilities, primary amenorrhea, ovarian dysgenesis, absence of secondary sex characteristics, coarctation of the aorta, horseshoe kidney, and aortic stenosis.

d. Fragile X syndrome

(1) Incidence is 1 in 1,250 male live births.

(2) Common characteristics

(a) Pale blue irides, long narrowed facies, large protruding ears, large protruding jaw, flat feet, and hyperextensible fingers

(b) Prepubertal large gonads

(c) Autism and/or moderate to severe mental retardation with disorganized speech patterns

(d) Mitral valve prolapse

(e) Female carriers exhibit mild learning disabilities

e. Beckwith–Wiedemann syndrome (chromosome 11p15)

(1) Incidence is 1 in 15,000 live births.

(2) Common characteristics

(a) Large-for-gestational-age infants, hypoglycemia during infancy, creases and pits in earlobes, asymmetric limbs, organomegaly, and large tongue

(b) At risk for Wilms' tumor and hepatoblastoma

f. Prader–Willi syndrome (chromosome 15q11)

(1) Incidence is 1 in 25,000 live births.

(2) Common characteristics

(a) Infants are often small-for-gestational-age and exhibit hypogonadism, small hands and feet, almond-shaped eyes, and hypotonia.

(b) Mental retardation, short stature, polyphagia, and eventually obesity are characteristic.

(c) Diabetes and Pickwickian syndrome are common complications.

g. Angelman's syndrome (chromosome 15)

(1) Incidence is unknown but estimated at between 1 in 15,000 and 1 in 30,000 live births.

(2) Common characteristics

(a) Severe mental retardation, marked developmental delay, poor language skills, paroxysmal laughter, and tongue thrusting

(b) Prognathism, seizures, and abnormal gait and posturing

C. Common dysmorphic syndromes

1. General considerations

a. Dysmorphic syndromes may result from a chromosomal anomaly or single-gene defects. Some are multifactorial; others may result from a combination of genetics and environment.

b. Characteristics of these chromosomal or genetic anomalies include

(1) Multiple anomalies are common.

(2) Abnormal growth patterns, both pre- and postnatally, are seen.

(3) Child typically exhibits characteristics not seen in parents or siblings.

(4) Infant may present with mental retardation, abnormal muscle tone, seizures, sensory deficits, as well as motor and speech delay.

    c. Testing is specific for the syndrome under consideration.

    d. Treatment involves detailed genetic counseling and, in some cases, surgical intervention.

  2. Common dysmorphic syndromes

    a. Ehlers–Danlos syndrome is primarily an autosomal dominant condition (10 syndromes or clinical types are known).

      (1) The primary defect involves collagen, resulting in joint laxity, hyperelastic skin, pectus deformity, and excessive bruising.

      (2) Death often results from ruptured aneurysm.

    b. Marfan syndrome is an autosomal dominant mutation.

      (1) The primary defect involves a connective tissue protein, resulting in tall, lanky stature, joint laxity, high arched palate, long digits, and myopia.

      (2) Complications result from mitral valve prolapse, aortic root dilation, aortic insufficiency, aneurysms, and spontaneous pneumothorax.

    c. Fetal alcohol syndrome is related to maternal alcohol use.

      (1) These children are born small and may remain small. Characteristics involving the head and facies include microcephaly, long and smooth philtrum, thin upper lip, small palpebral fissures, and small distal phalanges.

      (2) This syndrome is complicated by developmental delay, hyperactivity, moderate retardation, and involvement of internal organs (congenital heart disease, cleft lip/palate, and renal anomalies).

    d. Neural tube defects

      (1) Causes may include genetics and environment.

      (2) Defects may be as severe as anencephaly or as mild as a small spina bifida.

      (3) Folic acid supplementation prior to and throughout pregnancy may be protective.

    e. Cleft lip and palate

      (1) Typically, the cause is multifactorial, but cleft lip and palate may result from autosomal dominant, autosomal recessive, or X-linked disorders.

      (2) Various degrees of severity are seen, involving specific deformities of the lip, hard palate, and soft palate.

      (3) Look for other malformations because, in many cases, this will not be an isolated defect.

      (4) Many cases are amenable to surgery.

    f. Osteogenesis imperfecti

      (1) This autosomal dominant defect involves type 1 collagen, resulting in bone fragility and pathologic fractures.

      (2) Some cases result in blue-tinted sclera and varying degree of deafness.

      (3) In its severest form, fetal demise may occur.

V. FAILURE TO THRIVE, GROWTH DELAY, AND SELECTED NUTRITIONAL DISORDERS OF CHILDHOOD

A. Failure to thrive

  1. General characteristics

    a. Failure to thrive is defined as a child aged 2 years or younger with weight plotting below the fifth percentile for age on more than one occasion or whose weight crosses two major percentiles downward on a standardized growth grid.

    b. Exceptions to this definition are genetic short stature, small-for-gestational-age infants, preterm infants, Asian infants, and overweight infants with decreased rate of weight gain and increased rate of height gain.

    c. Failure-to-thrive presentation affects approximately 10% of infants and children. It is most commonly associated with environmental and/or behavioral factors, followed by organic causes such as reflux, renal tubular acidosis, and acute or chronic infections.

  2. Specific causes to be considered include:

    a. Lack of appetite (caused by anemia, psychosocial problems, central nervous system [CNS] pathology, chronic infection, or gastrointestinal [GI] disorder)

    b. Difficulty with ingestion (caused by psychosocial problems, cerebral palsy or other CNS disorders, dyspnea, craniofacial abnormalities, myopathies, or congenital syndromes)

    c. Unavailability of food (consider inappropriate feeding techniques, inadequate volume of food, inappropriate food for age, abuse, or neglect)

    d. Vomiting (caused by reflux, obstruction of the intestinal tract, or increased intracranial pressure)

    e. Malabsorption (cystic fibrosis, biliary disease, disorders of metabolism, immune deficiency, inflammatory bowel disease, or celiac disease)

    f. Diarrhea (caused by bacterial gastroenteritis, parasitic infection, or starvation)

    g. Inadequate absorption of calories (caused by hepatitis or Hirschsprung's disease)

    h. Increased metabolism/increased use of calories (chronic or recurrent infection [most common is urinary tract infection], chronic pulmonary insufficiency, congenital or acquired heart disease, neoplasm, lead poisoning, chronic anemia, or endocrinopathies)

    i. Defective use of calories (inborn errors of metabolism, renal tubular acidosis [uncommon], cyanotic heart disease)

3. Laboratory tests

    a. Investigation centers on uncovering any known cause.

    b. Observation by a team or in a hospital setting is desired if a behavioral or psychosocial cause is suspected.

    c. Specific laboratory testing is needed as per history and physical examination. Initial laboratory should include:

        (1) CBC with differential and erythrocyte sedimentation rate (ESR)

        (2) Urinalysis with culture and sensitivity

        (3) Serum electrolytes, blood urea nitrogen (BUN), and creatinine

        (4) Thyroid-stimulating hormone (TSH) with a thyroxine (T_4)

        (5) Tuberculin skin test

        (6) Radiography of wrists for bone age

4. Treatment

    a. Treat the underlying cause.

    b. Remove the child from the home if necessary.

    c. Increase feedings for infants from 100 to 150 kcal/kg/day.

B. Selected causes of growth delay

  1. Familial short stature

    a. General characteristics

        (1) Familial short stature is apparent before the second year of life and manifests as a deceleration in height.

        (2) Height is hereditary and closely matches parental height.

    b. Physical examination: The child has normal development without other signs or symptoms of disease.

    c. Special testing

        (1) Further testing to rule out other causes may include CBC; ESR; urinalysis; BUN and creatinine; serum electrolytes, including calcium and phosphorus; examination of stool for fat content; karyotype; and intrinsic growth factor (IGF)-1 and IGF-binding protein 3.

        (2) Radiography of the distal radius will reveal bone age equal to chronological age.

    d. Treatment: Reassure parents that deceleration is normal and expected, especially if both parents are short.

  2. Constitutional growth delay

    a. General characteristics

        (1) The child is often called a "late bloomer" and may have a family history of delayed growth.

        (2) Family members may be of normal height.

        (3) Skeletal bone age will lag behind chronological age.

        (4) Puberty may be delayed.

    b. Physical examination: Except for height, development is normal for age.

    c. Selected testing

        (1) Further testing is driven by the history and physical examination findings; testing is done to rule out other causes as mentioned earlier.

        (2) Radiography of the distal radius reveals chronological age greater than bone age.

    d. Treatment: Growth is delayed, but eventually the child will reach his or her expected height.

3. Growth hormone (GH) deficiency
   a. General characteristics
      (1) The anterior pituitary produces GH under stimulation from GH-releasing hormone (GHRH) and suppression of somatostatin.
      (2) GH deficiency may be an isolated disorder or may occur as a result of other pituitary hormone deficiencies. The most likely cause is idiopathic; other diagnoses to consider include congenital (empty sella syndrome) and acquired (craniopharyngioma).
      (3) Growth failure caused by GH deficiency may occur during infancy or appear later in childhood and is largely dependent on the underlying cause.
      (4) Laron syndrome is dwarfism that results from a mutation in the GH receptor.
   b. Physical examination
      (1) Decline in growth velocity or subnormal growth is characteristic.
      (2) Children with dwarfism have distinctive facial features.
      (3) Truncal obesity may be present, because GH also promotes lipolysis.
      (4) Impaired peripheral vision with optic chiasm tumors is frequent.
      (5) Delayed puberty and webbed neck are seen in cases of Turner's syndrome.
      (6) Disproportionately short limbs compared to trunk suggest a skeletal dysplasia.
   c. Testing
      (1) Testing should be as suggested by the history and physical examination and to rule out other causes, as mentioned earlier.
      (2) Radiography of the distal radius should be performed for bone age.
      (3) When other causes are ruled out and GH status is equivocal, more provocative studies are warranted.
      (4) In some cases, a trial of human GH may be warranted and may confirm the diagnosis.
   d. Treatment
      (1) Human GH has been approved for specific causes, such as Prader–Willi syndrome, Turner's syndrome, children born small for gestational age who fail to grow, and chronic renal failure.
      (2) Referral to a pediatric endocrinologist is recommended, because tests for GH deficiency often are difficult to interpret and treatment for other causes is controversial.

C. Selected nutritional disorders
   1. General considerations
      a. Nutritional deficiencies may result from internal causes (e.g., blood loss, malabsorption, chronic disease) or external causes (e.g., inappropriate feeding, psychosocial distress, inability to take in sufficient nutrition).
      b. The ideal source of infant nutrition is breast milk because it contains a perfect mix of nutrients as well as protein, lipids, and carbohydrates; promotes bonding; and strengthens the infant's immune system. Infant formulas today come very close to matching breast milk in terms of providing energy and nutrition.
      c. The typical infant diet should consist of breast milk or formula until 4 months of age. Cereal may be introduced at 4 months, fruit at 5 months, vegetables at 6 months, and complex proteins in the months that follow. Cow's milk with low fat content should be initiated no earlier than 1 year of age.
   2. Calcium, fluoride, vitamin K, protein, and carbohydrate deficiencies (Table 17-10)

VI. IMMUNIZATION OF INFANTS AND CHILDREN (FIG. 17-1)

A. General considerations
   1. Combination products (one syringe containing multiple vaccines) are preferred and have not been found to diminish immune response or to increase the rate of adverse events.
   2. Premature infants are immunized just as term newborns in regard to amount and timing. An exception is hepatitis B vaccine, which is recommended for premature infants weighing 2 kg or more.
   3. There are few contraindications to vaccines.
      a. Anaphylactic reaction to previous vaccine or component of a vaccine:
         (1) Neomycin and streptomycin are common preservatives in MMR (measles, mumps, and rubella vaccine) and IPV (inactivated polio vaccine) and have caused allergic reactions and anaphylaxis.
         (2) Baker's yeast allergy: Avoid hepatitis B vaccine.

| | **Risk Factors for** | | **Laboratory** | |
Nutrient	**Development**	**Signs and Symptoms**	**Examinations**	**Treatment**
Protein	Body cannot store protein, so a daily supply is needed Severe skin disease and burns Cystic fibrosis	Impaired growth velocity Severest form is kwashiorkor, resulting in lethargy, irritability, impaired growth velocity, edema, and hepatomegaly	Chemistry panel (may suggest decreased albumin) CBC (may reveal other deficiencies)	Adjust diet; increase daily intake of protein
Carbohydrate	Daily supply is required because of the body's limited ability to store excess Galactosemia (inborn error of metabolism) Diarrhea Malabsorption Improper diet Excess intake results in obesity and increased risk of type 2 diabetes mellitus	Impaired growth velocity Obesity Marasmus is a severe form of malnutrition resulting from multiple dietary deficiencies, including lack of carbohydrates	Chemistry panel (electrolyte imbalances likely) CBC	Dietary adjustment
Vitamin K	Aids in formulation of coagulation proteins Newborns Breast-fed newborns who do not receive vitamin K prophylactically at birth	Hemorrhagic purpura involving skin, internal organs, and CNS, which may be fatal	Vitamin K levels Prolonged prothrombin time	IM vitamin K injection
Fluoride	Fluoride is incorporated into the tooth matrix, increasing resistance to dental caries This element is contained in most public water sources	Increased number of dental caries In case of fluoridosis, look for undermineralization and discolored teeth	Dental examinations	Consider supplementation after 6 months of age when the water source does not contain fluoride
Iron	Breast-fed infants Untreated maternal anemia Prematurity Blood loss during the neonatal period	Asymptomatic when mild Pallor Fatigue Impaired cognitive and motor development Pica	CBC with differential Serum ferritin Serum iron Total iron-binding capacity Reticulocyte count	Food with high iron content Supplementation For breast-fed infants, introduce iron-fortified cereals at 4–6 months

TABLE 17-10 **Selected Nutritional Disorders**

CBC, complete blood count; IM, intramuscular; CNS, central nervous system.

(3) Allergy to eggs: Avoid influenza vaccine.

(4) Gelatin allergy: Avoid varicella vaccine.

b. History of encephalopathy within 7 days of giving DTaP or DTP (diphtheria, tetanus, and pertussis vaccine).

c. Pregnancy: Avoid live vaccines, such as MMR and varicella, and live attenuated influenza vaccine.

d. Avoid MMR and varicella vaccine if immunocompromised.

4. Precautions should be taken with the following vaccines under certain circumstances:

a. Consider rescheduling any vaccine in the presence of moderate to severe illness and/or fever ($\geq$102.5°F/39.0°C)

b. Postpone MMR and varicella vaccine until 3 to 6 months after administration of immunoglobulin.

Recommended Immunization Schedule for Persons Aged 0 Through 6 Years—United States • 2009

For those who fall behind or start late, see the catch-up schedule

Vaccine ▼ Age ►	Birth	1 month	2 months	4 months	6 months	12 months	15 months	18 months	19–23 months	2–3 years	4–6 years	
Hepatitis B[1]	HepB	HepB		see footnote 1	HepB							Range of recommended ages
Rotavirus[2]			RV	RV	RV[2]							
Diphtheria, Tetanus, Pertussis[3]			DTaP	DTaP	DTaP	see footnote 3	DTaP				DTaP	
Haemophilus influenzae type b[4]			Hib	Hib	Hib[4]	Hib						
Pneumococcal[5]			PCV	PCV	PCV	PCV				PPSV		Certain high-risk groups
Inactivated Poliovirus			IPV	IPV		IPV					IPV	
Influenza[6]						Influenza (Yearly)						
Measles, Mumps, Rubella[7]						MMR		see footnote 7			MMR	
Varicella[8]						Varicella		see footnote 8			Varicella	
Hepatitis A[9]						HepA (2 doses)				HepA Series		
Meningococcal[10]										MCV		

This schedule indicates the recommended ages for routine administration of currently licensed vaccines, as of December 1, 2008, for children aged 0 through 6 years. Any dose not administered at the recommended age should be administered at a subsequent visit, when indicated and feasible. Licensed combination vaccines may be used whenever any component of the combination is indicated and other components are not contraindicated and if approved by the Food and Drug Administration for that dose of the series. Providers should consult the relevant Advisory Committee on Immunization Practices statement for detailed recommendations, including high-risk conditions: http://www.cdc.gov/vaccines/pubs/acip-list.htm. Clinically significant adverse events that follow immunization should be reported to the Vaccine Adverse Event Reporting System (VAERS). Guidance about how to obtain and complete a VAERS form is available at http://www.vaers.hhs.gov or by telephone, 800-822-7967.

1. Hepatitis B vaccine (HepB). *(Minimum age: birth)*
At birth:
• Administer monovalent HepB to all newborns before hospital discharge.
• If mother is hepatitis B surface antigen (HBsAg)-positive, administer HepB and 0.5 mL of hepatitis B immune globulin (HBIG) within 12 hours of birth.
• If mother's HBsAg status is unknown, administer HepB within 12 hours of birth. Determine mother's HBsAg status as soon as possible and, if HBsAg-positive, administer HBIG (no later than age 1 week).
After the birth dose:
• The HepB series should be completed with either monovalent HepB or a combination vaccine containing HepB. The second dose should be administered at age 1 or 2 months. The final dose should be administered no earlier than age 24 weeks.
• Infants born to HBsAg-positive mothers should be tested for HBsAg and antibody to HBsAg (anti-HBs) after completion of at least 3 doses of the HepB series, at age 9 through 18 months (generally at the next well-child visit).
4-month dose:
• Administration of 4 doses of HepB to infants is permissible when combination vaccines containing HepB are administered after the birth dose.

2. Rotavirus vaccine (RV). *(Minimum age: 6 weeks)*
• Administer the first dose at age 6 through 14 weeks (maximum age: 14 weeks 6 days). Vaccination should not be initiated for infants aged 15 weeks or older (i.e., 15 weeks 0 days or older).
• Administer the final dose in the series by age 8 months 0 days.
• If Rotarix® is administered at ages 2 and 4 months, a dose at 6 months is not indicated.

3. Diphtheria and tetanus toxoids and acellular pertussis vaccine (DTaP). *(Minimum age: 6 weeks)*
• The fourth dose may be administered as early as age 12 months, provided at least 6 months have elapsed since the third dose.
• Administer the final dose in the series at age 4 through 6 years.

4. Haemophilus influenzae type b conjugate vaccine (Hib). *(Minimum age: 6 weeks)*
• If PRP-OMP (PedvaxHIB® or Comvax® [HepB-Hib]) is administered at ages 2 and 4 months, a dose at age 6 months is not indicated.
• TriHiBit® (DTaP/Hib) should not be used for doses at ages 2, 4, or 6 months but can be used as the final dose in children aged 12 months or older.

5. Pneumococcal vaccine. *(Minimum age: 6 weeks for pneumococcal conjugate vaccine [PCV]; 2 years for pneumococcal polysaccharide vaccine [PPSV])*
• PCV is recommended for all children aged younger than 5 years. Administer 1 dose of PCV to all healthy children aged 24 through 59 months who are not completely vaccinated for their age.

• Administer PPSV to children aged 2 years or older with certain underlying medical conditions (see *MMWR* 2000;49[No. RR-9]), including a cochlear implant.

6. Influenza vaccine. *(Minimum age: 6 months for trivalent inactivated influenza vaccine [TIV]; 2 years for live, attenuated influenza vaccine [LAIV])*
• Administer annually to children aged 6 months through 18 years.
• For healthy nonpregnant persons (i.e., those who do not have underlying medical conditions that predispose them to influenza complications) aged 2 through 49 years, either LAIV or TIV may be used.
• Children receiving TIV should receive 0.25 mL if aged 6 through 35 months or 0.5 mL if aged 3 years or older.
• Administer 2 doses (separated by at least 4 weeks) to children aged younger than 9 years who are receiving influenza vaccine for the first time or who were vaccinated for the first time during the previous influenza season but only received 1 dose.

7. Measles, mumps, and rubella vaccine (MMR). *(Minimum age: 12 months)*
• Administer the second dose at age 4 through 6 years. However, the second dose may be administered before age 4, provided at least 28 days have elapsed since the first dose.

8. Varicella vaccine. *(Minimum age: 12 months)*
• Administer the second dose at age 4 through 6 years. However, the second dose may be administered before age 4, provided at least 3 months have elapsed since the first dose.
• For children aged 12 months through 12 years the minimum interval between doses is 3 months. However, if the second dose was administered at least 28 days after the first dose, it can be accepted as valid.

9. Hepatitis A vaccine (HepA). *(Minimum age: 12 months)*
• Administer to all children aged 1 year (i.e., aged 12 through 23 months). Administer 2 doses at least 6 months apart.
• Children not fully vaccinated by age 2 years can be vaccinated at subsequent visits.
• HepA also is recommended for children older than 1 year who live in areas where vaccination programs target older children or who are at increased risk of infection. See *MMWR* 2006;55(No. RR-7).

10. Meningococcal vaccine. *(Minimum age: 2 years for meningococcal conjugate vaccine [MCV] and for meningococcal polysaccharide vaccine [MPSV])*
• Administer MCV to children aged 2 through 10 years with terminal complement component deficiency, anatomic or functional asplenia, and certain other high-risk groups. See *MMWR* 2005;54(No. RR-7).
• Persons who received MPSV 3 or more years previously and who remain at increased risk for meningococcal disease should be revaccinated with MCV.

The Recommended Immunization Schedules for Persons Aged 0 Through 18 Years are approved by the Advisory Committee on Immunization Practices (www.cdc.gov/vaccines/recs/acip), the American Academy of Pediatrics (http://www.aap.org), and the American Academy of Family Physicians (http://www.aafp.org).
DEPARTMENT OF HEALTH AND HUMAN SERVICES • CENTERS FOR DISEASE CONTROL AND PREVENTION

FIGURE 17-1   Recommended immunization schedule for persons aged 0 to 6 years. Available along with schedules for ages 7 to 18 years and catch-up at: http://www.cdc.gov/vaccines/recs/schedules/child-schedule.htm.

c. Carefully consider readministration of DTaP or DTP when serious or severe side effects, such as high fever (40.5°C/104.5°F), shock-like state, seizure, prolonged and inconsolable crying, or Guillain–Barré syndrome, have occurred with any dose.

d. Pregnant females should avoid exposure to IPV.

e. Consider postponing MMR with current or recent history of thrombocytopenic purpura.

f. Patients immunized with varicella vaccine should avoid family members with immunodeficiency.

5. Personal or family history of seizures, mild illness with or without fever (≤102.5°F/39.0°C), breast-feeding, recent positive tuberculin skin testing and use of antibiotics are not reasons to postpone vaccines.

B. Thimerosal

1. Routine childhood vaccines are now manufactured without the use of thimerosal.

2. Multidose vials of injectable influenza vaccine contain thimerosal, whereas single-dose preparations are free of the mercury-based preservative.

3. Numerous large studies have failed to link thimerosal or vaccines to autism, as was initially reported in one study.

VII. COMMON PEDIATRIC POISONINGS

A. General considerations

1. Each year, 85% of all poisonings occur in children under the age of 5 years; they generally are accidental and unwitnessed.

2. Mortality rates are low and likely to involve analgesics, household cleaning products, iron, hydrocarbons, and illicit drugs.

3. Adolescent ingestions likely are intentional and result from suicide attempts or use of illicit drugs and are 15-fold more fatal than accidental ingestions in small children.

4. Commonly ingested substances include cosmetic/hygiene products, cleaning products, analgesics, plants, cough/cold preparations, pesticides, vitamins, and hydrocarbons.

B. History and physical examination

1. Obtain a history of the what, when, and how of the ingestion.

2. If available, the offending substance should be brought to the emergency department.

3. Inventories of household products as well as over-the-counter and prescription medicines should be conducted.

4. History may reveal the substance in 90% of cases.

5. Physical examination (Table 17-11)

a. Note any unusual breath odors (arsenic and organophosphates produce garlic breath).

b. Check skin for excessive dryness, sweating, discoloration, and fever (anticholinergics cause warm, dry, skin, whereas organic phosphates produce salivation and urination).

c. Pupillary size as well as lacrimation should be noted.

d. Vomiting or excessive salivation should be noted.

e. Neurologic changes, such as agitation, ataxia, tremors, convulsion, and coma, often are encountered.

f. Tachycardia, tachypnea, and dysrhythmias (tricyclic antidepressants are notorious for causing prolonged QRS complexes) may occur in some settings.

C. Laboratory testing (Table 17-11)

1. Calculate the anion and osmolar gaps (alcohol causes an anion gap; methanol causes an osmolar gap).

2. Perform initial and ongoing electrocardiography.

3. When substance is unknown, standard emergency department toxin panels may provide the diagnosis.

4. Order specific toxicology screens, such as diuretics, ethylene glycol, lithium, aromatic hydrocarbons, and cyanide, as warranted.

5. Abdominal radiographs, as a rule, are not helpful, because very few agents are radiodense (e.g., heavy metals, iodine, enteric-coated tablets).

D. Management (Table 17-11)

1. Airway, breathing, and circulation should be the first concern.

2. Additional management is predicated on the type of ingestion.

TABLE 17-11	**Common Toxidromes**		
Toxin	**Physical Findings**	**Special Tests**	**Antidotes/Management**
Hydrocarbons (benzene, gasoline, petroleum distillates)	Mucosal irritation Vomiting, bloody diarrhea Cyanosis, respiratory distress Tachycardia Fever CNS depression	CXR Urinalysis ECG	Avoid emetics and lavage Oxygen with mist Antibiotics if pneumonia develops
Caustics (toilet bowel cleaners)	Skin, mucosal burns Hematemesis Abdominal pain Respiratory distress Convulsions, coma	EGD to determine the degree of esophageal injury ECG	Small amounts of water or milk Avoid vomiting Supportive care
Bases (Clorox, Drano)	Irritated mucous membranes Respiratory distress secondary to edematous epiglottis Perforation of stomach or esophagus	EGD to determine the degree of damage to larynx, esophagus, and stomach	Small amounts of water as dilutant Avoid vomiting Supportive care
Acetaminophen	Hepatotoxic	Monitor APAP plasma concentration (use specific nomogram)	Acetylcysteine is the specific antidote
Aspirin (salicylates)	Vomiting Hyperapnea Fever Encephalopathy, convulsions, coma Renal failure Pulmonary edema	Check serum salicylate level Look for metabolic acidosis and decreased K^+ Elevated or reduced serum glucose	Induce emesis Charcoal to bind drug Correct dehydration Hemodialysis
Antihistamines	Agitation and hallucinations Miosis Red eye, dry skin Fever Respiratory failure CV collapse	EC6 ligase chains Pulse oximetry	Activated charcoal Whole-bowel irrigation Physostigmine
Organophosphates (chlorthion, diazinon)	Salivation, lacrimation Diaphoresis Urination, diarrhea Miosis Pulmonary congestion Twitching, convulsions, coma	Measure red cell cholinesterase levels Blood glucose levels	ABCs Decontamination of skin Atropine plus pralidoxime
Iron (vitamins, prenatal vitamins)	Intestinal bleeding Impaired coagulation Acidosis Shock Coma Red urine	Blood indices Metabolic panel Monitor urine output for renal damage Blood type and cross-match LFTs	Evoke emesis Gastric lavage Whole-bowel irrigation Desferoxamine Dialysis

CXR, chest radiography; ECG, electrocardiography; CNS, central nervous system; EGD, esophagogastroduodensoscopy; APAP, *N*-acetyl-*P*-aminophenol; CV, cardiovascular; ABCs, airway, breathing, circulation; LFTs, liver function tests.

3. General principles of management

    a. Induced vomiting and/or gastric lavage are no longer recommended.

    b. Activated charcoal is used to promote GI decontamination. It is the current first-line treatment for most ingested poisons.

    c. Use of sorbitol or other cathartics may accelerate elimination.

    d. Whole-bowel irrigation, dialysis, and hemoperfusion rarely are necessary.

    e. Antidotes exist for specific ingestions. Check with local poison control center.

VIII. COMMON PEDIATRIC DISORDERS

For further information and other disorders, please see appropriate chapters.

A. Foreign bodies

    1. Infants and children often place objects in orifices. Common objects include beads, buttons, nuts, foodstuff, and toy parts.

    2. Ear, nose, and throat (ENT)

        a. Unilateral purulent rhinitis, persistent sinusitis, or a blocked nasal passage should prompt consideration of a foreign body in the nose.

        b. Ear pain, drainage, and hearing loss accompany foreign bodies in the ear.

        c. If the object is visible, remove it using a curette, forceps, or catheter. Be sure the child is restrained, and do not blindly probe.

    3. Respiratory tract

        a. Upper airway: Obstruction causes abrupt onset of cough, stridor, choking, and cyanosis; complete obstruction leads to inability to cough or choke.

        b. Lower airway: Obstruction causes acute to subacute cough, unilateral persistent wheezing, and recurrent pneumonia; complete obstruction may cause a ball valve effect, resulting in distal hyperinflation and mediastinal shift, which is most apparent on expiratory films.

        c. Attempt the Heimlich maneuver if respiratory distress is apparent and rigid bronchoscopy if the object is lodged in the lower airway.

    4. GI tract

        a. Most objects will pass through the GI tract. Large or irregularly shaped objects may become lodged; sharp objects, such as pins, may cause mucosal tearing.

        b. Removal by esophagogastroscopy is recommended for caustic (e.g., batteries), sharp, or lodged objects.

B. Functional (innocent) murmurs

    1. Approximately 40% to 45% of children have an innocent murmur at some point in their childhood.

    2. Still's murmur is the most common innocent murmur of childhood.

        a. It usually is apparent from 2 years of age through preadolescence.

        b. It is loudest in the apex and left sternal border. It typically is a grade I–III musical or vibratory, high-pitched, early systolic murmur that diminishes with sitting, standing, or Valsalva maneuvers, and it will accentuate with fever.

    3. Venous hum

        a. Grade I or II musical hum is heard best in the left and right infraclavicular areas and usually is louder on the right.

        b. It typically appears after 2 years of age.

        c. Best heard with the child sitting; diminishes with turning of the head, jugular compression, or supine position.

    4. Innominate or carotid bruits

        a. This is typically found in older chldren and adolescents.

        b. A grade II or III, harsh, systolic ejection murmur is characteristic.

    5. Pulmonary ejection murmur is a common innocent murmur of older children.

        a. It typically first appears around 3 years of age and continues through adolescence.

        b. Grade I or II, soft, systolic ejection murmur well localized to the upper left sternal border is heard.

        c. It typically becomes louder with the patient supine and diminishes with Valsalva maneuver.

    6. Echocardiography is recommended to rule out pathologic murmurs; other testing should be selected based on patient history, physical examination, and echocardiography results.

    7. The most important components of management are establishing the correct diagnosis and reassuring the parents.

C. Infectious diseases

1. Coxsackievirus

   a. Herpangina

      (1) There is acute onset of fever and posterior pharyngeal vesicles.

      (2) Vesicles are grayish white and quickly form ulcers with erythematous halos. Lesions may be linearly arranged on the palate, uvula, and tonsillar pillars.

      (3) Dysphagia, fever, vomiting, and anorexia occur. The child will be irritable secondary to pain.

      (4) Treatment is supportive (e.g., fluids, antipyretics, topical lidocaine).

   b. Hand–foot–mouth disease

      (1) Red papules or vesicles occur on the tongue, oral mucosa, hands, feet, and buttocks.

      (2) Fever, sore throat, and malaise usually are mild.

      (3) Treatment is supportive.

2. Kawasaki disease (mucocutaneous lymph node syndrome)

   a. Etiology is unknown, but a viral cause is suggested.

   b. Most patients are younger than 5 years.

   c. Fever (>5 days) plus at least four of the following symptoms are needed to make a diagnosis: conjunctivitis; lip cracking and fissuring, strawberry tongue, or inflammation of the oral mucosa; cervical lymphadenopathy, usually unilateral; polymorphous exanthem; or redness and swelling of the hands and feet with subsequent desquamation.

   d. Cardiovascular manifestations are worrisome; myocarditis, pericarditis, valvular heart disease, and coronary arteritis and aneurysms are possible. Two-dimensional echocardiography or angiography is recommended in all patients suspected of having Kawasaki's disease.

   e. Treatment is with IV immunoglobulin and high-dose aspirin; early treatment will reduce the chance of cardiac events. Patients with cardiac disease should receive long-term aspirin therapy and annual follow-up.

   f. Patients should be monitored through serial electrocardiography, chest radiography, and echocardiography until they have recovered.

3. Viral exanthems: Table 17-12 depicts the characteristics of some common viral exanthems.

TABLE 17-12	**Common Viral Exanthems**				
	Varicella (Chicken Pox)	**Erythema Infectiosum (Fifth Disease, Slapped Cheek)**	**Roseola (Roseola Infantum, Exanthem Subitum)**	**Measles (Rubeola)**	**Rubella (German Measles)**
Etiology	A human herpes virus	Human parvovirus B19	Human herpes virus 6 or 7	Measles virus	Rubella virus
Incubation period	10–21 days	4–14 days	10–14 days	8–14 days	14–21 days
Prodrome	Fever, respiratory symptoms (1–3 days)	None	Fever (4 days)	Fever, cough, anorexia, coryza (1–3 days)	None
Rash	Vesicular erythematous, torso and face to extremities (dew drop on rose petal)	Red face ("slapped cheek"); lacy, pink, macular rash on torso	Pink, macular rash	Maculopapular, face to extremities; Koplik's spots in mouth	Maculopapular, from head to toe
Comments	Pruritic		Fever resolves before rash		Teratogenic

Index

Page numbers followed by f indicate figure; those followed by t indicate table.